Chronic Rhinosinusitis

Luo Zhang • Claus Bachert
Editors

Chronic Rhinosinusitis

The Mucosal Concept

PEOPLE'S MEDICAL PUBLISHING HOUSE
PMPH

Springer

Editors
Luo Zhang
Department of Otorhinolaryngology
Beijing Tongren Hospital
Beijing, China

Claus Bachert
Department of Otolaryngology
Ghent University
Ghent, Belgium

ISBN 978-981-16-0783-7 ISBN 978-981-16-0784-4 (eBook)
https://doi.org/10.1007/978-981-16-0784-4

This Springer imprint is published by the registered company Springer Nature Singapore Pte Ltd.
The registered company address is: 152 Beach Road, #21-01/04 Gateway East, Singapore 189721, Singapore

Preface

Chronic rhinosinusitis (CRS) is a common disease, causing symptoms and impacting on quality of life of patients. Since 1980s, we have learned to understand CRS as a physical problem, a problem of drainage and ventilation, of ciliary activity to clean the sinuses. The proposed surgical approach by Messerklinger and Stammberger as well as Wigand and Hosemann incorporated these ideas, and many authors and guidelines adopted it. This approach was right in great parts, but did not yet appreciate the fact that sinus disease is so variable, and immunology does play a significant role much more than anticipated at that time point. It is clear today that the Messerklinger technique does not work in severe type 2 nasal polyposis, and one needs a better understanding of the immunology of the disease—and consequently the recognition of endotypes—to be able to address the diversity of CRS disease and tailor management and therapy to a variety of very different disease endotypes. Our understanding of the pathophysiology of CRS has developed from a physical problem to a mucosal problem.

Today, with the advent of biologics specifically for type 2 disease and specific surgical approaches for severe recurrent nasal polyposis, a differentiation of CRS into endotypes is overly due. These approaches are currently tailored for the severe nasal polyp patient, who so far found no or little support in the current guidelines for diagnosis, understanding of disease, let alone treatment. This will change within very few years, as we saw in severe asthma with great benefits for the patients formerly left untreated due to lack of understanding but also availability of treatment approaches. Today, we do see the benefits of biologics, offering great advantages to severe airway disease patients when properly endotyped; for asthma, these medications are life-saving and allowing the patient to live a normal life without limitations and the society to regain an active member. It is due time to adapt these principles also for CRS, often characterized by comorbidities such as asthma, but often by itself limiting the performance of patients and their quality of life to a great deal. The adaptation of endotypes should make a great difference to this dilemma. Surgical techniques responding to those needs also need to be further developed, adopted for the different needs of the patients according to their pheno- but specifically endotype. In any case, the ENT surgeon will need to learn immunology, to understand disease endotypes, to master diagnosis and advanced treatment options for a larger spectrum of disease. The biologics will support this development, by supporting the endotyping and offering so far unexperienced treatment possibilities for the patients most suffering at the moment and hopeless so far. For them with the highest unmet needs, the new development will bring the long-awaited relief.

This "mucosal concept" is the reason to write a new book for guidance of our colleagues who struggle to cure and appropriately treat our severe CRS patients.

Ghent, Belgium Claus Bachert
Beijing, China Luo Zhang

9 June 2020

Contents

1 **Introduction** 1
Claus Bachert and Luo Zhang

2 **Epidemiology** 3
Xiangdong Wang, Ming Zheng, and Luo Zhang

3 **Quality of Life and Psychological Burden** 9
Eduardo Lehrer, Mauricio López-Chacón, Isam Alobid, and Joaquim Mullol

4 **Genetics and Epigenetics** 19
Jingyun Li, Luo Zhang, and Yuan Zhang

5 **Involvement of the Immune System in Airways Disease** 31
Wei Wang and Ying Sun

6 **T Cells and Group 2 Innate Lymphoid Cells 2** 37
Atsushi Kato and Robert P. Schleimer

7 **B Cells and Plasma Cells** 47
Siobhan Ward, Zeynep Celebi Sözener, and Mübeccel Akdis

8 **Eosinophils** 57
Elien Gevaert

9 **Neutrophils** 69
Elien Gevaert

10 **Remodeling Features** 81
Lili Shi and Zheng Liu

11 **Nasal Mucociliary Clearance** 89
Jian Jiao and Luo Zhang

12 **Sinonasal Epithelium** 97
Michael Soyka and Cezmi A. Akdis

13 **Microbiology** 107
Mahboobeh Mahdavinia and Robert P. Schleimer

14 ***Staphylococcus aureus* and Its Proteins** 121
Goran Abdurrahman and Barbara M. Bröker

15 **Viruses** 133
Feng Lan and Luo Zhang

16 **Environmental and Allergic Triggers** 139
Changyu Qiu and Lei Cheng

17 **Dysfunctional Immune Regulatory System** 147
Jinmei Xue, Pingchang Yang, and Changqing Zhao

18 **Chronic Rhinosinusitis with and Without Nasal Polyps** 157
Bradley F. Marple

19 **Allergic Fungal Sinusitis** 167
Fenghong Chen, Matthew W. Ryan, and Bradley F. Marple

20 **Type 2 Immune Reactions and Consequences** 175
Claus Bachert

21 **Regional Difference** 181
Kun Du and Xiangdong Wang

22 **Multimorbidities** 187
David Bedoya, Cristóbal Langdon, Isam Alobid, José Antonio Castillo, and Joaquim Mullol

23 **Clinical Diagnosis and Phenotypes** 201
Kevin Hur and Robert C. Kern

24 **Imaging the Anatomic Landmarks for Safe FESS** 211
Simion James Zinreich and Sachin K. Gujar

25 **Olfactory Function Assessment** 227
Meritxell Valls-Mateus, Franklin Mariño-Sánchez, Isam Alobid, Concepció Marin, and Joaquim Mullol

26 **Local and Systemic Biomarkers** 239
Nan Zhang

27 **Benign Tumors of the Nose and Sinuses** 247
Manuel Bernal-Sprekelsen

28 **Sinonasal Inverted Papilloma** 253
Chengshuo Wang, Siyuan Ma, and Luo Zhang

29 **Malignant Tumors of the Nose and Sinuses** 259
Manuel Bernal-Sprekelsen and Isam Alobid

30 **Pediatric Chronic Rhinosinusitis: View from Europe** 267
Thibaut van Zele

31 **Pediatric Chronic Sinusitis: View from China** 277
Jingying Ma and Bing Zhou

32 Wegener's Granulomatosis 287
Jichao Sha and Dongdong Zhu

33 IgG4-Related Disorders 291
Yingshi Piao

34 Eosinophilic Granulomatosis with Polyangiitis 299
Yujie Cao and Huabin Li

35 Oral Corticosteroids 303
Chengshuo Wang, Yifan Meng, and Luo Zhang

36 Nasal Spray Corticosteroids 309
Yujie Cao, Huabin Li, and Dehui Wang

37 Nebulization Corticosteroids 313
Chengshuo Wang, Yifan Meng, and Luo Zhang

38 Steroid-Eluting Stent Placement 317
Chengshuo Wang, Longgang Yu, and Luo Zhang

39 Steroid Infiltrated Packing Materials 325
Yueqi Sun and Jianbo Shi

40 Corticosteroids Resistance 329
Yujie Cao, Dehui Wang, and Huabin Li

41 Leukotriene Receptor Antagonists 333
Rui Zheng, Tian Yuan, and Qintai Yang

42 Antihistamine 337
Hongfei Lou, Yanran Huang, and Luo Zhang

43 Antibiotics 341
Dawei Wu and Yongxiang Wei

44 Decongestant and Nasal Irrigation 355
Xiaoping Lai and Gehua Zhang

45 Probiotics, Bacterial Lysates, and Proton Pump Inhibitors 361
Luping Zhu and Lei Cheng

46 Impact of Endotyping on the Indication for Surgery 369
Claus Bachert

47 Surgical Procedures 371
Ashleigh Halderman and Bradley F. Marple

48 Reboot Surgery 383
Claus Bachert

49 Complications of Endoscopic Sinus Surgery 389
Yi Dong and Bing Zhou

50 Peri-operative Management 399
Jian Li and Weiping Wen

51 Surgery Outcome and Predictors 403
Fenghong Chen and Jianbo Shi

52 Biologics in Chronic Rhinosinusitis with Nasal Polyps 411
Claus Bachert

53 Integrated Care Pathways 423
Claus Bachert and Nan Zhang

54 Unmet Needs 437
Luo Zhang and Claus Bachert

Correction to: Staphylococcus aureus and Its Proteins. C1
Goran Abdurrahman and Barbara M. Bröker

Index. 439

Contributors

Goran Abdurrahman, PhD Institute of Immunology, University Medicine Greifswald, Greifswald, Germany

Cezmi A. Akdis, PhD Swiss Institute of Allergy and Asthma Research (SIAF), University Zurich, Davos, Switzerland

Christine Kühne Center for Allergy Research and Education, Davos, Switzerland

Mübeccel Akdis, MD, PhD Swiss Institute of Allergy and Asthma Research (SIAF), University of Zurich, Davos, Switzerland

Isam Alobid, MD, PhD Rhinology Unit & Smell Clinic, Department of Otorhinolaryngology, Hospital Clínic, Universitat de Barcelona, Barcelona, Catalonia, Spain

Clinical & Experimental Respiratory Immunoallergy, Institut d'Investigacions, Biomèdiques August Pi i Sunyer (IDIBAPS), Barcelona, Catalonia, Spain

CIBER of Respiratory Diseases (CIBERES), Barcelona, Catalonia, Spain

Claus Bachert, MD, PhD Upper Airways Research Laboratory and Department of Oto-Rhino-Laryngology, Ghent University, Ghent, Belgium

Division of ENT Diseases, CLINTEC, Karolinska Institute, University of Stockholm, Stockholm, Sweden

First Affiliated Hospital, Sun Yat-sen University, International Upper Airway Research Centre, Guangzhou, China

David Bedoya, MD Rhinology Unit and Smell Clinic, Department of Otorhinolaryngology, Hospital Clínic, Universitat de Barcelona, Barcelona, Catalonia, Spain

Clinical & Experimental Respiratory Immunoallergy, IDIBAPS, Barcelona, Catalonia, Spain

Sinonasal Inflammatory and Olfactory Research Group (INGENIO), IRCE, IDIBAPS, Barcelona, Catalonia, Spain

Manuel Bernal-Sprekelsen, MD, PhD Hospital Clinic, University of Barcelona, Barcelona, Spain

Barbara Bröker, PhD Department of Immunology, University Medicine Greifswald, Greifswald, Germany

Yujie Cao, MD, PhD Department of Otolaryngology, Head and Neck Surgery, Affiliated Eye and ENT Hospital, Fudan University, Shanghai, China

José Antonio Castillo, MD Clinical & Experimental Respiratory Immunoallergy, IDIBAPS, Barcelona, Catalonia, Spain

Respiratory Department, Hospital Universitario Quirón Dexeus, Barcelona, Catalonia, Spain

Rhinitis Group, SEPAR, Barcelona, Catalonia, Spain

Fenghong Chen, MD Otorhinolaryngology Hospital, First Affiliated Hospital Sun Yat-sen University, Guangzhou, Guangdong, China

Lei Cheng, MD, PhD Department of Otorhinolaryngology and Clinical Allergy Center, The First Affiliated Hospital, Nanjing Medical University, Nanjing, China

International Centre for Allergy Research, Nanjing Medical University, Nanjing, China

Yi Dong, MD Department of Otolaryngology, Head and Neck Surgery, Beijing Tongren Hospital, Capital Medical University, Beijing, China

Kun Du, MD Department of Otolaryngology, Head and Neck Surgery, Beijing Tongren Hospital, Capital Medical University, Beijing, China

Elien Gevaert, PhD Upper Airways Research Laboratory and Department of Oto-Rhino-Laryngology, Ghent University, Ghent, Belgium

Sachin K. Gujar, MBBS The Russel H. Morgan Department of Radiology, The Johns Hopkins Medical Institutions, Baltimore, MD, USA

Department of Otorhinolaryngology, Head and Neck Surgery, The Johns Hopkins Medical Institutions, Baltimore, MD, USA

Ashleigh Halderman, MD Southwestern Medical Center, Department of Otolaryngology, Head and Neck Surgery, University of Texas, Dallas, TX, USA

Yanran Huang, MD Department of Otolaryngology, Head and Neck Surgery, Beijing Tongren Hospital, Capital Medical University, Beijing, China

Kevin Hur, MD Department of Otolaryngology, Head and Neck Surgery, Feinberg School of Medicine, Northwestern University, Chicago, IL, USA

Jian Jiao, PhD Department of Otolaryngology, Head and Neck Surgery, Beijing Tongren Hospital, Capital Medical University, Beijing, China

Beijing Key Laboratory of Nasal Disease, Beijing Institute of Otolaryngology, Beijing, China

Atsushi Kato, PhD Division of Allergy and Immunology, Department of Medicine, Northwestern University Feinberg School of Medicine, Chicago, IL, USA

Department of Otolaryngology, Northwestern University Feinberg School of Medicine, Chicago, IL, USA

Robert C. Kern, MD Department of Otolaryngology, Head and Neck Surgery, Feinberg School of Medicine, Northwestern University, Chicago, IL, USA

Xiaoping Lai, MD Department of Otorhinolaryngology, The Third Affiliated Hospital of Sun Yat-sen University, Guangzhou, China

Feng Lan, PhD Beijing Key Laboratory of Nasal Disease, Beijing Institute of Otolaryngology, Beijing, China

Cristóbal Langdon, MD Rhinology Unit and Smell Clinic, Department of Otorhinolaryngology, Hospital Clínic, Universitat de Barcelona, Barcelona, Catalonia, Spain

Clinical & Experimental Respiratory Immunoallergy, IDIBAPS, Barcelona, Catalonia, Spain

Sinonasal Inflammatory and Olfactory Research Group (INGENIO), IRCE, IDIBAPS, Barcelona, Catalonia, Spain

Centre for Biomedical Research on Respiratory Diseases (CIBERES), Madrid, Spain

Eduardo Lehrer, MD Rhinology Unit & Smell Clinic, Department of Otorhinolaryngology, Hospital Clínic, Universitat de Barcelona, Barcelona, Catalonia, Spain

Clinical & Experimental Respiratory Immunoallergy, Institut d'Investigacions, Biomèdiques August Pi i Sunyer (IDIBAPS), Barcelona, Catalonia, Spain

Huabin Li, MD, PhD Department of Otolaryngology, Head and Neck Surgery, Affiliated Eye and ENT Hospital, Fudan University, Shanghai, China

Jingyun Li, MD, PhD Department of Otolaryngology, Head and Neck Surgery, Beijing Tongren Hospital, Capital Medical University, Beijing, China

Beijing Key Laboratory of Nasal Diseases, Beijing Institute of Otolaryngology, Beijing, China

Zheng Liu, MD, PhD Department of Otolaryngology, Head and Neck Surgery, Tongji Hospital, Tongji Medical College, Huazhong University of Science and Technology, Wuhan, China

Mauricio López-Chacón, MD Rhinology Unit & Smell Clinic, Department of Otorhinolaryngology, Hospital Clínic, Universitat de Barcelona, Barcelona, Catalonia, Spain

Clinical & Experimental Respiratory Immunoallergy, Institut d'Investigacions, Biomèdiques August Pi i Sunyer (IDIBAPS), Barcelona, Catalonia, Spain

Hongfei Lou, MD, PhD Department of Otolaryngology, Head and Neck Surgery, Beijing Tongren Hospital, Capital Medical University, Beijing, China

Beijing Key Laboratory of Nasal Diseases, Beijing Institute of Otolaryngology, Beijing, China

Jingying Ma, MD Department of Otolaryngology, Head and Neck Surgery, Beijing Tongren Hospital, Capital Medical University, Beijing, China

Siyuan Ma, MD Department of Otolaryngology, Head and Neck Surgery, Beijing Tongren Hospital, Capital Medical University, Beijing, China

Beijing Key Laboratory of Nasal Diseases, Beijing Institute of Otolaryngology, Beijing, China

Mahboobeh Mahdavinia, MD, PhD Division of Allergy-Immunology, Internal Medicine Department, Rush University Medical Center, Chicago, IL, USA

Concepció Marin, MD, PhD INGENIO, Immunoal.lèrgia Respiratòria Clínica i Experimental (IRCE), Institut d'Investigacions Biomèdiques August Pi i Sunyer (IDIBAPS), Barcelona, Catalonia, Spain

CIBER de Enfermedades Respiratorias (CIBERES), Barcelona, Catalonia, Spain

Unitat de Rinologia i Clinica de l'Olfacte, Servei d'Otorinolaringologia, Hospital Clínic Barcelona, Universitat de Barcelona, Barcelona, Catalonia, Spain

Franklin Mariño-Sánchez, MD, PhD Unidad de Rinología y Cirugía de Base de Cráneo, Servicio de Otorrinolaringología. Hospital Universitario Ramón y Cajal, Madrid, Spain

Bradley F. Marple, MD University of Texas, Southwestern Medical Center, Department of Otolaryngology, Head and Neck Surgery, Dallas, TX, USA

Yifan Meng, MD, PhD Department of Otolaryngology, Head and Neck Surgery, Beijing Tongren Hospital, Capital Medical University, Beijing, China

Joaquim Mullol, MD, PhD Rhinology Unit & Smell Clinic, Department of Otorhinolaryngology, Hospital Clínic, Universitat de Barcelona, Barcelona, Catalonia, Spain

Clinical & Experimental Respiratory Immunoallergy, Institut d'Investigacions, Biomèdiques August Pi i Sunyer (IDIBAPS), Barcelona, Catalonia, Spain

CIBER of Respiratory Diseases (CIBERES), Barcelona, Catalonia, Spain

Yingshi Piao, MD, PhD Department of Pathology, Beijing Tongren Hospital, Capital Medical University, Beijing, China

Changyu Qiu, MSc International Centre for Allergy Research, Nanjing Medical University, Nanjing, China

Matthew W. Ryan, MD Department of Otolaryngology, The University of Texas Southwestern Medical Center, Dallas, TX, USA

Robert P. Schleimer, PhD Division of Allergy and Immunology, Department of Medicine, Northwestern University Feinberg School of Medicine, Chicago, IL, USA

Department of Otolaryngology, Northwestern University Feinberg School of Medicine, Chicago, IL, USA

Jichao Sha, MD, PhD Department of Otolaryngology, Head and Neck Surgery, China-Japan Union Hospital of Jilin University, Changchun, China

Jianbo Shi, MD, PhD Otorhinolaryngology Hospital, The First Affiliated Hospital, Sun Yat-sen University, Guangzhou, China

Lili Shi, MD, PhD Department of Otolaryngology, Head and Neck Surgery, Tongji Hospital, Tongji Medical College, Huazhong University of Science and Technology, Wuhan, China

Michael Soyka, MD, PhD Department of Otorhinolaryngology, Head and Neck Surgery, University Hospital Zurich, Zurich, Switzerland

Zeynep Celebi Sözener, MD Swiss Institute of Allergy and Asthma Research (SIAF), University of Zurich, Davos, Wolfgang, Switzerland

Department of Chest Disease, Division of Allergy and Clinical Immunology, Ankara University School of Medicine, Ankara, Turkey

Ying Sun, MD, PhD Department of Immunology, School of Basic Medical Sciences, Capital Medical University, Beijing, China

Yueqi Sun, MD, PhD Department of Otolaryngology, The Seventh Affiliated Hospital, Sun Yat-sen University, Shenzhen, China

Otorhinolaryngology Hospital, The First Affiliated Hospital, Sun Yat-sen University, Guangzhou, China

Meritxell Valls-Mateus, MD, PhD Servei d'Otorinolaringologia, Hospital Universitari Son Espases, Palma de Mallorca, Illes Balears, Spain

Chengshuo Wang, MD, PhD Department of Otolaryngology, Head and Neck Surgery, Beijing Tongren Hospital, Capital Medical University, Beijing, China

Beijing Key Laboratory of Nasal Diseases, Beijing Institute of Otolaryngology, Beijing, China

Department of Allergy, Beijing Tongren Hospital, Capital Medical University, Beijing, China

Dehui Wang, MD, PhD Department of Otolaryngology, Head and Neck Surgery, Affiliated Eye and ENT Hospital, Fudan University, Shanghai, China

Wei Wang, MD, PhD Department of Immunology, School of Basic Medical Sciences, Capital Medical University, Beijing, China

Xiangdong Wang, MD, PhD Department of Otorhinolaryngology, Head and Neck Surgery, Beijing Tongren Hospital, Capital Medical University, Beijing, China

Beijing Key Laboratory of Nasal Diseases, Beijing Institute of Otorhinolaryngology, Beijing, China

Siobhan Ward, MD Swiss Institute of Allergy and Asthma Research (SIAF), University of Zurich, Davos, Wolfgang, Switzerland

Cristine Kühne-Center for Allergy Research and Education, Davos, Wolfgang, Switzerland

Yongxiang Wei, MD, PhD Department of Otorhinolaryngology, Head and Neck Surgery, Beijing Anzhen Hospital, Capital Medical University, Beijing, China

Department of Otorhinolaryngology, Head and Neck Surgery, Capital Institute of Pediatrics, Beijing, China

Weiping Wen, MD, PhD Otorhinolaryngology Department, The First Affiliated Hospital of Sun Yat-sen University, Guangzhou, China

Dawei Wu, MD, PhD Department of Otorhinolaryngology, Head and Neck Surgery, Beijing Anzhen Hospital, Capital Medical University, Beijing, China

Jinmei Xue, MD, PhD Department of Otolaryngology, Head and Neck Surgery, The Second Hospital, Shanxi Medical University, Taiyuan, China

Pingchang Yang, MD, PhD Research Center of Allergy and Immunology, Shenzhen University School of Medicine, Shenzhen, China

Qintai Yang, MD, PhD Department of Otorhinolaryngology, Head and Neck Surgery, The Third Affiliated Hospital, Sun Yat-sen University, Guangzhou, China

Longgang Yu, MD Department of Otolaryngology, Head and Neck Surgery, The Affiliated Hospital of Qingdao University, Qingdao, China

Tian Yuan, MD, PhD Department of Otorhinolaryngology, Head and Neck Surgery, The Third Affiliated Hospital, Sun Yat-sen University, Guangzhou, China

Thibaut van Zele, MD, PhD Upper Airways Research Laboratory and Department of Oto-Rhino-Laryngology, Ghent University, Ghent, Belgium

Gehua Zhang, MD, PhD Department of Otorhinolaryngology, The Third Affiliated Hospital of Sun Yat-sen University, Guangzhou, China

Luo Zhang, MD, PhD Department of Otorhinolaryngology, Head and Neck Surgery, Beijing Tongren Hospital, Capital Medical University, Beijing, China

Beijing Key Laboratory of Nasal Diseases, Beijing Institute of Otorhinolaryngology, Beijing, China

Department of Allergy, Beijing Tongren Hospital, Capital Medical University, Beijing, China

Nan Zhang, MD, PhD Upper Airways Research Laboratory, Ghent University, Ghent, Belgium

Yuan Zhang, MD, PhD Department of Otolaryngology, Head and Neck Surgery, Beijing Tongren Hospital, Capital Medical University, Beijing, China

Beijing Key Laboratory of Nasal Diseases, Beijing Institute of Otolaryngology, Beijing, China

Department of Allergy, Beijing Tongren Hospital, Capital Medical University, Beijing, China

Changqing Zhao, MD, PhD Department of Otolaryngology, Head and Neck Surgery, The Second Hospital, Shanxi Medical University, Taiyuan, China

Ming Zheng, MD, PhD Department of Otorhinolaryngology, Head and Neck Surgery, Beijing Tongren Hospital, Capital Medical University, Beijing, China

Rui Zheng, MD, PhD Department of Otorhinolaryngology, Head and Neck Surgery, The Third Affiliated Hospital, Sun Yat-sen University, Guangzhou, China

Bing Zhou, MD Department of Otolaryngology, Head and Neck Surgery, Beijing Tongren Hospital, Capital Medical University, Beijing, China

Dongdong Zhu, MD, PhD Department of Otolaryngology, Head and Neck Surgery, China-Japan Union Hospital of Jilin University, Changchun, China

Luping Zhu, MD, PhD Department of Otorhinolaryngology, The Second Affiliated Hospital, Nanjing Medical University, Nanjing, China

Simion James Zinreich, MD The Russel H. Morgan Department of Radiology, The Johns Hopkins Medical Institutions, Baltimore, MD, USA

Department of Otorhinolaryngology, Head and Neck Surgery, The Johns Hopkins Medical Institutions, Baltimore, MD, USA

Introduction

1

Claus Bachert and Luo Zhang

With the growing understanding of immune cells, their functions and communication pathways, and finally their role in different immune reactions, each orchestrated by specific adaptive immunity T cells and their innate counterparts, the innate lymphocyte cells (ILCs), a new complicated world was discovered within the nasal and sinus mucosa that served various purposes. First of all, these immune reactions were important to keep the airway mucosa healthy, able to form a living barrier with the outer epithelial lining, and reinforced by the microbiome, thousands of bacteria living together in a balance and preventing pathogens to colonize the mucosal surface. Second, the epithelial barrier also represents a warning and alarm system, composed of cells which are able to sense attack and damage, and report down to sensitive ILCs and dendritic cells and their cytokine networks. Depending on these sensitive cells, the response of the mucosa to the alarm will be different, and may be adequate or insufficient, thus allowing suppressing or developing a pathologic reaction. A virus can be such an acute stimulus, and would be under normal circumstances most likely be efficiently eliminated within a few days. Repeated virus infections, however, possibly in combination with the effects of smoking, pollution, and drugs to traumatize the mucosa further, may result one day into persistent changes of the mucosal immune reaction, which gives raise to chronic pathology or inflammation.

Chronic inflammation then translates into remodeling of the mucosa, a condition we call chronic rhinosinusitis (CRS) with or without nasal polyps; polyps are a clear sign of mucosal remodeling, with cross-linked fibrin deposition and edema formation driven by a persistent immune reaction. The deposition of collagen on the other hand is typically observed in CRS without nasal polyps, making the mucosa thick and stiff. Underneath this remodeling there always is inflammation, which can be differentiated into separate immune reactions, which we nowadays abbreviate as "type 1" to "type 3" reactions. The type of immune reaction can be read using cells or cytokines as markers (Table 1.1).

C. Bachert
Upper Airways Research Laboratory and Department of Oto-Rhino-Laryngology, Ghent University, Ghent, Belgium

Division of ENT Diseases, CLINTEC, Karolinska Institute, University of Stockholm, Stockholm, Sweden
e-mail: claus.bachert@ugent.be

L. Zhang (✉)
Department of Otorhinolaryngology, Head and Neck Surgery, Beijing Tongren Hospital, Capital Medical University, Beijing, China

Beijing Key Laboratory of Nasal Diseases, Beijing Institute of Otorhinolaryngology, Beijing, China

Department of Allergy, Beijing Tongren Hospital, Capital Medical University, Beijing, China

L. Zhang, C. Bachert (eds.), *Chronic Rhinosinusitis*, https://doi.org/10.1007/978-981-16-0784-4_1

Table 1.1 Inflammatory signatures of type 1 to type 3 immune reactions

	T helper cells Innate lymphocytes	Typical cytokines	Typical cells involved
Type 1	Th1, ILC1	IFN-gamma, TNF	Neutrophils, NK cells
Type 2	Th2, ILC2	IL-4, -5, -10, -13	IgE-producing B cells, eosinophils
Type 3	Th17, ILC3	IL-17, -22	Neutrophils

Although the inflammatory signatures are not strictly linked to a specific remodeling pattern in each individual patient, and a mixture of several signature may be found within the mucosa of one diseased subject, there are general rules that allow us to estimate the inflammatory signature from the remodeling pattern. Typically, CRS without nasal polyps (CRSsNP) is associated with a type 1 or type 3 immune reaction, with neutrophils and collagen deposition being prominent, whereas in a central European CRS with (w)NP patient, a type 2 immune reaction is found in more than 80% of subjects, with tissue eosinophilia and increased IgE production. However, in type 2 CRSwNP, there regularly also is a neutrophilic inflammation; this condition is orchestrated by type 3 cytokines in less severe CRSwNP, but by eosinophil products such as eosinophil products—independent from type 3 cytokines—including Charcot–Leyden crystals (CLCs) in severe polyp disease.

How does this new knowledge help us to optimize the care for our CRS patients? In fact, we learn how inflammation translates into clinical traits, such as asthma comorbidity, which is clearly associated with a type 2 immune reaction of the sinus mucosa. Further, the natural course of disease and the chance of recurrence are determined also by the immune reaction, and a type 2 immune reaction will much more likely result in disease recurrence even after an adequate surgical procedure. Type 2 often is also referred to as endotype 2, and determination of the inflammatory type as endotyping. Thus, we all need to be highly knowledgeable and skilled surgeons; there is no way of underestimating the importance of these skills, and each of us needed many years to develop those surgical skills! However, we still fail when we do not understand the underlying inflammation.

This new knowledge recently was translated into new therapeutic approaches, referred to as "biologics" or "humanized monoclonal antibodies." Biologics targeting type 2 cytokines—as indicated above, these cytokines and their products are orchestrating the most severe inflammatory reactions and associated clinical traits—are just gaining momentum and will within short time change our management of severe CRSwNP disease. The extent of surgery or better the completeness of removal of diseased sinus mucosa from all sinuses—but preserving the nasal mucosa and turbinates—the "Reboot" surgery concept, may offer solutions to those patients with type 2 immune reactions in whom conventional endoscopic surgery fails to control disease. And monoclonal antibodies will be used in patients in whom pharmacotherapy and surgical procedures failed to control disease, and will from there expand to first choices at the same level as or even before surgery, We would predict. Latest then, the importance of the mucosal composition and its inflammation is evident as a new concept with clinical consequences—the mucosal concept.

2 Epidemiology

Xiangdong Wang, Ming Zheng, and Luo Zhang

Key Points

- Chronic rhinosinusitis (CRS) is a highly prevalent respiratory disorder throughout the world, and has a great impact on individuals and society.
- Disparities in the prevalence of CRS are often attributed to the different diagnostic criteria used in clinical practice and epidemiological surveys.
- The risk factors for CRS have been the focus of discussions and arguments, but remain ambiguous.

2.1 Introduction

As an important heterogeneous disease, chronic rhinosinusitis (CRS) is a very common inflammatory condition of the paranasal sinuses in the respiratory system, and can be divided into two distinct phenotypic subtypes: chronic rhinosinusitis without nasal polyps (CRSsNP) and chronic rhinosinusitis with nasal polyps (CRSwNP). When diagnosed according to European and American clinical practice guidelines, CRSsNP accounts for >66% of CRS cases and CRSwNP accounts for <33% of cases [1, 2]. At present, CRS creates a substantial health and economic burden on both sufferers and society, and adversely affects a person's quality of life. As the second most frequent disorder and one of the "top ten" physical health problems affecting businesses in the USA [3, 4], medical complaints due to CRS lead to more than 18 million outpatient visits by adults and 5.6 million visits by individuals aged 0–20 years old each year [5, 6]. Consequently, approximately 4.5% of all U.S. health-care expenditure are devoted to CRS patients annually [7]. In Germany, the Institute of Medical Statistics reported that CRS was diagnosed 2.6 million times, and 2.2 million CRS patients consulted a doctor for medical assistance in the year 2002 [8]. Recently, a study conducted by the Asia-Pacific Burden of Respiratory Diseases (APBORD) investigated consecutive adult patients who were seeking care for a respiratory disease in six Asian countries. That study revealed that rhinosinusitis was diagnosed in 9% of 13,902 patients with different airway problems. Based on diagnostic criteria in the International Classification of Diseases, 10th revision (ICD-10), the rates of CRS diagnosis ranged from 2.4% in Thailand to 10.7% in

X. Wang · L. Zhang (✉)
Department of Otorhinolaryngology, Head and Neck Surgery, Beijing Tongren Hospital, Capital Medical University, Beijing, China

Beijing Key Laboratory of Nasal Diseases, Beijing Institute of Otorhinolaryngology, Beijing, China

M. Zheng
Department of Otorhinolaryngology, Head and Neck Surgery, Beijing Tongren Hospital, Capital Medical University, Beijing, China

L. Zhang, C. Bachert (eds.), *Chronic Rhinosinusitis*, https://doi.org/10.1007/978-981-16-0784-4_2

Singapore [9]. When taking into consideration the vast global population distribution, reliable and ample epidemiologic studies are absolutely essential for accurately assessing the prevalence and risk factors for CRS. The results of those studies could be used to formulate public health policies and provide medical resources required to meet the needs of CRS patients.

2.2 Variations in the Worldwide Prevalence of CRS

There are enormous international and inter-regional variations in the reported prevalence of CRS throughout the world. Some potential reasons for these variations include the answers given by different surveyed populations (e.g., a general population vs. residents listed in an administrative database), the use of different survey methods (e.g., a postal questionnaire vs. a face to face interview), and the criteria used for diagnosing CRS. Due to a lack of generally accepted diagnostic criteria for CRS that could apply to different situations, the Academy of Allergy and Clinical Immunology (EAACI) and the European Rhinology Society (ERS) initiated and approved the European Position Paper on Rhinosinusitis and Nasal Polyps (EPOS) in 2007 [1]. The EPOS document contains a consensus opinion on the epidemiological definition of CRS. That new definition has high degrees of diagnostic sensitivity and specificity, is based on self-reported major symptoms, and takes into account a combination of subjective symptoms and objective evidence of inflammation as confirmed by nasal endoscopy or a sinus computed tomography (CT).

Currently, estimates of CRS prevalence based on diagnostic criteria in the EPOS document have been extensively accepted and are increasing used in studies. Figure 2.1 shows the current worldwide prevalence of CRS as based on the epidemiological definition of CRS contained in the EPOS document. In 2008, the Global Allergy and Asthma European Network (GA^{2}LEN) began to conduct a trans-European collaborative survey that used a postal questionnaire to gather information. The questionnaire was sent to 57,128 people who were 15 to 75 years old at 19 centres in 12 European countries [10]. The results showed that the overall prevalence of CRS in Europe was

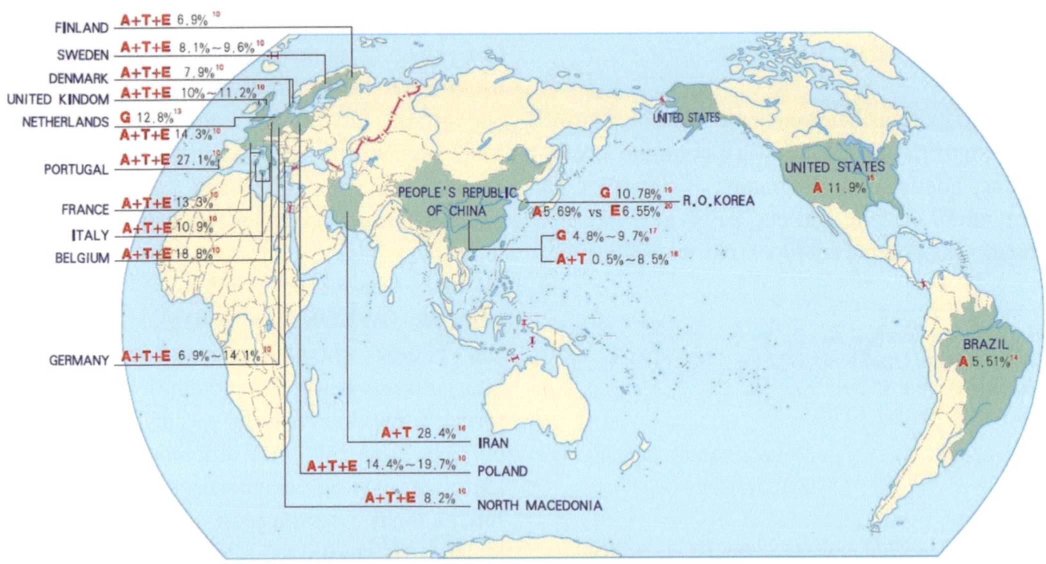

Fig. 2.1 Published data concerning the prevalence of CRS in different countries based on the epidemiological definition of CRS recommended by EPOS

10.9%; ranging from 6.9% in Helsinki, Finland to 27.1% in Coimbra, Portugal. This suggested that CRS was more prevalent in warmer regions than in colder regions. A similar geographic variation was observed in the USA, where the highest prevalence of CRS (17.2%) was in the southern region and the lowest prevalence (12.9%) was in northeast region. However, in that survey, the occurrence of CRS was based on a self-reported doctor's diagnosis, which was completely different from the epidemiological criteria outlined in the EPOS [11]. A single centre survey from the United Kingdom showed the prevalence of CRS was 24.9% among 2000 residents of Farnborough, England who were selected by using a stratified randomization procedure. Farnborough was surveyed because the age-range, ethnic distribution, and birth-place distribution of its population closely reflect the national averages [12]. Similarly, it was recently reported that the prevalence of CRS among the general population of Amsterdam was 12.8%. That estimate was based on the EPOS definition of CRS, as well as the prevalence of 3.0% or 6.4% calculated based on various clinical criteria (depending on the cut-off point of the imaging scoring system) [13]. In South America, the prevalence of CRS was determined to be 5.51% in Sao Paulo, Brazil, based on information provided during face-to-face interviews with >2000 individuals [14]. On the other hand, Hirsch found that 11.9% of respondents >18 years old in Pennsylvania could be diagnosed as CRS by using the EPOS criteria, which was the first time in the USA [15]. Meanwhile, an increasing amount of data from Asian countries is also become available. A survey of 5201 volunteers in Bushehr, Iran that was conducted using a random sampling method showed that the overall prevalence of CRS was 28.4% [16]. In mainland China, the mean overall prevalence of adult CRS was 8% in seven cities (range, 4.8–9.7%) and 2.1% in eighteen cities (range, 0.5–8.5%). Those data were obtained from two separate multicentre studies. The first study included 10,636 subjects who participated in face-to-face interviews, and the second study included 36,577 subjects who were interviewed by telephone [17, 18]. Due to the Korean National Health and Nutrition Examination Survey, sufficient epidemiological information is now available for Korea. Kim [19] reported that the prevalence of CRS in the general population of Korea was 10.78%. That estimate was based on information gathered from 7394 randomly selected individuals who were representative of the general population of South Korea in 2009, and CRS being diagnosed according to EPOS criteria [19]. Recent data gathered by KNHANES [20] showed that the prevalence of CRS was 5.88% among general adults, but was significantly higher in a population of 5590 elderly individuals (6.55%, ≥65 years old) when compared to a population of 19,939 younger individuals (5.69%, 19–64 years old). However, a symptom-based diagnosis of CRS probably cannot be used to predict the precise prevalence of CRS in the real world, even though it was broadly recommended for use in a large-scale epidemiological survey conducted by EPOS, because of inherent shortcomings of an overestimation. Endoscopic and radiographic evidence are difficult to obtain in population research studies, due to their high cost and the need for highly skilled professional technicians. In 2009, Kim [19] reported that the prevalence of CRS was 1.2%, as determined by endoscopic examinations and using the clinical definition of CRS. In another study, approximately 200 otorhinolaryngologists performed nasal endoscopy on 28,912 individuals aged ≥20 years old. The results showed that the overall prevalence of CRS was 8.4% (2.6% for CRSwNP versus 5.8% for CRSsNP), based on the clinical definition of CRS in the EPOS [21].

2.3 Risk Factors for CRS

Gaining a comprehensive understanding of the various risk factors (social, environmental, occupational, etc.) for CRS could allow for preventive intervention and help to alleviate the initiation or aggravation of the disorder. However, the risk factors for CRS have been examined and argued about for decades, due to the ambiguous or conflicting results obtained from different studies.

Among all the potential risk factors, tobacco is thought to play the most critical role in CRS development. The GA^2LEN study showed that active smokers had a higher odds ratio of suffering from CRS when compared with non-smokers, and the relationship was dose-dependent. Furthermore, current smokers of 50 pack years were nearly 50% more likely to report suffering from CRS [10]. Lee [22] discovered that each additional year of smoking resulted in a 1.5% increase in CRS prevalence. Moreover, passive smoking was found to be an independent risk factor for CRS and contribute to its sinonasal symptoms [17, 23]. Results from the USA and Canada showed that people with lower socioeconomic status had a higher prevalence of CRS [24, 25]. In contrast, a recent case-control study from the UK reported there was no significant difference of socioeconomic status between CRS patients and control subjects [26]. Results of a cross-sectional questionnaire study conducted by Smith [27] suggested that children from lower income families in the USA experienced CRS less often than a control group of children. Kilty [25] pointed out that a low educational level was associated with a worse CRS symptom burden, and Kim [23] suggested that a lower educational level was related to a higher CRS prevalence [23]. More specifically, a multivariable regression analysis found that a lower educational level was a risk factor for CRSwNP, but not for CRSsNP [21]. Nevertheless, Shi [17] observed an inverse U-shaped relationship between CRS and a person's educational degree. The prevalence of CRS was lower among people who were illiterate and had only a primary or secondary school education, than among people who had a college diploma. When compared to white collar workers, blue collar workers were more likely to suffer from CRS, possibly due to an increased exposure to gasses, fumes, dust, or smoke [28]. Another study revealed that the prevalence of CRS was usually higher among manual workers, and especially among machine operators, assemblers, and elementary workers [29]. Besides atmospheric pollution present in cities (carbon monoxide, sulphur dioxide, and particulate matter), a poor indoor environment (e.g., use of air conditioning in the summer, dampness in the house and having a house pet) was also found to be directly associated with CRS [30]. Interestingly, several studies have identified obesity as the important risk factor for CRS [31, 32].

2.4 Translation into Future Daily Practice

- Extensive and accurate epidemiological surveys specific for CRS can be used to help formulate and promote public health policies that meet unmet needs of the healthcare system. In the future, comprehensive, multicentre, collaborative, large-scale epidemiological studies involving multiple regions and nations will be able to supply more reliable and comparative data by using the same diagnostic criteria for CRS and the same method of investigation. Although a few studies have reported about trends in the prevalence of CRS in East Asia and North America, the results were contradictory due to different social and environmental backgrounds [33, 34]. Therefore, additional longitudinal studies will be required to reveal the actual tendency of CRS prevalence in different areas.
- It has to be admitted that the self-reported CRS symptom criteria can significantly overestimate the true prevalence of CRS because it fails to distinguish different disorders of the nasal cavity and sinus. However, an objective evaluation of inflammation by a sinus CT scan or endoscopy is difficult to incorporate into a population-based epidemiologic survey, because of the high cost and complexity of those procedures. Consequently, any reconstruction of the diagnostic definition of CRS should involve parameters that can be easily measured by methods that are easy to use. Especially, the diagnostic criteria for CRS based on subjective symptoms still need to be optimized with higher sensitivity and specificity in order to improve the consistency of a CRS diagnosis based on objective findings. It has recently been reported that some symptoms might serve as strong predictors of CRS [35].

- Nowadays, it has to admit that the internet is increasingly connected with people's daily life. Therefore, internet search might reflect the disease burden of various chronic disorders including CRS in the real world. The study of related search terms from analysis of internet user's search behaviour and medical needs will open a new era of epidemiological monitoring and recognizing of clinical feature of CRS. Moreover, the big data research based on extensively used internet search engines, such as Google, could serve as the predictor for potential CRS patients and discover the temporal and spatial distribution characteristics of CRS, which helps to understand CRS deeper and more comprehensive.

References

1. Fokkens W, Lund V, Mullol J. EP3OS 2007: European position paper on rhinosinusitis and nasal polyps 2007. A summary for otorhinolaryngologists. Rhinology. 2007;45(2):97–101.
2. Meltzer EO, Hamilos DL, Hadley JA, Lanza DC, Marple BF, Nicklas RA, et al. Rhinosinusitis: establishing definitions for clinical research and patient care. J Allergy Clin Immunol. 2004;114(6 Suppl):155–212. https://doi.org/10.1016/j.jaci.2004.09.029.
3. Collins JG. Prevalence of selected chronic conditions: United States, 1990–1992. Vital and health statistics Series 10, Data from the National Health Survey. 1997(194):1–89.
4. Goetzel RZ, Hawkins K, Ozminkowski RJ, Wang S. The health and productivity cost burden of the "top 10" physical and mental health conditions affecting six large U.S. employers in 1999. J Occup Environ Med. 2003;45(1):5–14. https://doi.org/10.1097/00043764-200301000-00007.
5. Benninger MS, Ferguson BJ, Hadley JA, Hamilos DL, Jacobs M, Kennedy DW, et al. Adult chronic rhinosinusitis: definitions, diagnosis, epidemiology, and pathophysiology. Otolaryngol Head Neck Surg. 2003;129(3 Suppl):S1–32. https://doi.org/10.1016/s0194-5998(03)01397-4.
6. Gilani S, Shin JJ. The burden and visit prevalence of pediatric chronic rhinosinusitis. Otolaryngol Head Neck Surg. 2017;157(6):1048–52. https://doi.org/10.1177/0194599817721177.
7. DeConde AS, Smith TL. Classification of chronic rhinosinusitis-working toward personalized diagnosis. Otolaryngol Clin N Am. 2017;50(1):1–12. https://doi.org/10.1016/j.otc.2016.08.003.
8. Stuck BA, Bachert C, Federspil P, Hosemann W, Klimek L, Mösges R, et al. Rhinosinusitis guidelines – unabridged version: S2 guidelines from the German society of otorhinolaryngology, head and neck surgery. HNO. 2012;60(2):141–62. https://doi.org/10.1007/s00106-011-2396-7.
9. Wang Y, Cho SH, Lin HC, Ghoshal AG, Bin Abdul Muttalif AR, Thanaviratananich S, et al. Practice patterns for chronic respiratory diseases in the Asia-Pacific region: a cross-sectional observational study. Int Arch Allergy Immunol. 2018;177(1):69–79. https://doi.org/10.1159/000489015.
10. Hastan D, Fokkens WJ, Bachert C, Newson RB, Bislimovska J, Bockelbrink A, et al. Chronic rhinosinusitis in Europe – an underestimated disease. A GA^{2}LEN study. Allergy. 2011;66(9):1216–23. https://doi.org/10.1111/j.1398-9995.2011.02646.x.
11. Pleis JR, Lethbridge-Cejku M. Summary health statistics for U.S. adults: National Health Interview Survey, 2006. Vital and health statistics Series 10, Data from the National Health Survey. 2007(235):1–153.
12. Sami AS, Scadding GK, Howarth P. A UK community-based survey on the prevalence of rhinosinusitis. Clin Otolaryngol. 2018;43(1):76–89. https://doi.org/10.1111/coa.12902.
13. Dietz de Loos D, Lourijsen ES, Wildeman MAM, Freling NJM, Wolvers MDJ, Reitsma S, et al. Prevalence of chronic rhinosinusitis in the general population based on sinus radiology and symptomatology. J Allergy Clin Immunol. 2019;143(3):1207–14. https://doi.org/10.1016/j.jaci.2018.12.986.
14. Pilan RR, Pinna FR, Bezerra TF, Mori RL, Padua FG, Bento RF, et al. Prevalence of chronic rhinosinusitis in Sao Paulo. Rhinology. 2012;50(2):129–38. https://doi.org/10.4193/Rhino11.256.
15. Hirsch AG, Stewart WF, Sundaresan AS, Young AJ, Kennedy TL, Scott Greene J, et al. Nasal and sinus symptoms and chronic rhinosinusitis in a population-based sample. Allergy. 2017;72(2):274–81. https://doi.org/10.1111/all.13042.
16. Ostovar A, Fokkens WJ, Vahdat K, Raeisi A, Mallahzadeh A, Farrokhi S. Epidemiology of chronic rhinosinusitis in Bushehr, southwestern region of Iran: a GA2LEN study. Rhinology. 2019;57(1):43–8. https://doi.org/10.4193/Rhin18.061.
17. Shi JB, Fu QL, Zhang H, Cheng L, Wang YJ, Zhu DD, et al. Epidemiology of chronic rhinosinusitis: results from a cross-sectional survey in seven Chinese cities. Allergy. 2015;70(5):533–9. https://doi.org/10.1111/all.12577.
18. Wang XD, Zheng M, Lou HF, Wang CS, Zhang Y, Bo MY, et al. An increased prevalence of self-reported allergic rhinitis in major Chinese cities from 2005 to 2011. Allergy. 2016;71(8):1170–80. https://doi.org/10.1111/all.12874.
19. Kim JH, Cho C, Lee EJ, Suh YS, Choi BI, Kim KS. Prevalence and risk factors of chronic rhinosinusitis in South Korea according to diagnostic criteria. Rhinology. 2016;54(4):329–35. https://doi.org/10.4193/Rhin15.157.
20. Hwang CS, Lee HS, Kim SN, Kim JH, Park DJ, Kim KS. Prevalence and risk factors of chronic rhi-

nosinusitis in the elderly population of Korea. Am J Rhinol Allergy. 2019;33(3):240–6. https://doi.org/10.1177/1945892418813822.
21. Ahn JC, Kim JW, Lee CH, Rhee CS. Prevalence and risk factors of chronic rhinosinusitus, allergic rhinitis, and nasal septal deviation: results of the Korean National Health and Nutrition Survey 2008–2012. JAMA Otolaryngol Head Neck Surg. 2016;142(2):162–7. https://doi.org/10.1001/jamaoto.2015.3142.
22. Lee WH, Hong SN, Kim HJ, Ahn S, Rhee CS, Lee CH, et al. Effects of cigarette smoking on rhinologic diseases: Korean National Health and Nutrition Examination Survey 2008–2011. Int Forum Allergy Rhinol. 2015;5(10):937–43. https://doi.org/10.1002/alr.21553.
23. Kim YS, Kim NH, Seong SY, Kim KR, Lee GB, Kim KS. Prevalence and risk factors of chronic rhinosinusitis in Korea. Am J Rhinol Allergy. 2011;25(3):117–21. https://doi.org/10.2500/ajra.2011.25.3630.
24. Chen Y, Dales R, Lin M. The epidemiology of chronic rhinosinusitis in Canadians. Laryngoscope. 2003;113(7):1199–205. https://doi.org/10.1097/00005537-200307000-00016.
25. Kilty SJ, McDonald JT, Johnson S, Al-Mutairi D. Socioeconomic status: a disease modifier of chronic rhinosinusitis? Rhinology. 2011;49(5):533–7. https://doi.org/10.4193/Rhino10.298.
26. Philpott C, Erskine S, Hopkins C, Coombes E, Kara N, Sunkareneni V, et al. A case-control study of medical, psychological and socio-economic factors influencing the severity of chronic rhinosinusitis. Rhinology. 2016;54(2):134–40. https://doi.org/10.4193/Rhin15.272.
27. Smith DF, Ishman SL, Tunkel DE, Boss EF. Chronic rhinosinusitis in children: race and socioeconomic status. Otolaryngol Head Neck Surg. 2013;149(4):639–44. https://doi.org/10.1177/0194599813498206.
28. Thilsing T, Rasmussen J, Lange B, Kjeldsen AD, Al-Kalemji A, Baelum J. Chronic rhinosinusitis and occupational risk factors among 20- to 75-year-old Danes-A GA(2) LEN-based study. Am J Ind Med. 2012;55(11):1037–43. https://doi.org/10.1002/ajim.22074.
29. Koh DH, Kim HR, Han SS. The relationship between chronic rhinosinusitis and occupation: the 1998, 2001, and 2005 Korea National health and nutrition examination survey (KNHANES). Am J Ind Med. 2009;52(3):179–84. https://doi.org/10.1002/ajim.20665.
30. Gao WX, Ou CQ, Fang SB, Sun YQ, Zhang H, Cheng L, et al. Occupational and environmental risk factors for chronic rhinosinusitis in China: a multicentre cross-sectional study. Respir Res. 2016;17(1):54. https://doi.org/10.1186/s12931-016-0366-z.
31. Chung SD, Chen PY, Lin HC, Hung SH. Comorbidity profile of chronic rhinosinusitis: a population-based study. Laryngoscope. 2014;124(7):1536–41. https://doi.org/10.1002/lary.24581.
32. Bhattacharyya N. Associations between obesity and inflammatory sinonasal disorders. Laryngoscope. 2013;123(8):1840–4. https://doi.org/10.1002/lary.24019.
33. Beule A. Epidemiology of chronic rhinosinusitis, selected risk factors, comorbidities, and economic burden. GMS current topics in otorhinolaryngology, head and neck surgery. 2015;14:Doc11. https://doi.org/10.3205/cto000126.
34. Xu Y, Quan H, Faris P, Garies S, Liu M, Bird C, et al. Prevalence and incidence of diagnosed chronic rhinosinusitis in Alberta, Canada. JAMA Otolaryngol Head Neck Surg. 2016;142(11):1063–9. https://doi.org/10.1001/jamaoto.2016.2227.
35. Park DY, Lee EJ, Kim JH, Kim YS, Jung CM, Kim KS. Correlation between symptoms and objective findings may improve the symptom-based diagnosis of chronic rhinosinusitis for primary care and epidemiological studies. BMJ Open. 2015;5(12):e009541. https://doi.org/10.1136/bmjopen-2015-009541.

3 Quality of Life and Psychological Burden

Eduardo Lehrer, Mauricio López-Chacón, Isam Alobid, and Joaquim Mullol

Key Points

- Chronic rhinosinusitis impairs daily functioning and quality of life in a very negative way comparatively as chronic illnesses such as angina, chronic cardiac failure, asthma, or back pain.
- A thorough evaluation of a patient with chronic rhinosinusitis must include the evaluation of quality of life.
- Patient reported outcomes show deleterious effect on quality of life that reverts after adequate treatment.

E. Lehrer · M. López-Chacón
Rhinology Unit & Smell Clinic, Department of Otorhinolaryngology, Hospital Clínic, Universitat de Barcelona, Barcelona, Catalonia, Spain

Clinical & Experimental Respiratory Immunoallergy, Institut d'Investigacions, Biomèdiques August Pi i Sunyer (IDIBAPS), Barcelona, Catalonia, Spain
e-mail: elehrer@clinic.cat; lochacon@clinic.cat

I. Alobid · J. Mullol (✉)
Rhinology Unit & Smell Clinic, Department of Otorhinolaryngology, Hospital Clínic, Universitat de Barcelona, Barcelona, Catalonia, Spain

Clinical & Experimental Respiratory Immunoallergy, Institut d'Investigacions, Biomèdiques August Pi i Sunyer (IDIBAPS), Barcelona, Catalonia, Spain

CIBER of Respiratory Diseases (CIBERES), Barcelona, Catalonia, Spain
e-mail: JMULLOL@clinic.cat

3.1 Introduction

The conception of quality of life (QoL) carries an effort to comprise what is felt as well-being. From a health-related perspective, it could be outlined as the subject's perception of its situation in life considering the cultural background and value system in which it is, and in relation with its expectations, goals, standards, and interests.

The assessment of QoL in chronic rhinosinusitis (CRS) with (CRSwNP) or without (CRSsNP) nasal polyps focuses on the health status from the perspective of the patient. This fact has been considered by rhinologists over last decades as a very valuable outcome. The term health-related quality of life (HRQoL) covers every aspect that could impact on well-being such as physical, social, emotional, psychological, sexual, cognitional, or economical features. Nowadays, it is well-known how CRS very negatively affects HRQoL and how treatment options can revert that situation.

Patient reported outcomes (PRO) consist of self-administered measures (i.e. questionnaires, visual scales, grading systems) given to patients, or in selected cases by proxies, that reflect disease severity and the effect of the treatment.

Classically, PRO have been divided into two main types: those designed to determine a general health status, named generic PRO, and those

L. Zhang, C. Bachert (eds.), *Chronic Rhinosinusitis*, https://doi.org/10.1007/978-981-16-0784-4_3

directed to a specific disease or treatment, named specific PRO. Generic PRO allow to analyse the burden of CRS among the rest of diseases to subsequently inform commissioning decisions while specific questionnaires provide details on the distinct disease domains [1].

CRS burden greatly depend upon the selected population, this being reflected by selected symptoms as bothersome or severe (Fig. 3.1). The disease severity could be influenced by gender or cultural beliefs. Recent studies revealed that females are inclined to express more severity

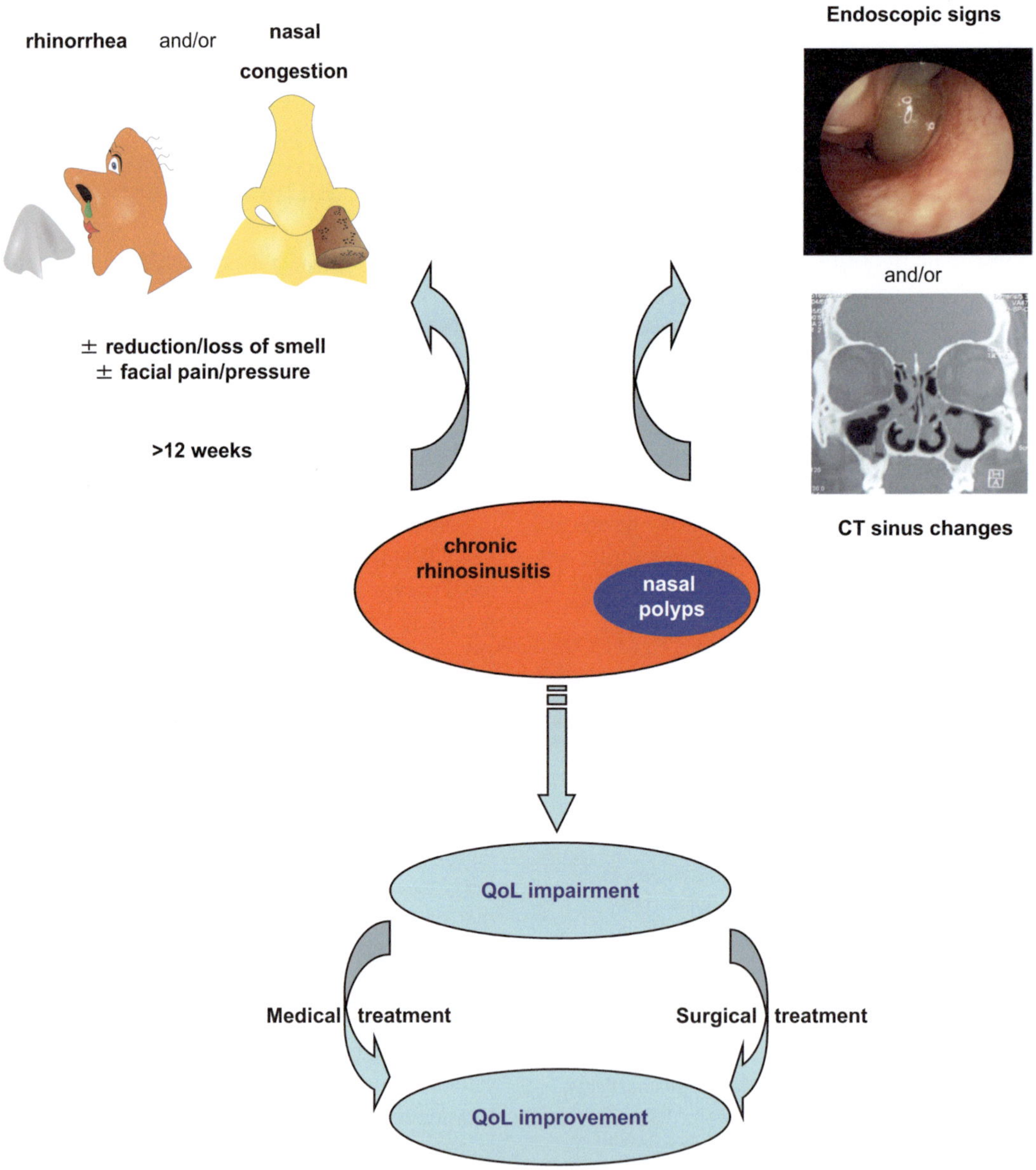

Fig. 3.1 Scheme of the chronic rhinosinusitis (Source: adopted with courtesy for EPOS2020). Chronic rhinosinusitis, including nasal polyps, lead to negatively impact patients' quality of life, which offset by both medical (including biologicals) and/or surgical treatment

than males, thus it reflects more influence on their HRQoL [1, 2]. Concomitant disorders such as depression or any social feature could enhance negatively the impact on HRQoL.

3.2 Psychometric Properties

The most important psychometric characteristics that must be covered in any QoL PRO are validity, reliability, and responsiveness. Moreover, when PRO are to be delivered in different language other than the original, forward-backward translations to confirm the original meaning as well as revalidation of the outcomes to ensure the same psychometric properties are required.

3.2.1 Validity

It refers to the level to which evidence supports the interpretations of test scores. Validity is *convergent* when the level to which two measures concepts theoretically related are empirically related, or *discriminant* when measurements theoretically unrelated are unrelated [3].

3.2.2 Reliability

There are two procedures applied to PRO to confirm that they are reliable.

3.2.2.1 Test–Retest

Test–retest is executed by employing the same PRO after a specific treatment in two time points. Period between measurements is critical, as it will determine the degree of correlation between constructs.

3.2.2.2 Internal Consistency

It measures at one time several items that are proposed to measure a same general characteristic to generate similar values. It is calculated by the Cronbach's alpha coefficient in a range from 0 to 1. When the coefficient is ≥0.7 it is contemplated as reliable for group level comparisons; or ≥0.9 at individual level. When the set of items are displayed to measure more than one characteristic, the hierarchical omega coefficient is more appropriate [4].

3.2.3 Responsiveness

Responsiveness is the aptitude of an implement to notice meaningful changes in an accurate way. *Internal responsiveness* indicates the aptitude of a measure to adapt in a period of time. Internal responsiveness is often studied before and after treatment. On the other hand, *external responsiveness* reflects how much there is a variation in a measure adjusted to other measures of health situation [5].

3.3 Patient Reported Outcomes (PRO) in CRS

3.3.1 Generic Questionnaires

Short Form-36 Health Survey (SF-36), Short Form-12 Health Survey (SF-12), EuroQol-5D (EQ-5D), McGill Pain Questionnaire (MPQ) are some of the most used and published generic questionnaires in CRS (Table 3.1). Most of them are mainly designed to be filled during interviews, in daily clinical practice, or in clinical research. Only in the paediatric population they are often delivered to proxies. Concepts as mental or physical status, pain, self-care, mobility, or anxiety are delimited by these PRO. Most of these PRO have been validated into several languages. Depending on the selected questionnaire, there are normative values for general population as for patients suffering diseases as CRS.

CRS has shown great changes compared to healthy population when general PRO have been applied. Significant differences have been found

Table 3.1 Most used patient reported outcomes in CRS (adapted from Lehrer et al. 2013 [6])

Category	Questionnaire	Number of concepts	Items	Score range	Fill-in time (min)
Generic	SF-36	8	36	0 to 100	<20
	SF-12	8	12	0 to 100	<10
	EQ-5D	5	15	0 to 100	<10
	MPQ	20	78	0 to78	<20
	GBI	3	18	−100 to 100	<10
	CHQ-PF50	14	50	0 to 100	<20
Specific	RSOM-31	7	31	0 to 155	<20
	SNOT-22	–	22	0 to 110	<5
	SNOT-20	–	20	0 to 100	<5
	SNOT-16	–	16	0 to 48	<5
	RhinoQoL	3	17	0 to 100	<10
	SN-5	–	5	5 to 35	<5
	SOQ	5	26	0 to 130	<10
	RQLQ	7	28	0 to 168	<15
	CSS	2	6	0 to 100	<5

CRS chronic rhinosinusitis, *SF-36* Short Form-36 Health Survey, *SF-12* Short Form-12 Health Survey, *EQ-5D* EuroQoL-5D, *MPQ* McGill Pain Questionnaire, *GBI* Glasgow Benefit Inventory, *CHQ-PF50* Child Health Questionnaire Parent Form-50, *RSOM* Rhinosinusitis Outcome Measure, *SNOT-16/20/22* Sino-Nasal Outcome Test-16/20/22, *RhinoQoL* Rhinosinusitis Quality of Life questionnaire, *SN-5* Sino-Nasal 5, *SOQ* Sinusitis Outcome Questionnaire, *RQLQ* Rhinoconjunctivitis Quality of Life Questionnaire, *CSS* Chronic Sinusitis Survey

Table 3.2 Representative studies assessing HRQoL in CRS using generic questionnaires

Survey	Patients included (n)	Subject of analysis	Generic PRO used	QoL evaluation	Level of evidence
Alobid et al. [7]	78	CRSwNP vs. CRSsNP	SF-36	CRS impairs QoL, QoL improves after treatment	1b
Guilemany et al. [8]	80	CRSwNP with bronchiectasis	SF-36	CRSwNP impairs QoL	2b
Dudvarski et al. [9]	88	CRS with or without asthma	SF-36	CRS with asthma and CRS alone respond similar to treatment	2a
Gevaert et al. [10]	24	CRSwNP with asthma	SF-36	CRSwNP improves after treatment	1b
Ek et al. [11]	605	Healthy individuals, CRS alone and CRS with asthma	EQ-5D	CRS with or without asthma impairs QoL	2b
Campbell et al. [12]	350	CRS with or without asthma	EQ-5D	CRS with or without asthma impairs QoL	2b
Hoehle et al. [13]	203	CRS	EQ-5D	CRS impairs QoL	2b
Khan et al. [14]	445	CRSwNP	SF-36	CRSwNP impairs QoL	2a

HRQoL health-related quality of life, *CRS* chronic rhinosinusitis, with (CRSwNP) or without (CRSsNP) nasal polyps, *PRO* patient reported outcomes, *QoL* quality of life, *CSF-36* Short Form-36 Health Survey, *EQ-5D* EuroQoL-5D

applying generic PRO in all of their domains according to last decade publications (Table 3.2). CRS has demonstrated to have a big impact on social functioning similar to other very limiting illnesses such as angina, chronic cardiac failure, asthma, or back pain [15].

3.3.2 Specific Questionnaires

Specific questionnaires were thought to detect precise details in terms of QoL variations under a specific situation or disease. They are addressed to measure health status and effectiveness of treatment. Several specific PRO are available for CRS (Table 3.1). The instrument selection must be done depending on the specific outcome that is desired to analyse. Currently, Sino-Nasal Outcome Test-22 is by far the most employed QoL questionnaire in CRS. Other PRO widely used are the Rhinoconjunctivitis Quality of Life Questionnaire or the Chronic Sinusitis Survey Score.

Specific questionnaires lead to neatly describe CRS symptomatology. Nasal congestion, obstruction, and nasal discharge plus facial ache, and alteration in sense of smell are considered as the main manifestations in CRS; and these symptoms alter negatively the HRQoL. Treatment of CRS, even medical or surgical, has shown to improve in a significant way HRQoL.

3.3.2.1 SNOT-22: A Measure of Severity

The SNOT-22, validated in 2009, is a modified form of SNOT-20 and the RSOM, that contains 22 entries related to general symptoms, nose, and paranasal sinuses [16]. The revision included the addition of one question on loss of smell and taste and another on nasal obstruction; besides, it was also modified to make the scale easier to use. Patients are also asked to identify the five most important items. Big amounts of published trials provide data on the implementation of SNOT-22 and in all publications a greater score indicates a greater QoL problem [16, 17].

Hopkins et al. showed that SNOT-22 is able to distinguish between healthy controls and patients with CRS. SNOT-22 is capable of recognizing differences in specific clusters of patients with CRS, such as CRS patients with history of revision surgery, those with symptoms for less than one year, with asthma or aspirin sensitivity, or patients who were smokers [16].

Although SNOT-22 is able to quantify QoL in patients with CRS, only faint correlations between objective CRS parameters and SNOT-22 total scores, such as computed tomography (CT) and endonasal polyp scores have been observed. Still, a significant correlation between before/after surgery SNOT-22 total scores motivated by the "*nasal symptoms*" domain has been observed [18]. A recent meta-analysis has insinuated that patient-specific factors may affect the degree of SNOT-22 change after treatment [19]. These factors included age and gender.

Some authors debated on the need of grouping items in different domains for a better interpretation of the test. Feng et al. evaluated the instrument in 177 non-European patients with history of CRS and proposed grouping the items of the SNOT-22 in four domains based on major module analysis. These domains were "nasal symptoms", "otologic symptoms", "sleep symptoms", and "emotional symptoms". The authors argued that this modification may allow the test to become a reference composition for European CRS patients [20].

A recent study has led to the discussion that there might be cultural biases in patients with CRS that should be considered when trying to group the items in domains [21].

3.3.2.2 SNOT-22: A Measure of Response to Medical Treatment

The minimally clinically important difference (MCID), the smallest variation in symptom, or QoL following a specific intervention that can be detected and is clinically important for the patient, has been defined as the reduction of 8.9 points on the global SNOT-22 result [16]. Therefore, patients who have a reduction of less than nine points after receiving treatment are unlikely to perceive any real benefit.

Lidder et al. studied the response to treatment in adult CRS patients which had started medical therapy (MT) using SNOT-22 and symptom VAS at baseline and after three months post-treatment. The authors observed that the two measured PRO showed response to treatment although not in every item were equally reactive. Especially, responsiveness metrics showed that SNOT-22 main items were the most responsive [22]. Hence, the manifestation of non-responsive items and others related to general QoL might diminish SNOT-22 overall responsiveness, whereas discovering valuable variations just after treatments with bigger effects, such as endoscopic sinus surgery (ESS). A recent publication showed that the SNOT-22 MCID is rather specific than sensitive for detecting individuals experiencing important CRS symptom changes [23]. The authors detected that, subjects with less than 1 MCID difference (sub-MCID) in the SNOT-22 who reported an improvement in one nasal symptom but not in CRS symptoms out of the nose, they also showed improvement of their CRS manifestations by VAS. However, it is still imprecise why some subjects with less than one MCID difference in SNOT-22 result inform so manifest improvement.

Regarding to subjects who experience difficult-to-treat CRS, Dejaco et al. compared the outcomes of patients who received at least one course of maximal medical therapy (MMT) using four standardized treatments with patients who received intranasal steroids and irrigation (cNSI) in an uninterrupted way, reiterated MMT, intranasal corticosteroid, or ESS [24]. The authors determined that standard interventions improved SNOT-22 results in patients with recalcitrant CRS. The trial exposed patients with CRSwNP and CRSsNP that improved their scores evaluated by SNOT-22, yet the measured effects were less intense among those with CRSsNP. ESS patients manifested fewer symptoms than medically treated patients at the first year of follow-up. Those cases of recalcitrant CRS did not get any benefit from additional courses of MMT when they were compared to those who were just treated with cNSI.

3.3.2.3 SNOT-22: A Measure of Response to Surgical Treatment

Several studies have reported a failure to correlate the degree of sinonasal inflammation measured by CT scan or nasal endoscopy to the magnitude of symptoms that could be experienced [15]. Therefore, numerous studies have evaluated the use of SNOT-22 as a tool to determine which patients could be candidates for surgical treatment and also to evaluate their post-surgical response [18].

SNOT-22 applicability has increased over the years as PRO are progressively being used in daily practice. However, due to the heterogeneity in the methodological design of the published studies, it is difficult to determine the differences between surgical and medical treatment.

The SNOT-22 has the advantage of combining items that are specific to sinonasal complaints with other general health topics, which may be evaluated alone or combined, before and after surgery [16]. In a multicentric cohort trial, 382 CRS patients, in whom the medical treatment had previously failed, total SNOT-22 score and productivity loss were assessed using five age clusters. Discriminant analysis identified three out of five clusters that improved SNOT-22 results after surgery when were contrasted with medical treatment. These differences persisted at 18 months after surgery. The two clusters left had similar outcomes after surgery or medical treatment [18].

Some studies indicate that subjects with a pre-surgical SNOT-22 result over 40 have more than 75% likelihood of reaching MCID and in average 40% of improving their QoL after ESS [19]. In a recent meta-analysis, the authors studied 40 individual cohorts ($n = 5547$ patients) and found that the mean variation in SNOT-22 within all reports was 24.4 (95% CI: 22.0–26.8) [18]. Reports with higher mean preoperative SNOT-22 results and superior asthma occurrence were linked to larger variations in SNOT-22 after surgery, while reports with longer mean follow-up had reduced changes. The authors observed that the extent dimension was fairly variable and seemed to be induced by several features including baseline SNOT-22 result, asthma occurrence, and follow-up length [19].

3.3.2.4 SNOT-22: A Measure of Response to Biologic Treatment

Is currently on debate if monoclonal antibodies are a logical substitute to primary ESS [25]. As more studies have been developed, biologics have been increasingly considered. In this sense, HRQoL evaluation has played a major role.

Up to the present time, one report showed in patients with CRSwNP and asthma that omalizumab compared to ESS leads to similar effects reducing SNOT-22 [10]. In an asthma trial evaluating the effects of dupilumab, each participant completed the SNOT-22 at baseline and after 12 weeks [26]. Results favoured dupilumab in some nasal items of SNOT-22 including the sense of smell. This information allowed to study the effects of dupilumab on severe CRSwNP, which were then evaluated thoroughly in two international multicentre trial of phase II and III, respectively [27, 28]. These trials had as objective to measure changes in nasal polyps as in its symptoms. Dupilumab was very superior to placebo in terms of symptoms measured by means of VAS and SNOT-22. The trials showed significant improvements in the sense of smell, nasal congestion, morning rhinorrhoea, or nocturnal awakenings.

Later, in another randomized, double-blind, placebo-controlled trial, the authors showed by means of objective and subjective measures a consistent reduction in the demand of ESS on the selected population [29]. Symptoms significantly improved after 9 weeks of administration of mepolizumab in subjects with refractory nasal polyposis, and the effect remained until the end of treatment after 25 weeks.

3.4 Translation into the Future Daily Practice

PRO altogether have been extensively employed to assess the CRS burden on QoL. These outcomes are as useful in the daily clinical practice as in clinical trials. Generic and specific questionnaires have shown that CRS affects negatively the HRQoL while the appropriate therapy reverts the situation by improving QoL (Fig. 3.1).

In the last decade, the most commonly used generic questionnaires to measure changes in QoL in patients with CRS are the SF-36 and the EQ-5d. In terms of specific questionnaires, SNOT-22 won this role by including important CRS symptoms, for example, nasal obstructions and the sense of smell and taste.

All these outcomes must always be in consonance with the current guidelines in order to show appropriate psychometric properties to assess CRS.

Current mobile technology allows the enhancement of patient empowerment via education and self-management. This technology can be very useful in the assessment of chronic illnesses such as CRS. EUFOREA recently developed and implemented an instrument to monitor the CRS symptoms in such patients. The digital support platform provides patients with trustworthy medical material about their conditions and possible cares. The use of this platform could also generate authentic data, which could help to endorse clinical trials, patient classification and increase the understanding of the CRS-related socioeconomic burden [30]. All these tools may help the physician to provide treatment information or recommend the patient to the platform which could be time saving. Moreover, it could help to detect those CRS patients who will potentially require additional medical, surgical, or biological treatment.

References

1. Remenschneider AK, Scangas G, Meier JC, Gray ST, Holbrook EH, Gliklich RE, et al. EQ-5D-derived health utility values in patients undergoing surgery for chronic rhinosinusitis. Laryngoscope. 2015;125(5):1056–61. https://doi.org/10.1002/lary.25054.
2. Fu QL, Ma JX, Ou CQ, Guo C, Shen SQ, Xu G, et al. Influence of self-reported chronic rhinosinusitis on health-related quality of life: a population-based survey. PLoS One. 2015;10(5):e0126881. https://doi.org/10.1371/journal.pone.0126881.
3. Aaronson N, Alonso J, Burnam A, Lohr KN, Patrick DL, Perrin E, et al. Assessing health status and quality-of-life instruments: attributes and review criteria. Qual Life Res Int J Qual Life Asp Treat Care Rehab. 2002;11(3):193–205. https://doi.org/10.1023/a:1015291021312.
4. Zinbarg RE, Revelle W, Yovel I, Li W. Cronbach's α, Revelle's β, and Mcdonald's ωH: their relations with each other and two alternative conceptualizations of reliability. Psychometrika. 2005;70(1):123–33. https://doi.org/10.1007/s11336-003-0974-7.
5. Husted JA, Cook RJ, Farewell VT, Gladman DD. Methods for assessing responsiveness: a critical review and recommendations. J Clin Epidemiol. 2000;53(5):459–68. https://doi.org/10.1016/s0895-4356(99)00206-1.
6. Lehrer E, Mariño-Sánchez F, Alobid I, Mullol J. Quality of life measures in patients on rhinosinusitis trials. Clin Investig (Lond). 2013;3(3):251–63.

https://doi.org/10.4155/CLI.13.5.
7. Alobid I, Benítez P, Bernal-Sprekelsen M, Roca J, Alonso J, Picado C, et al. Nasal polyposis and its impact on quality of life: comparison between the effects of medical and surgical treatments. Allergy. 2005;60(4):452–8. https://doi.org/10.1111/j.1398-9995.2005.00725.x.
8. Guilemany JM, Angrill J, Alobid I, Centellas S, Prades E, Roca J, et al. United airways: the impact of chronic rhinosinusitis and nasal polyps in bronchiectasic patient's quality of life. Allergy. 2009;64(10):1524–9. https://doi.org/10.1111/j.1398-9995.2009.02011.x.
9. Dudvarski Z, Djukic V, Janosevic L, Tomanovic N, Soldatovic I. Influence of asthma on quality of life and clinical characteristics of patients with nasal polyposis. Eur Arch Otorhinolaryngol. 2013;270(4):1379–83. https://doi.org/10.1007/s00405-012-2242-x.
10. Gevaert P, Calus L, Van Zele T, Blomme K, De Ruyck N, Bauters W, et al. Omalizumab is effective in allergic and nonallergic patients with nasal polyps and asthma. J Allergy Clin Immunol. 2013;131(1):110–6.e1. https://doi.org/10.1016/j.jaci.2012.07.047.
11. Ek A, Middelveld RJ, Bertilsson H, Bjerg A, Ekerljung L, Malinovschi A, et al. Chronic rhinosinusitis in asthma is a negative predictor of quality of life: results from the Swedish GA(2)LEN survey. Allergy. 2013;68(10):1314–21. https://doi.org/10.1111/all.12222.
12. Campbell AP, Phillips KM, Hoehle LP, Gaudin RA, Caradonna DS, Gray ST, et al. Association between asthma and chronic rhinosinusitis severity in the context of asthma control. Otolaryngol Head Neck Surg. 2018;158(2):386–90. https://doi.org/10.1177/0194599817728920.
13. Hoehle LP, Phillips KM, Speth MM, Caradonna DS, Gray ST, Sedaghat AR. Responsiveness and minimal clinically important difference for the EQ-5D in chronic rhinosinusitis. Rhinology. 2019;57(2):110–6. https://doi.org/10.4193/Rhin18.122.
14. Khan A, Huynh TMT, Vandeplas G, Joish VN, Mannent LP, Tomassen P, et al. The GALEN rhinosinusitis cohort: chronic rhinosinusitis with nasal polyps affects health-related quality of life. Rhinology. 2019;57(5):343–51. https://doi.org/10.4193/Rhin19.158.
15. Fokkens WJ, Lund VJ, Mullol J, Bachert C, Alobid I, Baroody F, et al. European Position Paper on Rhinosinusitis and Nasal Polyps 2012. Rhinology Supplement. 2012;23:3 p preceding table of contents, 1–298.
16. Hopkins C, Gillett S, Slack R, Lund VJ, Browne JP. Psychometric validity of the 22-item sinonasal outcome test. Clin Otolaryngol. 2009;34(5):447–54. https://doi.org/10.1111/j.1749-4486.2009.01995.x.
17. Soler ZM, Hyer JM, Ramakrishnan V, Smith TL, Mace J, Rudmik L, et al. Identification of chronic rhinosinusitis phenotypes using cluster analysis. Int Forum Allergy Rhinol. 2015;5(5):399–407. https://doi.org/10.1002/alr.21496.
18. Soler ZM, Jones R, Le P, Rudmik L, Mattos JL, Nguyen SA, et al. Sino-Nasal outcome test-22 outcomes after sinus surgery: a systematic review and meta-analysis. Laryngoscope. 2018;128(3):581–92. https://doi.org/10.1002/lary.27008.
19. Soler ZM, Hyer JM, Rudmik L, Ramakrishnan V, Smith TL, Schlosser RJ. Cluster analysis and prediction of treatment outcomes for chronic rhinosinusitis. J Allergy Clin Immunol. 2016;137(4):1054–62. https://doi.org/10.1016/j.jaci.2015.11.019.
20. Feng AL, Wesely NC, Hoehle LP, Phillips KM, Yamasaki A, Campbell AP, et al. A validated model for the 22-item Sino-Nasal Outcome Test subdomain structure in chronic rhinosinusitis. Int Forum Allergy Rhinol. 2017;7(12):1140–8. https://doi.org/10.1002/alr.22025.
21. Dejaco D, Riedl D, Huber A, Moschen R, Giotakis AI, Bektic-Tadic L, et al. The SNOT-22 factorial structure in European patients with chronic rhinosinusitis: new clinical insights. Eur Arch Otorhinolaryngol. 2019;276(5):1355–65. https://doi.org/10.1007/s00405-019-05320-z.
22. Lidder AK, Detwiller KY, Price CP, Kern RC, Conley DB, Shintani-Smith S, et al. Evaluating metrics of responsiveness using patient-reported outcome measures in chronic rhinosinusitis. Int Forum Allergy Rhinol. 2017;7(2):128–34. https://doi.org/10.1002/alr.21866.
23. Phillips KM, Hoehle LP, Caradonna DS, Gray ST, Sedaghat AR. Determinants of noticeable symptom improvement despite sub-MCID change in SNOT-22 score after treatment for chronic rhinosinusitis. Int Forum Allergy Rhinol. 2019;9(5):508–13. https://doi.org/10.1002/alr.22269.
24. Dejaco D, Riedl D, Giotakis A, Bektic-Tadic L, Kahler P, Riechelmann H. Treatment outcomes in chronic rhinosinusitis refractory to maximal medical therapy: a prospective observational study under real-world conditions. Ear Nose Throat J 2019:145561319849421. https://doi.org/10.1177/0145561319849421.
25. Fokkens WJ, Lund V, Bachert C, Mullol J, Bjermer L, Bousquet J, et al. EUFOREA consensus on biologics for CRSwNP with or without asthma. Allergy. 2019;74(12):2312–9. https://doi.org/10.1111/all.13875.
26. Wenzel SE, Wang L, Pirozzi G. Dupilumab in persistent asthma. N Engl J Med. 2013;369(13):1276. https://doi.org/10.1056/NEJMc1309809.
27. Bachert C, Mannent L, Naclerio RM, Mullol J, Ferguson BJ, Gevaert P, et al. Effect of subcutaneous dupilumab on nasal polyp burden in patients with chronic sinusitis and nasal polyposis: a randomized clinical trial. JAMA. 2016;315(5):469–79. https://doi.org/10.1001/jama.2015.19330.
28. Bachert C, Han JK, Desrosiers M, Hellings PW, Amin N, Lee SE, et al. Efficacy and safety of dupilumab in

patients with severe chronic rhinosinusitis with nasal polyps (LIBERTY NP SINUS-24 and LIBERTY NP SINUS-52): results from two multicentre, randomised, double-blind, placebo-controlled, parallel-group phase 3 trials. Lancet (London, England). 2019;394(10209):1638–50. https://doi.org/10.1016/s0140-6736(19)31881-1.
29. Bachert C, Sousa AR, Lund VJ, Scadding GK, Gevaert P, Nasser S, et al. Reduced need for surgery in severe nasal polyposis with mepolizumab: randomized trial. J Allergy Clin Immunol. 2017;140(4):1024–31.e14. https://doi.org/10.1016/j.jaci.2017.05.044
30. Seys SF, Bousquet J, Bachert C, Fokkens WJ, Agache I, Bernal-Sprekelsen M, et al. mySinusitisCoach: patient empowerment in chronic rhinosinusitis using mobile technology. Rhinology. 2018;56(3):209–15. https://doi.org/10.4193/Rhin17.253.

4 Genetics and Epigenetics

Jingyun Li, Luo Zhang, and Yuan Zhang

Key Points

- CRS has a complex genetic architecture with heritability of 13–53%.
- Candidate gene association studies in CRS patients have investigated the genes for CRS related to immunity, inflammatory, and airway remodelling related molecules.
- Genome-wide association studies have shown that CRS shares genetic susceptibility loci with allergic and immunological diseases and traits.
- Some epigenetic marks (DNA methylation, histone modifications, and noncoding RNAs) have important roles and therapeutic potentialities in CRS.

4.1 Heritability of CRS

The inconsistent findings from early studies in twins suggest that both genetic and environmental factors contribute to the pathogenesis of CRS. The genetic architecture of CRS is complex, and the heritability for CRS has been shown to range from 13% to 53% [1–3]; the highest heritability shown in the triad of aspirin intolerance, nasal polyposis, and asthma [2]. The mutations in cystic fibrosis transmembrane conductance regulator (*CFTR*) gene [4] and in dynein axonemal heavy chain 5 (*DNAH5*) gene [5], which have been identified for cystic fibrosis (CF) and primary ciliary dyskinesia (PCD), respectively, exhibit similar features with CRS, and thus provide further evidence for the role of a genetic component in the aetiology of CRS.

4.2 Genetics of CRS

Sequencing the whole human genome completely in 2002 has made it possible to perform population-based association studies on a large scale to elucidate the susceptibility genes or loci associated with some common diseases, including upper and lower airway diseases.

J. Li
Department of Otolaryngology, Head and Neck Surgery, Beijing Tongren Hospital, Capital Medical University, Beijing, China

Beijing Key Laboratory of Nasal Diseases, Beijing Institute of Otolaryngology, Beijing, China

L. Zhang · Y. Zhang (✉)
Department of Otolaryngology, Head and Neck Surgery, Beijing Tongren Hospital, Capital Medical University, Beijing, China

Beijing Key Laboratory of Nasal Diseases, Beijing Institute of Otolaryngology, Beijing, China

Department of Allergy, Beijing Tongren Hospital, Capital Medical University, Beijing, China

L. Zhang, C. Bachert (eds.), *Chronic Rhinosinusitis*, https://doi.org/10.1007/978-981-16-0784-4_4

4.2.1 Candidate Gene Association Studies of CRS

Candidate gene or pathway approaches, which focus on single nucleotide polymorphisms (SNPs) in specific genes that have been shown to be involved in the pathogenesis of specific diseases, have commonly been employed in the identification of genetic component/s implicated in CRS. Most susceptibility genes for CRS have been shown to be associated with immunity, inflammatory, and airway remodelling related molecules. Table 4.1 summarizes the candidate genes which have been shown to be elucidated in CRS patients of different ethnicity. HLA loci were found to be the most hot spot loci in earlier candidate gene association studies for CRS due to the vital function of antigen presentation [6–14]. Several alleles of HLA-DR and HLA-DQ have been shown to be linked with CRS in different ethnicity groups. Two functional SNPs in IL1A (rs17561) [15–17] and TNFA (rs1800629) [16, 22, 23] genes associated with CRSwNP have been replicated in distinct populations of European descent. Interestingly, variants in bitter taste receptors (T2Rs) have been proposed to be associated with upper respiratory diseases, including CRS [58]. In particular, three common SNPs located in TASR38 gene (Pro49Ala, Ala262Val, Val296Ile) have been shown to affect the activity of T2R. These SNPs segregate together and form two more common haplotypes, of which one is the functional allele composed of proline, alanine, and valine (PAV) and the other is the non-functional allele composed of alanine, valine, and isoleucine (AVI). Recent genetic investigations have demonstrated that the PAV/PAV genotype was associated not only with CRS, but also with CRS related factors including comorbidities, bacterial infection, surgical intervention, and outcomes [51–55]. One recent study has demonstrated that a SNP in the GLCCI1 (rs37973) is related to postoperative recovery from CRS for individual sensitivity to glucocorticoids (Liu et al. 2018b). However, because the relatively small sample size of cohort leads to the study being underpowered and genetic heterogeneity among the cohort, candidate gene association studies suffer from inconsistent results and lack of replicability.

4.2.2 Genome-Wide Association Studies of CRS

Genome-wide association studies (GWAS) do not depend on any specific gene driven hypotheses, but screen the whole genome to find any associations between susceptibility loci and disease. To date a total of four GWAS have been carried out for genetic predisposition to CRS phenotypes.

The first GWAS study of CRS was performed using a DNA pooling-based technique and identified 600 significant SNPs ($P < 0.05$) from 445 genes among 210 CRS patients and 189 controls from a Caucasian population [59]. The top 10 CRS-associated genes were shown to be linked with interactions at the level of basement membrane and extracellular matrix (LAMA2 and LAMB1), mitochondrial function (PARS2), and lipopolysaccharide degradation (AOAH). Zhang and colleagues [60] showed that 17 of these CRS-associated genes were replicated in a Han Chinese population. Furthermore, the rs4504543 polymorphism in AOAH gene was markedly associated with CRS. However, another replication study reported rs2873551 in PARS2 to be significantly associated with CRS in a Caucasian population [25].

Using the same pooling-based strategy, another GWAS involving 408 CRS patients and 190 control subjects from a Caucasian population reported 23 SNPs ($P < 0.05$) to be associated with *S. aureus* colonization in CRS patients [61]. These SNPs were located within or near 21 genes reported to be implicated in endocytic internalization and bacterial recognition.

A recent family-based GWAS has identified 5 CRSwNP susceptible loci, including HLA-DRA, HLCS, BICD2, VSIR, and SLC5A1; of which only HLA-DRA has been reported in previous candidate gene association studies [62].

More recently, a large-scale meta-analysis of GWAS for NP and CRS was performed in two large European cohorts: one from deCODE

Table 4.1 Candidate gene association studies in CRS

Gene	Polymorphism	Population	Phenotype	Reference
HLA	HLA-A1B8	European	CRSwNP, asthma, ASA	[6]
	HLA-A74	European	CRSwNP	[7]
	HLA-DR7-DQA1*0201, HLA-DQB1*0202, HLA-DR5	European	CRSwNP, asthma, aspirin sensitivity	[8]
	HLA-DQB*03	American	Allergic fungal rhinosinusitis, hypertrophic sinus disease	[9]
	HLA-DRB1*03, HLA-DRB1*04, HLA-DRB1*08	Mexican	CRSwNP	[10]
	HLA-DQA*0201	Mexican	CRSwNP	[11]
	HLA-DR16, HLA-DQ8, HLA-DQ9	Chinese	CRSwNP	[12]
	HLA-B*07, -B*57, HLA-Cw*12, -Cw*04, HLA-A*24, HLA-DRB*04	Turkish	CRSwNP, asthma, acetylsalicylic acid triad	[13]
	HLA-DRA (rs9268644, rs3129878)	Korean	Asthma with CRSwNP	[14]
IL1A	rs17561	Finnish Caucasian	Asthma with CRSwNP	[15]
	rs17561	Turkish	CRSwNP	[16]
	rs17561, rs2856838, rs2048874	Canadian	CRSwNP	[17]
IL1RN	5 Variable number tandem repeat	Chinese	CRS	[18]
IL1B	rs16944	Turkish	CRSwNP	[16]
	rs16944	Polish	CRSwNP	[19]
IL1RL1	rs10204137, rs10208293, rs13431828, rs2160203, rs4988957	Canadian	CRS	[20]
IRAK4	rs1461567, rs4251513, rs4251559	Canadian	Total serum IgE in CRS	[21]
TNFA	rs361525, rs1800629	Turkish	CRSwNP	[16]
	rs1800629	American	CRSwNP	[22]
	rs1800629	European	CRSwNP	[23]
TGFB	rs11466315	Korean	AIA, CRS	[24]
	rs1800469	Caucasian	CRS	[25]
TNFAIP3	rs3757173, rs5029938	Canadian	CRS	[26]
IL4	C-590T	Korean	CRSwNP	[27]
IL10	rs1800896	Korean	AIA and CRSwNP	[28]
IL22RA1	rs4292900, rs4648936, rs16829225	Canadian	Severe CRS	[29]
	rs11579657	Caucasian	CRS	[25]
IL33	rs3939286	Belgian	CRSwNP	[30]
TSLP	rs252706, rs764917	Chinese	CRSwNP	[31]
CD8A	rs3810831	Canadian	CRS and severity factors	[32]
TAPBP	rs2282851	Canadian	CRS	[32]
EBI3	rs428253	Chinese	CRS	[33]
FOXP3	rs2232365, rs3761548	Chinese	CRS	[33]
ADRB2	Arg16Gly	European	CRSwNP	[34]
MET	rs38850	Canadian	CRS	[35]
	C-14G	Polish	CRSwNP	[36]
COX2	G-765C	Polish	CRSwNP	[36]
ALOX5	rs3780894	Canadian	CRS	[37]
ALOX5AP	rs17612127	Canadian	CRS	[37]
	rs17238773	Caucasian	CRS	[25]
CYSTLR1	rs321090	Canadian	CRS	[37]
SERPINA1	rs1243168, rs4900229	Canadian	CRS unresponsive to medical therapy	[38]
TP73	rs3765731	Canadian	CRS	[39]

(continued)

Table 4.1 (continued)

Gene	Polymorphism	Population	Phenotype	Reference
TLR2	rs3804099, rs3804100	Korean	CRS	[40]
NOS1	rs1483757, rs9658281	Canadian	Severe CRS	[41]
	rs1483757	Caucasian	CRS	[25]
iNOS	C-277T	Turkish	Eosinophilic and non-eosinophilic CRSwNP	[42]
CAT	A-21T	Turkish	Eosinophilic and non-eosinophilic CRSwNP	[42]
MMP9	rs3918242	Turkish	CRSwNP with aspirin-induced asthma	[43]
	rs3918242, rs2274756	Chinese	CRSwNP	[44]
MMP1	-1607insG	Polish	CRSwNP	[45]
CACNG6	rs192808	Korean	AIA, CRSwNP	[46]
EMID2	rs6945102-rs4729697-rs221-rs1043533 haplotype	Korean	CRSwNP with asthma	[47]
DCBLD2	rs828618	Korean	CRSwNP with asthma	[48]
	rs828618	Caucasian	CRS	[25]
LF	140A/G	Polish	CRSwNP	[49]
OSF-2	-33C/G	Polish	CRSwNP	[49]
FCERIA	rs2427827	Indian	Total serum IgE in CRSwNP	[50]
TAS2R38	Pro49Ala-Ala262Val-Val296Ile haplotype (PAV/AVI)	American	CRS necessitating surgical intervention	[51]
	PAV/AVI	American	CRS requiring sinus surgery	[52]
	rs10246939	Canadian	Refractory CRS, CRSwNP	[53]
	PAV/AVI	American	Surgical outcome in CRSsNP	[54]
	PAV/AVI	Italian	Gram-negative infections with CRSwNP	[55]
TAS2R13	rs1015443, rs12226919	Canadian	Refractory CRS	[53]
CDHR3	rs6967330	Non-Hispanic white	CRS	[56]
GLCCI1	rs37973	Chinese	Sensitivity to glucocorticoids in CRS	[57]

CRS chronic rhinosinusitis, *CRSwNP* chronic rhinosinusitis with nasal polyps, *AIA* aspirin-intolerant asthma

genetics in Iceland (1175 cases vs. 309,305 controls) and the other from UK Biobank (3191 cases and 405,376 controls) [63]. A total of 27 variants were found to be associated with NP susceptibility, of which, 17 variants were associated with eosinophil count, 7 with CRS and 13 with asthma. It is noteworthy that a low frequency (0.025) missense variant p.Thr560Met (rs34210653) in ALOX15 contributed to a 68% reduction of risk of NP and 36% reduction of risk of CRS. ALOX15 encodes 15-lipoxygenase (15-LO), which is involved in inflammatory and immune processes and is elevated in NP tissue [64]. The variant p.Thr560Met affects hydrogen bonding network of the active sites leading to near-null variant of the enzyme [65]. However, the variant p.Thr560Met shows an extremely low frequency in Asian and African populations (South Asian, 0.0097; East Asian, 0; African, 0.0036) in ExAC database. NP association signals in ALOX15 may lead to linkage disequilibrium (LD) differences between populations. Therefore, it is necessary to access LD variations in subsequent replication and fine-mapping studies in other populations.

4.3 Epigenetics of CRS

The term "epigenetics" refers to external modifications to DNA that turn genes "on" or "off" without changing the actual DNA sequence.

Epigenetic modifications work in cooperation with other components of the transcription machinery to regularize the temporal and spatial levels of gene expression rather than to alter the DNA sequence. While some epigenetic markers are inherited like genetic variants, some are more dynamic and change in response to environmental factors. Three main forms of epigenetic modifications involve DNA methylation, histone modifications, and noncoding RNAs.

4.3.1 DNA Methylation in CRS

DNA methylation is one of the most investigated and crucial form of epigenetic modifications, and involves covalently bonding a methyl group at the fifth carbon of cytosine (C) residue, mostly within the context of CG dinucleotide (CpG), in the DNA molecule. In general, hypermethylation of CpG sites results in transcriptional silencing, and conversely hypomethylation results in transcriptional activation.

Two studies have examined the genome-wide changes in markers of methylation in CRS using Illumina 450k BeadChip, the most common array platform. Cheong and colleagues [66] investigated the genome-wide DNA methylation in NP tissues and peripheral blood cells from 5 patients with aspirin-intolerant asthma (AIA) and 4 patients with aspirin-tolerant asthma (ATA), and found that changes in methylation in 337 genes were important features in NP of AIA patients. Pathway enrichment analysis further demonstrated that hypomethylated genes were involved in immune responses and cytokine and inflammation-related pathways, whereas hypermethylated genes were enriched in pathways of ectoderm development, wounding healing, and oxidoreductase activity. Another study by Zheng and colleagues [67] identified 198 genes, which had important methylation changes in the promoter in NP tissues compared with inferior turbinate mucosa from controls. The authors evaluated the top 4 genes and found that DNA methylation in COL18A1 gene promoter in NP group was significantly increased. A more recent study employed the methyl-CpG-binding domain sequencing technique and found that 40 genes had altered methylation in NP tissues compared with controls, and that the top four genes were keratin 19 (KRT19), nuclear receptor subfamily 2 group F member 2 (NR2F2), a disintegrin-like and metallopeptidase with thrombospondin type 1 motif 1 (ADAMTS1), and zinc finger protein 222 (ZNF222) [68].

Pyrosequencing is commonly used for detecting methylation of a small number of CpG sites in candidate DNA segments. Employing this technique Kidoguchi and colleagues [69] investigated the methylation levels of three different CpG sites (-618, -121, and -105 bp from transcription start site) in the proximal promoter of tissue-type plasminogen activator (PLAT) gene by bisulfite pyrosequencing in NP tissues, and showed that hypermethylation of PLAT promoter may contribute to NP development. More recently, Li and colleagues [70] compared DNA methylation of proximal promoter of IL8 gene in nasal epithelial cells (NECs) of patients with CRSsNP, CRSwNP, and control subjects from two independent cross-sectional Chinese cohorts (total 187 CRSwNP, 89 CRSsNP and 57 controls). The authors found that DNA methylation at CpG sites -116, -106, and -31 bp from transcription start site was significantly reduced in the NECs from patients with CRSwNP compared to CRSsNP patients and control subjects [70]. Furthermore, ex vivo and in vitro experiments showed that methylation levels of the IL8 gene were correlated negatively with tissue IL-8, ECP (eosinophils) and MPO (neutrophils) concentrations; and elevated IL8 expression in primary NECs was accompanied by decreased methylation of CpG3 site (-31) in cells stimulated with IL-1β and TNF-α. Additionally, change of methylation at CpG3 site effected the binding of octamer-binding transcription factor-1 (Oct-1) and nuclear factor-kappa B (NF-κB).

4.3.2 Histone Modifications in CRS

Histone modifications comprise methylation, acetylation, phosphorylation, ubiquitylation, and other modifications at specific amino residues of histone tails. Histone modifications control gene expression by regulating DNA accessibility to the transcription machinery and chromatin spatial organization. For example, monomethylation or trimethylation of lysine 4 of H3 histone (H3K4me1 or H3K4me3) is markedly linked to transcriptional activation, while trimethylation of lysine 27 of H3 histone (H3K27me3) is mostly linked to transcriptional silencing.

Methylation modifications at histone tails are dynamic and reversible processes that are controlled by histone methyltransferases and demethylases. Liu and colleagues [71] found that the global level of H3K4me3 is increased in NP patients compared with control. Furthermore, IL-13 was shown to upregulate the level of H3K4me3 and the methyltransferase genes (MLL1, MLL2, MLL3, MLL4, MLL5) and downregulate demethylase JARID1B in NECs. The lysine-specific demethylase 2b (KDM2B), which demethylates H3K4me3 and H3K36me2, were also found to be significantly reduced in CRSwNP and involved in inflammatory response of poly(I:C) treated NECs.

Likewise, acetylation of histone tails by histone acetyltransferases relates to active gene transcription, while deacetylation by histone deacetylases relates to repressive gene transcription. Indeed, one previous study has demonstrated that both transcriptional and protein expression levels of histone deacetylase 2 (HDAC2) were significantly elevated in NP tissues compared to normal inferior turbinate tissues [72]. Another study has demonstrated that the levels of acetylation of lysine27 of H3 histone (H3K27ac) of prostaglandin E receptor 2 (PTGER2) were variable and significantly associated with PTGER2 mRNA expression on nasal fibroblasts from the NP patients with aspirin-exacerbated respiratory disease (AERD) [73].

4.3.3 Noncoding RNA in CRS

RNA that does not encode for protein is termed as noncoding RNA. Two classes of noncoding RNA, long and short RNAs, are well recognized and most have an effect on chromatin structuring and transcriptional regulation.

MicroRNAs (miRNAs) are one of the most widely studied members of short noncoding RNAs (18–22 nucleotides in length). They can influence posttranscriptional gene expression via binding to the 3′untranslated regions (3′UTR) of targeted mRNA, which results in mRNA degradation or inhibition of protein translation. Some miRNAs have important roles and therapeutic potential in CRS of which miR-125b is the most frequently investigated differentially expressed miRNA in studies involving the pathogenesis of CRS [74–77]. Zhang and colleagues [74] first used miRNA microarray to identify the miRNA expression profiles in distinct phenotypes of CRS and found that 31 differentially expressed miRNA in eosinophilic CRSwNP and 4 differentially expressed miRNA in CRSsNP compared to control subjects. Of these, miR-125b was found to be the only miRNA that was over-expressed in eosinophilic CRSwNP, which facilitated type I interferon expression by supressing EIF4E-binding protein1 expression in NECs, and thus appears to be involved in innate antiviral immunity and eosinophilic inflammation. Another study has indicated that different phenotypes of CRS have distinct expression profiles of miRNAs in peripheral mature dendritic cells (DCs), suggesting that miRNAs might mediate the core pathogenesis of CRS through regulating dendritic cells and thus may also serve as potential therapeutic targets for CRS [75]. A more recent study has demonstrated that differentially expressed miRNAs in tissues of CRSwNP are significantly enriched in mucin type O-glycan biosynthesis and transforming growth factor-beta (TGF-β) pathways implicated in the aetiology of CRS [77]. The mechanisms involved in miRNAs-mediated immune and inflammatory responses in CRS have also started to be explored [78, 79].

Similarly, long noncoding RNAs (lncRNAs), a class of noncoding RNAs longer than 200 nucleotides, are also being followed with interest as key links of transcriptional and posttranscriptional regulation. Wang and colleagues [80] have performed next generation RNA sequencing and integrated bioinformatics analyses to feature the mRNAs and lncRNAs expression profiles in patients with eosinophilic and non-eosinophilic

CRSwNP and demonstrated that eosinophilic and non-eosinophilic CRSwNP show distinct transcriptome profiles. Furthermore, lncRNA XLOC_010280 was specifically expressed in eosinophilic CRSwNP and may modulate eosinophilic inflammation by affecting CCL18 expression.

4.4 Translation into Future Daily Practice

CRS is a complex disease, and although identification of genetic and epigenetic markers provide some insight into the genetic mechanisms underlying CRS, the identified markers have small effects and can explain only little amount of biological function. Moreover, the effects of heterogeneity within the population and differences in inflammatory endo/phenotypes of CRS are of great importance and need to be considered for better understanding and design of genetic and epigenetic studies in the future. The huge challenge is how the genetic and epigenetic biomarkers will be applied to clinical reality. In this regard, a more recent study has developed the priority index (Pi) pipeline for human genetics and drug discovery [81], providing a useful tool of how genetic data can be harnessed to promote the clinical translatability of genetic findings. Future research should thus systematically integrate omics data (genomic, epigenomics, transcriptome, proteomics, metabolomics, and microbiome), phenotyping of diverse inflammatory patterns and ancestral populations, and environmental factors, as well as develop "big data" handling tools to resolve the clinical complexity of CRS.

References

1. Alexiou A, Sourtzi P, Dimakopoulou K, Manolis E, Velonakis E. Nasal polyps: heredity, allergies, and environmental and occupational exposure. J Otolaryngol Head Neck Surg. 2011;40(1):58–63.
2. Cohen NA, Widelitz JS, Chiu AG, Palmer JN, Kennedy DW. Familial aggregation of sinonasal polyps correlates with severity of disease. Otolaryngol Head Neck Surg. 2006;134(4):601–4. https://doi.org/10.1016/j.otohns.2005.11.042.
3. Rugina M, Serrano E, Klossek JM, Crampette L, Stoll D, Bebear JP, et al. Epidemiological and clinical aspects of nasal polyposis in France; the ORLI group experience. Rhinology. 2002;40(2):75–9.
4. Wang X, Moylan B, Leopold DA, Kim J, Rubenstein RC, Togias A, et al. Mutation in the gene responsible for cystic fibrosis and predisposition to chronic rhinosinusitis in the general population. JAMA. 2000;284(14):1814–9. https://doi.org/10.1001/jama.284.14.1814.
5. Qiu Q, Peng Y, Zhu Z, Chen Z, Zhang C, Ong HH, et al. Absence or mislocalization of DNAH5 is a characteristic marker for motile ciliary abnormality in nasal polyps. Laryngoscope. 2018;128(3):E97–E104. https://doi.org/10.1002/lary.26983.
6. Moloney JR, Oliver RT. HLA antigens, nasal polyps and asthma. Clin Otolaryngol Allied Sci. 1980;5(3):183–9.
7. Luxenberger W, Posch U, Berghold A, Hofmann T, Lang-Loidolt D. HLA patterns in patients with nasal polyposis. Eur Arch Otorhinolaryngol. 2000;257(3):137–9.
8. Molnar-Gabor E, Endreffy E, Rozsasi A. HLA-DRB1, -DQA1, and -DQB1 genotypes in patients with nasal polyposis. Laryngoscope. 2000;110(3 Pt 1):422–5. https://doi.org/10.1097/00005537-200003000-00017.
9. Schubert MS, Hutcheson PS, Graff RJ, Santiago L, Slavin RG. HLA-DQB1 *03 in allergic fungal sinusitis and other chronic hypertrophic rhinosinusitis disorders. J Allergy Clin Immunol. 2004;114(6):1376–83. https://doi.org/10.1016/j.jaci.2004.08.029.
10. Ramirez-Anguiano J, Yamamoto-Furusho JK, Barquera R, Beltran O, Granados J. Association of HLA-DR3 and HLA-DR4 with sinonasal polyposis in Mexican Mestizos. Otolaryngol Head Neck Surg. 2006;135(1):90–3. https://doi.org/10.1016/j.otohns.2006.01.009.
11. Fajardo-Dolci G, Solorio-Abreu J, Romero-Alvarez JC, Zavaleta-Villa B, Cerezo-Camacho O, Jimenez-Lucio R, et al. DQA1 and DQB1 association and nasal polyposis. Otolaryngol Head Neck Surg. 2006;135(2):243–7. https://doi.org/10.1016/j.otohns.2006.03.034.
12. Zhai L, Sun Y, Tang L, Liu H. Polymorphism between loci for human leukocyte antigens DR and DQ in patients with nasal polyps. Ann Otol Rhinol Laryngol. 2007;116(1):66–8. https://doi.org/10.1177/000348940711600111.
13. Keles B, Cora T, Acar H, Arbag H, Inan Z, Ozturk K, et al. Evaluation of HLA-A, -B, -Cw, and -DRB1 alleles frequency in Turkish patients with nasal polyposis. Otolaryngol Head Neck Surg. 2008;139(4):580–5. https://doi.org/10.1016/j.otohns.2008.07.002.
14. Kim JH, Park BL, Cheong HS, Pasaje CF, Bae JS, Park JS, et al. HLA-DRA polymorphisms associated with risk of nasal polyposis in asthmatic patients. Am J Rhinol Allergy. 2012;26(1):12–7. https://doi.org/10.2500/ajra.2012.26.3692.

15. Karjalainen J, Joki-Erkkila VP, Hulkkonen J, Pessi T, Nieminen MM, Aromaa A, et al. The IL1A genotype is associated with nasal polyposis in asthmatic adults. Allergy. 2003;58(5):393–6.
16. Erbek SS, Yurtcu E, Erbek S, Atac FB, Sahin FI, Cakmak O. Proinflammatory cytokine single nucleotide polymorphisms in nasal polyposis. Arch Otolaryngol Head Neck Surg. 2007;133(7):705–9. https://doi.org/10.1001/archotol.133.7.705.
17. Mfuna Endam L, Cormier C, Bosse Y, Filali-Mouhim A, Desrosiers M. Association of IL1A, IL1B, and TNF gene polymorphisms with chronic rhinosinusitis with and without nasal polyposis: a replication study. Arch Otolaryngol Head Neck Surg. 2010;136(2):187–92. https://doi.org/10.1001/archoto.2009.219.
18. Cheng YK, Lin CD, Chang WC, Hwang GY, Tsai SW, Wan L, et al. Increased prevalence of interleukin-1 receptor antagonist gene polymorphism in patients with chronic rhinosinusitis. Arch Otolaryngol Head Neck Surg. 2006;132(3):285–90. https://doi.org/10.1001/archotol.132.3.285.
19. Mrowicka M, Zielinska-Blizniewska H, Milonski J, Majsterek I, Olszewski J. Association of IL1beta and IL4 gene polymorphisms with nasal polyps in a Polish population. Mol Biol Rep. 2014;41(7):4653–8. https://doi.org/10.1007/s11033-014-3336-x.
20. Castano R, Bosse Y, Endam LM, Desrosiers M. Evidence of association of interleukin-1 receptor-like 1 gene polymorphisms with chronic rhinosinusitis. Am J Rhinol Allergy. 2009;23(4):377–84. https://doi.org/10.2500/ajra.2009.23.3303.
21. Tewfik MA, Bosse Y, Lemire M, Hudson TJ, Vallee-Smejda S, Al-Shemari H, et al. Polymorphisms in interleukin-1 receptor-associated kinase 4 are associated with total serum IgE. Allergy. 2009;64(5):746–53. https://doi.org/10.1111/j.1398-9995.2008.01889.x.
22. Bernstein JM, Anon JB, Rontal M, Conroy J, Wang C, Sucheston L. Genetic polymorphisms in chronic hyperplastic sinusitis with nasal polyposis. Laryngoscope. 2009;119(7):1258–64. https://doi.org/10.1002/lary.20239.
23. Batikhan H, Gokcan MK, Beder E, Akar N, Ozturk A, Gerceker M. Association of the tumor necrosis factor-alpha −308 G/A polymorphism with nasal polyposis. Eur Arch Otorhinolaryngol. 2010;267(6):903–8. https://doi.org/10.1007/s00405-009-1167-5.
24. Kim SH, Park HS, Holloway JW, Shin HD, Park CS. Association between a TGFbeta1 promoter polymorphism and rhinosinusitis in aspirin-intolerant asthmatic patients. Respir Med. 2007;101(3):490–5. https://doi.org/10.1016/j.rmed.2006.07.002.
25. Henmyr V, Vandeplas G, Hallden C, Sall T, Olze H, Bachert C, et al. Replication study of genetic variants associated with chronic rhinosinusitis and nasal polyposis. J Allergy Clin Immunol. 2014;133(1):273–5. https://doi.org/10.1016/j.jaci.2013.08.011.
26. Cormier C, Bosse Y, Mfuna L, Hudson TJ, Desrosiers M. Polymorphisms in the tumour necrosis factor alpha-induced protein 3 (TNFAIP3) gene are associated with chronic rhinosinusitis. J Otolaryngol Head Neck Surg. 2009;38(1):133–41.
27. Yea SS, Yang YI, Park SK, Jang WH, Lee SS, Seog DH, et al. Interleukin-4 C-590T polymorphism is associated with protection against nasal polyps in a Korean population. Am J Rhinol. 2006;20(5):550–3.
28. Kim SH, Yang EM, Lee HN, Cho BY, Ye YM, Park HS. Combined effect of IL-10 and TGF-beta1 promoter polymorphisms as a risk factor for aspirin-intolerant asthma and rhinosinusitis. Allergy. 2009;64(8):1221–5. https://doi.org/10.1111/j.1398-9995.2009.01989.x.
29. Endam LM, Bosse Y, Filali-Mouhim A, Cormier C, Boisvert P, Boulet LP, et al. Polymorphisms in the interleukin-22 receptor alpha-1 gene are associated with severe chronic rhinosinusitis. Otolaryngol Head Neck Surg. 2009;140(5):741–7. https://doi.org/10.1016/j.otohns.2008.12.058.
30. Buysschaert ID, Grulois V, Eloy P, Jorissen M, Rombaux P, Bertrand B, et al. Genetic evidence for a role of IL33 in nasal polyposis. Allergy. 2010;65(5):616–22. https://doi.org/10.1111/j.1398-9995.2009.02227.x.
31. Zhang Y, Wang X, Zhang W, Han D, Zhang L, Bachert C. Polymorphisms in thymic stromal lymphopoietin gene demonstrate a gender and nasal polyposis-dependent association with chronic rhinosinusitis. Hum Immunol. 2013;74(2):241–8. https://doi.org/10.1016/j.humimm.2012.11.004.
32. Alromaih S, Mfuna-Endam L, Bosse Y, Filali-Mouhim A, Desrosiers M. CD8A gene polymorphisms predict severity factors in chronic rhinosinusitis. Int Forum Allergy Rhinol. 2013;3(8):605–11. https://doi.org/10.1002/alr.21174.
33. Zhang Y, Wang C, Zhao Y, Zhang L. Some polymorphisms in Epstein-Barr virus-induced gene 3 modify the risk for chronic rhinosinusitis. Am J Rhinol Allergy. 2013;27(2):91–7. https://doi.org/10.2500/ajra.2013.27.3851.
34. Bussu F, Tiziano FD, Giorgio A, Pinto AM, De Corso E, Angelozzi C, et al. Argl6gly polymorphism of the beta2-adrenoceptor gene (ADRBeta2) as a susceptibility factor for nasal polyposis. Am J Rhinol. 2007;21(3):378–82.
35. Castano R, Bosse Y, Endam LM, Filali-Mouhim A, Desrosiers M. c-MET pathway involvement in chronic rhinosinusitis: a genetic association analysis. Otolaryngol Head Neck Surg. 2010;142(5):665–71 e1–2. https://doi.org/10.1016/j.otohns.2010.01.004.
36. Sitarek P, Zielinska-Blizniewska H, Dziki L, Milonski J, Przybylowska K, Mucha B, et al. Association of the -14C/G MET and the -765G/C COX-2 gene polymorphisms with the risk of chronic rhinosinusitis with nasal polyps in a Polish population. DNA Cell Biol. 2012;31(7):1258–66. https://doi.org/10.1089/dna.2011.1453.
37. Al-Shemari H, Bosse Y, Hudson TJ, Cabaluna M, Duval M, Lemire M, et al. Influence of leukotriene gene polymorphisms on chronic rhinosinusitis. BMC Med Genet. 2008;9:21. https://doi.org/10.1186/1471-2350-9-21.

38. Kilty SJ, Bosse Y, Cormier C, Endam LM, Desrosiers MY. Polymorphisms in the SERPINA1 (Alpha-1-Antitrypsin) gene are associated with severe chronic rhinosinusitis unresponsive to medical therapy. Am J Rhinol Allergy. 2010;24(1):e4–9. https://doi.org/10.2500/ajra.2010.24.3429.
39. Tournas A, Mfuna L, Bosse Y, Filali-Mouhim A, Grenier JP, Desrosiers M. A pooling-based genome-wide association study implicates the p73 gene in chronic rhinosinusitis. J Otolaryngol Head Neck Surg. 2010;39(2):188–95.
40. Park CS, Cho JH, Park YJ. Toll-like receptor 2 gene polymorphisms in a Korean population: association with chronic rhinosinusitis. Otolaryngol Head Neck Surg. 2011;144(1):96–100. https://doi.org/10.1177/0194599810390881.
41. Zhang Y, Endam LM, Filali-Mouhim A, Bosse Y, Castano R, Desrosiers M. Polymorphisms in the nitric oxide synthase 1 gene are associated with severe chronic rhinosinusitis. Am J Rhinol Allergy. 2011;25(2):e49–54. https://doi.org/10.2500/ajra.2011.25.3588.
42. Akyigit A, Keles E, Etem EO, Ozercan I, Akyol H, Sakallioglu O, et al. Genetic polymorphism of antioxidant enzymes in eosinophilic and non-eosinophilic nasal polyposis. Eur Arch Otorhinolaryngol. 2017;274(1):267–73. https://doi.org/10.1007/s00405-016-4259-z.
43. Erbek SS, Yurtcu E, Erbek S, Sahin FI. Matrix metalloproteinase-9 promoter gene polymorphism (-1562C>T) in nasal polyposis. Am J Rhinol Allergy. 2009;23(6):568–70. https://doi.org/10.2500/ajra.2009.23.3371.
44. Wang LF, Chien CY, Tai CF, Kuo WR, Hsi E, Juo SH. Matrix metalloproteinase-9 gene polymorphisms in nasal polyposis. BMC Med Genet. 2010;11:85. https://doi.org/10.1186/1471-2350-11-85.
45. Molga P, Fendler W, Borowiec M, Pietruszewska W. Impact of −1607 1G/2G MMP1 gene polymorphism on the morbidity and clinical course of chronic rhinosinusitis with nasal polyps. Otolaryngol Pol. 2016;70(1):24–33. https://doi.org/10.5604/00306657.1193692.
46. Lee JS, Kim JH, Bae JS, Kim JY, Park TJ, Pasaje CF, et al. Association of CACNG6 polymorphisms with aspirin-intolerance asthmatics in a Korean population. BMC Med Genet. 2010;11:138. https://doi.org/10.1186/1471-2350-11-138.
47. Pasaje CF, Bae JS, Park BL, Cheong HS, Kim JH, Jang AS, et al. Possible role of EMID2 on nasal polyps pathogenesis in Korean asthma patients. BMC Med Genet. 2012;13:2. https://doi.org/10.1186/1471-2350-13-2.
48. Pasaje CF, Bae JS, Park BL, Cheong HS, Kim JH, Jang AS, et al. DCBLD2 gene variations correlate with nasal polyposis in Korean asthma patients. Lung. 2012;190(2):199–207. https://doi.org/10.1007/s00408-011-9354-8.
49. Zielinska-Blizniewska H, Sitarek P, Milonski J, Dziki L, Przybylowska K, Olszewski J, et al. Association of the -33C/G OSF-2 and the 140A/G LF gene polymorphisms with the risk of chronic rhinosinusitis with nasal polyps in a Polish population. Mol Biol Rep. 2012;39(5):5449–57. https://doi.org/10.1007/s11033-011-1345-6.
50. Dar SA, Rai G, Ansari MA, Akhter N, Gupta N, Sharma S, et al. FcεR1α gene polymorphism shows association with high IgE and anti-FcεR1α in chronic rhinosinusitis with nasal polyposis. J Cell Biochem. 2018;119(5):4142–9. https://doi.org/10.1002/jcb.26619.
51. Adappa ND, Howland TJ, Palmer JN, Kennedy DW, Doghramji L, Lysenko A, et al. Genetics of the taste receptor T2R38 correlates with chronic rhinosinusitis necessitating surgical intervention. Int Forum Allergy Rhinol. 2013;3(3):184–7. https://doi.org/10.1002/alr.21140.
52. Adappa ND, Zhang Z, Palmer JN, Kennedy DW, Doghramji L, Lysenko A, et al. The bitter taste receptor T2R38 is an independent risk factor for chronic rhinosinusitis requiring sinus surgery. Int Forum Allergy Rhinol. 2014;4(1):3–7. https://doi.org/10.1002/alr.21253.
53. Mfuna Endam L, Filali-Mouhim A, Boisvert P, Boulet LP, Bosse Y, Desrosiers M. Genetic variations in taste receptors are associated with chronic rhinosinusitis: a replication study. Int Forum Allergy Rhinol. 2014;4(3):200–6. https://doi.org/10.1002/alr.21275.
54. Adappa ND, Farquhar D, Palmer JN, Kennedy DW, Doghramji L, Morris SA, et al. TAS2R38 genotype predicts surgical outcome in nonpolypoid chronic rhinosinusitis. Int Forum Allergy Rhinol. 2016;6(1):25–33. https://doi.org/10.1002/alr.21666.
55. Cantone E, Negri R, Roscetto E, Grassia R, Catania MR, Capasso P, et al. In vivo biofilm formation, gram-negative infections and TAS2R38 polymorphisms in CRSw NP patients. Laryngoscope. 2018;128(10):E339–E45. https://doi.org/10.1002/lary.27175.
56. Chang EH, Willis AL, McCrary HC, Noutsios GT, Le CH, Chiu AG, et al. Association between the CDHR3 rs6967330 risk allele and chronic rhinosinusitis. J Allergy Clin Immunol. 2017;139(6):1990–2 e2. https://doi.org/10.1016/j.jaci.2016.10.027.
57. Liu S, Che N, Fan K, Xu F, Qin M, Zhang R, et al. Impact of genetic variants of GLCCI1 on operational therapy in Chinese chronic rhinosinusitis patients. Int Forum Allergy Rhinol. 2018;8(11):1356–62. https://doi.org/10.1002/alr.22220.
58. Lee RJ, Xiong G, Kofonow JM, Chen B, Lysenko A, Jiang P, et al. T2R38 taste receptor polymorphisms underlie susceptibility to upper respiratory infection. J Clin Invest. 2012;122(11):4145–59. https://doi.org/10.1172/JCI64240.

59. Bosse Y, Bacot F, Montpetit A, Rung J, Qu HQ, Engert JC, et al. Identification of susceptibility genes for complex diseases using pooling-based genome-wide association scans. Hum Genet. 2009;125(3):305–18. https://doi.org/10.1007/s00439-009-0626-9.
60. Zhang Y, Endam LM, Filali-Mouhim A, Zhao L, Desrosiers M, Han D, et al. Polymorphisms in RYBP and AOAH genes are associated with chronic rhinosinusitis in a Chinese population: a replication study. PLoS One. 2012;7(6):e39247. https://doi.org/10.1371/journal.pone.0039247.
61. Cormier C, Mfuna Endam L, Filali-Mouhim A, Boisvert P, Boulet LP, Boulay ME, et al. A pooling-based genome wide association study identifies genetic variants associated with *Staphylococcus aureus* colonization in chronic rhinosinusitis patients. Int Forum Allergy Rhinol. 2014;4(3):207–15. https://doi.org/10.1002/alr.21276.
62. Bohman A, Juodakis J, Oscarsson M, Bacelis J, Bende M, Torinsson NA. A family-based genome-wide association study of chronic rhinosinusitis with nasal polyps implicates several genes in the disease pathogenesis. PLoS One. 2017;12(12):e0185244. https://doi.org/10.1371/journal.pone.0185244.
63. Kristjansson RP, Benonisdottir S, Davidsson OB, Oddsson A, Tragante V, Sigurdsson JK, et al. A loss-of-function variant in ALOX15 protects against nasal polyps and chronic rhinosinusitis. Nat Genet. 2019;51(2):267–76. https://doi.org/10.1038/s41588-018-0314-6.
64. Dineen-Griffin S, Garcia-Cardenas V, Rogers K, Williams K, Benrimoj SI. Evaluation of a collaborative protocolized approach by community pharmacists and general medical practitioners for an australian minor ailments scheme: protocol for a cluster randomized controlled trial. JMIR Res Protoc. 2019;8(8):e13973. https://doi.org/10.2196/13973.
65. Schurmann K, Anton M, Ivanov I, Richter C, Kuhn H, Walther M. Molecular basis for the reduced catalytic activity of the naturally occurring T560M mutant of human 12/15-lipoxygenase that has been implicated in coronary artery disease. J Biol Chem. 2011;286(27):23920–7. https://doi.org/10.1074/jbc.M110.211821.
66. Cheong HS, Park SM, Kim MO, Park JS, Lee JY, Byun JY, et al. Genome-wide methylation profile of nasal polyps: relation to aspirin hypersensitivity in asthmatics. Allergy. 2011;66(5):637–44. https://doi.org/10.1111/j.1398-9995.2010.02514.x.
67. Zheng YB, Zhao Y, Yue LY, Lin P, Liu YF, Xian JM, et al. Pilot study of DNA methylation in the pathogenesis of chronic rhinosinusitis with nasal polyps. Rhinology. 2015;53(4):345–52. https://doi.org/10.4193/Rhin14.086.
68. Kim JY, Kim DK, Yu MS, Cha MJ, Yu SL, Kang J. Role of epigenetics in the pathogenesis of chronic rhinosinusitis with nasal polyps. Mol Med Rep. 2018;17(1):1219–27. https://doi.org/10.3892/mmr.2017.8001.
69. Kidoguchi M, Noguchi E, Nakamura T, Ninomiya T, Morii W, Yoshida K, et al. DNA methylation of proximal PLAT promoter in chronic rhinosinusitis with nasal polyps. Am J Rhinol Allergy. 2018;32(5):374–9. https://doi.org/10.1177/1945892418782236.
70. Li J, Jiao J, Wang M, Gao Y, Li Y, Wang Y, et al. Hypomethylation of the IL8 promoter in nasal epithelial cells of patients with chronic rhinosinusitis with nasal polyps. J Allergy Clin Immunol. 2019;144(4):993–1003 e12. https://doi.org/10.1016/j.jaci.2019.06.042.
71. Liu CC, Sun C, Zheng X, Zhao MQ, Kong F, Xu FL, et al. Regulation of KDM2B and Brg1 on inflammatory response of nasal mucosa in CRSwNP. Inflammation. 2019;42(4):1389–400. https://doi.org/10.1007/s10753-019-01000-6.
72. Cho JS, Moon YM, Park IH, Um JY, Moon JH, Park SJ, et al. Epigenetic regulation of myofibroblast differentiation and extracellular matrix production in nasal polyp-derived fibroblasts. Clin Exp Allergy. 2012;42(6):872–82. https://doi.org/10.1111/j.1365-2222.2011.03931.x.
73. Cahill KN, Raby BA, Zhou X, Guo F, Thibault D, Baccarelli A, et al. Impaired E Prostanoid2 expression and resistance to Prostaglandin E2 in nasal polyp fibroblasts from subjects with aspirin-exacerbated respiratory disease. Am J Respir Cell Mol Biol. 2016;54(1):34–40. https://doi.org/10.1165/rcmb.2014-0486OC.
74. Zhang XH, Zhang YN, Li HB, Hu CY, Wang N, Cao PP, et al. Overexpression of miR-125b, a novel regulator of innate immunity, in eosinophilic chronic rhinosinusitis with nasal polyps. Am J Respir Crit Care Med. 2012;185(2):140–51. https://doi.org/10.1164/rccm.201103-0456OC.
75. Ma ZX, Tan X, Shen Y, Ke X, Yang YC, He XB, et al. MicroRNA expression profile of mature dendritic cell in chronic rhinosinusitis. Inflamm Res. 2015;64(11):885–93. https://doi.org/10.1007/s00011-015-0870-5.
76. Xia G, Bao L, Gao W, Liu S, Ji K, Li J. Differentially expressed miRNA in inflammatory mucosa of chronic rhinosinusitis. J Nanosci Nanotechnol. 2015;15(3):2132–9. https://doi.org/10.1166/jnn.2015.9161.
77. Xuan L, Luan G, Wang Y, Lan F, Zhang X, Hao Y, et al. MicroRNAs regulating mucin type O-glycan biosynthesis and transforming growth factor beta signaling pathways in nasal mucosa of patients with chronic rhinosinusitis with nasal polyps in Northern China. Int Forum Allergy Rhinol. 2019;9(1):106–13. https://doi.org/10.1002/alr.22230.
78. Ma Z, Shen Y, Zeng Q, Liu J, Yang L, Fu R, et al. MiR-150-5p regulates EGR2 to promote the development of chronic rhinosinusitis via the DC-Th axis. Int Immunopharmacol. 2018;54:188–97. https://doi.org/10.1016/j.intimp.2017.11.011.

79. Liu CC, Xia M, Zhang YJ, Jin P, Zhao L, Zhang J, et al. Micro124-mediated AHR expression regulates the inflammatory response of chronic rhinosinusitis (CRS) with nasal polyps. Biochem Biophys Res Commun. 2018;500(2):145–51. https://doi.org/10.1016/j.bbrc.2018.03.204.
80. Wang W, Gao Z, Wang H, Li T, He W, Lv W, et al. Transcriptome analysis reveals distinct gene expression profiles in eosinophilic and noneosinophilic chronic rhinosinusitis with nasal polyps. Sci Rep. 2016;6:26604. https://doi.org/10.1038/srep26604.
81. Fang H, Consortium U-D, De Wolf H, Knezevic B, Burnham KL, Osgood J, et al. A genetics-led approach defines the drug target landscape of 30 immune-related traits. Nat Genet. 2019;51(7):1082–91. https://doi.org/10.1038/s41588-019-0456-1.

Involvement of the Immune System in Airways Disease

5

Wei Wang and Ying Sun

Key Points

- Immunity, both innate and adaptive plays an important role in airways disease.
- Both innate and adaptive immunity are likely independently involved in the pathogenesis of airways disease.
- Each of these facets of immunity interacts with, and influences the others, as if a symphony orchestra.
- Airways disease is the final outcome of interactions between innate and adaptive immunity and many other factors.

As with any site in the body, the immune system in the airways and lungs comprises of two parts, namely innate immunity and adaptive immunity. The former exists in the absence of challenge to the immune system and includes physical, epithelial barriers (such as the cough reflex, mucociliary clearance, humoral factors including surface active substances, the complement system, antibacterial peptides, etc.) while the latter is initiated by various cells involved in triggering and sustaining specific immune responses (epithelial cells, macrophages, monocytes, plasmacytoid and lymphoid dendritic cells, granulocytes, natural killer (NK) cells, natural killer T (NKT) cells, innate lymphoid cells (ILC), and mast cells) [1]. The adaptive immune cells mainly include the subsets of T lymphocytes, B lymphocytes, and plasma cells [2].

In the respiratory tract, respiratory epithelial cells are the first line of defence against environmental damage, especially from inhaled pathogens, harmful irritants, and allergens. They are not, however, simply a physical barrier hindering the ingress of potentially harmful substances, but also play a key role in regulating fluid balance, the metabolism and clearance of inhaled particles, and regulating innate and adaptive immune responses by secreting mediators involved in inflammation, recruitment, and activation of other immune cells [3]. If the epithelial barrier is inadequate to withstand potentially harmful environmental invasion, innate immune mechanisms may be activated, such as direct recruitment of granulocytes, particularly neutrophils, and monocytes either directly in response to the inhaled irritant itself or as a result of production of cytokines and chemokines by activated and/or damaged epithelial cells (see below). If this response is still inadequate, adaptive immune responses may be called into play, mediated mainly by activation of specific T cell subsets and the production of specific antibodies by plasma cells. The polymorphonuclear leucocyte (PMN, neutrophil) is an important effector cell in innate immunity and is ideally designed to circulate the body and

W. Wang · Y. Sun (✉)
Department of Immunology, School of Basic Medical Sciences, Capital Medical University, Beijing, China
e-mail: wy_robin@ccmu.edu.cn; ying.sun@ccmu.edu.cn

L. Zhang, C. Bachert (eds.), *Chronic Rhinosinusitis*, https://doi.org/10.1007/978-981-16-0784-4_5

accumulate rapidly at sites of acute inflammation. Under normal conditions, they reach the tissue ready to ingest and kill invading microorganisms, and then leave quietly by programmed cell death. PMN-derived signals regulate local inflammation and stimulate adaptive immune responses, providing a broader role for PMN in host defence [1]. Once blood monocytes are recruited into local tissues, they differentiate into airways or alveolar macrophages and add to the resident population. Normally, resident alveolar macrophages also regulate alveolar inflammation and activation of adaptive immunity. The innate immune system has evolved to protect the airways and lungs from environmentally acquired microbes and other inhaled substances as well as host-derived adverse stressors such as unwanted inflammation. From this point of view, innate immune protection in the lung is not the result of individual cell-specific responses, but rather represents a coordinated response and collective cooperation between resident and recruited lung cell types. These coordinated events result in homeostasis of the airways and alveoli, tolerance to innocuous inhalants, and ability to respond to harmful pathogenic microorganisms. In addition, innate immune mechanisms act swiftly to resolve damage and restore lung function.

From the nose to the alveoli, the respiratory epithelium, resident macrophages, recruited PMNs, and monocytes have evolved diverse, sophisticated and partially overlapping mechanisms to distinguish between harmful and harmless inhaled substances. Such cross talk between epithelial cells and innate immune cells acts to maintain an anti-inflammatory and immunosuppressive environment in the upper and lower airways and the lung parenchyma. In contrast, the adaptive immune system acts more slowly but more specifically in normal homeostasis, and more so in abnormal circumstances. This equilibrium of innate and adaptive immunity is critical to maintain physiological homeostasis and protect the host from disease. Despite this, however, it is considered that derangement of this equilibrium of innate and adaptive immunity is the basis for many diseases, including chronic diseases of the upper respiratory tract (such as rhinitis and chronic rhinosinusitis) and the lower respiratory tract (such as asthma, bronchitis, chronic obstructive pulmonary disease, and pulmonary fibrosis). For example, it is generally accepted that chronic rhinosinusitis (CRS) is a disease caused by a disordered immune response to external stimuli, although whether or not this results, at least in part, from heritable deficiencies in the homeostatic response of the upper airways to these stimuli remains to be clarified. Thus, impairment of innate immune functions provided by the airways epithelium in CRS patients might result in failure to resist microbial agents, with local invasiveness and tissue irritation resulting in further recruitment of other innate and adaptive immune cells, resulting in chronic inflammation [4]. It has been found that patients with CRSwNP (CRS with nasal polyps) are characterized by abnormalities of their nasal epithelial cells, including tight junctional rupture or sinusoidal defects, presumably provoked by external stimuli and/or inflammatory mediators, and finally resulting in epithelial dysfunction [5].

In addition, environmental cellular damage and/or activation of signaling pathways (such as those mediated by Toll-like receptors) in epithelial cells may cause production of epithelium-derived alarmins (such as thymic stromal lymphopoietin, TSLP, interleukin-25, IL-25, and IL-33), which mediate a critical link between innate and adaptive immunity [6, 7]. Elevated local expression of IL-25, IL-33, and TSLP has been found in the diseased nasal tissue of patients with CRSwNP [8–10], which might contribute to local activation of Th0 lymphocytes to activated, Th2 cells as well as activation of type 2, innate lymphocytes (ILC2s), accounting for predominant local production of Th2 cytokines such as IL-4, IL-5, and IL-13 [11–13]. This scenario is consistent with the observation of increased numbers and activity of ILC2s in CRSwNP alongside activation of dendritic cells and Th2-type T cells [6]. Furthermore, it has been shown that IL-33 plays a role in the additional recruitment of neutrophils in the pathogenesis of CRSwNP by inducing production of Th1/Th17 cytokines [14].

ILC2s are a type of innate lymphoid cell, which not only protect against parasites but also contribute to a variety of inflammatory airways diseases by producing type 2 cytokines, some of which induce the production, maturation, and activation of eosinophils [15, 16]. In addition, these cytokines might also activate other target cells expressing T cell adhesion molecules, chemokines, and differential factors [15, 17]. Aside from ILC2s and granulocytes, various subpopulations of dendritic cells (DCs) and macrophages have been implicated in the pathogenesis of various phenotypes and endotypes of CRS [18, 19]. The data suggest that these subtypes of DC may be functionally different. For example, DCs isolated from eosinophilic CRSwNP primarily trigger Th2 cells, while DCs from non-eosinophilic CRSwNP primarily induce Th1/Th17 cell differentiation [18]. In some cases, the IL-13 secreted by ILC2s and Th2 cells activates $CD11b^+$ DCs and drives their migration to local lymph nodes, where they in turn drive the differentiation of naïve CD4 T cells into effector Th2 cells. Accordingly, M2 macrophages are the major macrophages in CRSwNP patients. These M2 macrophages can produce the chemokine CCL18, counting for the further chemoattraction of DC and Th2 cells. In contrast, M1 macrophages are the predominant phenotype in patients with CRS without nasal polyps [20]. It is generally accepted that eosinophils in CRSwNP are important effector cells in the associated type 2 inflammation and tissue damage [21], while the number of local basophils and mast cells is usually associated with local eosinophilia in CRSwNP [22].

Not only innate but also adaptive immune cells, including T and B cells participate in the pathogenesis of CRS. For example, subtypes of T helper cells, through expression of their relevant cytokines, may be associated with different phenotypes and endotypes of CRS. Specifically, it has been shown that Th1 cells predominate in the nasal tissues of patients with CRS without nasal polyps (CRSsNP), while Th2 cells are found predominantly in the tissues of patients with CRSwNP and less frequent seen in the absence of polyps [20, 23, 24]. Patients originating from Europe with CRSwNP typically have local inflammation characterized by eosinophilic infiltration and Th2-type inflammation primarily, which, however, also results in neutrophilic inflammation [24, 25]. In contrast Asian patients, and especially the Chinese, tend to display a mixed pattern of infiltration of various inflammatory cells, including neutrophils and Th1-type and/or Th17 cytokines [26], although co-existence of both patterns, with infiltration of both neutrophils and eosinophils has been described in some patients with CRSwNP [27, 28]. Although regulatory T cells (Treg) have been suggested to play an important role in the downregulation of many immune-mediated diseases, the role of these cells in CRSwNP tissues remains controversial [2, 29].

It has been also noted that the numbers of B cells, plasma cells, and lymphoid follicles are elevated in nasal polyps from CRSwNP subjects, possibly associated with upregulation of expression of B cell activating factor (BAFF) by DCs and other types of cells in local tissues. Under some circumstances, local B cells may be activated and further differentiate into memory B cells or plasma cells synthesizing immunoglobulins IgM, IgG, IgA, and IgE after undergoing somatic hypermutation and/or class switch recombination [2, 30]. It is interesting to note that administration of anti-IgE antibody afforded some clinical benefit, at least in some patients with CRSwNP disease [17, 31]. Other classes of antibody may contribute to local inflammation and responses to infectious agents through neutralization or activation of the classic pathway of complement activation [32], which might also cause tissue damage. It is worth noting that autoantibodies have also been detected in polyp tissues, including anti-nuclear antibodies, anti-dsDNA antibodies, anti-neutrophil cytoplasmic antibodies, and others [2, 33], although their possible roles in the pathogenesis of CRS remain to be explored. The underlying mechanisms associated with asthma, rhinitis, and CRS are shown in Fig. 5.1.

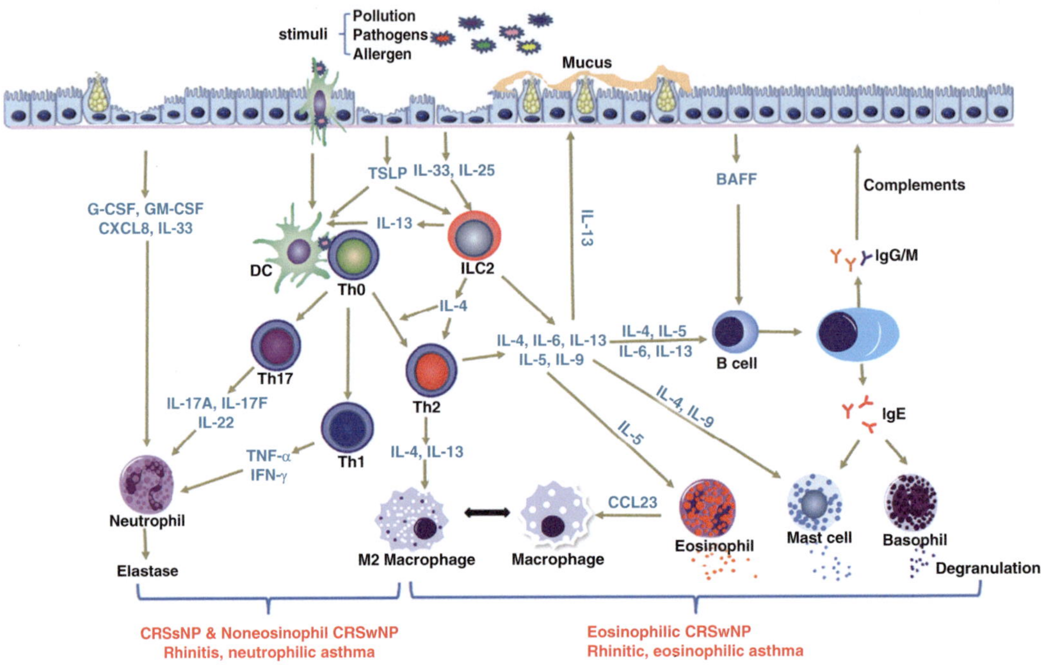

Fig. 5.1 Potential immune cells and mediators involved in the pathogenesis of airways diseases. *TSLP* thymic stromal lymphopoietin, *BAFF* B cell activating factor, *CCL23* CC chemokine 23, also called macrophage inflammatory protein 3

5.1 Conclusions

Increasing evidence suggests that the interaction of both innate and adaptive immune processes makes a significant contribution to the pathogenesis of airways diseases, which are further supported by some efficacy of treatment with some biological agents specific targeting IgE, IL-5, IL-4, and IL-13. However, CRS is a heterogeneous disease, while many factors might be associated with the occurrence of disease, including external risk factors, host factors, epigenetic modification and nasal microenvironment, etc. Under the influence of all of the factors, the immune cells and their subsets may be variable and transformed to perform different biological functions, which might contribute to clinical phenotypes and endotypes. It is certain, therefore, that further clarification of the precise roles of innate and adaptive immunity in airways mucosal diseases, as well as identification of new molecular biomarkers and targets will enlighten their clinical management, in terms of both treatment and prophylaxis.

References

1. Riches DWH, Martin TR. Overview of innate lung immunity and inflammation. Methods Mol Biol. 2018;1809:17–30. https://doi.org/10.1007/978-1-4939-8570-8_2.
2. Tan BK, Min JY, Hulse KE. Acquired immunity in chronic rhinosinusitis. Curr Allergy Asthma Rep. 2017;17(7):49. https://doi.org/10.1007/s11882-017-0715-0.
3. Heffler E, Malvezzi L, Boita M, Brussino L, De Virgilio A, Ferrando M, et al. Immunological mechanisms underlying chronic rhinosinusitis with nasal polyps. Expert Rev Clin Immunol. 2018;14(9):731–7. https://doi.org/10.1080/1744666x.2018.1512407.
4. Hariri BM, Cohen NA. New insights into upper airway innate immunity. Am J Rhinol Allergy. 2016;30(5):319–23. https://doi.org/10.2500/ajra.2016.30.4360.
5. Soyka MB, Wawrzyniak P, Eiwegger T, Holzmann D, Treis A, Wanke K, et al. Defective epithelial barrier in chronic rhinosinusitis: the regulation of tight

junctions by IFN-γ and IL-4. J Allergy Clin Immunol. 2012;130(5):1087–96.e10. https://doi.org/10.1016/j.jaci.2012.05.052.
6. Kim DW, Cho SH. Emerging endotypes of chronic rhinosinusitis and its application to precision medicine. Allergy Asthma Immunol Res. 2017;9(4):299–306. https://doi.org/10.4168/aair.2017.9.4.299.
7. Wang W, Li Y, Lv Z, Chen Y, Li Y, Huang K, et al. Bronchial allergen challenge of patients with atopic asthma triggers an alarmin (IL-33, TSLP, and IL-25) response in the airways epithelium and submucosa. J Immunol (Baltimore, Md: 1950). 2018;201(8):2221–31. https://doi.org/10.4049/jimmunol.1800709.
8. Lam EP, Kariyawasam HH, Rana BM, Durham SR, McKenzie AN, Powell N, et al. IL-25/IL-33-responsive TH2 cells characterize nasal polyps with a default TH17 signature in nasal mucosa. J Allergy Clin Immunol. 2016;137(5):1514–24. https://doi.org/10.1016/j.jaci.2015.10.019.
9. Dogan M, Sahin M, Yenisey C. Increased TSLP, IL-33, IL-25, IL-19, IL 21 and amphiregulin (AREG) levels in chronic rhinosinusitis with nasal polyp. Eur Arch Otorhinolaryngol. 2019;276(6):1685–91. https://doi.org/10.1007/s00405-019-05379-8.
10. Nagata Y, Maruoka S, Gon Y, Mizumura K, Kishi H, Nomura Y, et al. Expression of IL-25, IL-33, and thymic stromal lymphopoietin in nasal polyp gland duct epithelium in patients with chronic rhinosinusitis. Am J Rhinol Allergy. 2019;33(4):378–87. https://doi.org/10.1177/1945892419835333.
11. Patel NN, Kohanski MA, Maina IW, Workman AD, Herbert DR, Cohen NA. Sentinels at the wall: epithelial-derived cytokines serve as triggers of upper airway type 2 inflammation. Int Forum Allergy Rhinol. 2019;9(1):93–9. https://doi.org/10.1002/alr.22206.
12. Symowski C, Voehringer D. Interaction between innate lymphoid cells and cells of the innate and adaptive immune system. Front Immunol. 2017;8:1422.
13. Nagarkar DR, Poposki JA, Tan BK, Comeau MR, Peters AT, Hulse KE, et al. Thymic stromal lymphopoietin activity is increased in nasal polyps of patients with chronic rhinosinusitis. J Allergy Clin Immunol. 2013;132(3):593–600.e12. https://doi.org/10.1016/j.jaci.2013.04.005.
14. Kim DK, Jin HR, Eun KM, Mo JH, Cho SH, Oh S, et al. The role of interleukin-33 in chronic rhinosinusitis. Thorax. 2017;72(7):635–45. https://doi.org/10.1136/thoraxjnl-2016-208772.
15. Poposki JA, Klingler AI, Tan BK, Soroosh P, Banie H, Lewis G, et al. Group 2 innate lymphoid cells are elevated and activated in chronic rhinosinusitis with nasal polyps. Immun Inflamm Dis. 2017;5(3):233–43. https://doi.org/10.1002/iid3.161.
16. Gevaert P, Calus L, Van Zele T, Blomme K, De Ruyck N, Bauters W, et al. Omalizumab is effective in allergic and nonallergic patients with nasal polyps and asthma. J Allergy Clin Immunol. 2013;131(1):110–6.e1. https://doi.org/10.1016/j.jaci.2012.07.047.
17. Gurram RK, Zhu J. Orchestration between ILC2s and Th2 cells in shaping type 2 immune responses. Cell Mol Immunol. 2019;16(3):225–35. https://doi.org/10.1038/s41423-019-0210-8.
18. Shi LL, Song J, Xiong P, Cao PP, Liao B, Ma J, et al. Disease-specific T-helper cell polarizing function of lesional dendritic cells in different types of chronic rhinosinusitis with nasal polyps. Am J Respir Crit Care Med. 2014;190(6):628–38. https://doi.org/10.1164/rccm.201402-0234OC.
19. Poposki JA, Peterson S, Welch K, Schleimer RP, Hulse KE, Peters AT, et al. Elevated presence of myeloid dendritic cells in nasal polyps of patients with chronic rhinosinusitis. Clin Exp Allergy. 2015;45(2):384–93. https://doi.org/10.1111/cea.12471.
20. Scheckenbach K, Wagenmann M. Cytokine patterns and endotypes in acute and chronic rhinosinusitis. Curr Allergy Asthma Rep. 2016;16(1):3. https://doi.org/10.1007/s11882-015-0583-4.
21. Hulse KE, Stevens WW, Tan BK, Schleimer RP. Pathogenesis of nasal polyposis. Clin Exp Allergy. 2015;45(2):328–46. https://doi.org/10.1111/cea.12472.
22. Mahdavinia M, Carter RG, Ocampo CJ, Stevens W, Kato A, Tan BK, et al. Basophils are elevated in nasal polyps of patients with chronic rhinosinusitis without aspirin sensitivity. J Allergy Clin Immunol. 2014;133(6):1759–63. https://doi.org/10.1016/j.jaci.2013.12.1092.
23. Derycke L, Eyerich S, Van Crombruggen K, Pérez-Novo C, Holtappels G, Deruyck N, et al. Mixed T helper cell signatures in chronic rhinosinusitis with and without polyps. PLoS One. 2014;9(6):e97581. https://doi.org/10.1371/journal.pone.0097581.
24. Delemarre T, Holtappels G, De Ruyck N, Zhang N, Nauwynck H, Bachert C, et al. Type 2 inflammation in chronic rhinosinusitis without nasal polyps: another relevant endotype. J Allergy Clin Immunol. 2020;146(2):337–43.e6. https://doi.org/10.1016/j.jaci.2020.04.040.
25. Delemarre T, Holtappels G, De Ruyck N, Zhang N, Nauwynck H, Bachert C, et al. A substantial neutrophilic inflammation as regular part of severe type 2 chronic rhinosinusitis with nasal polyps. J Allergy Clin Immunol. 2020;146(2):337–343.e6. https://doi.org/10.1016/j.jaci.2020.08.036.
26. Van Zele T, Claeys S, Gevaert P, Van Maele G, Holtappels G, Van Cauwenberge P, et al. Differentiation of chronic sinus diseases by measurement of inflammatory mediators. Allergy. 2006;61(11):1280–9. https://doi.org/10.1111/j.1398-9995.2006.01225.x.
27. Wang X, Zhang N, Bo M, Holtappels G, Zheng M, Lou H, et al. Diversity of T(H) cytokine profiles in patients with chronic rhinosinusitis: a multicenter study in Europe, Asia, and Oceania. J Allergy Clin Immunol. 2016;138(5):1344–53. https://doi.org/10.1016/j.jaci.2016.05.041.
28. Cao PP, Wang ZC, Schleimer RP, Liu Z. Pathophysiologic mechanisms of chronic rhinosi-

nusitis and their roles in emerging disease endotypes. Ann Allergy Asthma Immunol. 2019;122(1):33–40. https://doi.org/10.1016/j.anai.2018.10.014.

29. Hulse KE. Immune mechanisms of chronic rhinosinusitis. Curr Allergy Asthma Rep. 2016;16(1):1. https://doi.org/10.1007/s11882-015-0579-0.
30. Hulse KE, Norton JE, Suh L, Zhong Q, Mahdavinia M, Simon P, et al. Chronic rhinosinusitis with nasal polyps is characterized by B-cell inflammation and EBV-induced protein 2 expression. J Allergy Clin Immunol 2013;131(4):1075–1083, 83.e1–7. doi:https://doi.org/10.1016/j.jaci.2013.01.043
31. Gurrola J II, Borish L. Chronic rhinosinusitis: endotypes, biomarkers, and treatment response. J Allergy Clin Immunol. 2017;140(6):1499–508. https://doi.org/10.1016/j.jaci.2017.10.006.
32. Van Roey GA, Vanison CC, Wu J, Huang JH, Suh LA, Carter RG, et al. Classical complement pathway activation in the nasal tissue of patients with chronic rhinosinusitis. J Allergy Clin Immunol. 2017;140(1):89–100.e2. https://doi.org/10.1016/j.jaci.2016.11.015.
33. Tan BK, Li QZ, Suh L, Kato A, Conley DB, Chandra RK, et al. Evidence for intranasal antinuclear autoantibodies in patients with chronic rhinosinusitis with nasal polyps. J Allergy Clin Immunol. 2011;128(6):1198–206.e1. https://doi.org/10.1016/j.jaci.2011.08.037.

T Cells and Group 2 Innate Lymphoid Cells 2

6

Atsushi Kato and Robert P. Schleimer

Key Points

- Type 2 inflammation is the most common inflammatory endotype in CRS.
- Biologics that target type 2 cytokines and their receptors including the IL-4 receptor, IL-5, and the IL-5 receptor as well as IgE are becoming available for treatment with allergic and type 2 inflammatory diseases.
- Type 2 cytokines (IL-4, IL-5, and IL-13) and the major type 2 cytokine producing cells include Th2 cells and ILC2s primarily.

6.1 Introduction

Chronic rhinosinusitis (CRS) is a heterogeneous disease characterized by local inflammation of the paranasal sinuses and nose lasting at least 12 weeks [1–3]. CRS is frequently divided into the two main phenotypes: CRS with nasal polyps (CRSwNP) and CRS without nasal polyps (CRSsNP). The inflammatory response in CRS is well known to be controlled by $CD4^+$ T helper cell associated cytokines including a Th1 cytokine (IFN-γ), Th2 cytokines (IL-4, IL-5, and IL-13) and Th17 cytokines (IL-17A and IL-22). Recent studies indicate that these T helper cytokines are not only produced from T cells but also from innate lymphoid cells (ILCs). Unlike T cells, ILCs lack antigen receptors but produce high levels of T helper cytokines after activation via antigen-independent stimuli including cytokines and lipid mediators. ILC can be classified into three major subsets; group 1 ILC (ILC1), ILC2, and ILC3, based on the function and production of cytokines [4, 5]. ILC1s are characterized by the production of the Th1 cytokine IFN-γ. ILC2s produce Th2 cytokines, IL-4, IL-5, and IL-13. ILC3s are characterized by the production of Th17 cytokines, IL-17A and IL-22. Currently, ILCs are viewed as an innate counterpart of T helper cells in that ILC1s, ILC2s, and ILC3s mirror Th1 cells, Th2 cells, and Th17 cells, respectively. Since both T helper cells and ILCs release the same cytokines, many groups now call IFN-γ a type 1 cytokine, IL-4, IL-5, and IL-13 type 2 cytokines and IL-17A and IL-22 type 3 (or 17) cytokines (Fig. 6.1a). Similarly, inflammation caused by these cytokines is called type 1, 2, and 3 (or 17) inflammation, respectively [4, 5, 8]. We will use the above terminology in this chapter.

A. Kato · R. P. Schleimer (✉)
Division of Allergy and Immunology, Department of Medicine, Northwestern University Feinberg School of Medicine, Chicago, IL, USA

Department of Otolaryngology, Northwestern University Feinberg School of Medicine, Chicago, IL, USA
e-mail: a-kato@northwestern.edu; rpschleimer@northwestern.edu

L. Zhang, C. Bachert (eds.), *Chronic Rhinosinusitis*, https://doi.org/10.1007/978-981-16-0784-4_6

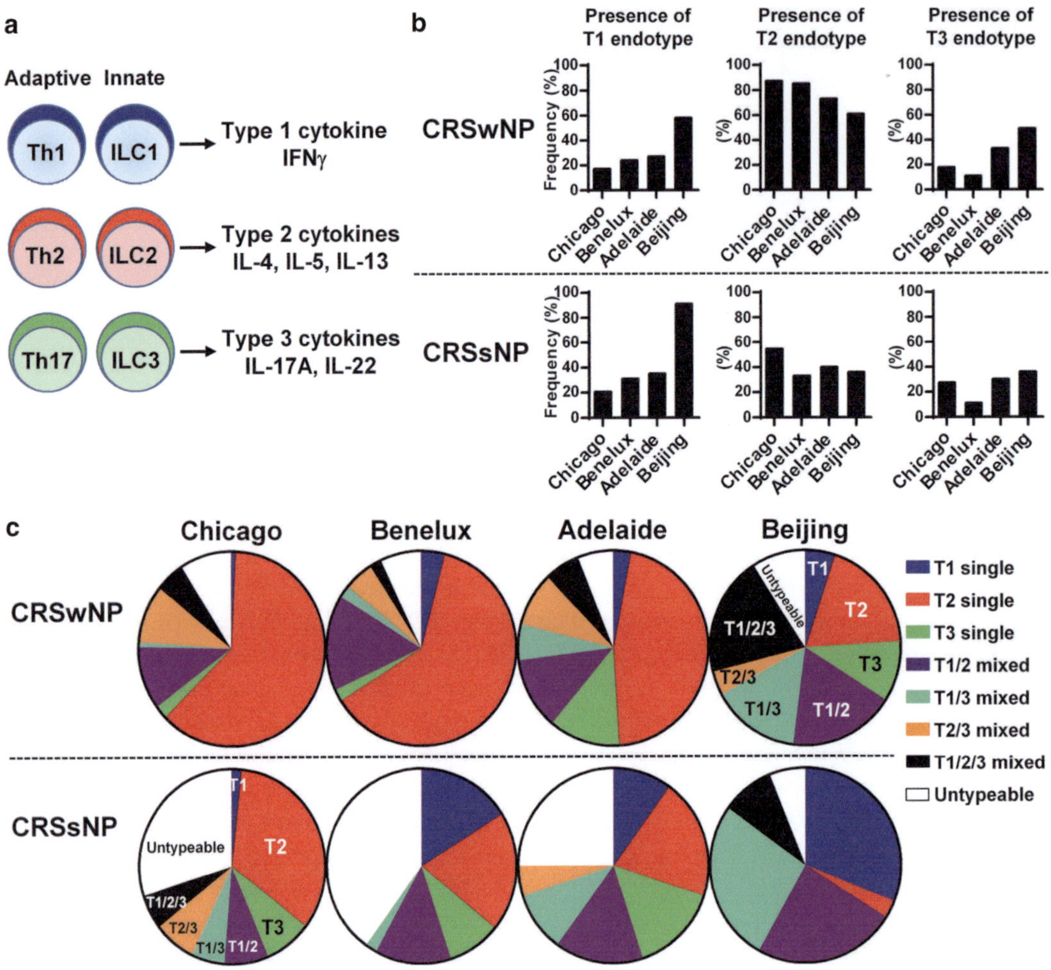

Fig. 6.1 Inflammatory endotypes in CRS. Definition of T helper and innate lymphoid cells based on production of type 1, type 2, and type 3 cytokines is shown in (**a**). The frequency of having any T1, T2 or T3 inflammation in sinonasal tissue samples from patients with CRSsNP [Chicago (n = 121), Benelux (n = 45), Adelaide (n = 20), and Beijing (n = 33)] and CRSwNP [Chicago (n = 134), Benelux (n = 45), Adelaide (n = 33), and Beijing (n = 95)] is shown in B. The overall frequency of having single or mixed endotype in Chicago, Benelux, and Beijing is shown by pie charts in (**c**). All results in (**b**) and (**c**) were adapted from published studies by Stevens et al. [6] and Wang et al. [7]

6.2 Inflammatory Endotypes of CRS

CRSwNP is well known to be characterized by type 2 inflammation with pronounced eosinophilia in Western countries [1–3]. Recently, two groups, including our own, performed larger scale endotyping studies in CRS [6, 7, 9, 10]. Although there was no consistent protocol to define endotypes between the two research groups, these studies confirmed the current knowledge, showing that 70–90% of CRSwNP patients show type 2 inflammation in the US (Chicago), Europe (Benelux), and Oceana (Adelaide) (Fig. 6.1b) [6, 7]. In contrast to Western countries, earlier studies suggested that type 2 inflammation with eosinophilia in CRSwNP was less common in East Asia including China, Korea, and Japan [3, 11–13]. In these countries, CRS was therefore frequently divided into two phenotypes, eosinophilic CRS (ECRS) and non-eosinophilic CRS. However, recent studies indicated that the prevalence of ECRS has dramatically increased in East Asia over the past 20 years [3, 14, 15]. Indeed, Wang et al. found in their recent endotype study that the most common endotype in CRSwNP patients in China (Beijing) was now type 2 inflammation, although the frequency of the type 2 endotype in China was less than in the US and Europe (Fig. 6.1b) [7]. Interestingly, type 2 single endotype was less common in patients with CRSwNP in China and actually many Chinese patients had mixed endotypes (e.g. type 2 with type 1 and/or type 3) (Fig. 6.1c) [7]. In contrast to CRSwNP, the mechanism of inflammation in CRSsNP has been understudied, despite the fact that 75–90% of all CRS patients have this phenotype [1, 2]. Although initial studies suggested that CRSsNP is characterized by type 1 inflammation [16–18] recent endotyping studies suggested that inflammation in CRSsNP is much more heterogeneous than in CRSwNP and only Chinese patients showed type 1 dominant inflammation in CRSsNP (Fig. 6.1b) [6, 7, 9, 10]. Surprisingly, type 2 inflammation is also common in CRSsNP patients, and 30–55% of them were found to show this inflammation worldwide (Fig. 6.1b) [6, 7]. This suggests that type 2 inflammation is the most common inflammation type in all CRS and influences a wider range of CRS patients than previously believed, especially in the US and Europe. Thus, we further focus on type 2 cytokines and the cells that produce them, including Th2 cells and ILC2s.

6.3 Type 2 Cytokine-Induced Inflammation in Nasal Polyps

Type 2 cytokines, including IL-4, IL-5, and IL-13, play key roles in type 2 inflammatory and allergic diseases. In the case of CRS and NPs, IL-5 and IL-13 are well known to be elevated in NPs but expression of IL-4 in NPs is generally very low and consequently the reports regarding IL-4 have been inconsistent in past studies [3, 16, 19]. IL-5 is a key cytokine that controls eosinophil development, activation, and survival and therefore primarily induces eosinophilia in NPs. Indeed, recent clinical trials of biologics targeting IL-5 (Mepolizumab and Reslizumab) and the IL-5 receptor (Benralizumab) showed a strong reduction of peripheral blood and sinus tissue eosinophils in patients with CRSwNP [20–23]. IL-4 and IL-13 are key factors that control IgE responses in B cells and plasma cells, mucus production and remodeling in epithelial cells and the activation of M2 macrophages [3]. IL-4 and IL-13 are also involved in eosinophil recruitment by inducing eosinophil chemokines including eotaxins (CCL11, CCL24, and CCL26) from epithelial cells, fibroblasts, and endothelial cells [3]. Fibrin deposition is also a key feature of NPs and is controlled at least in part by type 2 cytokines IL-4 and IL-13 [24]. Our group found that IL-4 and IL-13 reduced epithelial cell production of tissue plasminogen activator, an enzyme that promotes fibrin degradation [24]. IL-4 and IL-13 also induced expression of factor XIII-A in macrophages, an enzyme that induces fibrin crosslinking and deposition [25]. Importantly, tissue plasminogen activator is reduced and factor XIII-A is increased in NPs [24, 25]. These findings suggest that IL-4 and IL-13 may have a broader range of inflammatory roles in NPs than IL-5, which primarily modulates eosinophilia. Importantly, a monoclonal antibody against IL-4Ra (Dupilumab) that blocks both IL-4- and IL-13-mediated signals reduced nasal polyp size, sinus opacification, and severity of symptoms, and this drug has been recently approved for treatment of CRSwNP by the FDA [26, 27]. These clinical studies confirm the importance of type 2 cytokines including IL-4, IL-5, and IL-13 in CRSwNP.

6.4 Th2 Cells

Type 2 cytokines can be induced by both antigen specific and antigen-independent stimuli; antigen specific type 2 inflammation is controlled mainly by Th2 cells. Th2 cells are differentiated from naive $CD4^+$ T cells through activation of T cell receptor (TCR)-mediated signaling, costimulation, and cytokine signals, and currently GATA3 is known to be a key transcription factor that controls differentiation of Th2 cells and production of type 2 cytokines [28–30]. Th2 cells can be identified by flow cytometry in several ways: the cell surface expression of the prostaglandin D2 receptor CRTH2 (also known as DP2), intracellular GATA3 staining or intracellular type 2 cytokine staining after stimulation in the presence of a protein transport inhibitor, within the $CD4^+$ T cell population. In the case of CRS, earlier studies by Van Zele et al. and Van Bruaene et al. showed elevation of CD3, GATA3, and IL-5 in NP tissue, suggesting that Th2 cells are elevated in NPs [16, 17]. Following these observations, Derycke et al. and Lam et al. reported the elevation of Th2 cells in NPs by flow cytometry in Belgium and the United Kingdom, respectively [31, 32]. Shi et al. also found an elevation of Th2 cells in eosinophilic NPs but not in non-eosinophilic NPs in China [33]. These results suggest that Th2 cells are highly elevated in CRSwNP patients who have type 2 inflammation around the world.

Recent studies have suggested that Th2 cells display functional heterogeneity [28–30]. Several groups identified Th2 subsets that produce type 2 cytokines and are involved in the pathogenesis of allergic diseases. They named these populations as pathogenic Th2 (Tpath2), pathogenic effector Th2 (peTh2), and proallergic Th2 (Th2A) [34–36]. Importantly, all groups showed that these Th2 subsets have high levels of innate cytokine receptors including the IL-25 receptor (IL-17RB), IL-33 receptor (ST2; IL-1RL1), and thymic stromal lymphopoietin receptor (TSLPR; CRLF2), at least comparing mRNA levels with those in conventional Th2 cells. Furthermore, two groups demonstrated that high cell surface expression of CD161 was a marker of pathogenic Th2 cells [35, 36]. These results suggest that Tpath2, peTh2, and Th2A may be the same or very similar Th2 subsets and therefore we refer to all of them together as pathogenic Th2 cells in this chapter. We now can identify pathogenic Th2 cells as $CD161^{high}$ $CD4^+$ $CRTH2^+$ T cells by flow cytometry.

The numbers of pathogenic Th2 cells are known to be highly elevated in allergic and type 2 inflammatory diseases including allergic asthma, atopic dermatitis, and eosinophilic gastrointestinal disease [28, 35, 36]. In the case of CRS, Endo et al. first found evidence supporting accumulation of pathogenic Th2 cells in ECRS; expression of mRNAs for IL-4, IL-13, IL-1RL1, and GATA3 in memory $CD4^+$ T cells was significantly higher in patients with ECRS compared to non-eosinophilic CRS patients in Japan [37]. Lam et al. in the United Kingdom then found that $IL\text{-}17RB^+$ $IL\text{-}1RL1^+$ Th2 cells were elevated in NPs compared to normal nasal mucosa and that $IL\text{-}17RB^+$ $IL\text{-}1RL1^+$ Th2 cells made high levels of type 2 cytokines [32]. These studies suggest that pathogenic Th2 cells are highly elevated in CRSwNP patients who have type 2 inflammation and contribute to high levels of type 2 cytokines in this disease.

Th2 cells can be activated by mainly three types of stimuli, antigens, superantigens, and innate cytokines in NPs in vivo. Antigen-mediated activation is believed to be a key pathway for the expansion, activation, and production of type 2 cytokines in Th2 cells in NPs. Indeed, pathogenic Th2 cells that were elevated in NPs were identified as allergen-specific Th2 cells [35, 36] and 40–65% of CRSwNP patients had atopy to at least one of the common allergens in the US and Europe [6, 7], although specific allergens that are directly linked with CRS have not been identified yet. The second pathway is superantigen-mediated activation. Certain enterotoxins released from bacteria can bind between the alpha chain of class II MHC and a particular family of Vβ region on the T cell receptor and then activate T cells. Since this enterotoxin-mediated activation of T cells does not require antigen specificity, they are called superantigens. Importantly, CRSwNP is characterized by high rates of *Staphylococcus aureus* colonization, staphylococcal superantigens including SEA, SEB, and TSST-1 are frequently detected in NPs and *Staphylococcus aureus* enterotoxin-specific IgE is known to be elevated in NPs [7, 38–40]. This suggests that superantigens may play a significant role on both conventional and pathogenic Th2-mediated type 2 inflammation in CRSwNP. The last pathway is cytokine-mediated signaling. Unlike conventional Th2 cells, pathogenic Th2 cells have receptors for innate epithelial-derived cytokines, TSLP, IL-25, and IL-33 and release type 2 cytokines upon stimulation with these cytokines [35–37]. Lam et al. found that nasal polyp-derived IL-17RB$^+$ IL-1RL1$^+$ pathogenic Th2 cells responded to IL-25 and IL-33 and then expressed IL-5 and IL-13 [32]. This suggests that innate cytokines, especially IL-25 and IL-33, may play an important role in pathogenic Th2 cell-mediated type 2 inflammation in CRSwNP. However, since there is no consistent evidence that either IL-25 or IL-33 are elevated in CRSwNP [41], the importance of IL-25 and IL-33 to Th2-mediated inflammation in CRSwNP will need further careful studies.

6.5 ILC2s

Antigen-independent type 2 inflammation is mainly controlled by ILC2s, although pathogenic Th2 cells can also participate (see above). All ILCs develop from ILC precursors (ILCPs) which are differentiated from the common lymphoid progenitors (CLPs) [42, 43]. CLPs are also able to differentiate into lymphocytes including T cells and B cells. ILC2s are further differentiated from ILCPs by the expression of transcription factors GATA3 and RORα [42, 43]. Human ILC2s can be identified by flow cytometry as CD45$^+$ lymphoid cells that are Lineage (CD1a, CD3, CD4, CD16, CD19, CD34, CD94, CD303, FcRI) negative and CD127$^+$CD161$^+$CRTH2$^+$ [4, 5]. Importantly, NPs are one of the first tissues in which human ILC2s were discovered [44] and many groups have confirmed the accumulation of ILC2s in NP tissue [5, 45–48]. Our group recently characterized the presence of all major ILC subsets in CRS tissues and found that ILC2s are the predominant ILCs in NPs and are 100-fold elevated in NPs compared to sinus mucosa of control subjects [48]. Tojima et al. found that ILC2s are elevated in eosinophilic NPs but not in non-eosinophilic NPs in Japan [47]. These studies suggest that not only pathogenic Th2 cells but also ILC2s are highly elevated in CRSwNP patients who have type 2 inflammation. Although patients with CRSsNP with type 2 endotype have the same type 2 cytokines, our initial study could not detect elevation of ILC2s in CRSsNP based on variability with a small sample size [48]. Future studies are clearly required to examine whether ILC2s and pathogenic Th2 cells are elevated in the type 2 endotype of CRSsNP patients.

In addition to the accumulation of ILC2s in NPs, our group also found that ILC2s are activated and release type 2 cytokines in NPs in vivo [48]. However, factors that activate ILC2s in vivo in NPs are still not fully understood since ILC2s can be activated by many pathways. Epithelial-derived innate cytokines IL-25, IL-33, and TSLP were initially identified as key type 2 cytokine inducers for ILC2s and receptors for IL-25 (IL-17RA and IL-17RB), IL-33 (IL-1RL1 and IL-1RAP), and TSLP (IL-7Ra and CRLF2) are highly expressed on human ILC2s. Especially in combination with each other, these epithelial cytokines potently induce production of type 2 cytokines in ILC2s. In addition to epithelial-derived cytokines, receptors for pro-inflammatory cytokines including IL-1β and IL-18 and members of the TNF superfamily (TNFSF) including TNF (also known as TNFα, [TNFSF2]), receptor activator of NF-κB ligand (RANK-L [TNFSF11]), TNF-like cytokine 1A (TL1A [TNFSF15]), and glucocorticoid-induced TNF-related ligand (GITR-L [TNFSF18]) are expressed on human ILC2s and these cytokines are able to induce production of type 2 cytokines from ILC2s [5, 49–52]. Although human ILC2s also have receptors for other cytokines including IL-2, IL-7, and IL-9, and these cytokines are involved in proliferation and survival of ILC2s, they do not directly induce production of type 2 cytokines [5]. In addition to cytokines, lipid mediators (leukotriene C4 [LTC4], LTD4, LTE4, and prostaglandin D2 [PGD2]), inducible T cell costimulator ligand (ICOS-L), complement C3a and neuropeptides including neuromedin U (NMU), vasoactive intestinal peptide (VIP), and calcitonin gene-related peptide (CGRP) are all known to activate ILC2s [5, 53–59]. These studies showed that C3a, NMU and VIP directly promote production of type 2 cytokines while ICOS-L and CGRP may play a costimulatory role in ILC2-mediated type 2 inflammation. To date, the role of C3a and neuropeptides in human ILC2s has not been investigated yet and future studies are still required in humans.

In the case of epithelial cytokines (IL-25, IL-33, and TSLP), only TSLP consistently showed significant elevation in NPs [41]. However, TSLP alone does not induce type 2 cytokines in human ILC2s but acts as a potent enhancer of type 2 cytokines in the presence of other ILC2 activators [60]. Our group recently screened other potential ILC2 activators in NPs and found that RANK-L was significantly elevated in NPs and RANK-L enhanced production of IL-5 and IL-13 in NP-derived ILC2s [52]. We also found that TSLP significantly and synergistically enhanced RANK-L-mediated production of type 2 cytokines in human ILC2s [52]. In addition to RANK-L and TSLP, several groups found elevation of lipid mediators including LTC4 and PDG2 in NPs, especially in patients with aspirin-exacerbated respiratory disease (AERD, which has a triad of symptoms; CRSwNP, asthma and sensitivity to COX1 inhibitors) [61, 62]. These studies suggest that TSLP, RANK-L, and lipid mediators may play a significant role in ILC2-mediated type 2 inflammation in CRSwNP.

Although we found that IL-33 is detected but not elevated in NPs in the US, some groups found elevation of IL-33 in NPs [41]. In addition, IL-33 is known to act in synergy with other elevated factors on NPs including TSLP and lipid mediators [53, 60]. This implies the possibility that IL-33 together with TSLP and/or lipid mediators may play a role in type 2 inflammation in CRSwNP even if IL-33 is not elevated [5]. In the case of IL-25, many Asian groups showed elevation of IL-25 in NPs, although IL-25 was almost undetectable in whole NP tissue in our cohort in Chicago in the US [41]. This suggests that the mechanisms of ILC2-mediated type 2 inflammation may be different between Asian and Western countries and that IL-25 may be involved in Asian NPs. Recently, Kohanski et al. found that IL-25 is expressed in a minor subset of epithelial cells called solitary chemosensory cells and these cells are increased in NPs in the US [63]. This may suggest that IL-25 plays a role on the activation of ILC2s in a specific epithelial area of NP tissue even in Western countries. Further studies require examination of the direct role of IL-25 and IL-33 in CRSwNP.

6.6 ILC2-Th2 Interaction in NPs

Our studies showed that both Th2 cells and ILC2s sorted from NP tissue released IL-5 and IL-13 without additional stimulation in *in vitro* culture [48, 49, 52, 60]. This suggests that both Th2 cells and ILC2s are activated in NPs *in vivo* and both cell types contribute to production of type 2 cytokines in CRSwNP. Recent studies suggest that T cells are able to directly interact with ILC2s through the ligation of ICOS/ICOS-L, programmed cell death 1 (PD-1)/PD-1 ligand 1, OX40/OX40-ligand, and RANK/RANK-L [52, 55, 64, 65]. These studies raise the possibility that Th2 cells and ILC2s may also interact in NPs in vivo, further enhancing Th2 cell- and/or ILC2-mediated type 2 inflammation. Indeed, our recent study showed that the co-culture of ILC2s with Th2 cells significantly enhanced the production of IL-5 and IL-13 (5.0-fold and 4.2-fold, respectively) compared to the sum of individual cultures [52]. Importantly, a neutralizing antibody against RANK-L almost completely abolished the enhancement of type 2 cytokine production in the ILC2-Th2 cell co-culture indicating that it is mainly via the RANK-L/RANK-mediated pathway. We further found that RANK-L was expressed on Th2 cells in NPs, RANK was expressed on both NP Th2 cells and ILC2s and RANK-L much more effectively induced IL-13 in ILC2s than in Th2 cells [52]. These results suggest that the direct interaction of ILC2s and Th2 cells enhances type 2 cytokine responses and that the enhancement activity is mainly controlled by a RANK-L dependent activation of ILC2s by Th2 cells in NPs. The direct role of ICOS-, PD-1-, and OX40-mediated pathways in Th2-ILC2 interaction in NPs will require further investigation.

6.7 Conclusion and Translation into Future Daily Practice

Increasing evidence suggests that pathogenic Th2 cells, ILC2s and their activators are highly accumulated in CRSwNP patients with the type 2 endotype; and that Th2 cells and ILC2s significantly contribute to type 2 inflammation via the production of type 2 cytokines including IL-5 and IL-13 in this disease. Although there is currently almost no Th2- and ILC2-targeting therapy, monoclonal antibodies against downstream molecules of these cell types, including type 2 cytokines and their receptors, such as IL-5, IL-5Rα and IL-4Rα, have been developed and anti-IL-4Ra (Dupilumab) is already approved for treatment of CRSwNP [20, 23, 26, 27, 66, 67]. Although these drugs will be useful to treat CRSwNP patients, they only target those who have type 2 inflammation. Clearly, the generation of a simple identification protocol for the type 2 endotype in CRS will be useful for the future design of more precise and personal medicine strategies that effectively prevent or treat disease in CRS patients. Although it is now clear that type 2 inflammation is also common in patients with CRSsNP, the mechanisms and composition of inflammatory cells and these activators in CRSsNP with type 2 endotype is still largely unclear. This area will require active investigation in the future.

Acknowledgments
The authors acknowledge Ms. Julie Poposki for proofreading of this review.

This research was supported in part by NIH grants, R01 AI104733, R01 AI137174, R37 HL068546, U19 AI106683 and P01 AI145818 and by grant from the Ernest S. Bazley Foundation.

References

1. Fokkens WJ, Lund VJ, Mullol J, Bachert C, Alobid I, Baroody F, et al. European position paper on rhinosinusitis and nasal polyps 2012. Rhinol Suppl. 2012;23:3 p preceding table of contents, 1–298.
2. Orlandi RR, Kingdom TT, Hwang PH, Smith TL, Alt JA, Baroody FM, et al. International consensus statement on allergy and rhinology: rhinosinusitis. Int Forum Allergy Rhinol. 2016;6(Suppl 1):S22–209. https://doi.org/10.1002/alr.21695.
3. Kato A. Immunopathology of chronic rhinosinusitis. Allergol Int. 2015;64(2):121–30. https://doi.org/10.1016/j.alit.2014.12.006.
4. Vivier E, Artis D, Colonna M, Diefenbach A, Di Santo JP, Eberl G, et al. Innate lymphoid cells: 10 years on. Cell. 2018;174(5):1054–66. https://doi.org/10.1016/j.cell.2018.07.017.
5. Kato A. Group 2 innate lymphoid cells in airway diseases. Chest. 2019;156(1):141–9. https://doi.org/10.1016/j.chest.2019.04.101.
6. Stevens WW, Peters AT, Tan BK, Klingler AI, Poposki JA, Hulse KE, et al. Associations between inflammatory endotypes and clinical presentations in chronic rhinosinusitis. J Allergy Clin Immunol Pract. 2019;7(8):2812–20.e3. https://doi.org/10.1016/j.jaip.2019.05.009.
7. Wang X, Zhang N, Bo M, Holtappels G, Zheng M, Lou H, et al. Diversity of T(H) cytokine profiles in patients with chronic rhinosinusitis: a multicenter study in Europe, Asia, and Oceania. J Allergy Clin Immunol. 2016;138(5):1344–53. https://doi.org/10.1016/j.jaci.2016.05.041.
8. Annunziato F, Romagnani C, Romagnani S. The 3 major types of innate and adaptive cell-mediated effector immunity. J Allergy Clin Immunol. 2015;135(3):626–35. https://doi.org/10.1016/j.jaci.2014.11.001.
9. Tomassen P, Vandeplas G, Van Zele T, Cardell LO, Arebro J, Olze H, et al. Inflammatory endotypes of chronic rhinosinusitis based on cluster analysis of biomarkers. J Allergy Clin Immunol. 2016;137(5):1449–56.e4. https://doi.org/10.1016/j.jaci.2015.12.1324.
10. Tan BK, Klingler AI, Poposki JA, Stevens WW, Peters AT, Suh LA, et al. Heterogeneous inflammatory patterns in chronic rhinosinusitis without nasal polyps in Chicago, Illinois. J Allergy Clin Immunol. 2017;139(2):699–703.e7. https://doi.org/10.1016/j.jaci.2016.06.063.
11. Zhang N, Van Zele T, Perez-Novo C, Van Bruaene N, Holtappels G, DeRuyck N, et al. Different types of T-effector cells orchestrate mucosal inflammation in chronic sinus disease. J Allergy Clin Immunol. 2008;122(5):961–8. https://doi.org/10.1016/j.jaci.2008.07.008.
12. Kim JW, Hong SL, Kim YK, Lee CH, Min YG, Rhee CS. Histological and immunological features of non-eosinophilic nasal polyps. Otolaryngol Head Neck Surg. 2007;137(6):925–30. https://doi.org/10.1016/j.otohns.2007.07.036.
13. Tokunaga T, Sakashita M, Haruna T, Asaka D, Takeno S, Ikeda H, et al. Novel scoring system and algorithm for classifying chronic rhinosinusitis: the JESREC Study. Allergy. 2015;70(8):995–1003. https://doi.org/10.1111/all.12644.

14. Kim SJ, Lee KH, Kim SW, Cho JS, Park YK, Shin SY. Changes in histological features of nasal polyps in a Korean population over a 17-year period. Otolaryngol Head Neck Surg. 2013;149(3):431–7. https://doi.org/10.1177/0194599813495363.
15. Katotomichelakis M, Tantilipikorn P, Holtappels G, De Ruyck N, Feng L, Van Zele T, et al. Inflammatory patterns in upper airway disease in the same geographical area may change over time. Am J Rhinol Allergy. 2013;27(5):354–60. https://doi.org/10.2500/ajra.2013.27.3922.
16. Van Zele T, Claeys S, Gevaert P, Van Maele G, Holtappels G, Van Cauwenberge P, et al. Differentiation of chronic sinus diseases by measurement of inflammatory mediators. Allergy. 2006;61(11):1280–9. https://doi.org/10.1111/j.1398-9995.2006.01225.x.
17. Van Bruaene N, Pérez-Novo CA, Basinski TM, Van Zele T, Holtappels G, De Ruyck N, et al. T-cell regulation in chronic paranasal sinus disease. J Allergy Clin Immunol. 2008;121(6):1435–41, 41.e1–3. https://doi.org/10.1016/j.jaci.2008.02.018.
18. Cao PP, Li HB, Wang BF, Wang SB, You XJ, Cui YH, et al. Distinct immunopathologic characteristics of various types of chronic rhinosinusitis in adult Chinese. J Allergy Clin Immunol. 2009;124(3):478–84, 84.e1–2. https://doi.org/10.1016/j.jaci.2009.05.017.
19. Stevens WW, Ocampo CJ, Berdnikovs S, Sakashita M, Mahdavinia M, Suh L, et al. Cytokines in chronic rhinosinusitis. Role in eosinophilia and aspirin-exacerbated respiratory disease. Am J Respir Crit Care Med. 2015;192(6):682–94. https://doi.org/10.1164/rccm.201412-2278OC.
20. Bachert C, Sousa AR, Lund VJ, Scadding GK, Gevaert P, Nasser S, et al. Reduced need for surgery in severe nasal polyposis with mepolizumab: randomized trial. J Allergy Clin Immunol. 2017;140(4):1024–31.e14. https://doi.org/10.1016/j.jaci.2017.05.044.
21. Stevens WW, Staudacher AG, Peters AT, Suh LA, Carter RG, Fischer SR, et al. Effects of reslizumab on nasal polyp inflammation in aspirin exacerbated respiratory disease. J Allergy Clin Immunol. 2018;141(2) https://doi.org/10.1016/j.jaci.2017.12.963.
22. Tsurumaki H, Matsuyama T, Ezawa K, Koga Y, Yatomi M, Aoki-Saito H, et al. Rapid effect of benralizumab for hypereosinophilia in a case of severe asthma with eosinophilic chronic rhinosinusitis. Medicina (Kaunas, Lithuania). 2019;55(7):336. https://doi.org/10.3390/medicina55070336.
23. Kartush AG, Schumacher JK, Shah R, Patadia MO. Biologic agents for the treatment of chronic rhinosinusitis with nasal polyps. Am J Rhinol Allergy. 2019;33(2):203–11. https://doi.org/10.1177/1945892418814768.
24. Takabayashi T, Kato A, Peters AT, Hulse KE, Suh LA, Carter R, et al. Excessive fibrin deposition in nasal polyps caused by fibrinolytic impairment through reduction of tissue plasminogen activator expression. Am J Respir Crit Care Med. 2013;187(1):49–57. https://doi.org/10.1164/rccm.201207-1292OC.
25. Takabayashi T, Kato A, Peters AT, Hulse KE, Suh LA, Carter R, et al. Increased expression of factor XIII-A in patients with chronic rhinosinusitis with nasal polyps. J Allergy Clin Immunol. 2013;132(3):584–92.e4. https://doi.org/10.1016/j.jaci.2013.02.003.
26. Bachert C, Han JK, Desrosiers M, Hellings PW, Amin N, Lee SE, et al. Efficacy and safety of dupilumab in patients with severe chronic rhinosinusitis with nasal polyps (LIBERTY NP SINUS-24 and LIBERTY NP SINUS-52): results from two multicentre, randomised, double-blind, placebo-controlled, parallel-group phase 3 trials. Lancet (London, England). 2019;394(10209):1638–50. https://doi.org/10.1016/s0140-6736(19)31881-1.
27. Laidlaw TM, Mullol J, Fan C, Zhang D, Amin N, Khan A, et al. Dupilumab improves nasal polyp burden and asthma control in patients with CRSwNP and AERD. J Allergy Clin Immunol Pract. 2019;7(7):2462–5.e1. https://doi.org/10.1016/j.jaip.2019.03.044.
28. Nakayama T, Hirahara K, Onodera A, Endo Y, Hosokawa H, Shinoda K, et al. Th2 cells in health and disease. Annu Rev Immunol. 2017;35:53–84. https://doi.org/10.1146/annurev-immunol-051116-052350.
29. Zhu J. T helper 2 (Th2) cell differentiation, type 2 innate lymphoid cell (ILC2) development and regulation of interleukin-4 (IL-4) and IL-13 production. Cytokine. 2015;75(1):14–24. https://doi.org/10.1016/j.cyto.2015.05.010.
30. Walker JA, McKenzie ANJ. T(H)2 cell development and function. Nat Rev Immunol. 2018;18(2):121–33. https://doi.org/10.1038/nri.2017.118.
31. Derycke L, Eyerich S, Van Crombruggen K, Pérez-Novo C, Holtappels G, Deruyck N, et al. Mixed T helper cell signatures in chronic rhinosinusitis with and without polyps. PLoS One. 2014;9(6):e97581. https://doi.org/10.1371/journal.pone.0097581.
32. Lam EP, Kariyawasam HH, Rana BM, Durham SR, McKenzie AN, Powell N, et al. IL-25/IL-33-responsive TH2 cells characterize nasal polyps with a default TH17 signature in nasal mucosa. J Allergy Clin Immunol. 2016;137(5):1514–24. https://doi.org/10.1016/j.jaci.2015.10.019.
33. Shi LL, Song J, Xiong P, Cao PP, Liao B, Ma J, et al. Disease-specific T-helper cell polarizing function of lesional dendritic cells in different types of chronic rhinosinusitis with nasal polyps. Am J Respir Crit Care Med. 2014;190(6):628–38. https://doi.org/10.1164/rccm.201402-0234OC.
34. Endo Y, Iwamura C, Kuwahara M, Suzuki A, Sugaya K, Tumes DJ, et al. Eomesodermin controls interleukin-5 production in memory T helper 2 cells through inhibition of activity of the transcription factor GATA3. Immunity. 2011;35(5):733–45. https://doi.org/10.1016/j.immuni.2011.08.017.
35. Mitson-Salazar A, Yin Y, Wansley DL, Young M, Bolan H, Arceo S, et al. Hematopoietic prostaglandin D synthase defines a proeosinophilic pathogenic effector human T(H)2 cell subpopulation

with enhanced function. J Allergy Clin Immunol. 2016;137(3):907–18.e9. https://doi.org/10.1016/j.jaci.2015.08.007.
36. Wambre E, Bajzik V, DeLong JH, O'Brien K, Nguyen QA, Speake C, et al. A phenotypically and functionally distinct human T(H)2 cell subpopulation is associated with allergic disorders. Sci Transl Med. 2017;9(401):eaam9171. https://doi.org/10.1126/scitranslmed.aam9171.
37. Endo Y, Hirahara K, Iinuma T, Shinoda K, Tumes DJ, Asou HK, et al. The interleukin-33-p38 kinase axis confers memory T helper 2 cell pathogenicity in the airway. Immunity. 2015;42(2):294–308. https://doi.org/10.1016/j.immuni.2015.01.016.
38. Gevaert P, Holtappels G, Johansson SG, Cuvelier C, Cauwenberge P, Bachert C. Organization of secondary lymphoid tissue and local IgE formation to Staphylococcus aureus enterotoxins in nasal polyp tissue. Allergy. 2005;60(1):71–9. https://doi.org/10.1111/j.1398-9995.2004.00621.x.
39. Seiberling KA, Conley DB, Tripathi A, Grammer LC, Shuh L, Haines GK III, et al. Superantigens and chronic rhinosinusitis: detection of staphylococcal exotoxins in nasal polyps. Laryngoscope. 2005;115(9):1580–5. https://doi.org/10.1097/01.mlg.0000168111.11802.9c.
40. Ou J, Wang J, Xu Y, Tao ZZ, Kong YG, Chen SM, et al. Staphylococcus aureus superantigens are associated with chronic rhinosinusitis with nasal polyps: a meta-analysis. Eur Arch Otorhinolaryngol. 2014;271(10):2729–36. https://doi.org/10.1007/s00405-014-2955-0.
41. Ogasawara N, Klingler AI, Tan BK, Poposki JA, Hulse KE, Stevens WW, et al. Epithelial activators of type 2 inflammation: elevation of thymic stromal lymphopoietin, but not IL-25 or IL-33, in chronic rhinosinusitis with nasal polyps in Chicago, Illinois. Allergy. 2018;73(11):2251–4. https://doi.org/10.1111/all.13552.
42. Lim AI, Li Y, Lopez-Lastra S, Stadhouders R, Paul F, Casrouge A, et al. Systemic human ILC precursors provide a substrate for tissue ILC differentiation. Cell. 2017;168(6):1086–100.e10. https://doi.org/10.1016/j.cell.2017.02.021.
43. Scoville SD, Freud AG, Caligiuri MA. Cellular pathways in the development of human and murine innate lymphoid cells. Curr Opin Immunol. 2019;56:100–6. https://doi.org/10.1016/j.coi.2018.11.003.
44. Mjösberg JM, Trifari S, Crellin NK, Peters CP, van Drunen CM, Piet B, et al. Human IL-25- and IL-33-responsive type 2 innate lymphoid cells are defined by expression of CRTH2 and CD161. Nat Immunol. 2011;12(11):1055–62. https://doi.org/10.1038/ni.2104.
45. Shaw JL, Fakhri S, Citardi MJ, Porter PC, Corry DB, Kheradmand F, et al. IL-33-responsive innate lymphoid cells are an important source of IL-13 in chronic rhinosinusitis with nasal polyps. Am J Respir Crit Care Med. 2013;188(4):432–9. https://doi.org/10.1164/rccm.201212-2227OC.
46. Walford HH, Lund SJ, Baum RE, White AA, Bergeron CM, Husseman J, et al. Increased ILC2s in the eosinophilic nasal polyp endotype are associated with corticosteroid responsiveness. Clin Immunol (Orlando, Fla). 2014;155(1):126–35. https://doi.org/10.1016/j.clim.2014.09.007.
47. Tojima I, Kouzaki H, Shimizu S, Ogawa T, Arikata M, Kita H, et al. Group 2 innate lymphoid cells are increased in nasal polyps in patients with eosinophilic chronic rhinosinusitis. Clin Immunol (Orlando, Fla). 2016;170:1–8. https://doi.org/10.1016/j.clim.2016.07.010.
48. Poposki JA, Klingler AI, Tan BK, Soroosh P, Banie H, Lewis G, et al. Group 2 innate lymphoid cells are elevated and activated in chronic rhinosinusitis with nasal polyps. Immun Inflamm Dis. 2017;5(3):233–43. https://doi.org/10.1002/iid3.161.
49. Ogasawara N, Poposki JA, Klingler AI, Tan BK, Hulse KE, Stevens WW, et al. TNF induces production of type 2 cytokines in human group 2 innate lymphoid cells. J Allergy Clin Immunol. 2020;145(1):437–40.e8. https://doi.org/10.1016/j.jaci.2019.09.001.
50. Yu X, Pappu R, Ramirez-Carrozzi V, Ota N, Caplazi P, Zhang J, et al. TNF superfamily member TL1A elicits type 2 innate lymphoid cells at mucosal barriers. Mucosal Immunol. 2014;7(3):730–40. https://doi.org/10.1038/mi.2013.92.
51. Galle-Treger L, Sankaranarayanan I, Hurrell BP, Howard E, Lo R, Maazi H, et al. Costimulation of type-2 innate lymphoid cells by GITR promotes effector function and ameliorates type 2 diabetes. Nat Commun. 2019;10(1):713. https://doi.org/10.1038/s41467-019-08449-x.
52. Ogasawara N, Poposki JA, Klingler AI, Tan BK, Hulse KE, Stevens WW, et al. Role of RANK-L as a potential inducer of ILC2-mediated type 2 inflammation in chronic rhinosinusitis with nasal polyps. Mucosal Immunol. 2020;13(1):86–95. https://doi.org/10.1038/s41385-019-0215-8.
53. Salimi M, Stöger L, Liu W, Go S, Pavord I, Klenerman P, et al. Cysteinyl leukotriene E(4) activates human group 2 innate lymphoid cells and enhances the effect of prostaglandin D(2) and epithelial cytokines. J Allergy Clin Immunol. 2017;140(4):1090–100.e11. https://doi.org/10.1016/j.jaci.2016.12.958.
54. Xue L, Salimi M, Panse I, Mjösberg JM, McKenzie AN, Spits H, et al. Prostaglandin D2 activates group 2 innate lymphoid cells through chemoattractant receptor-homologous molecule expressed on TH2 cells. J Allergy Clin Immunol. 2014;133(4):1184–94. https://doi.org/10.1016/j.jaci.2013.10.056.
55. Maazi H, Patel N, Sankaranarayanan I, Suzuki Y, Rigas D, Soroosh P, et al. ICOS:ICOS-ligand interaction is required for type 2 innate lymphoid cell function, homeostasis, and induction of airway hyperreactivity. Immunity. 2015;42(3):538–51. https://doi.org/10.1016/j.immuni.2015.02.007.
56. Gour N, Smole U, Yong HM, Lewkowich IP, Yao N, Singh A, et al. C3a is required for ILC2 function in

allergic airway inflammation. Mucosal Immunol. 2018;11(6):1653–62. https://doi.org/10.1038/s41385-018-0064-x.

57. Cardoso V, Chesné J, Ribeiro H, García-Cassani B, Carvalho T, Bouchery T, et al. Neuronal regulation of type 2 innate lymphoid cells via neuromedin U. Nature. 2017;549(7671):277–81. https://doi.org/10.1038/nature23469.
58. Nussbaum JC, Van Dyken SJ, von Moltke J, Cheng LE, Mohapatra A, Molofsky AB, et al. Type 2 innate lymphoid cells control eosinophil homeostasis. Nature. 2013;502(7470):245–8. https://doi.org/10.1038/nature12526.
59. Sui P, Wiesner DL, Xu J, Zhang Y, Lee J, Van Dyken S, et al. Pulmonary neuroendocrine cells amplify allergic asthma responses. Science (New York, NY). 2018;360(6393):eaan8546. https://doi.org/10.1126/science.aan8546.
60. Ogasawara N, Poposki JA, Klingler AI, Tan BK, Weibman AR, Hulse KE, et al. IL-10, TGF-β, and glucocorticoid prevent the production of type 2 cytokines in human group 2 innate lymphoid cells. J Allergy Clin Immunol. 2018;141(3):1147–51.e8. https://doi.org/10.1016/j.jaci.2017.09.025.
61. Eastman JJ, Cavagnero KJ, Deconde AS, Kim AS, Karta MR, Broide DH, et al. Group 2 innate lymphoid cells are recruited to the nasal mucosa in patients with aspirin-exacerbated respiratory disease. J Allergy Clin Immunol. 2017;140(1):101–8.e3. https://doi.org/10.1016/j.jaci.2016.11.023.
62. Cahill KN, Bensko JC, Boyce JA, Laidlaw TM. Prostaglandin D2: a dominant mediator of aspirin-exacerbated respiratory disease. J Allergy Clin Immunol. 2015;135(1):245–52. https://doi.org/10.1016/j.jaci.2014.07.031.
63. Kohanski MA, Workman AD, Patel NN, Hung LY, Shtraks JP, Chen B, et al. Solitary chemosensory cells are a primary epithelial source of IL-25 in patients with chronic rhinosinusitis with nasal polyps. J Allergy Clin Immunol. 2018;142(2):460–9.e7. https://doi.org/10.1016/j.jaci.2018.03.019.
64. Schwartz C, Khan AR, Floudas A, Saunders SP, Hams E, Rodewald HR, et al. ILC2s regulate adaptive Th2 cell functions via PD-L1 checkpoint control. J Exp Med. 2017;214(9):2507–21. https://doi.org/10.1084/jem.20170051.
65. Halim TYF, Rana BMJ, Walker JA, Kerscher B, Knolle MD, Jolin HE, et al. Tissue-restricted adaptive type 2 immunity is orchestrated by expression of the costimulatory molecule OX40L on group 2 innate lymphoid cells. Immunity. 2018;48(6):1195–207.e6. https://doi.org/10.1016/j.immuni.2018.05.003.
66. Weinstein SF, Katial RK, Bardin P, Korn S, McDonald M, Garin M, et al. Effects of reslizumab on asthma outcomes in a subgroup of eosinophilic asthma patients with self-reported chronic rhinosinusitis with nasal polyps. J Allergy Clin Immunol Pract. 2019;7(2):589–96.e3. https://doi.org/10.1016/j.jaip.2018.08.021.
67. Bleecker ER, Wechsler ME, FitzGerald JM, Menzies-Gow A, Wu Y, Hirsch I, et al. Baseline patient factors impact on the clinical efficacy of benralizumab for severe asthma. Eur Respir J. 2018;52(4):1800936. https://doi.org/10.1183/13993003.00936-2018.

7 B Cells and Plasma Cells

Siobhan Ward, Zeynep Celebi Sözener,
and Mübeccel Akdis

Key Points

- There are elevated numbers of B cells, plasma cells, and antibodies in CRSwNP tissue.
- Increased levels of chemokines and cytokines in nasal polyp tissue, specifically BAFF, IL-6, CXCL12, CXCL13, that may play a role in the recruitment of B cells into nasal polyp tissue, and their activation, differentiation, and survival.
- B cells may be activated via extra follicular mechanisms, with increased expression of EBI2 being found in nasal polyp tissue and on plasma blasts in nasal polyp tissue.
- There is evidence of tertiary lymphoid structures in nasal polyp tissue with an increased formation of these structures being associated with increased previous surgeries, suggesting an association of tertiary lymphoid structures with recalcitrant disease.
- B cells may be activated and undergo class switching locally in nasal polyp tissue.
- Autoreactive antibodies have been found in nasal polyp tissue, particularly IgG and IgG to nuclear antigens.

7.1 Introduction

B lymphocytes, often referred to as B cells, are a type of white blood cell that form an integral part of the humoral adaptive immune response. They are responsible for the production of antigen specific Immunoglobulin (Ig), known as antibodies, that are directed against invasive pathogens. In addition to producing antibodies, they perform critical immune functions including generating immunological memory, antigen presentation, and regulatory cytokine production [1].

Recent findings suggest that B cells, plasma cells, and antibodies may play a key role in chronic rhinosinusitis (CRS). In order to better understand the mechanisms by which B cells, plasma cells, and antibodies are involved in CRS, we must first give a brief overview of B cell development and B cell activation.

S. Ward
Swiss Institute of Allergy and Asthma Research (SIAF), University of Zurich, Davos Wolfgang, Switzerland

Cristine Kühne-Center for Allergy Research and Education, Davos Wolfgang, Switzerland

Z. C. Sözener
Swiss Institute of Allergy and Asthma Research (SIAF), University of Zurich, Davos Wolfgang, Switzerland

Department of Chest Disease, Division of Allergy and Clinical Immunology, Ankara University School of Medicine, Ankara, Turkey

M. Akdis (✉)
Swiss Institute of Allergy and Asthma Research (SIAF), University of Zurich, Davos, Switzerland
e-mail: akdism@siaf.uzh.ch

L. Zhang, C. Bachert (eds.), *Chronic Rhinosinusitis*, https://doi.org/10.1007/978-981-16-0784-4_7

7.2 B Cell

7.2.1 B Cell Development

B cells arise from common lymphoid progenitor (CLP) cells in the bone marrow [1]. B cells possess Ig receptors on their cell surface. During B cell development the Ig receptor undergoes extensive recombination, finally producing a complete and functional B cell receptor [1]. To prevent auto-reactivity immature B cells which encounter self-antigen that is capable of binding to the B cell receptor are eliminated. Immature B cells then migrate to the spleen where they differentiate through transitional B cell stages T1 and T2 to form either mature follicular (FO) or marginal zone (MZ) B cells [1].

MZ B cells are polyreactive and capable of T-dependent and independent activation. They are located mainly in the marginal sinus of the spleen. This position allows them to rapidly initiate an immune response against blood borne pathogens, particularly encapsulated bacteria [2]. In humans MZ B cells may also be found in the blood and are able to recirculate through secondary lymphoid organs [2, 3]. However, the number of B cells that develop into MZ B cells is relatively small in comparison to FO B cells [3, 4].

FO B cells participate in T cell-dependent antibody responses. When FO B cells are activated, they differentiate either into short lived plasma cells or enter a germinal center response in which long lived plasma cells and memory B cells are produced [1] (Fig. 7.1). This process will be outlined below.

7.2.2 B Cell Activation-Response to Antigen

Mature FO B cells circulate between secondary lymphoid organs in search of antigen. Secondary lymphoid organs such as the spleen, lymph nodes, tonsils, adenoids, and Peyer's patches are where the antigen is localized, where it can encounter a mature B cell and initiate an adaptive immune response. In contrast, primary lymphoid organs are locations where immature lymphocytes develop, and include the thymus and bone marrow.

Upon encountering an antigen that binds to the B cell antibody receptor, B cells are activated. The development possibilities of the activated B cell is dependent on a number of factors including the presence or absence of T cell help. B cells may differentiate either into plasmablasts, plasma cells or memory B cells [1]. The initial response results in the activation of antigen specific B cells, local expansion and the generation of short lived plasma cells. This response is known as the extrafollicular immune response, as it occurs outside the B cell follicles. Short lived plasma cells provide a rapid initial response to antigen.

Subsequently, activated B cells migrate into the B cell follicle forming a germinal center. A germinal center is a specialized structure in which B cells undergo proliferation, affinity maturation and class switching and differentiate into long lived plasma cells or memory B cells [1] (Fig. 7.1). Memory B cells are able to survive in a quiescent state for great lengths of time. Upon re-exposure to an antigen, these memory B cells are able to produce a rapid and enhanced response to the antigen [1]. Plasma cells are terminally differentiated antibody-secreting cells.

Affinity maturation is the process by which B cells producing antibodies that bind to antigen with increased affinity are selected for survival and proliferation, resulting in the B cell response being dominated by high-affinity antibodies (Fig. 7.1). Class switching is the process by which B cells change their immunoglobulin isotype allowing for the generation of different antibodies with different effector functions. In total there are five varying isotypes of antibodies; IgA, IgD, IgE, IgG, and IgM [1]. Only IgA (A1 and A2) and IgG (G1, G2, G3, and G4) have subclasses as well. These can exist both as cell surface receptors (IgD and IgM serve as B cell receptor) or as secreted antibodies in the serum or in nasal secretions. Different isotypes of antibodies do not change the specific antigen recognition, but rather influences the nature of the biological response triggered after antibody binds to antigen.

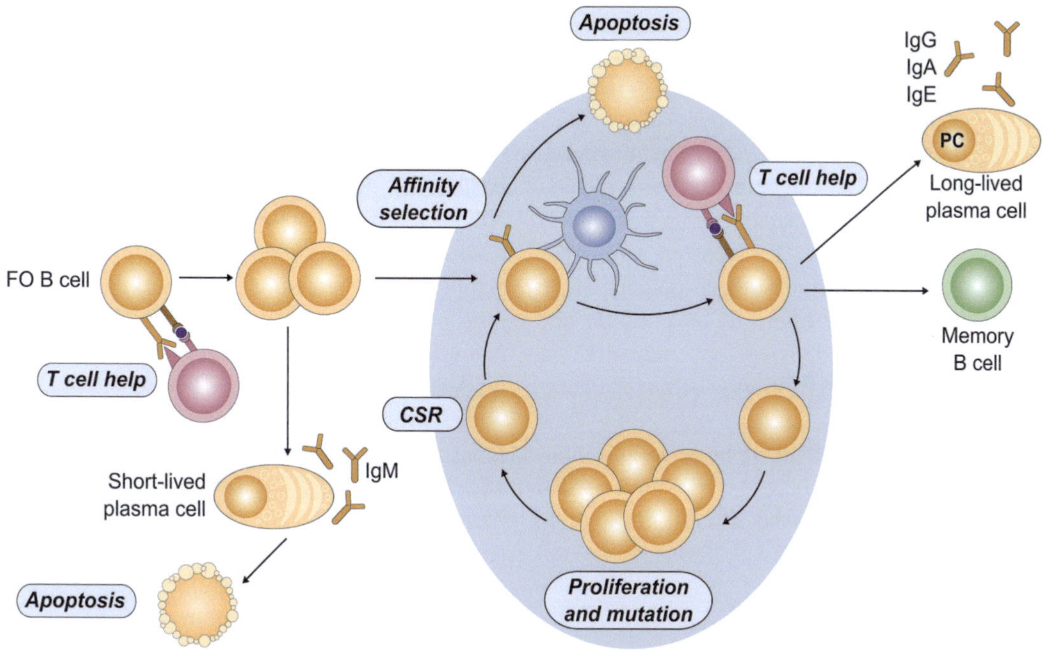

Fig. 7.1 B cell responses to antigen

7.2.3 Role of B Cells and Plasma Cells in CRS

Increased levels of B cells and plasma cells have been found in the inflammatory infiltrate of CRS [5]. Following this, recent studies have begun evaluating the mechanism of action of such B cells with findings suggesting that B cells may play a critical role in the pathogenesis of disease in CRS. While further studies aiming for a better understanding of the B cell associated mechanisms that may drive disease in CRS are still ongoing, this chapter will attempt to provide the current most up to date knowledge.

CRS is often divided into two classifications based on endoscopic examination findings, this being CRS with Nasal Polyps (CRSwNP) and CRS without nasal polyps (CRSsNP) [6]. Similarly, we may look at the role of B cells being different between these two groups in the pathogenesis of disease. CRSwNP patients generally have more severe disease radiographically and have an increased risk of recurrence after surgery [7]. While extensive study is ongoing in both CRSwNP and CRSsNP, it must be noted that CRSwNP forms the majority of the current new findings and developments in relation to B cells in CRS. As such, this chapter will focus mainly on B cells and their role in CRSwNP.

7.3 CRSsNP

Non-polyp CRS (CRSsNP) is characterized by an insufficient immune response permitting recurrent and chronic infections. Deficient or inadequate B cell response can result in increased infections in the nose, causing chronic or recurrent acute infections, potentially resulting in CRSsNP.

Immunodeficiencies that have been found to be associated with CRSsNP are:

- Selective IgA deficiency.
- Specific antibody deficiency.
- Common variable immunodeficiency (CVID).

CVID is the most common symptomatic antibody deficiency and typically involves the reduction in at least two of three major

Immunoglobulin's; IgG, IgA, and/or IgM [8]. Recurrent infections of the upper and lower respiratory tract are common in CVID, and although symptoms often appear many years before diagnosis, CVID is often not diagnosed until later in life [8]. In cohort studies screening patients for immunodeficiency, approximately 5–6% of patients with CRS have been found to have CVID [9, 10]. Further, patients with CRSsNP were more likely to have CVID and specific antibody deficiencies compared to patients with CRSwNP [9]. As such, it is important for healthcare professionals who treat patients with rhinosinusitis to be aware of immunodeficiencies and to consider them when encountering patients who do not respond to treatment [9, 11].

7.4 CRSwNP

Overall, it has been shown that B cells, plasma cell, and antibodies are highly elevated locally in CRSwNP tissue, and it is thought that B cells may play a key role in the pathophysiology of CRSwNP. Below we will outline the current key findings and knowledge in relation to B cells in CRSwNP. However, more studies must be undertaken to further fully understand the mechanisms by which B cells contribute to the pathogenesis of CRSwNP.

7.4.1 Elevated B Cell Population in CRSwNP

B cells, plasma cells, and antibodies are all highly elevated in the polyp tissue of patients with CRSwNP. This was first found with immunohistology demonstrating elevated expression of B cell marker CD19 and plasma cell marker CD138 in CRSwNP tissue [5]. Following this, the presence of B cells and plasma cells in CRSwNP tissue was confirmed via flow cytometry, with results showing elevated levels of B cells and plasma cells in CRSwNP tissue compared to control [12]. Further, studies indicate that B cells are highly activated, may switch isotypes and secrete a large amount of antibodies locally within nasal polyps, with the local production of antibodies being thought to form an essential part of the pathophysiology behind the development of nasal polyps [13]. Among the B cell subpopulations present in polyp tissue, B regulatory cells and mature B cells are significantly lower, while memory B cells are significantly higher and represent the main subpopulation in CRSwNP tissue compared to peripheral blood in the same patients [14]. In relation to antibodies present, antibodies of all isotypes except IgG3 have been found in nasal polyp tissue [15, 16]. The specificity and pathogenic potential of these B cells has recently been studied. It has been reported that B cell activation that occurs in CRSwNP is highly distinct from the classical activation mechanisms observed in germinal centers, as outlined above, and this may be important for the overall increased levels of activated B cell subsets found in CRSwNP [17, 18].

7.4.2 Activation Mechanisms

There is currently mixed views by which activation of B cells occurs in nasal polyp tissue. While there is large evidence and support for B cell activation in CRSwNP being similar to the extra follicular response that is known to occur in lymph nodes and the spleen, contrasting studies have evidence to support the formation of tertiary lymphoid structures. Further, chemokines and cytokines have been shown to play a role. All in all, it is likely that a variety of mechanisms together contribute to the activation of B cells in CRSwNP.

- **Presence of Tertiary Lymphoid Structures in CRSwNP**
- Evidence of the formation of tertiary lymphoid structures in nasal polyp tissue has been found, suggesting that the activation of B cells may occur in such structures [19, 20]. Tertiary lymphoid structures are ectopic lymphoid organs that develop in non-lymphoid tissues at

sites of chronic inflammation [21]. Further, it has also been found that an increased number of tertiary lymphoid structures is associated with a higher number of previous surgeries suggesting that their formations may be associated with recalcitrant disease [19].

- **Activation via extrafollicular mechanisms in CRSwNP**
- In contrast, studies suggest that local activation of B cells may occur in nasal polyp tissue, with data demonstrating that the B cell activation pathway is very different from the activation pathway that occurs in the germinal centers, as outlined above [18]. It is suggested that the local B cell response in nasal polyps may be similar to the extra follicular response that is known to occur in lymph nodes and the spleen. Epstein–Barr virus-induced protein G coupled receptor 2 (EBI2), a chemotactic receptor, plays a critical role in guiding B cells away from germinal centers towards extra follicular regions in secondary lymphoid organs, facilitating B cell differentiation into extrafollicular plasmablasts [22]. As such EBI2 is a marker for extra follicular plasma blasts, this being B cells that are activated outside germinal centers. EBI2 has been found to be highly elevated in nasal polyp tissue extracts [22]. Further, plasma blasts in nasal polyps show a higher frequency of expression of EBI2 [18]. As such, given increased EBI2 expression it seems that some B cells in nasal polyps may be activated via extra follicular mechanisms [18, 23, 24]. Further to this, group 2 innate lymphoid cells (ILC2s) are known to be elevated in nasal polyp tissue. ILC2s can directly induce EBI2 expression on B cells, suggesting that they may play a role in the induction of these extra follicular B cell responses occurring in nasal polyps during chronic inflammation in the airways [18].
- ***Increased expression of chemokines and cytokines in nasal polyp tissue***
- Nasal polyp tissue from CRSwNP patients show elevation in a variety of inflammatory mediators known to play a role in activation, survival, and recruitment of B cells. Studies have demonstrated the elevated expression of B cell attracting chemokines CXCL12 and CXCL13 in nasal polyps, with chemokines being a potent inducer of cell migration and recruitment of cells to inflamed tissues [23–25]. Further, B cell activating factor of the TNF family (BAFF), a cytokine, which plays an important role in B cell activation, differentiation, survival in secondary lymphoid organs and class switch recombination has been shown to be highly elevated in nasal polyp tissue, in comparison to that seen in the tissue from patients with CRSsNP and control subjects [26]. Further, increased expression of BAFF in patients with CRSwNP was associated with increased levels of B cells, plasma cells and increased production of IgA [27]. BAFF is thought to mainly be produced by activated epithelium and dendritic cells but has been shown to be produced by eosinophils in nasal polyp tissue [26]. Increased levels of BAFF have also been reported in the setting of asthma and chronic obstructive pulmonary disease (COPD) further indicating its likely important role in the pathogenesis of airway inflammatory diseases [28, 29]. Moreover, APRIL, a proliferation inducing ligand that is produced by eosinophils, is very homogenous to BAFF has an important role in the survival of long lived plasma cells in the bone marrow and has been found to be elevated in CRSwNP tissue [30]. IL-6, a key cytokine involved in the survival and activation of B cells, is once again elevated in nasal polyp tissue [31]. Further IL-6 in also known to induce B cell proliferation, differentiation of B cells into plasma cells and has the ability to induce class switch recombination. This information indicates that the increased levels of chemokines CXCL12 and CXCL13 may contribute to the initial recruitment of B-lineage cells into nasal polyp tissue, while cytokines BAFF, APRIL, and IL-6 may be involved in the proliferation, activation, and survival of B-lineage cells in nasal polyp tissue, and may be responsible for the increase in plasma cells and antibodies that have been reported in nasal polyp tissue.

7.5 Antibodies and Class Switching

7.5.1 Class Switching

Antibodies of almost every isotype have been found to be elevated in nasal polyp tissue but not in sinus tissue from patients with CRSsNP. Further, local antibody production may play an important role in the pathogenesis of CRSwNP [22]. Evidence suggests that some antibody-secreting B cells may be directly activated to undergo class switching within nasal polyps. There is known to be an increased expression of type 2 cytokines, IL-5 and IL-13, in nasal polyp tissue [32]. IL-13 is known to be able to directly act on B cells and promote class switching, particular to IgE [33]. Elevated levels of both IgE and findings of ε-germline gene transcripts for IgE have been found in nasal polyp tissue [34]. This suggests that IgE class switching and B cell differentiation into IgE-secreting plasma cells can occur within nasal polyps, and that IL-13 may play a role in these events [34].

7.5.2 Autoreactive Antibodies

The overall specificity of antibodies found in CRS is currently unknown. However, evidence has found that most nasal polyp tissue shows a polyclonal antibody response [35]. Polyclonal antibodies are antibodies that come from different B cell lineages, in comparison to monoclonal antibodies that arise from the same B cell lineage. Within the polyclonal antibody response there has been found to be elevated levels of autoreactive antibodies. Autoreactive antibodies are antibodies that are able to recognize and attack self-antigen. Autoreactive antibodies found include IgA and IgG to nuclear antigens including double stranded DNA (dsDNA) and basement membrane components, with increased levels of anti-BP180 IgG autoantibodies being found in nasal polyp tissue [35–37]. BP180 is a transmembrane glycoprotein that maintains adhesion of the stratified epithelia to the basement membrane, and the findings of this autoantibody may play a role in the loss of the epithelial barrier function that is seen in nasal polyps [36]. These autoantibodies are present at a locally increased levels in nasal polyp tissue in comparison to control nasal tissue and inflamed tissue from patients with CRSsNP [35]. Further, in nasal polyp tissue obtained from patients undergoing revision surgery for recurrence of CRSwNP, frequently higher levels of anti-dsDNA IgG were found in comparison to the polyp tissue obtained during primary surgery, suggesting that increased levels of anti-dsDNA IgG is associated with recurrent disease [35]. This local increase in autoreactive antibodies is unlikely to correlate with systemic autoimmune response given the lack of systemic manifestation of autoimmunity in patients with CRS. The above information suggests that the microenvironment of a nasal polyp may promote the expansion of self-reactive B cell clones.

Recently, the presence of local anti-cytokine autoantibodies in nasal secretions of CRS patients has been found. IgA autoantibodies against IL-1β, IL-2, IL-5, and IL-8 were interestingly found in patients with CRS, including CRSsNP and CRSsNP, however, the highest levels of anti-IL-5 and anti-IL-17A autoantibodies were detected only in patients with CRSwNP [38].

7.5.3 IgE to *Staphylococcus aureus*

Staphylococcus aureus and its super antigens are known to be implicated in the intense inflammatory processes of the upper and lower airways in patients with allergic diseases. These super antigens, particularly *Staphylococcus aureus* enterotoxins have been found to be strongly associated with CRSwNP, with evidence that some of the IgE found in nasal polyps being specific to enterotoxins produced by *Staphylococcus aureus [15, 39, 40]*. Further, increased colonization of nasal polyps with *Staphylococcus aureus* has been reported combined with a local immune response consisting of IgE formation and eosinophilic inflammation [20, 41]. Interestingly, this is rarely found in CRSsNP [41]. This topic regarding the effect of *Staphylococcus aureus* and its proteins on CRS will be discussed in more detail in the following sections.

7.6 Conclusion

In conclusion, there is emerging evidence that B cells and plasma cells play a key role in the pathogenesis of CRS. Deficient or inadequate B cell responses may result in increased risk of infections, leading to chronic CRS and is typically associated with CRSsNP. Contrasting this, CRSwNP is associated with increased numbers of B cells, plasma cells, and antibodies in polyp tissue. Further, in tissue of CRSwNP high levels of BAFF, a potent stimulator of B cell proliferation and class switching, has been found in addition to high levels of cytokines such as IL-6 and chemokines such as CXCL12 and CXCL13 which are known to play a role in B cell recruitment and plasma cell differentiation. It is proposed that these findings, coupled with the findings of germinal center like structures may contribute to the high numbers of B cells and plasma cells in nasal polyp tissue and thus resulting in the chronic inflammation at the site. Further understanding of the B cells mechanisms in CRSwNP and CRSsNP is ongoing, and will provide large insights into the pathogenesis of the varying forms of CRS. From a clinical perspective, better understanding of the B cell mechanisms contributing to CRS provides an avenue to improving the diagnosis and treatment of the disease.

B Cell Glossary of Terms

Plasmablasts The precursors of plasma cells. Plasmablasts have the capacity to divide and have migratory potential.

Plasma cells Terminally differentiated antibody-secreting cells of the B cell lineage.

Memory B cells B cells that are antigen-experienced and express high-affinity antibodies. Upon re-exposure to an antigen, they are able to quickly differentiate into plasma cells to produce a rapid response to antigen.

Affinity maturation The somatic mutation process by which B cells are selected for on the basis of their increased affinity for antigen.

Class switch recombination (CSR) The process by which B cells change their immunoglobulin isotype to generate antibodies with different effector functions.

Tertiary Lymphoid Structures Ectopic lymphoid organs that develop in non-lymphoid tissues at sites of chronic inflammation.

References

1. Abbas AK. In: Lichtman AH, Pillai S, editors. Cellular and molecular immunology. 8th ed. Philadelphia, PA: Elsevier Saunders; 2015.
2. Weill J-C, Weller S, Reynaud C-A. Human marginal zone b cells. Annu Rev Immunol. 2009;27(1):267–85. https://doi.org/10.1146/annurev.immunol.021908.132607.
3. Shiv P, Annaiah C. The follicular versus marginal zone B lymphocyte cell fate decision. Nat Rev Immunol. 2009;9(11):767. https://doi.org/10.1038/nri2656.
4. Kato AHK, Tan BK, Schleimer RP. B-lymphocyte lineage cells and the respiratory system. J Allergy Clin Immunol. 2013;131:933–57.
5. Stoop AE, van Der Heijden HA, Biewenga J, van Der Baan S. Lymphocytes and nonlymphoid cells in human nasal polyps. J Allergy Clin Immunol. 1991;87(2):470. https://doi.org/10.1016/0091-6749(91)90004-8.
6. Orlandi RR, Kingdom TT, Hwang PH, Smith TL, Alt JA, Baroody FM, et al. International consensus statement on allergy and rhinology: rhinosinusitis. Int Forum Allergy Rhinol. 2016;6(Suppl 1):S22–209. https://doi.org/10.1002/alr.21695.
7. Tokunaga T, Sakashita M, Haruna T, Asaka D, Takeno S, Ikeda H, et al. Novel scoring system and algorithm for classifying chronic rhinosinusitis: the JESREC Study. Allergy. 2015;70(8):995–1003. https://doi.org/10.1111/all.12644.
8. Akdis CA, Hellings PW, Agache I. Global atlas of allergic rhinitis and chronic rhinosinusitis. In: Akdis CA, Hellings PW, Agache I, editors. Zurich: European Academy of Allergy and Clinical Immunology; 2015.
9. Bonilla FA, Barlan I, Chapel H, Costa-Carvalho BT, Cunningham-Rundles C, de La Morena MT, et al. International consensus document (ICON): common variable immunodeficiency disorders. J Allergy Clin Immunol Pract. 2016;4(1):38. https://doi.org/10.1016/j.jaip.2015.07.025.
10. Benjamin MR, Stevens WW, Li N, et al. Clinical characteristics of patients with chronic rhinosinusitis without nasal polyps in an academic setting. J Allergy Clin Immunol Pract. 2019;7(3):1010–16. https://doi.org/10.1016/j.jaip.2018.10.014.

11. Kashani S, Carr T, Grammer L, Schleimer R, Hulse K, Kato A, et al. Clinical characteristics of adults with chronic rhinosinusitis and specific antibody deficiency. J Allergy Clin Immunol Pract. 2015;3(2):236–42. https://doi.org/10.1016/j.jaip.2014.09.022.
12. Van Zele T, Claeys S, Gevaert P, Van Maele G, Holtappels G, Van Cauwenberge P, et al. Differentiation of chronic sinus diseases by measurement of inflammatory mediators. Allergy. 2006;61(11):1280–9. https://doi.org/10.1111/j.1398-9995.2006.01225.x.
13. Ho J, Bailey M, Zaunders J, Mrad N, Sacks R, Sewell W, et al. Cellular comparison of sinus mucosa vs polyp tissue from a single sinus cavity in chronic rhinosinusitis. Int Forum Allergy Rhinol. 2015;5(1):14–27. https://doi.org/10.1002/alr.21417.
14. Ickrath P, Kleinsasser N, Ding X, Ginzkey C, Beyersdorf N, Kerkau T, et al. Impact and modulations of peripheral and edaphic B cell subpopulations in chronic rhinosinusitis with nasal polyposis. Clin Exp Otorhinolaryngol. 2018;11(2):133–40. https://doi.org/10.21053/ceo.2017.01389
15. Bachert C, Gevaert P, Holtappels G, Johansson SG, van Cauwenberge P. Total and specific IgE in nasal polyps is related to local eosinophilic inflammation. J Allergy Clin Immunol. 2001;107(4):607. https://doi.org/10.1067/mai.2001.112374.
16. Van Zele T, Gevaert P, Holtappels G, Van Cauwenberge P, Bachert C. Local immunoglobulin production in nasal polyposis is modulated by superantigens. Clin Exp Allergy. 2007;37(12):1840–7. https://doi.org/10.1111/j.1365-2222.2007.02838.x.
17. Tan BK, Min JY, Hulse KE. Acquired immunity in chronic rhinosinusitis. Curr Allergy Asthma Rep. 2017;17(7):49. https://doi.org/10.1007/s11882-017-0715-0.
18. Feldman S, Kasjanski R, Poposki J, Hernandez D, Chen JN, Norton JE, et al. Chronic airway inflammation provides a unique environment for B cell activation and antibody production. Clin Exp Allergy. 2017;47(4):457–66. https://doi.org/10.1111/cea.12878.
19. Lau A, Lester S, Moraitis S, Ou J, Psaltis AJ, McColl S, et al. Tertiary lymphoid organs in recalcitrant chronic rhinosinusitis. J Allergy Clin Immunol. 2017;139(4):1371. https://doi.org/10.1016/j.jaci.2016.08.052.
20. Gevaert P, Holtappels G, Johansson SG, Cuvelier C, Cauwenberge P, Bachert C. Organization of secondary lymphoid tissue and local IgE formation to Staphylococcus aureus enterotoxins in nasal polyp tissue. Allergy. 2005;60(1):71–9. https://doi.org/10.1111/j.1398-9995.2004.00621.x.
21. Sautès-Fridman C, Petitprez F, Calderaro J. Tertiary lymphoid structures in the era of cancer immunotherapy. Nat Rev Cancer. 2019;19(6):307–25. https://doi.org/10.1038/s41568-019-0144-6.
22. Hulse KE, Norton JE, Suh L, Zhong Q, Mahdavinia M, Simon P, et al. Chronic rhinosinusitis with nasal polyps is characterized by B-cell inflammation and EBV-induced protein 2 expression. J Allergy Clin Immunol 2013;131(4):1075–1083, 83.e1–7. doi:https://doi.org/10.1016/j.jaci.2013.01.043
23. Tan BK, Peters AT, Schleimer RP, Hulse KE. Pathogenic and protective roles of B cells and antibodies in patients with chronic rhinosinusitis. J Allergy Clin Immunol. 2018;141(5):1553. https://doi.org/10.1016/j.jaci.2018.03.002.
24. Hulse KE. Immune mechanisms of chronic rhinosinusitis. Curr Allergy Asthma Rep. 2016;16(1):1. https://doi.org/10.1007/s11882-015-0579-0.
25. Min J-Y, Hulse KE, Tan BK. B-cells and antibody-mediated pathogenesis in chronic rhinosinusitis with nasal polyps. In: Rhinosinusitis with nasal polyposis, vol. 79. Basel: Karger; 2016. p. 48–57.
26. Kato APA, Suh L, Carter R, Harris KE, Chandra R, et al. Evidence of a role for B cell-activating factor of the TNF family in the pathogenesis of chronic rhinosinusitis with nasal polyps. J Allergy Clin Immunol. 2008;121:1385–92.
27. Yoon YH, Jin J, Kwon KR, Kim SH, Rha KS, Kim YM. The role of B cell Activating Factor (BAFF) expression on pathogenesis of nasal polyp in chronic rhinosinusitis with nasal polyposis. Rhinology. 2014;52(4):390–6. https://doi.org/10.4193/Rhin13.154.
28. Kato A, Xiao H, Chustz RT, Liu MC, Schleimer RP. Local release of B cell-activating factor of the TNF family after segmental allergen challenge of allergic subjects. J Allergy Clin Immunol. 2009;123(2):369. https://doi.org/10.1016/j.jaci.2008.11.022.
29. Polverino F, Baraldo S, Bazzan E, Agostini S, Turato G, Lunardi F, et al. A novel insight into adaptive immunity in chronic obstructive pulmonary disease: B cell activating factor belonging to the tumor necrosis factor family. Am J Respir Crit Care Med. 2010;182(8):1011. https://doi.org/10.1164/rccm.200911-1700OC.
30. Chu VT, Berek C. The establishment of the plasma cell survival niche in the bone marrow. Immunol Rev. 2013;251(1):177–88.
31. Peters AT, Kato A, Zhang N, Conley DB, Suh L, Tancowny B, et al. Evidence for altered activity of the IL-6 pathway in chronic rhinosinusitis with nasal polyps. J Allergy Clin Immunol. 2010;125(2):397–403.e10.
32. Stevens WW, Ocampo CJ, Berdnikovs S, Sakashita M, Mahdavinia M, Suh L, et al. Cytokines in chronic rhinosinusitis. Role in eosinophilia and aspirin-exacerbated respiratory disease. Am J Respir Crit Care Med. 2015;192(6):682–94. https://doi.org/10.1164/rccm.201412-2278OC.
33. Cocks BG, de Waal Malefyt R, Galizzi JP, de Vries JE, Aversa G. IL-13 induces proliferation and differentiation of human B cells activated by the CD40 ligand. Int Immunol. 1993;5:657–63.
34. Gevaert P, Nouri-Aria KT, Wu H, Harper CE, Takhar P, Fear DJ, et al. Local receptor revision and class switching to IgE in chronic rhinosinusitis with nasal polyps. Allergy. 2013;68(1):55–63. https://doi.org/10.1111/all.12054.

35. Tan BKLQ, Suh L, Kato A, Conley DB, Chandra RK, et al. Evidence for intranasal antinuclear autoantibodies in patients with chronic rhinosinusitis with nasal polyps. J Allergy Clin Immunol. 2011;128:1198–206.
36. Jeffe JS, Seshadri S, Hamill KJ, Huang JH, Carter R, Suh L, et al. A role for anti-BP180 autoantibodies in chronic rhinosinusitis. Laryngoscope. 2013;123(9):2104–11. https://doi.org/10.1002/lary.24016.
37. De Schryver E, Calus L, Bonte H, Natalie DR, Gould H, Donovan E, et al. The quest for autoreactive antibodies in nasal polyps. J Allergy Clin Immunol. 2016;138(3):893–5.e5. https://doi.org/10.1016/j.jaci.2016.03.040.
38. Tsybikov NN, Egorova EV, Kuznik BI, Fefelova EV, Magen E. Anticytokine autoantibodies in chronic rhinosinusitis. Allergy Asthma Proc. 2015;36(6):473–80.
39. Bachert CZN, Holtappels G, De Lobel L, van Cauwenberge P, Liu S, Lin P, Bousquet J, Van Steen K. Presence of IL-5 protein and IgE antibodies to staphylococcal enterotoxins in nasal polyps is associated with comorbid asthma. J Allergy Clin Immunol. 2010;126(5):962–8.
40. Chen JBJL, Davies AM, Wu YB, Rimmer J, Lund VJ, et al. Antibodies and superantibodies in patients with chronic rhinosinusitis with nasal polyps. J Allergy Clin Immunol. 2017;139:1195–204.
41. Van Zele T, Gevaert P, Watelet J-B, Claeys G, Holtappels G, Claeys C, et al. Staphylococcus aureus colonization and IgE antibody formation to enterotoxins is increased in nasal polyposis. J Allergy Clin Immunol. 2004;114(4):981. https://doi.org/10.1016/j.jaci.2004.07.013.

8 Eosinophils

Elien Gevaert

Key Points

- Eosinophilia is an indicator of severe CRS with a high chance of recurrence.
- Caucasian nasal polyps are mostly associated with eosinophilia, but the rate of eosinophilic nasal polyp is increasing in Asia.
- Eosinophils use different mechanisms to attack and kill bacteria in CRS, but can also have immunomodulatory functions.
- Glucocorticoids and novel biologics directly target eosinophils in a very effective way.

8.1 Clinical Manifestations and Diagnosis of Eosinophilic CRS

Eosinophilic CRS patients represent a subtype of CRS that is typically characterized by symptoms such as loss of smell, thick mucus production, secondary bacterial infections, long-term nasal congestion, and a poor treatment response [1, 2]. From clinical point of view CRS is nowadays subdivided by CRS with nasal polyps (CRSwNP) and CRS without nasal polyps (CRSsNP). In the Caucasian population, a minority of the CRSsNP patients has tissue eosinophilia, but the majority of the CRSwNP patients (about 80%) are characterized by tissue eosinophilia. This is substantially higher than the percentage of CRSwNP patients in Asian populations, where percentages with tissue eosinophilia range from 20 to 60%. However, the percentage of type 2 signature disease in patients with CRS is dramatically increased over the last 20 years, implying an ongoing "eosinophilic shift" in several Asian countries. To determine the role of the different environmental and/or lifestyle factors in the observed eosinophilic shift will require additional research [3, 4].

While Chinese patients have in general a more moderated degree of eosinophilia than Caucasian patients, higher recurrence rates and appearance of comorbid asthma is associated with eosinophilia in both populations. Other studies have linked eosinophilia with more extensive sinus disease and higher post-operative symptom scores [5, 6]. In addition, tissue eosinophil counts are found directly associated with loss of olfactory function in CRSwNP, independent of disease severity [7]. In general, the manifestation of eosinophils is troublesome for the course of the disease with multiple studies indicating it as a risk factor for disease recurrence hampering the improvement in both general and disease-specific quality of life of the patient [5–9]. These features imply that eosinophils are either biomarkers of the disease or the key responsible in driving the disease.

E. Gevaert (✉)
Upper Airways Research Laboratory and Department of Oto-Rhino-Laryngology, Ghent University, Ghent, Belgium
e-mail: elien.gevaert@ugent.be

L. Zhang, C. Bachert (eds.), *Chronic Rhinosinusitis*, https://doi.org/10.1007/978-981-16-0784-4_8

Some studies have reported that blood eosinophilia is correlated with their infiltration in the polyps and the severity of paranasal cavity computed tomography (CT) findings of CRSwNP patients [6, 8–11]. These studies suggest that blood eosinophil counts or determination of eosinophilic specific markers (like ECP concentrations) in the blood could be a diagnostic maker for eosinophilic CRSwNP. However, it is important to realize that this approach rather indicates an ongoing type 2-driven disease, such as asthma and allergy, and might therefore not unambiguously identify eosinophilic CRS. This is in contrast to the identification of tissue eosinophilia which can be diagnosed by histopathology (Fig. 8.1) or via quantification of eosinophilic proteins like eosinophilic cationic protein (ECP) or Major Basic Protein (MBP) in the tissue. However, there is a lack of clear guidelines and cut-off values to discriminate between eosinophilic and non-eosinophilic CRSwNP. For diagnostic purposes and the introduction of precision medicine in CRS, there is a clear need for validated and continent/country- specific eosinophil related biomarkers in the future [12].

Several environmental stimuli have been proposed to play a role in the pathophysiology and the recruitment of eosinophils in CRS. Eosinophils have been recognized as a central feature in the response to infection with large and multicellular parasites like helminths.

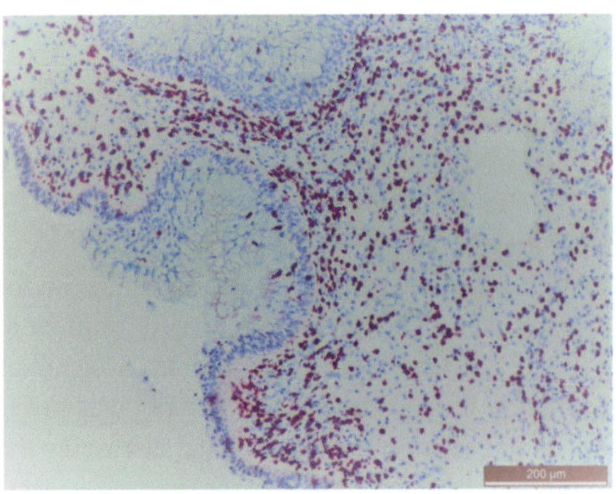

Fig. 8.1 Immunohistochemistry stain for MBP (pink) and DNA (purple) in nasal polyps

Along these lines, the fungal hypothesis, implying a prominent role for fungi or at least fungal allergens at the basis of eosinophilic CRS pathology, was proposed. Some groups observed the intranasal presence of fungi along with eosinophil and eosinophil-degraded products and mucus [13, 14]. Further evidence in favor of this hypothesis was provided by experiments showing that nasal mucus or tissue from patients could trigger eosinophil migration, that blood mononuclear cells of CRS patients responded to fungal antigens with increased IL-5 and IL13-production in vitro, and the observation that *Alternaria* fungi are able induce eosinophil degranulation via activation of the protease-activated receptor (PAR) [15–17]. However, others reported the absence of hyper-responsiveness to fungal antigens in CRS and topical antifungal treatment failed to show any efficacy in a clinical trial setting [18–21]. Despite the fact that the fungal hypothesis is potentially valid in some specific patients, it is rather controversial and doubtful that it is a the base of eosinophilic CRS pathology.

Another hypothesis points to *S. aureus* and its produced toxins. Colonization of the nasal mucosa with *S. aureus* is far more prominent in CRSwNP patients than in healthy controls with reported frequencies up to 90% of the patients. Staphylococcal super antigens can directly drive a type2 inflammatory response with eosinophilic inflammation as a consequence [22–24]. In addition, it was shown that exposure of nasal epithelium to *S. aureus* can induce eosinophil migration and that *S. aureus* can activate specific defense mechanisms in eosinophils as discussed below [25]. Staphylococcal super antigens can also act as allergens, demonstrated by the finding of functional IgE antibodies directed against *S. aureus* antigens in the nasal polyp tissue tissue [26, 27]. Bacterial infections are prominent in eosinophilic CRS patients, and it is clear that other factors like (innate/temporary) defects in the immune barriers, possibly cause by eosinophils, could further contribute to the pathophysiology as it could make patients more susceptible to infection in general.

8.2 Eosinophil Development, Chemotaxis, and Activation in CRS

In 1879, Paul Ehrlich was the first to describe the existence of eosinophils as "cells with granules having an affinity for eosin and other acid dyes." Eosinophil-like cells are found in all vertebrates and are thus highly evolutionary conserved. For this reason, eosinophils must be more than troublemakers and are likely to play crucial, and possibly yet unidentified role in important processes. They originate from CD34+ hematopoietic stem cells in the bone marrow and develop from a common myeloid progenitor to an eosinophil lineage-committed progenitor. The latter exclusively gives rise to eosinophils and IL-3, IL-5 and Granulocyte Macrophage colony-stimulating factor (GM-CSF) are particularly important in regulating eosinophil development, differentiation, and maturation [28–30]. However, the crucial factors seems to be IL-5, a it was found necessary and sufficient for the development of eosinophilia [31]. Other cytokines including IL-3 and GM-CSF synergize with IL-5 in this process [32–34]. In humans, IL-5 receptor expression is unique to eosinophils and basophils, which enables IL5 to work very specifically on those cells to promote maturation, activation, and survival [35, 36]. Once eosinophils have entered the blood, also mediated by IL-5, they have a short half-life, ranging from 8 to 18 h [35].

After circulating in the blood, eosinophils migrate into the nasal mucosa, which is a process mediated by the synergistic influence of cellular adhesion and chemotaxis. Eosinophil adhesion to the endothelium in a type 2 inflammatory context is mediated by VCAM1 and P-selectin in polyp tissue [37, 38]. The type 2 cytokines IL-4 and IL-13 seem of crucial importance for induction of these proteins [39]. Proof for the role of other adhesion molecules in the specific recruitment of eosinophils like L-selectin, MadCAM1, and I-CAM in CRS is rather implicit [40, 41].

The chemotaxis of eosinophils into the tissue is mainly mediated by ligands of the C-C chemokine receptor 3 (CCR3). The importance of this receptor was demonstrated by a study showing that polyp tissue fluid exhibited strong chemotactic activity for eosinophils that was significantly inhibited by blocking CCR3 [42]. While many endogenous ligands are identified for this receptor, eotaxin 1–3, RANTES, monocyte-chemotactic protein (MCP) 1–4 are of particular interest for directing eosinophil chemotaxis. In nasal polyps, eotaxin 1–2, MCP-1, MCP-4, and RANTES levels were found significantly increased [42–46]. A crucial role in guiding eosinophil chemotaxis is attributed to the epithelium, as it is the main source of many of these factors. This role of the epithelium in the chemotaxis is further illustrated by the subepithelial localization of eosinophil often observed in polyps [25, 47]. A link between *S. aureus* colonization and eosinophil accumulation has been proposed. Indeed, *S. aureus* and its super antigen SEB can induce eosinophil migration by inducing eotaxin 1–3 expression. In addition SEB can also induce RANTES and MCP-1 in epithelial cells [42, 48]. However, in nasal polyps it appears that eotaxin, rather than RANTES, in cooperation with IL-5, plays a key role in chemoattraction and activation of eosinophils in NP tissue [49].

Many other factors like complement factors C5a and C3a, platelet-activating factor (PAF), eicosanoids like the CysLTs, SCF, and IL33 might contribute to the chemotaxis, priming, and activation of eosinophils in the nasal polyps [43, 50]. In addition, to their role in eosinophil development, IL-5 and GM-CSF also play a crucial role in eosinophil priming, maturation, and increasing their survival in the tissue. As a consequence, the life span of eosinophils is extended and ranges from 2 to 5 days once migrated in the tissue [51]. *S. aureus* also contributes to the prolonged survival as supernatant of SEB treated epithelial cells was shown to increase eosinophil survival in vitro [44]. Another factor contributing to increased eosinophil survival could be an impairment of NK cell-mediated eosinophil apoptosis in chronic rhinosinusitis likely attributed to deregulated prostaglandin D2 production [52].

It was hypothesized that initial eosinophil recruitment occurs in response to the release of one or more small molecule mediators of inflammation (e.g. DAMPs) due to localized bursts of cell death. The tissue immune microenvironment would subsequently determine the downstream immune consequences mediated by eosinophil effector functions. As a consequence, this would lead to exacerbations of local immune responses (Type 2 -Polarized Microenvironment), suppression of these site-specific immune responses (Type 1/Type 17-Polarized Microenvironment), or essentially little to no modulations of local immune responses (Immune-Neutral Microenvironment). As a consequence, the immune microenvironment present upon eosinophil recruitment would be key as to direct the predominance of specific eosinophil activities and would define the final functional roles of eosinophils. From this perspective the released mediators, action and consequences of eosinophils would be highly dependent on the environment [53]. Additionally the existence of innate eosinophil heterogeneity and tissue resident, immune-regulatory eosinophils have been proposed but more research is required in humans, and to date it is unclear as to what extend this is relevant in CRS [54].

8.3 Functions of Eosinophils in CRS

8.3.1 Effector Functions

A key role for eosinophils in the development of nasal polyps has been proposed by a study on early-phase polyps showing subepithelial presence of eosinophils at the upper surface of the early polyp outgrowth. The polyp formation was associated with the deposition of fibronectin, albumin (pointing to a vascular leak), and extracellular matrix protein and the process was found to correlate to IL-5 and eotaxin-2 tissue levels. This study pointed to a possible central role for eosinophils in polyp formation in the very early stages [51]. Apart from their possible key role in polyp development, eosinophils are also known to play multiple roles in the chronic and established polyps. As described in the previous part, eosinophils accumulate rapidly in polyps where they are primed, activated, synthesize and release lipid mediators, enzymes and proteins that can exert a wide variety of actions.

Eosinophil are characterized by the bilobed nucleus and the cytoplasmic storage of granules (Fig. 8.2). These granules store and secrete cationic proteins and an array of cytokines and chemokines. Eosinophilic granules are not simply storage depots of preformed proteins. It is well-established that differential release of cytokines occurs in response to specific stimuli. Eosinophils can secrete mediators via de novo synthesis following the classical pathway of secretion or can secrete their preformed granule content by exocytosis (or “degranulation”), piecemeal degranulation or cytolysis. In nasal polyps, it was found that 30.7% of the eosinophils seems inactive, 27.5% of the eosinophils undergo cytolysis, and 41.7% of the eosinophils undergo piecemeal degranulation [55, 56].

The most reported role of eosinophils in polyps is associated with the degranulation and release of the highly basic and cytotoxic granule proteins such as ECP, MBP, and eosinophil-derived neurotoxin (EDN) that are released during degranulation or cytolysis. While they play an

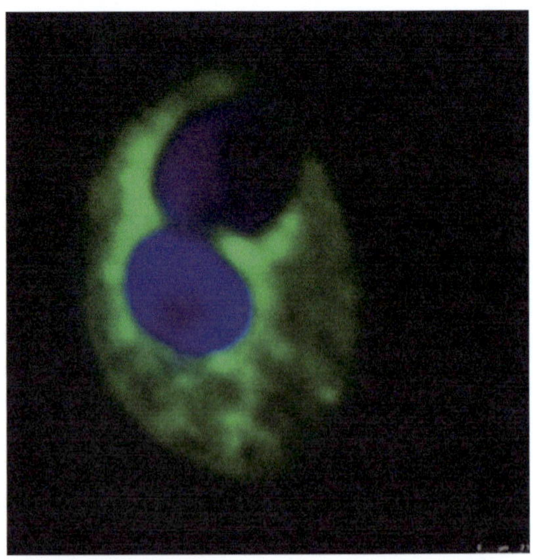

Fig. 8.2 Eosinophil in CRSwNP. Immunofluorescent stain for MBP (green) and DAPI (blue) shows the characteristic bilobed nucleus and granular cytoplasmatic structures

important role in innate immune defense and pathogen elimination, they can be very harmful to the host when they are excessively released. In mucus and CRSwNP tissue the deposition of MBP is described and found associated with epithelial damage [51, 57]. Major basic protein is toxic and causes erosion of the epithelium at concentrations less than 10 μg/ml. Because concentrations of MBP are merely exceeding this concentration in the mucus, it was suggested that epithelial damage might arise from the mucus, rather than the tissue [51]. ECP is a cytotoxic ribonuclease and often used as a marker of eosinophil activity and to monitor disease progression. Interestingly, ECP is dependent on its RNAse activity to exert neurotoxic and antiviral actions, while their antibacterial and antihelminthic effects are independent of this activity. Another RNAse and powerful neurotoxin is EDN. This protein can promote an allergic reaction via dendritic cell activation and it may play an important role in allergic disease [58]. One study showed that EDN enhances airway remodeling in chronic rhinosinusitis and correlates with disease severity [59]. However, only few studies have shown a clear association between EDN and CRSwNP. Beside their well-known antibacterial properties, additional functionalities have been attributed to these eosinophilic proteins. For example, eosinophilic granule proteins such as ECP and EDN have been shown to suppress T cell proliferation in vitro [60]. The toxicity of MBP was shown to be regulated by crystallization and to stimulate histamine and leukotriene C4 release from basophils and to activate mast cells [61]. How and if these mechanism are also important in the pathophysiology of CRS is unclear.

Eosinophils are also an important source of lipid mediators. Nasal polyp tissue-derived eosinophils were shown to possess a specific phenotype with a dysregulated fatty acid metabolism [62]. In addition eicosanoid metabolism is found increased and correlated with ECP and IL5 in CRS [63]. In CRS, eosinophils are an important source of 5-LO and LTC4 synthase. Especially in patients with aspirin hypersensitivity this could play a role where the 5-lipoxygenase pathway is found activated [64].

8.3.2 Extracellular Trap Formation and Charcot–Leyden Crystal Deposition

In addition to degranulation, eosinophils contribute to antibacterial defense by the formation of the so-called eosinophilic extracellular traps (EETs). These extracellular traps can be generated by both viable eosinophils and by eosinophils undergoing extracellular formation associated cell death (EETosis) [65, 66]. While both viable EET formation and EETosis are regulated via different pathways, they are both dependent on NADPH activity and ROS production. In vitro, EET formation is evoked by a sequence of stimuli like adhesion molecules, IL-5, and interferon (IFN)-γ, complement factor 5a (C5a), LPS, TSLP, and eotaxin [65, 67]. While the exact pathways of EET formation are unknown, it is clear that EETs can bind and kill bacteria like *S. aureus*, *S. epidermidis*, and *E. coli*. In vitro, eosinophils generate EETs immediately after co-culture with *S. aureus* and without additional stimuli, while EET formation evoked with S. epidermidis required priming with TSLP [27, 67]. It seems that a different additional stimulus (like IL5, C5a, TSLP) is needed to cause EET formation, depending on the type of bacteria [15, 59]. Caucasian CRSwNP patients have elevated, IL-5, eotaxin, IL-33, and TSLP levels; and a consistent colonization with *S. aureus*. Interestingly, these are all possible triggers for EET formation.

A study in Caucasian CRSwNP patients showed that eosinophils are specifically recruited to sites of epithelial damage and form EETs to protect the host from infections with *S. aureus* and possibly other microorganisms [25]. Another study reported EETs in secretions of eosinophilic CRS patients contributing to the increased viscosity of the secretions [68]. Chinese patients with CRSwNP of the type 2 endotype (IL5+ polyps) displayed similar patterns with subepithelial recruitment of eosinophils and EET formation. In addition, EETs correlated positively with the presence of S aureus, but not with Pseudomonas aeruginosa, pan-fungi or Escherichia coli colonization pointing to a prominent role of *S. aureus*

[4]. These results show that the same mechanisms play a role in patients with CRSwNP with a dominant TH2 profile. Later, EETs were found associated with disease severity regardless of polyp status in Asian patients [64].

Beside their role in antibacterial defense, EETs can contribute to the properties of highly viscous eosinophilic mucin and impair its clearance in CRS patients. In addition, EETs can contain intact granules. These granules can cause long-lasting inflammation but could also have immune-regulatory roles [69]. Recently, the process of EETosis was linked to the formation of Charcot–Leyden crystals (CLCs) [70, 71]. CLCs are composed of galectin-10, a major auto-crystallizing granule protein of human eosinophils. CLCs were abundantly found in CRSwNP patient mucosa and mucus and have also been found frequently in the tenacious eosinophil-rich mucus of allergic fungal sinusitis patients [72]. In vivo, crystallization of endogenous proteins is often associated with pathological conditions that trigger an inflammatory response. In nasal polyp tissue, it was shown that CLCs, as a result of EETosis, cause a pro-inflammatory response, a secondary neutrophilic inflammation and NETosis [73]. Via various ways (e.g. intact granules or CLCs), eosinophils may thus possess ways to have post-postmortem impacts on innate immunity, local immune response, sterile inflammation, and tissue damage. An overview of the most important mechanisms and effector functions is depicted in Fig. 8.3.

8.3.3 Other Roles of Eosinophils

In addition to their granule proteins, eosinophils produce a remarkable number of pro-inflammatory cytokines and chemokines. The mediators can have pro-inflammatory (e.g. TNFα), anti-inflammatory (e.g. IL-10), tissue remodeling (e.g. TGFβ) or immunomodulatory effects (e.g. IL-4). In addition, they might damage epithelial cells, stimulate epithelial-to-mesenchymal transition, activate or suppress sensory nerves, modulate the activity of stem cells and plasma cells, and alter the mechanical response of airways [67, 68].

Eosinophilic indoleamine 2, 3 dioxygenase (IFNϒ inducible enzyme) was shown to act on the production of kynurenines (KYN) which is reported to induce apoptosis and inhibition of proliferation mainly of Type 1 cells, actively causing a Type 2 bias [74]. Eosinophils can also sustain their own survival and recruitment via the autocrine production of IL5, eotaxin, and GM-CSF. In addition, eosinophils were found to serve as antigen presenting cells in allergic upper airway disease and to express MHCII, costimulatory molecules, and to traffic to regional lymph nodes [75]. However, it is unknown as to what extend these effects are relevant in CRS patients. As previously described, the exact role of the eosinophil and the mediators released are likely dependent on the microenvironment and the specific context of the CRS endotype.

8.4 Treatment Considerations

Eosinophils are implicated in the pathogeneses of a large fraction of the CRSwNP patients. For these patients, the induction of their apoptosis and efficient clearance is crucial in the resolution of inflammation. Treatment with doxycycline can significantly reduce the polyp size and the level ECP in nasal secretions of CRSwNP patients [76]. In contrast to neutrophils, eosinophils are also an important target of glucocorticoids. Glucocorticoids can decrease eosinophilia in multiple ways. For example, they interfere with the recruitment by inhibiting expression for VCAM1, eotaxin, eotaxin-2, and MCP-4 [42]. Further, glucocorticoids can interfere with eosinophil adhesion, chemotaxis, activation and induce apoptosis [77].

Despite the multiple effects of steroid on eosinophils, current FDA approved treatment of intranasal steroids does not provide significant relief for many patients. For these patients monoclonal antibodies bring hope for an exciting new treatment option. In CRSwNP IL-5 is a key cytokine with a possible autocrine role for this cytokine in the activation of eosinophils, and a strong correlation with eosinophilic cationic protein (ECP). The key role of IL-5 was supported by the finding that treatment of eosin-

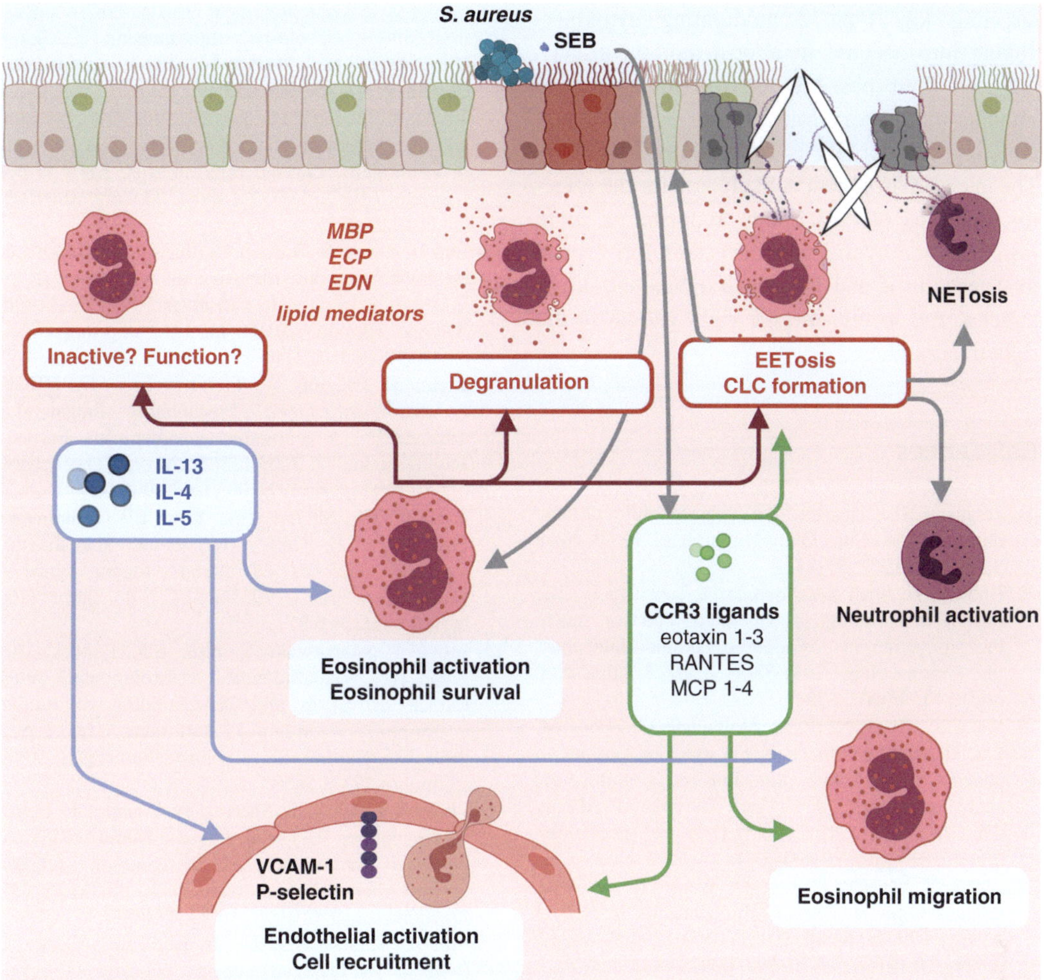

Fig. 8.3 Eosinophil chemotaxis, activation and effector functions in CRS

ophil-infiltrated polyp tissue with neutralizing anti-IL-5 monoclonal antibody, but not anti-IL-3 or anti-GM-CSF antibodies in vitro, resulted in eosinophil apoptosis and decreased tissue eosinophilia [49]. The monoclonal antibodies targetting IL5 signaling including reslizumab and mepolizumab (both anti IL-5), and benralizumab (anti IL-5Rα) directly target IL-5 in the pathophysiology of nasal polyposis (NP). Antibodies against IL5 or IL4/IL13 recepter alpha chain were shown to reduce eosinophils and shrink polyps, supporting a role of eosinophils in the pathogenesis [75, 76]. These drugs also restore olfactory function supporting the hypothesis that eosinophils mediate anosmia. Recently the FDA approved Dupilumab for the treatment of CRSwNP. Blocking IL4 and IL13 simultaneously affects a broad range of type 2 effector cells and affect eosinophil recruitment, chemotaxis and activation far upstream. These effects are likely to account for their great success.

8.5 Translation into Future Daily Practice

Eosinophilia is a key factor in Caucasian CRSwNP patients, but to date, it is not entirely clear if they are the main cause or rather a marker of the disease. While many reports point to a key role of these cells in the pathogenesis, targeting solely eosinophils seems less effective that targeting key type 2 modulating cytokines. Taking into account their post-mortem effects, but also their possible anti-inflammatory and immune-modulatory role it is a possibility that targeting eosinophils is not always beneficial. The microenvironment is likely key for the effector functions of eosinophils and gaining more insight by endotyping patients is therefore crucial to determine if and how eosinophils should be targeted and to allocate the right patient to the right treatment.

References

1. Ferguson BJ. Categorization of eosinophilic chronic rhinosinusitis. Curr Opin Otolaryngol Head Neck Surg. 2004;12(3):237–42.
2. Ishinaga H, Shah SA, Sakaida H, Takeuchi K. The role of transforming growth factor-alpha on mucin overproduction in eosinophilic chronic rhinosinusitis. Pharmacology. 2011;88(5–6):302–8. https://doi.org/10.1159/000333794.
3. Wang X, Zhang N, Bo M, Holtappels G, Zheng M, Lou H, et al. Diversity of TH cytokine profiles in patients with chronic rhinosinusitis: a multicenter study in Europe, Asia, and Oceania. J Allergy Clin Immunol. 2016;138(5):1344–53. https://doi.org/10.1016/j.jaci.2016.05.041.
4. Zhang Y, Gevaert E, Lou H, Wang X, Zhang L, Bachert C, et al. Chronic rhinosinusitis in Asia. J Allergy Clin Immunol. 2017;140(5):1230–9. https://doi.org/10.1016/j.jaci.2017.09.009.
5. Kountakis SE, Arango P, Bradley D, Wade ZK, Borish L. Molecular and cellular staging for the severity of chronic rhinosinusitis. Laryngoscope. 2004;114(11):1895–905. https://doi.org/10.1097/01.mlg.0000147917.43615.c0.
6. Szucs E, Ravandi S, Goossens A, Beel M, Clement PA. Eosinophilia in the ethmoid mucosa and its relationship to the severity of inflammation in chronic rhinosinusitis. Am J Rhinol. 2002;16(3):131–4.
7. Hauser LJ, Chandra RK, Li P, Turner JH. Role of tissue eosinophils in chronic rhinosinusitis-associated olfactory loss. Int Forum Allergy Rhinol. 2017;7(10):957–62. https://doi.org/10.1002/alr.21994.
8. Ishitoya J, Sakuma Y, Tsukuda M. Eosinophilic chronic rhinosinusitis in Japan. Allergol Int. 2010;59(3):239–45. https://doi.org/10.2332/allergolint.10-RAI-0231.
9. Sakuma Y, Ishitoya J, Komatsu M, Shiono O, Hirama M, Yamashita Y, et al. New clinical diagnostic criteria for eosinophilic chronic rhinosinusitis. Auris Nasus Larynx. 2011;38(5):583–8. https://doi.org/10.1016/j.anl.2011.01.007.
10. Ponikau JU, Sherris DA, Kephart GM, Kern EB, Congdon DJ, Adolphson CR, et al. Striking deposition of toxic eosinophil major basic protein in mucus: implications for chronic rhinosinusitis. J Allergy Clin Immunol. 2005;116(2):362–9. https://doi.org/10.1016/j.jaci.2005.03.049.
11. Takeda K, Takeno S, Hirakawa K, Ishino T. Expression and distribution of glucocorticoid receptor isoforms in eosinophilic chronic rhinosinusitis. Auris Nasus Larynx. 2010;37(6):700–7. https://doi.org/10.1016/j.anl.2010.03.005.
12. Lou H, Zhang N, Bachert C, Zhang L. Highlights of eosinophilic chronic rhinosinusitis with nasal polyps in definition, prognosis, and advancement. Int Forum Allergy Rhinol. 2018;8(11):1218–25. https://doi.org/10.1002/alr.22214.
13. Braun H, Buzina W, Freudenschuss K, Beham A, Stammberger H. 'Eosinophilic fungal rhinosinusitis': a common disorder in Europe? Laryngoscope. 2003;113(2):264–9. https://doi.org/10.1097/00005537-200302000-00013.
14. Ponikau JU, Sherris DA, Kern EB, Homburger HA, Frigas E, Gaffey TA, et al. The diagnosis and incidence of allergic fungal sinusitis. Mayo Clin Proc. 1999;74(9):877–84. https://doi.org/10.4065/74.9.877.
15. Inoue Y, Matsuwaki Y, Shin SH, Ponikau JU, Kita H. Nonpathogenic, environmental fungi induce activation and degranulation of human eosinophils. J Immunol (Baltimore, Md: 1950). 2005;175(8):5439–47. https://doi.org/10.4049/jimmunol.175.8.5439.
16. Shin SH, Ponikau JU, Sherris DA, Congdon D, Frigas E, Homburger HA, et al. Chronic rhinosinusitis: an enhanced immune response to ubiquitous airborne fungi. J Allergy Clin Immunol. 2004;114(6):1369–75. https://doi.org/10.1016/j.jaci.2004.08.012.
17. Wei JL, Kita H, Sherris DA, Kern EB, Weaver A, Ponikau JU. The chemotactic behavior of eosinophils in patients with chronic rhinosinusitis. Laryngoscope. 2003;113(2):303–6. https://doi.org/10.1097/00005537-200302000-00019.
18. Douglas R, Bruhn M, Tan LW, Ooi E, Psaltis A, Wormald PJ. Response of peripheral blood lymphocytes to fungal extracts and staphylococcal superantigen B in chronic rhinosinusitis. Laryngoscope. 2007;117(3):411–4. https://doi.org/10.1097/MLG.0b013e31802c0707.
19. Ebbens FA, Scadding GK, Badia L, Hellings PW, Jorissen M, Mullol J, et al. Amphotericin B nasal lavages: not a solution for patients with chronic rhinosinusitis. J Allergy Clin Immunol. 2006;118(5):1149–56. https://doi.org/10.1016/j.jaci.2006.07.058.
20. Isaacs S, Fakhri S, Luong A, Citardi MJ. A meta-analysis of topical amphotericin B for the treatment of chronic rhinosinusitis. Int Forum Allergy Rhinol. 2011;1(4):250–4. https://doi.org/10.1002/alr.20056.
21. Orlandi RR, Marple BF, Georgelas A, Durtschi D, Barr L. Immunologic response to fungus is not universally associated with rhinosinusitis. Otolaryngol Head Neck Surg. 2009;141(6):750–6.e1–2. https://doi.org/10.1016/j.otohns.2009.09.016.

22. Bachert C, Gevaert P, van Cauwenberge P. Staphylococcus aureus superantigens and airway disease. Curr Allergy Asthma Rep. 2002;2(3):252–8.
23. Bachert C, van Zele T, Gevaert P, De Schrijver L, Van Cauwenberge P. Superantigens and nasal polyps. Curr Allergy Asthma Rep. 2003;3(6):523–31.
24. Bernstein JM, Ballow M, Schlievert PM, Rich G, Allen C, Dryja D. A superantigen hypothesis for the pathogenesis of chronic hyperplastic sinusitis with massive nasal polyposis. Am J Rhinol. 2003;17(6):321–6.
25. Gevaert E, Zhang N, Krysko O, Lan F, Holtappels G, De Ruyck N, et al. Extracellular eosinophilic traps in association with Staphylococcus aureus at the site of epithelial barrier defects in patients with severe airway inflammation. J Allergy Clin Immunol. 2017;139(6):1849–60 e6. https://doi.org/10.1016/j.jaci.2017.01.019.
26. Van Zele T, Gevaert P, Watelet J-B, Claeys G, Holtappels G, Claeys C, et al. Staphylococcus aureus colonization and IgE antibody formation to enterotoxins is increased in nasal polyposis. J Allergy Clin Immunol. 2004;114(4):981. https://doi.org/10.1016/j.jaci.2004.07.013.
27. Perez-Novo CA, Kowalski ML, Kuna P, Ptasinska A, Holtappels G, van Cauwenberge P, et al. Aspirin sensitivity and IgE antibodies to Staphylococcus aureus enterotoxins in nasal polyposis: studies on the relationship. Int Arch Allergy Immunol. 2004;133(3):255–60. https://doi.org/10.1159/000076832.
28. Mori Y, Iwasaki H, Kohno K, Yoshimoto G, Kikushige Y, Okeda A, et al. Identification of the human eosinophil lineage-committed progenitor: revision of phenotypic definition of the human common myeloid progenitor. J Exp Med. 2009;206(1):183–93. https://doi.org/10.1084/jem.20081756.
29. Iwasaki H, Mizuno S, Mayfield R, Shigematsu H, Arinobu Y, Seed B, et al. Identification of eosinophil lineage-committed progenitors in the murine bone marrow. J Exp Med. 2005;201(12):1891–7. https://doi.org/10.1084/jem.20050548.
30. Lopez AF, Begley CG, Williamson DJ, Warren DJ, Vadas MA, Sanderson CJ. Murine eosinophil differentiation factor. An eosinophil-specific colony-stimulating factor with activity for human cells. J Exp Med. 1986;163(5):1085–99. https://doi.org/10.1084/jem.163.5.1085.
31. Sanderson CJ. Eosinophil differentiation factor (interleukin-5). Immunol Ser. 1990;49:231–56.
32. Clutterbuck E, Shields JG, Gordon J, Smith SH, Boyd A, Callard RE, et al. Recombinant human interleukin 5 is an eosinophil differentiation factor but has no activity in standard human B cell growth factor assays. Eur J Immunol. 1987;17(12):1743–50. https://doi.org/10.1002/eji.1830171210.
33. Clutterbuck EJ, Hirst EM, Sanderson CJ. Human interleukin-5 (IL-5) regulates the production of eosinophils in human bone marrow cultures: comparison and interaction with IL-1, IL-3, IL-6, and GMCSF. Blood. 1989;73(6):1504–12.
34. Clutterbuck EJ, Sanderson CJ. Regulation of human eosinophil precursor production by cytokines: a comparison of recombinant human interleukin-1 (rhIL-1), rhIL-3, rhIL-5, rhIL-6, and rh granulocyte-macrophage colony-stimulating factor. Blood. 1990;75(9):1774–9.
35. Hirai K, Yamaguchi M, Misaki Y, Takaishi T, Ohta K, Morita Y, et al. Enhancement of human basophil histamine release by interleukin 5. J Exp Med. 1990;172(5):1525–8. https://doi.org/10.1084/jem.172.5.1525.
36. Resnick MB, Weller PF. Mechanisms of eosinophil recruitment. Am J Respir Cell Mol Biol. 1993;8(4):349–55. https://doi.org/10.1165/ajrcmb/8.4.349.
37. Symon FA, Walsh GM, Watson SR, Wardlaw AJ. Eosinophil adhesion to nasal polyp endothelium is P-selectin-dependent. J Exp Med. 1994;180(1):371–6. https://doi.org/10.1084/jem.180.1.371.
38. Jahnsen FL, Haraldsen G, Aanesen JP, Haye R, Brandtzaeg P. Eosinophil infiltration is related to increased expression of vascular cell adhesion molecule-1 in nasal polyps. Am J Respir Cell Mol Biol. 1995;12(6):624–32. https://doi.org/10.1165/ajrcmb.12.6.7539273.
39. Bachert C, Gevaert P, Holtappels G, van Cauwenberge P. Mediators in nasal polyposis. Curr Allergy Asthma Rep. 2002;2(6):481–7.
40. Ebbens FA, Toppila-Salmi SK, Renkonen JA, Renkonen RL, Mullol J, van Drunen CM, et al. Endothelial L-selectin ligand expression in nasal polyps. Allergy. 2010;65(1):95–102. https://doi.org/10.1111/j.1398-9995.2009.01986.x.
41. Demoly P, Sahla M, Campbell AM, Bousquet J, Crampette L. ICAM-1 expression in upper respiratory mucosa is differentially related to eosinophil and neutrophil inflammation according to the allergic status. Clin Exp Allergy. 1998;28(6):731–8. https://doi.org/10.1046/j.1365-2222.1998.00308.x.
42. Jahnsen FL, Haye R, Gran E, Brandtzaeg P, Johansen FE. Glucocorticosteroids inhibit mRNA expression for eotaxin, eotaxin-2, and monocyte-chemotactic protein-4 in human airway inflammation with eosinophilia. J Immunol. 1999;163(3):1545–51.
43. Stevens WW, Ocampo CJ, Berdnikovs S, Sakashita M, Mahdavinia M, Suh L, et al. Cytokines in chronic rhinosinusitis. Role in eosinophilia and aspirin-exacerbated respiratory disease. Am J Respir Crit Care Med. 2015;192(6):682–94. https://doi.org/10.1164/rccm.201412-2278OC.
44. Huvenne W, Callebaut I, Reekmans K, Hens G, Bobic S, Jorissen M, et al. Staphylococcus aureus enterotoxin B augments granulocyte migration and survival via airway epithelial cell activation. Allergy. 2010;65(8):1013–20. https://doi.org/10.1111/j.1398-9995.2009.02313.x.
45. Beck LA, Stellato C, Beall LD, Schall TJ, Leopold D, Bickel CA, et al. Detection of the chemokine

RANTES and endothelial adhesion molecules in nasal polyps. J Allergy Clin Immunol. 1996;98(4):766–80. https://doi.org/10.1016/s0091-6749(96)70126-4.
46. Davidsson A, Danielsen A, Viale G, Olofsson J, Dell'Orto P, Pellegrini C, et al. Positive identification in situ of mRNA expression of IL-6, and IL-12, and the chemotactic cytokine RANTES in patients with chronic sinusitis and polypoid disease. Clinical relevance and relation to allergy. Acta Otolaryngol. 1996;116(4):604–10. https://doi.org/10.3109/00016489609137897.
47. Meyer JE, Bartels J, Gorogh T, Sticherling M, Rudack C, Ross DA, et al. The role of RANTES in nasal polyposis. Am J Rhinol. 2005;19(1):15–20.
48. Gu Z, Jin M, Cao Z. Role of eotaxin-3 in chronic rhinosinusitis with nasal polyps. Otolaryngol Head Neck Surg. 2011;145(2):324–6. https://doi.org/10.1177/0194599811403077.
49. European position paper on rhinosinusitis and nasal polyps. Rhinol Suppl. 2005;18:1–87.
50. Van Roey GA, Vanison CC, Wu J, Huang JH, Suh LA, Carter RG, et al. Classical complement pathway activation in the nasal tissue of patients with chronic rhinosinusitis. J Allergy Clin Immunol. 2017;140(1):89–100.e2. https://doi.org/10.1016/j.jaci.2016.11.015.
51. Simon HU, Yousefi S, Schranz C, Schapowal A, Bachert C, Blaser K. Direct demonstration of delayed eosinophil apoptosis as a mechanism causing tissue eosinophilia. J Immunol (Baltimore, Md: 1950). 1997;158(8):3902–8.
52. Kim JH, Choi GE, Lee BJ, Kwon SW, Lee SH, Kim HS, et al. Natural killer cells regulate eosinophilic inflammation in chronic rhinosinusitis. Sci Rep. 2016;6:27615. https://doi.org/10.1038/srep27615.
53. Lee JJ, Jacobsen EA, McGarry MP, Schleimer RP, Lee NA. Eosinophils in health and disease: the LIAR hypothesis. Clin Exp Allergy. 2010;40(4):563–75. https://doi.org/10.1111/j.1365-2222.2010.03484.x.
54. Mesnil C, Raulier S, Paulissen G, Xiao X, Birrell MA, Pirottin D, et al. Lung-resident eosinophils represent a distinct regulatory eosinophil subset. J Clin Invest. 2016;126(9):3279–95. https://doi.org/10.1172/JCI85664.
55. Armengot M, Garin L, Carda C. Eosinophil degranulation patterns in nasal polyposis: an ultrastructural study. Am J Rhinol Allergy. 2009;23(5):466–70. https://doi.org/10.2500/ajra.2009.23.3357.
56. Erjefalt JS, Greiff L, Andersson M, Adelroth E, Jeffery PK, Persson CG. Degranulation patterns of eosinophil granulocytes as determinants of eosinophil driven disease. Thorax. 2001;56(5):341–4. https://doi.org/10.1136/thorax.56.5.341.
57. Frigas E, Motojima S, Gleich GJ. The eosinophilic injury to the mucosa of the airways in the pathogenesis of bronchial asthma. Eur Respir J Suppl. 1991;13:123s–35s.
58. Kita H. Eosinophils: multifaceted biological properties and roles in health and disease. Immunol Rev. 2011;242(1):161–77. https://doi.org/10.1111/j.1600-065X.2011.01026.x.
59. Tsuda T, Maeda Y, Nishide M, Koyama S, Hayama Y, Nojima S, et al. Eosinophil-derived neurotoxin enhances airway remodeling in eosinophilic chronic rhinosinusitis and correlates with disease severity. Int Immunol. 2019;31(1):33–40. https://doi.org/10.1093/intimm/dxy061.
60. Peterson CG, Skoog V, Venge P. Human eosinophil cationic proteins (ECP and EPX) and their suppressive effects on lymphocyte proliferation. Immunobiology. 1986;171(1–2):1–13. https://doi.org/10.1016/s0171-2985(86)80013-4.
61. Soragni A, Yousefi S, Stoeckle C, Soriaga AB, Sawaya MR, Kozlowski E, et al. Toxicity of eosinophil MBP is repressed by intracellular crystallization and promoted by extracellular aggregation. Mol Cell. 2015;57(6):1011–21. https://doi.org/10.1016/j.molcel.2015.01.026.
62. Miyata J, Fukunaga K, Kawashima Y, Watanabe T, Saitoh A, Hirosaki T, et al. Dysregulated fatty acid metabolism in nasal polyp-derived eosinophils from patients with chronic rhinosinusitis. Allergy. 2019;74(6):1113–24. https://doi.org/10.1111/all.13726.
63. Pérez-Novo CA, Claeys C, Van Cauwenberge P, Bachert C. Expression of eicosanoid receptors subtypes and eosinophilic inflammation: implication on chronic rhinosinusitis. Respir Res. 2006;7(1):75. https://doi.org/10.1186/1465-9921-7-75.
64. Hwang CS, Park SC, Cho HJ, Park DJ, Yoon JH, Kim CH. Eosinophil extracellular trap formation is closely associated with disease severity in chronic rhinosinusitis regardless of nasal polyp status. Sci Rep. 2019;9(1):8061. https://doi.org/10.1038/s41598-019-44627-z.
65. Dworski R, Simon HU, Hoskins A, Yousefi S. Eosinophil and neutrophil extracellular DNA traps in human allergic asthmatic airways. J Allergy Clin Immunol. 2011;127(5):1260–6. https://doi.org/10.1016/j.jaci.2010.12.1103.
66. Yousefi S, Gold JA, Andina N, Lee JJ, Kelly AM, Kozlowski E, et al. Catapult-like release of mitochondrial DNA by eosinophils contributes to antibacterial defense. Nat Med. 2008;14(9):949–53. https://doi.org/10.1038/nm.1855.
67. Morshed M, Yousefi S, Stöckle C, Simon HU, Simon D. Thymic stromal lymphopoietin stimulates the formation of eosinophil extracellular traps. Allergy. 2012;67(9):1127–37. https://doi.org/10.1111/j.1398-9995.2012.02868.x.
68. Ueki S, Melo RC, Ghiran I, Spencer LA, Dvorak AM, Weller PF. Eosinophil extracellular DNA trap cell death mediates lytic release of free secretion-competent eosinophil granules in humans. Blood. 2013;121(11):2074–83. https://doi.org/10.1182/blood-2012-05-432088.
69. Ueki S, Tokunaga T, Fujieda S, Honda K, Hirokawa M, Spencer LA, et al. Eosinophil ETosis and DNA

traps: a new look at eosinophilic inflammation. Curr Allergy Asthma Rep. 2016;16(8):54. https://doi.org/10.1007/s11882-016-0634-5.
70. Persson EK, Verstraete K, Heyndrickx I, Gevaert E, Aegerter H, Percier JM, et al. Protein crystallization promotes type 2 immunity and is reversible by antibody treatment. Science. 2019;364(6442):eaaw4295. https://doi.org/10.1126/science.aaw4295.
71. Ueki S, Tokunaga T, Melo RCN, Saito H, Honda K, Fukuchi M, et al. Charcot-Leyden crystal formation is closely associated with eosinophil extracellular trap cell death. Blood. 2018;132(20):2183–7. https://doi.org/10.1182/blood-2018-04-842260.
72. Katzenstein AL, Sale SR, Greenberger PA. Allergic Aspergillus sinusitis: a newly recognized form of sinusitis. J Allergy Clin Immunol. 1983;72(1):89–93.
73. Gevaert E, Delemarre T, De Volder J, Zhang N, Holtappels G, De Ruyck N, et al. Charcot-Leyden crystals promote neutrophilic inflammation in patients with nasal polyposis. J Allergy Clin Immunol. 2019; https://doi.org/10.1016/j.jaci.2019.08.027.
74. Terness P, Bauer TM, Rose L, Dufter C, Watzlik A, Simon H, et al. Inhibition of allogeneic T cell proliferation by indoleamine 2,3-dioxygenase-expressing dendritic cells: mediation of suppression by tryptophan metabolites. J Exp Med. 2002;196(4):447–57. https://doi.org/10.1084/jem.20020052.
75. Akuthota P, Wang H, Weller PF. Eosinophils as antigen-presenting cells in allergic upper airway disease. Curr Opin Allergy Clin Immunol. 2010;10(1):14–9. https://doi.org/10.1097/ACI.0b013e328334f693.
76. Van Zele T, Gevaert P, Holtappels G, Beule A, Wormald PJ, Mayr S, et al. Oral steroids and doxycycline: two different approaches to treat nasal polyps. J Allergy Clin Immunol. 2010;125(5):1069–76.e4. https://doi.org/10.1016/j.jaci.2010.02.020.
77. Schleimer RP, Bochner BS. The effects of glucocorticoids on human eosinophils. J Allergy Clin Immunol. 1994;94(6 Pt 2):1202–13. https://doi.org/10.1016/0091-6749(94)90333-6.

Neutrophils

9

Elien Gevaert

Key Points

- Neutrophilia is usually associated with CRSsNP, Asian CRSwNP or CF nasal polyps.
- Different inflammatory patterns including type 2 inflammation can be associated with neutrophilia in CRS.
- A wide variety of mediators are capable of mediating neutrophil recruitment.
- Neutrophils are more than bystanders of inflammation and use a variety of mediators to modulate inflammation.
- The presentation of neutrophilia indicates a bad response to corticosteroids and macrolides or doxycycline might be a better treatment approach.
- The development of novel drugs targeting the activation and infiltration of neutrophils may offer a more efficient solution for patient with steroid resistant CRS, associated with neutrophilic inflammation.
- A better understanding of neutrophil biology in CRS combined with a solid endotyping of CRS patients will enable a more specialized treatment.

E. Gevaert (✉)
Upper Airways Research Laboratory and Department of Oto-Rhino-Laryngology, Ghent University, Ghent, Belgium
e-mail: elien.gevaert@ugent.be

9.1 Clinical Manifestations of Neutrophilia in CRS

Neutrophilia is considered a typical feature of type 1 or type 17 inflammation and has therefore been associated with CRSsNP, Asian CRSwNP, and cystic fibrosis polyp patients. While CRSwNP patients show a predominant type 2 inflammation with eosinophilia in a majority of the Caucasian population, polyps in Asian patients were associated with a rather type 1/17 inflammation and neutrophilia as described more than a decade ago [1]. The relative presentation of CRSwNP patients with type 2 inflammation in Asian populations is significantly increasing [2]. Currently 20% to 60% of Asian CRSwNP patients have a significant type 2 response, indicating a shift to type 2 inflammation [2, 3]. For long neutrophilic/eosinophilic inflammation in CRS has been presented as black and white, almost implying mutual exclusion. Also, the main focus for type 2 inflammation with eosinophilia, without a doubt the most severe patient group, has somehow distracted the attention from neutrophils. Interestingly, several studies over the last decade indicate the existence of a mixed inflammation in a substantial fraction of CRSwNP patients. A Chinese study of CRSwNP patients showed that 76.5% had an eosinophilic phenotype, 46.0% had a neutrophilic phenotype, and 35.8% had a mixed phenotype [4]. Other studies in Chinese populations also report a

L. Zhang, C. Bachert (eds.), *Chronic Rhinosinusitis*, https://doi.org/10.1007/978-981-16-0784-4_9

significant infiltration of neutrophils in CRSwNP compared to controls, with, however, a more pronounced neutrophilia in non-eosinophilic CRSwNP than in eosinophilic CRwNP patients [5–8]. Similarly, a prominent presence of neutrophils has been described in several studies of Caucasian CRSwNP patients [3, 9–11]. A recent cluster analysis of inflammatory endotypes indicates a markedly increased presence of neutrophilic marker proteins in the high type 2 clusters containing the most severe and difficult to treat CRSwNP patients [11]. While some reports claim that the number of neutrophils is elevated in CRSsNP compared to CRSwNP, other studies find that the numbers are comparable or elevated in CRSwNP [7, 12–14]. These contradicting results are more than likely attributed to the existence of different CRS endotypes of which some have a clear neutrophilic inflammation co-existing with eosinophilia [11]. Neutrophilia in CRS can be diagnosed by measurement of neutrophil specific proteins such as elastase or myeloperoxidase (MPO), or via immunohistochemistry against one of these proteins in the tissue (Fig. 9.1).

In severe asthma, the existence of a Type 2/Type 17 (predominant) subgroup of asthmatic patients was associated with more glucocorticoid resistance, the greatest airway obstruction and hyperactivity compared with the Type 2 (predominant) and Type 2/Type 17 (low) subgroups. These reports pointed to IL-17 as the main driving force to produce intense neutrophil infiltration and to exacerbate Type 2 cell-mediated eosinophilic airway inflammation and hyperresponsiveness [15–17]. Also in nasal polyps, increased neutrophilia was found associated with a reduced response to oral corticoid therapy. In addition, markers of severe or moderate neutrophilic inflammation were associated with elevated levels of IL-8 and high proportions of difficult-to-treat CRS [18]. However, unlike severe asthma, a significant role for IL-17 and the existence of a mixed type2/type17 could not be confirmed as the driving force for the mixed eosinophilia/neutrophilia in CRSwNP.

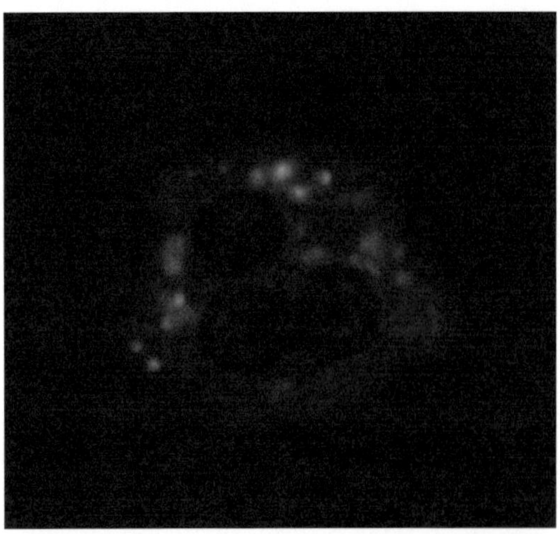

Fig. 9.1 Neutrophils in CRSwNP. Immunohistochemistry stain for elastase (pink) and DNA (purple)

9.2 Neutrophil Recruitment and Activation in CRS

Neutrophils are terminally differentiated cells that develop in the bone marrow. Under control of several key transcription factors, neutrophils develop from a common myeloid progenitor cell. While transcription factors C/EBP-α and PU.1 induce the progenitor to differentiate into monocytes and macrophages, acetylated C/EBP-ε, Gfi-1, and the lack of GATA-1 expression generate neutrophils [19]. The neutrophil receptor, CXC motif receptor (CXCR)-4 and CXCR-2 and their chemokines CXC motif ligands (CXCL)-12 and CXCL-2 regulate the release of neutrophils from the bone marrow [20].

Neutrophils represent the first line of cellular defense against invading microorganism and are able to rapidly move across the blood-endothelial cell barrier to exert their effector functions. Within minutes, neutrophil respond to soluble factor like chemokines and cytokines and are recruited to the site of infection. The first step of the neutrophil recruitment cascade involves interactions between neutrophils and endothelial cells via various adhesive modules [21]. The cell adhesion molecules P-selectin, VCAM, and ICAM-1 are known to play a role in the trans endothelial migration of neutrophils [22]. Increased I-CAM expression has been reported in both CRSwNP and CRSsNP [12, 23–25]. Interestingly, also nasal epithelial cells were shown to upregulate ICAM-1 and P-selectin under hypoxic conditions in vitro [26]. This can result in an increased migration and adherence of neutrophils. Another study confirmed that ICAM-1 was upregulated on epithelial cells from Caucasian CRSwNP patients, suggesting a mechanism for a neutrophil-epithelial cell interaction in nasal polyps [27].

To further guide neutrophil infiltration, a wide variety of chemokines and cytokines can play a role. CXCR expression on neutrophils, especially CXCR-1 and CXCR-2, is important in this process and CXCLs, like CXCL-1, CXCL-2, CXCL-5, and CXCL-8, can direct neutrophil migration through their engagement with the receptor. Both infiltrated immune cells (e.g. neutrophil and mast cells) and structural cells (e.g. epithelial cells and fibroblasts) engage in producing CXCL-1, CXCL-2, and CXCL-8 for neutrophil recruitment [28–30]. In China, two independent cluster analyses identified a neutrophilic CRS clusters associated with high CXCL-8, pointing to a key role of this cytokine in the recruitment of neutrophils [18, 31]. Other reports show that CXCL-8 indeed is upregulated in both CRSsNP and CRSwNP compared to controls in both Chinese and Caucasian populations [5, 32]. Nasal epithelial cells were indicated as a major source of CXCL-8 in response to inflammatory stimuli, bacteria and even diesel exhaust particles and seem a crucial compound in guiding neutrophil recruitment [33–35]. In addition to these chemokines and cytokines, lipid mediators also can direct neutrophil chemotaxis. Along these lines, leukotriene (LT) B4 is found secreted by nasal epithelial cells from CRSwNP in response to oxidative stress. LTB4 is sensed by the LTB4 receptor expressed on neutrophils and induces its migration [36]. Another study found that another lipid mediator, thromboxane A2 regulates CXCL-1 and CXCL-8 chemokine expression in nasal mucosa-derived fibroblasts of CRSsNP patients [29].

Once recruited in the tissue, neutrophils can be primed for further activity. Priming of neutrophils with a primary agonist can enhance or modulate the response to a secondary stimulus and can set the stage for further neutrophil adhesion, phagocytosis, superoxide production, degranulation, and survival. Stimuli like IL-1α, IL1-β, IL-6, IL-8, granulocyte colony-stimulating factor (G-CSF), GM-CSF, complement components C3a and C5a, and IFNϒ can prime or further activate the neutrophils in the tissue [37]. Once in the tissue, neutrophils might sustain their own recruitment, priming, and activation via production of factors like CXCL-1, CXCL-2, and CXCL-8, creating a positive feedback loop [5]. Many of these factors have been reported upregulated in one or another CRS subtype. As each factor and combinations of factors can influence neutrophil activity differently it is likely that the neutrophil specific activity is highly context dependent and therefore impossible to understand without a thorough endotyping of the patients.

As discussed in Sect. 9.1, the central role of IL-17 as driving force for neutrophilia in the different CRS endotypes is not always clear. However, in a majority of Chinese patients with nasal polyposis and in patients with nasal polyps suffering from cystic fibrosis (CF), described as a Type 17 biased diseases, it is likely that IL-17 is at the base of the observed neutrophilia [1, 38]. IL-17A causes release of chemokines like IL-6 and CXCL-8 that recruit neutrophils [33]. In addition, both IL-17A and IL-17F cause the upregulation of G-CSF, CXCL-1, and CXCL-2 [39]. Interestingly, a study showed that IL-17A has a direct impact on neutrophil survival in adult nasal polyp disease, but not in nasal polyps from CF patients [38]. As shortly addressed in Sect. 9.1, the link between IL-17 and increased tissue neutrophilia is less clear in a high type 2 inflammatory context. A cluster analysis for endotyping patients reported by Tomassen et al. showed that the subtypes with severe CRSwNP and comorbid asthma are characterized by high type 2 cytokines but also by high levels of neutrophil-associated cytokines or proteins like IL-6, CXCL-8, and MPO, but not IL-17 [11]. This points to a role for neutrophils in these subtypes without the involvement of IL-17. A possible explanation for this phenomenon came recently. In both Asian and

Causasian severe eosinophilic CRSwNP patients, eosinophils are described to undergo EETosis with the deposition of Charcot–Leyden crystals as a result [40, 41]. Recently it was shown that CLCs are more than just markers of eosinophilia and actively contribute to airway disease. In mouse models, CLCs can stimulate innate and adaptive immunity and act as a type 2 adjuvant, promoting key features of asthma [40]. In addition it was shown that they can activate the inflammasome in human macrophages in vitro [42]. In Caucasian CRSwNP patients it was shown that exposure to CLCs evokes a pro-inflammatory cytokine release resulting in neutrophilic inflammation [43].

As first-line defense cells, neutrophils are rapidly recruited in response to bacterial infection, a common problem in CRS. As a consequence their chemotaxis and activation can be directly induced by pathogen derived peptides such a formylated met-leu-ph (fMLF) [20]. One study showed that neutrophil recruitment is more prominent in CRS patients with bacterial biofilms than patients without, irrespective of the clinical subtype (CRSwNP or CRSsNP) [44]. However, it is known that CRSwNP is associated with higher rates of upper airway colonization with *Staphylococcus aureus* (*S. aureus*) and biofilm formation which correlate with more severe disease phenotypes [45, 46]. Supernatant of epithelial cells treated with Staphylococcus aureus enterotoxin B has chemotactic activity for neutrophils in vitro, while no effect on neutrophil survival was noticed [47]. Interestingly, *S. aureus* is one of the germs with an impressive arsenal of molecules to modulate neutrophil chemotaxis, adhesion and activation pointing to primary role for neutrophils in combatting *S. aureus* infections [37].

Another factor possibly contributing to neutrophilia in CRS is hypoxia. Local hypoxia can be caused by sinus occlusion and poor ventilation of the sinus but may lead to neutrophilic inflammation with overproduction of TGFβ2 and fibrosis [42, 43]. Under hypoxic conditions, nasal tissue-derived fibroblasts were found to produce chemokines such as CXCL-8 and CCL-11, which could further support neutrophil (and eosinophil) recruitment [42, 43]. Further evidence for the importance of hypoxia came from experiments with nasal epithelial cells showing increased expression of CXCL-8, CCL-2, CCL-4, CXCL-12, ICAM-1, and P-selectin under hypoxic conditions in vitro. In addition, hypoxia induced (HIF)-1alpa was found upregulated in CRSsNP and is positively correlated with the numbers of neutrophils [7, 44]. Whether hypoxia is a major component in CRSwNP or CRSsNP or both is matter of debate and requires further research.

9.3 Functions of Neutrophils in CRS

About 60% of the circulating white blood cells are neutrophils, making them the most abundant leukocytes in humans. In circulating blood, they are in a quiescent state, characterized by a circular shape. A mature neutrophil is characterized by a segmented nucleus and multiple cytoplasmic granules (Fig. 9.2). Neutrophils contain three types of granules. The primary (also called azurophilic) granules consist of MPO, cathepsin G, elastase and proteinase 3 and multiple defensins. Secondary granules contain antimicrobial peptides like lactoferrin, and the tertiary granules contain gelatinase proteins such as MMP9 [20] (Fig. 9.3).

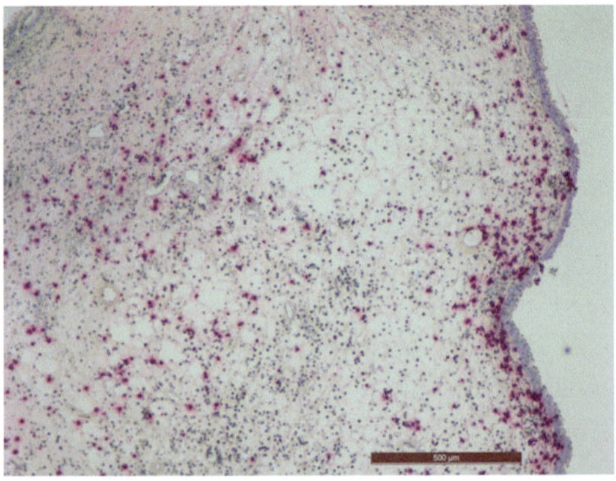

Fig. 9.2 Mature neutrophil in nasal polyp tissue. Immunofluorescent stain for Elastase (green) and DNA (red)

9.4 Antibacterial Defense

As first-line defense, neutrophils are specialized immune cells to protect the host from foreign invaders. Neutrophils can protect the host from bacteria through phagocytosis, degranulation or the formation of NETs. Neutrophils are professional phagocytes and, as such, express Fcγ receptors, C-type lectins and complement receptors that recognize opsonized invaders in the environment. Upon recognition, the opsonized invaders are bound and phagocytosed. In the resulting phagosome, the generation of ROS and fusion of the phagosome with primary and secondary granules cooperatively kill the invader in the phagosome [20]. Recent research revealed an $CD16^{high}$ $CD62L^{dim}$ neutrophil subset in CRwNP capable of phagocytosis and induction of ROS, indicating that these processes take place within the polyp [27]. Neutrophils are also able to release granule proteins or mediators in the extracellular environment through exocytosis or degranulation [5]. The released mediators have antimicrobial activity but are also highly cytotoxic.

Another mechanism to clear invaders is the formation of neutrophil extracellular trap NET formation. Those NETs can be formed via different processes but generally consist of neutrophil DNA associated with granule proteins such as

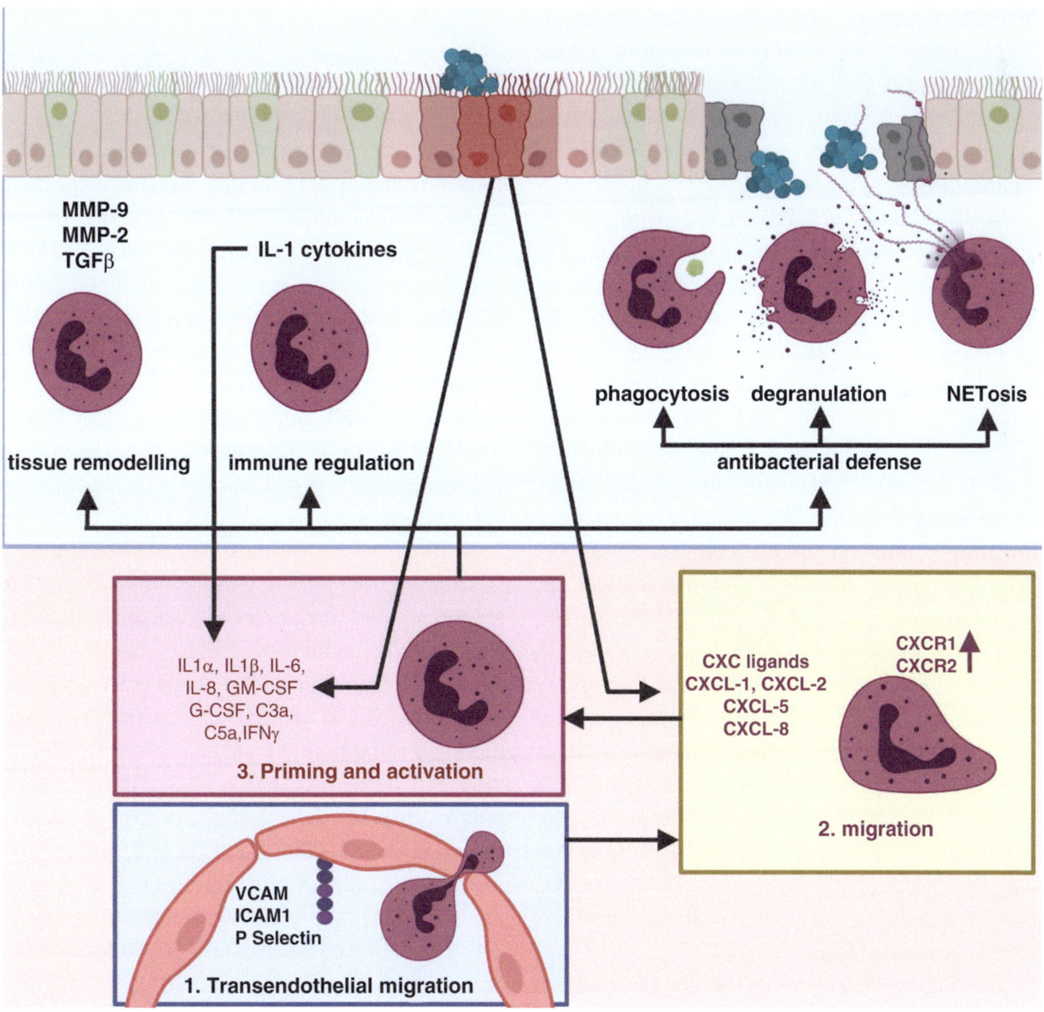

Fig. 9.3 Overview

neutrophil elastase (NE), cathepsin G, and metalloproteinase 9 (MMP-9) [48]. NETs were found in secretions of eosinophilic CRSwNP patients and in Chinese polyps. One study reported not to find NETS in Asian CRSwNP patients, while other studies found NETs in nasal secretions of eosinophilic CRSwNP patients [47–49]. In the tissue, NETs were located in the sub-epithelial layer of nasal polyps and LL-37 was shown to play a role in evoking neutrophil extracellular trap formation in Asian CRSwNP patients [49]. Recently, it was found that CLCs, like other crystals, evoke NETosis in vitro [43]. It is likely that the excessive CLC deposition in tissue and nasal secretions in CRSwNP patients evoke NETosis in the patients [43]. In addition, multiple of microorganisms, including bacteria, viruses, fungi, and parasites have been shown to induce NETs. Interestingly, the pathway of NET formation and outcome is highly dependent on the individual microorganism identity and additional stimuli [48].

In CRS the role of NETs on the pathophysiology is still poorly understood. However, it is clear that NETs play a dual role in host homeostasis. While they protect hosts from infectious diseases by killing bacteria; they are also likely causing pathologic alterations, much like is extensively reported in autoimmune and auto-inflammatory diseases [48]. Along these lines, autoantibodies against dsDNA, chromatin, and histone were found in nasal polyps [50]. However, if an autoimmune compound really contributes to the pathophysiology of CRS remains unclear. In secretions of eosinophilic CRSwNP patient, NETS (in addition to EETs) were found to increase viscosity of the secretions hampering clearing [51]. In line with these observations, it was found that the elevated production of NETs was associated with disease severity in CF patients. In addition, NETs could have pro-inflammatory effects on macrophages or stimulate remodeling of the extracellular matrix. However, if this is truly the case in CRS remains to be investigated [48].

The factors determining the choice between phagocytosis, netosis or degranulation is poorly understood and more than likely regulated by a complex interplay of different factors. One factor could be the size of the invader as neutrophils were reported to sense microbe size and to selectively release neutrophil extracellular traps in response to large pathogens [21]. In CRS, it should be shown if the size of the microbes or the crystals and the inability to be phagocytized is involved in turning on NETosis. Another factor driving NET formation could be prolonged survival as neutrophils of CF patients were reported to have a prosurvival phenotype that is associated increased NET production [47]. It is likely that different mechanisms are more or less important in different endotypes of CRS patients and it is clear that neutrophils should be regarded as much more than only bystander cells.

9.5 Immune Regulation and Tissue Remodeling

Recent research has revealed neutrophils as more sophisticated immune cells that are able to precisely regulate their granular enzymes release by ion fluxes and can release immunomodulatory cytokines and chemokines that interact with various components of the immune system [20]. Neutrophilic elastase activity was found increased in both CRSsNP and CRSwNP patient tissue, implying a role for elastase in host defense or immune regulation [5]. Interestingly, once in the extracellular environment, neutrophil proteases, including elastase, cathepsin G, and Proteinase 3, were found less effective in microbial killing but able to regulate the processing and activity of six IL-1 family cytokines (IL-1α, IL-1β, IL-33, IL-36α, IL-36β, and IL-36γ) in an extremely efficient way [52]. IL-1 and IL33 are important initiators of inflammation and can indirectly control type 2 cytokine production in eosinophilic nasal polyps [53]. In CRS, IL36y promotes the secretion of CXCL-1, CXCL-2, CXCL-8, and IL-17A from tissue neutrophils, reinforcing a positive feedback loop and their own recruitment [5]. In addition, neutrophilic elastase can induce mucus secretion and goblet cell metaplasia [53, 54].

CRSsNP, non-eosinophilic CRSwNP and eosinophilic CRSwNP each display distinct features of tissue remodeling. Neutrophil derived MMP-9 and MMP-2 was found elevated in both eosinophilic and non-eosinophilic CRSwNP, indicating a role for neutrophils in tissue remodeling [5, 7]. In CRSsNP and non-eosinophilic CRSwNP tissue, neutrophils were found to contribute to tissue remodeling via the production of TGF-β2, acting on tissue myofibroblasts and inducing the expression of fibronectin [7].

Increasing evidence has demonstrated a phenotypic heterogeneity or at least a functional versatility among neutrophils. Neutrophilic subsets based on maturation stage, activation state, potential to form NETS or based on phagocytic capacity have been described. In addition the existence, tissue resident, pro-inflammatory or "N1" neutrophils, and anti-inflammatory, or "N2," neutrophils has been proposed [54]. In CRS, neutrophil heterogeneity is gaining increasing interest, but progression is tackled by the difficulty to study activated neutrophils. Sub-setting of neutrophils revealed $CD16^{high}$ $CD62L^{dim}$ neutrophils in chronic rhinosinusitis with nasal polyps, indicating an activated phenotype [27]. Also in CRSwNP, neutrophils were found to be a major source of oncostatin M. A majority of those cells also expressed arginase 1, which is suggestive of a N2 phenotype [9]. Beside its role in neutrophil polarization, oncostatin M is also able to disrupt the epithelial barrier, implying a possible role for neutrophils in impairing barrier function [9]. IL-33 treatment of neutrophils resulted in a polarization of the neutrophil and to electively produce Type 2 cytokine like IL-4, IL-5, IL-9, and IL-13 [52, 55]. While neutrophil heterogeneity among the different CRS endotypes is an appealing possibility, more research is required in humans to come to a consensus on marker identification and to determine if the observed heterogeneity is caused by microenvironmental or tissue specific guided differences in activation, polarization or maturation state or if it is a truly intrinsically different subpopulation. In any way, the existence of heterogeneous neutrophils adds another layer of complexity in understanding these cells in the context of different disease endotypes.

9.6 Therapeutic Implications

For long, neutrophils have been considered as bystanders of inflammation. This point of view has started to shift over the last few years and research is starting to pay more and more attention to the possible role of neutrophils as effector cells in at least certain subtypes of CRS, as the presentation of neutrophilia can certainly affect treatment outcome of CRS patients.

The appearance of neutrophils, might be troublesome in specific CRS endotypes. Especially in severe type 2 CRSwNP patients as increased neutrophilia in nasal polyp reduces the response to oral corticosteroid therapy. Reports show that patients' symptoms improved after corticosteroid treatment. In addition, the numbers of eosinophils and levels of their mediators (IL-4 and IL-5) decreased, but the number of neutrophils and levels of their mediators (e.g. IL-8) remained unaltered. Despite the improvement of the symptoms, neutrophil-negative polyps had significantly greater reductions in bilateral polyp size scores, nasal congestion scores, and total nasal symptom scores compared to neutrophilic-positive patients [4]. In addition, the use of topical steroids did not seem to affect neutrophil activation state reflected by the expression of CD16, CD62L, CD11b or ICAM-1 in CRSwNP [27]. Also, dexamethasone treatment had no influence on LL-37 induced NET formation in Chinese CRSwNP patients [49]. Corticosteroid were even reported to prevent apoptosis of neutrophils and to promote neutrophilic inflammation [56, 57]. In general, significant neutrophilic inflammation is associated with difficulties in general guideline recommended, glucocorticoid and endoscopic surgery centered treatment, especially in eosinophilic CRSwNP patients but also in Chinese neutrophilic CRSwNP patients [4, 18].

There are conflicting results concerning the efficacy of macrolides in CRS. However, they are capable of decreasing the bacterial load and possibly biofilm formation and could, as such, diminish neutrophil recruitment in response to bacterial infection. In addition, they induce neutrophil apoptosis and long-term treatment with clarithromycin was shown to decrease CXCL8 and MPO levels in Chinese CRSsNP patients, implying to interfere with recruitment [58]. Another antibiotic, doxycycline can impair neutrophil migration, induce apoptosis, and modulate the oxidative burst of neutrophils [58, 59]. However, if this is truly the case in CRS patients remains to be investigated.

Other strategies to interfere with neutrophil recruitment and activation are being developed. The use of CXCR1 and CXCR2 antagonist and inhibition of IL-17A, IL-16ϒ, GM-CSF, and LTB4 is under clinical trial evaluation for diverse inflammatory pathologies [60]. Dual CXCR-1/CXCR-2 antagonist were effective in reducing neutrophil levels in mild atopic asthma subjects [61]. Anti IL-17A biologics have been approved by FDA for the treatment of psoriasis [62]. Monoclonal antibodies against GM-CSF, and a monoclonal antibody against GM-CSFRα have been developed. A phase II trial targeting GM-CSF was conducted in asthmatic patients that were poorly controlled with long-acting bronchodilators and or corticosteroids. If these can help in the treatment of CRS remains to be studied in the future [9].

A special case could be the high type 2 CRSwNP patients. In these severe CRSwNP patients, it was hypothesized that neutrophils driven by high amounts of CLCs found in CRSwNP mucosa and mucus can contribute to the persistence of severe airway disease, and may turn the inflammation non-responsive to GCS and possibly biologics CRSwNP [43]. A study in mice could prevent such CLC-evoked effects by antibody treatment causing the dissolution of the CLCs [40]. Although this is an interesting approach, appropriate studies are required to test this hypothesis in CRSwNP patients [43]. In addition, it is unclear if and how neutrophilia contributes to, and how it is affected by treatment with successful biologics targeting specific type 2 mediators such as dupilumab [63]. To summarize, targeting neutrophilia will be enabled in the future by variable approaches, but key will be the understanding of the crucial mediators in the different endotypes. This knowledge is needed to allocate the right therapeutic to the right patient in the future.

9.7 Translation into Future Daily Practice

The identification of neutrophils in CRS patients will likely evolve as one of the critical parameters in determining the treatment approach of CRS patients. More research is required to enhance the understanding on neutrophil heterogeneity and the role of the microenvironment. As the consequences of neutrophils in a type 17 environment might significantly differ of their appearance in a type 2 context, and research on heterogeneity will evolve, the identification of solid neutrophil (heterogeneity) biomarkers and a thorough endotyping of each patient will be key to determine the treatment strategy of those patients with significant neutrophilic inflammation.

References

1. Zhang N, Holtappels G, Claeys C, Huang G, van Cauwenberge P, Bachert C. Pattern of inflammation and impact of Staphylococcus aureus enterotoxins in nasal polyps from southern China. Am J Rhinol. 2006;20(4):445–50.
2. Zhang Y, Gevaert E, Lou H, Wang X, Zhang L, Bachert C, et al. Chronic rhinosinusitis in Asia. J Allergy Clin Immunol. 2017;140(5):1230–9. https://doi.org/10.1016/j.jaci.2017.09.009.
3. Wang X, Zhang N, Bo M, Holtappels G, Zheng M, Lou H, et al. Diversity of TH cytokine profiles in patients with chronic rhinosinusitis: a multicenter study in Europe, Asia, and Oceania. J Allergy Clin Immunol. 2016;138(5):1344–53. https://doi.org/10.1016/j.jaci.2016.05.041.
4. Wen W, Liu W, Zhang L, Bai J, Fan Y, Xia W, et al. Increased neutrophilia in nasal polyps reduces the response to oral corticosteroid therapy. J Allergy Clin Immunol. 2012;129(6):1522–8.e5. https://doi.org/10.1016/j.jaci.2012.01.079.
5. Wang H, Li ZY, Jiang WX, Liao B, Zhai GT, Wang N, et al. The activation and function of IL-36gamma in neutrophilic inflammation in chronic rhinosinusitis. J Allergy Clin Immunol. 2018;141(5):1646–58. https://doi.org/10.1016/j.jaci.2017.12.972.
6. Cao PP, Wang ZC, Schleimer RP, Liu Z. Pathophysiologic mechanisms of chronic rhinosinusitis and their roles in emerging disease endotypes. Ann Allergy Asthma Immunol. 2019a;122(1):33–40. https://doi.org/10.1016/j.anai.2018.10.014.
7. Shi LL, Xiong P, Zhang L, Cao PP, Liao B, Lu X, et al. Features of airway remodeling in different types of Chinese chronic rhinosinusitis are associated with

inflammation patterns. Allergy. 2013;68(1):101–9. https://doi.org/10.1111/all.12064.
8. Ma J, Shi LL, Deng YK, Wang H, Cao PP, Long XB, et al. CD8(+) T cells with distinct cytokine-producing features and low cytotoxic activity in eosinophilic and non-eosinophilic chronic rhinosinusitis with nasal polyps. Clin Exp Allergy. 2016;46(9):1162–75. https://doi.org/10.1111/cea.12758.
9. Pothoven KL, Norton JE, Suh LA, Carter RG, Harris KE, Biyasheva A, et al. Neutrophils are a major source of the epithelial barrier disrupting cytokine oncostatin M in patients with mucosal airways disease. J Allergy Clin Immunol. 2017;139(6):1966–78.e9. https://doi.org/10.1016/j.jaci.2016.10.039.
10. Bachert C, Zhang N, Holtappels G, De Lobel L, van Cauwenberge P, Liu S, et al. Presence of IL-5 protein and IgE antibodies to staphylococcal enterotoxins in nasal polyps is associated with comorbid asthma. J Allergy Clin Immunol. 2010;126(5):962–8, 8.e1–6. https://doi.org/10.1016/j.jaci.2010.07.007.
11. Tomassen P, Vandeplas G, Van Zele T, Cardell LO, Arebro J, Olze H, et al. Inflammatory endotypes of chronic rhinosinusitis based on cluster analysis of biomarkers. J Allergy Clin Immunol. 2016;137(5):1449–56.e4. https://doi.org/10.1016/j.jaci.2015.12.1324.
12. Polzehl D, Moeller P, Riechelmann H, Perner S. Distinct features of chronic rhinosinusitis with and without nasal polyps. Allergy. 2006;61(11):1275–9. https://doi.org/10.1111/j.1398-9995.2006.01132.x.
13. Soler ZM, Sauer D, Mace J, Smith TL. Impact of mucosal eosinophilia and nasal polyposis on quality-of-life outcomes after sinus surgery. Otolaryngol Head Neck Surg. 2010;142(1):64–71. https://doi.org/10.1016/j.otohns.2009.10.005.
14. Tokunaga T, Sakashita M, Haruna T, Asaka D, Takeno S, Ikeda H, et al. Novel scoring system and algorithm for classifying chronic rhinosinusitis: the JESREC Study. Allergy. 2015;70(8):995–1003. https://doi.org/10.1111/all.12644.
15. Irvin C, Zafar I, Good J, Rollins D, Christianson C, Gorska MM, et al. Increased frequency of dual-positive TH2/TH17 cells in bronchoalveolar lavage fluid characterizes a population of patients with severe asthma. J Allergy Clin Immunol. 2014;134(5):1175–86.e7. https://doi.org/10.1016/j.jaci.2014.05.038.
16. Wakashin H, Hirose K, Maezawa Y, Kagami S, Suto A, Watanabe N, et al. IL-23 and Th17 cells enhance Th2-cell-mediated eosinophilic airway inflammation in mice. Am J Respir Crit Care Med. 2008;178(10):1023–32. https://doi.org/10.1164/rccm.200801-086OC.
17. Wilson RH, Whitehead GS, Nakano H, Free ME, Kolls JK, Cook DN. Allergic sensitization through the airway primes Th17-dependent neutrophilia and airway hyperresponsiveness. Am J Respir Crit Care Med. 2009;180(8):720–30. https://doi.org/10.1164/rccm.200904-0573OC.
18. Liao B, Liu JX, Li ZY, Zhen Z, Cao PP, Yao Y, et al. Multidimensional endotypes of chronic rhinosinusitis and their association with treatment outcomes. Allergy. 2018;73(7):1459–69. https://doi.org/10.1111/all.13411.
19. Lawrence SM, Corriden R, Nizet V. The ontogeny of a neutrophil: mechanisms of granulopoiesis and homeostasis. Microbiol Mol Biol Rev. 2018;82(1):e00057-17. https://doi.org/10.1128/mmbr.00057-17.
20. Sheshachalam A, Srivastava N, Mitchell T, Lacy P, Eitzen G. Granule protein processing and regulated secretion in neutrophils. Front Immunol. 2014;5:448. https://doi.org/10.3389/fimmu.2014.00448.
21. Filippi MD. Neutrophil transendothelial migration: updates and new perspectives. Blood. 2019;133(20):2149–58. https://doi.org/10.1182/blood-2018-12-844605.
22. Kolaczkowska E, Kubes P. Neutrophil recruitment and function in health and inflammation. Nat Rev Immunol. 2013;13(3):159–75. https://doi.org/10.1038/nri3399.
23. Elmorsy S, El-Naggar MM, Abdel aal SM, Abou-elela MA. Sinus aspirates in chronic rhinosinusitis: fungal colonization of paranasal sinuses, evaluation of ICAM-1 and IL-8 and studying of immunological effect of long-term macrolide therapy. Rhinology. 2010;48(3):312–7. https://doi.org/10.4193/Rhin09.140.
24. Cao PP, Li HB, Wang BF, Wang SB, You XJ, Cui YH, et al. Distinct immunopathologic characteristics of various types of chronic rhinosinusitis in adult Chinese. J Allergy Clin Immunol. 2009;124(3):478–84, 84.e1–2. https://doi.org/10.1016/j.jaci.2009.05.017.
25. Demoly P, Sahla M, Campbell AM, Bousquet J, Crampette L. ICAM-1 expression in upper respiratory mucosa is differentially related to eosinophil and neutrophil inflammation according to the allergic status. Clin Exp Allergy. 1998;28(6):731–8. https://doi.org/10.1046/j.1365-2222.1998.00308.x.
26. Steinke JW, Woodard CR, Borish L. Role of hypoxia in inflammatory upper airway disease. Curr Opin Allergy Clin Immunol. 2008;8(1):16–20. https://doi.org/10.1097/ACI.0b013e3282f3f488.
27. Arebro J, Drakskog C, Winqvist O, Bachert C, Kumlien Georen S, Cardell LO. Subsetting reveals CD16(high) CD62L(dim) neutrophils in chronic rhinosinusitis with nasal polyps. Allergy. 2019; https://doi.org/10.1111/all.13919.
28. Coffelt SB, Wellenstein MD, de Visser KE. Neutrophils in cancer: neutral no more. Nat Rev Cancer. 2016;16(7):431–46. https://doi.org/10.1038/nrc.2016.52.
29. de Oliveira S, Rosowski EE, Huttenlocher A. Neutrophil migration in infection and wound repair: going forward in reverse. Nat Rev Immunol. 2016;16(6):378–91. https://doi.org/10.1038/nri.2016.49.
30. Tsai Y-J, Hao S-P, Chen C-L, Wu W-B. Thromboxane A2 regulates CXCL1 and CXCL8 chemokine expression in the nasal mucosa-derived fibroblasts of chronic rhinosinusitis patients. PLoS One. 2016;11(6):e0158438-e. https://doi.org/10.1371/journal.pone.0158438.

31. Wei B, Liu F, Zhang J, Liu Y, Du J, Liu S, et al. Multivariate analysis of inflammatory endotypes in recurrent nasal polyposis in a Chinese population. Rhinology. 2018;56(3):216–26. https://doi.org/10.4193/Rhin17.240.
32. Van Zele T, Claeys S, Gevaert P, Van Maele G, Holtappels G, Van Cauwenberge P, et al. Differentiation of chronic sinus diseases by measurement of inflammatory mediators. Allergy. 2006;61(11):1280–9. https://doi.org/10.1111/j.1398-9995.2006.01225.x.
33. Shiozawa A, Miwa M, Ono N, Homma H, Hirotsu M, Ikeda K. Comparative analysis of cytokine release from epithelial cell cultures of the upper airway. Rhinology. 2015;53(2):135–41. https://doi.org/10.4193/Rhin14.078.
34. Shimizu S, Kouzaki H, Kato T, Tojima I, Shimizu T. HMGB1-TLR4 signaling contributes to the secretion of interleukin 6 and interleukin 8 by nasal epithelial cells. Am J Rhinol Allergy. 2016;30(3):167–72. https://doi.org/10.2500/ajra.2016.30.4300.
35. Rammal A, Tewfik M, Rousseau S. Differences in RANTES and IL-6 levels among chronic rhinosinusitis patients with predominant gram-negative and gram-positive infection. J Otolaryngol Head Neck Surg. 2017;46(1):7. https://doi.org/10.1186/s40463-016-0183-x.
36. Jeanson L, Kelly M, Coste A, Guerrera IC, Fritsch J, Nguyen-Khoa T, et al. Oxidative stress induces unfolding protein response and inflammation in nasal polyposis. Allergy. 2012;67(3):403–12. https://doi.org/10.1111/j.1398-9995.2011.02769.x.
37. Guerra FE, Borgogna TR, Patel DM, Sward EW, Voyich JM. Epic immune battles of history: neutrophils vs. Staphylococcus aureus. Front Cell Infect Microbiol. 2017;7:286. https://doi.org/10.3389/fcimb.2017.00286.
38. Derycke L, Zhang N, Holtappels G, Dutre T, Bachert C. IL-17A as a regulator of neutrophil survival in nasal polyp disease of patients with and without cystic fibrosis. J Cyst Fibros. 2012;11(3):193–200. https://doi.org/10.1016/j.jcf.2011.11.007.
39. Fossiez F, Djossou O, Chomarat P, Flores-Romo L, Ait-Yahia S, Maat C, et al. T cell interleukin-17 induces stromal cells to produce proinflammatory and hematopoietic cytokines. J Exp Med. 1996;183(6):2593–603. https://doi.org/10.1084/jem.183.6.2593.
40. Persson EK, Verstraete K, Heyndrickx I, Gevaert E, Aegerter H, Percier JM, et al. Protein crystallization promotes type 2 immunity and is reversible by antibody treatment. Science. 2019;364(6442):eaaw4295. https://doi.org/10.1126/science.aaw4295.
41. Ueki S, Tokunaga T, Melo RCN, Saito H, Honda K, Fukuchi M, et al. Charcot-Leyden crystal formation is closely associated with eosinophil extracellular trap cell death. Blood. 2018;132(20):2183–7. https://doi.org/10.1182/blood-2018-04-842260.
42. Rodriguez-Alcazar JF, Ataide MA, Engels G, Schmitt-Mabmunyo C, Garbi N, Kastenmuller W, et al. Charcot-Leyden crystals activate the NLRP3 inflammasome and cause IL-1beta inflammation in human macrophages. J Immunol. 2019;202(2):550–8. https://doi.org/10.4049/jimmunol.1800107.
43. Gevaert E, Delemarre T, De Volder J, Zhang N, Holtappels G, De Ruyck N, et al. Charcot-Leyden crystals promote neutrophilic inflammation in patients with nasal polyposis. J Allergy Clin Immunol. 2019; https://doi.org/10.1016/j.jaci.2019.08.027.
44. Wang X, Du J, Zhao C. Bacterial biofilms are associated with inflammatory cells infiltration and the innate immunity in chronic rhinosinusitis with or without nasal polyps. Inflammation. 2014;37(3):871–9. https://doi.org/10.1007/s10753-013-9807-8.
45. Van Zele T, Gevaert P, Watelet J-B, Claeys G, Holtappels G, Claeys C, et al. Staphylococcus aureus colonization and IgE antibody formation to enterotoxins is increased in nasal polyposis. J Allergy Clin Immunol. 2004;114(4):981. https://doi.org/10.1016/j.jaci.2004.07.013.
46. Suh JD, Ramakrishnan V, Palmer JN. Biofilms. Otolaryngol Clin N Am. 2010;43(3):521–30, viii. https://doi.org/10.1016/j.otc.2010.02.010.
47. Huvenne W, Callebaut I, Reekmans K, Hens G, Bobic S, Jorissen M, et al. Staphylococcus aureus enterotoxin B augments granulocyte migration and survival via airway epithelial cell activation. Allergy. 2010;65(8):1013–20. https://doi.org/10.1111/j.1398-9995.2009.02313.x.
48. Delgado-Rizo V, Martínez-Guzmán MA, Iñiguez-Gutierrez L, García-Orozco A, Alvarado-Navarro A, Fafutis-Morris M. Neutrophil extracellular traps and its implications in inflammation: an overview. Front Immunol. 2017;8:81. https://doi.org/10.3389/fimmu.2017.00081.
49. Cao Y, Chen F, Sun Y, Hong H, Wen Y, Lai Y, et al. LL-37 promotes neutrophil extracellular trap formation in chronic rhinosinusitis with nasal polyps. Clin Exp Allergy. 2019b;49(7):990–9. https://doi.org/10.1111/cea.13408.
50. Tan BK, Li QZ, Suh L, Kato A, Conley DB, Chandra RK, et al. Evidence for intranasal antinuclear autoantibodies in patients with chronic rhinosinusitis with nasal polyps. J Allergy Clin Immunol. 2011;128(6):1198–206.e1. https://doi.org/10.1016/j.jaci.2011.08.037.
51. Ueki S, Melo RC, Ghiran I, Spencer LA, Dvorak AM, Weller PF. Eosinophil extracellular DNA trap cell death mediates lytic release of free secretion-competent eosinophil granules in humans. Blood. 2013;121(11):2074–83. https://doi.org/10.1182/blood-2012-05-432088.
52. Clancy DM, Sullivan GP, Moran HBT, Henry CM, Reeves EP, McElvaney NG, et al. Extracellular neutrophil proteases are efficient regulators of IL-1, IL-33, and IL-36 cytokine activity but poor effectors

of microbial killing. Cell Rep. 2018;22(11):2937–50. https://doi.org/10.1016/j.celrep.2018.02.062.
53. Kato A. Immunopathology of chronic rhinosinusitis. Allergol Int. 2015;64(2):121–30. https://doi.org/10.1016/j.alit.2014.12.006.
54. Silvestre-Roig C, Hidalgo A, Soehnlein O. Neutrophil heterogeneity: implications for homeostasis and pathogenesis. Blood. 2016;127(18):2173–81. https://doi.org/10.1182/blood-2016-01-688887.
55. Sun B, Zhu L, Tao Y, Sun HX, Li Y, Wang P, et al. Characterization and allergic role of IL-33-induced neutrophil polarization. Cell Mol Immunol. 2018;15(8):782–93. https://doi.org/10.1038/cmi.2017.163.
56. Cox G. Glucocorticoid treatment inhibits apoptosis in human neutrophils. Separation of survival and activation outcomes. J Immunol. 1995;154(9):4719–25.
57. Liles WC, Dale DC, Klebanoff SJ. Glucocorticoids inhibit apoptosis of human neutrophils. Blood. 1995;86(8):3181–8.
58. Moon A, Gil S, Gill SE, Chen P, Matute-Bello G. Doxycycline impairs neutrophil migration to the airspaces of the lung in mice exposed to intratracheal lipopolysaccharide. J Inflamm (Lond). 2012;9(1):31. https://doi.org/10.1186/1476-9255-9-31.
59. Takeshita S, Ono Y, Kozuma K, Suzuki M, Kawamura Y, Yokoyama N, et al. Modulation of oxidative burst of neutrophils by doxycycline in patients with acute myocardial infarction. J Antimicrob Chemother. 2002;49(2):411–3. https://doi.org/10.1093/jac/49.2.411.
60. Wang H, Pan L, Liu Z. Neutrophils as a protagonist and target in chronic rhinosinusitis. Clin Exp Otorhinolaryngol. 2019;12(4):337–47. https://doi.org/10.21053/ceo.2019.00654
61. Todd CM, Salter BM, Murphy DM, Watson RM, Howie KJ, Milot J, et al. The effects of a CXCR1/CXCR2 antagonist on neutrophil migration in mild atopic asthmatic subjects. Pulm Pharmacol Ther. 2016;41:34–9. https://doi.org/10.1016/j.pupt.2016.09.005.
62. Natsis NE, Gottlieb AB. Bimekizumab for the treatment of psoriatic disease. Expert Opin Biol Ther. 2018;18(12):1193–7. https://doi.org/10.1080/14712598.2018.1538351.
63. Bachert C, Han JK, Desrosiers M, Hellings PW, Amin N, Lee SE, et al. Efficacy and safety of dupilumab in patients with severe chronic rhinosinusitis with nasal polyps (LIBERTY NP SINUS-24 and LIBERTY NP SINUS-52): results from two multicentre, randomised, double-blind, placebo-controlled, parallel-group phase 3 trials. Lancet (London, England). 2019;394(10209):1638–50. https://doi.org/10.1016/s0140-6736(19)31881-1.

10 Remodeling Features

Lili Shi and Zheng Liu

Key Points

- Different types of chronic rhinosinusitis (CRS) show distinct remodeling patterns. Fibrosis is the main histopathological feature of CRSsNP, while edema is the featured tissue remodeling in CRSwNP, especially in eosinophilic type.
- Epithelial-mesenchymal transition (EMT)/transforming growth factor (TGF), matrix metalloproteinase (MMP)/tissue inhibitor of metalloproteinase (TIMP) imbalance, and coagulation system are involved in different types of tissue remodeling in CRS.
- Tissue remodeling is associated with inflammation patterns in CRS.

10.1 Introduction

Remodeling refers to the dynamic process leading to transient or permanent changes in tissue architecture that includes extracellular matrix production or degradation and epithelium changes. For chronic rhinosinusitis (CRS), this process may include one or several following events: loss of cilia, loss of epithelial integrity, goblet cell hyperplasia, basement membrane (BM) thickening, excessive deposition of collagen fibers and fibrin, and edema [1–3]. Tissue remodeling in CRS is regulated by numerous factors. So far, various cytokines, growth factors, proteases, and coagulation factors have been reported involved in the tissue remodeling in CRS [4].

L. Shi · Z. Liu (✉)
Department of Otolaryngology, Head and Neck Surgery, Tongji Hospital, Tongji Medical College, Huazhong University of Science and Technology, Wuhan, China

10.2 The Features of Tissue Remodeling in Different Types of CRS

According to the European Position Paper on Rhinosinusitis and Nasal Polyps (EPOS), CRS can be clinically divided into CRS with nasal polyps (CRSwNP) and CRS without nasal polyps (CRSsNP) [5]. These two subtypes of CRS show significant difference in remodeling pattern, although no specific cell type or protein expression can completely explain the distinct histologic changes noted in CRSwNP and CRSsNP. Four types of tissue remodeling can be found in CRS according to Hellquist's classification, including fibrosis type, edematous type, glandular type, and atypical type [6]. Although these types of tissue remodeling can occur simultaneously in CRS, different subtypes of CRS may be dominated by one kind of tissue remodeling. CRSsNP shows prominent fibrosis with thickening of the collagen fibers (fibrosis type), whereas

L. Zhang, C. Bachert (eds.), *Chronic Rhinosinusitis*, https://doi.org/10.1007/978-981-16-0784-4_10

CRSwNP generally demonstrates tissue edema with albumin deposition and pseudocyst formation (edematous type) [4, 7]. As a highly heterogeneous disorder, CRS is more heterogeneous than this clinical classification. In Caucasians, CRSsNP presents a type 1 response, whereas CRSwNP is dominated by eosinophilic inflammation with a skewed type 2 response. However, in East Asia, a considerable number of CRSwNP patients do not demonstrate eosinophilic inflammation [8, 9], and non-eosinophilic CRSwNP is characterized by a type 1/type 17 cytokine milieu and a more neutrophilic inflammation [8, 9]. Both eosinophilic and non-eosinophilic CRSwNP demonstrate obvious edema formation in lamina propria in comparison to the diseased mucosa tissues of CRSsNP. However, non-eosinophilic CRSwNP is less edematous and more fibrotic than eosinophilic CRSwNP [10]. In addition, both CRSsNP and CRSwNP demonstrate goblet cell hyperplasia within the epithelial lining, nevertheless CRSsNP additionally exhibits high density of subepithelial hyperplastic glands [11]. Hyperplasia of submucosal glands is common in CRSsNP but rare in CRSwNP, especially in the eosinophilic form. The atypical type is characterized by large, pleomorphic histiocytes, however, is rarely found in CRS.

10.3 The Mechanism of Tissue Remodeling in CRS

Tremendous efforts have been put in the researches on the underlying mechanisms of tissue remodeling in CRS. Until now, epithelial-mesenchymal transition (EMT)/transforming growth factor (TGF), matrix metalloproteinase (MMP)/tissue inhibitor of metalloproteinase (TIMP) imbalance, and coagulation system have been implicated in different types of tissue remodeling in CRS. TGF-β1 can induce EMT, which leads to transformation of epithelial cells to interstitial fibroblasts and production of extracellular matrix (ECM) [12]. Nevertheless, tissue remodeling is a dynamic process involving not only the deposition and production, but also the degradation of ECM. The balance of proteases and protease inhibitors [3], such as MMPs and TIMPs, play a critical role in the degradation of ECM. It has been shown that TGF-β and MMPs are critical pro-fibrotic cytokine and ECM-degrading protease involved in tissue remodeling in CRS, respectively [10, 13]. Upregulation of the coagulation cascade and downregulation of fibrinolysis may result in enhanced fibrin deposition in nasal mucosa, which retains water in lamina propria of nasal mucosa and promote edema formation [14, 15]. During this process, an important factor of regulating fibrin degradation, tissue plasminogen activator (t-PA), is decreased in CRSwNP. The downregulation of t-PA can be induced by both type 2 and type 1 cytokines. Therefore, t-PA downregulation may be a common mechanism for the edema formation in different phenotypic CRSwNP, such as eosinophilic and non-eosinophilic CRSwNP [15].

Fibrosis is the main histopathological feature of CRSsNP. CRSsNP shows increased fibrosis with high levels of TGF-β1 or TGF-β2 in diseased sinonasal mucosa. In addition, the upregulated TGF-β receptor I, TGF-β receptor II, and signal transducer Smad3 have been demonstrated in CRSsNP, reflecting the activation of TGF-β signaling pathway [16]. In contrast, compared to the diseased sinonasal mucosa from CRSsNP patients and normal nasal tissues, there are lower TGF-β1 protein concentration, downregulated TGF-βRII expression, and decreased number of pSmad 2-positive cells in CRSwNP, indicating a low level of TGF-β signaling activation and deficiency in tissue fibrosis in CRSwNP [13]. These findings are compatible with the contrary remodeling patterns observed in CRSsNP and CRSwNP, including the lack of collagen in CRSwNP, and excessive collagen production with thickening of the collagen fibers in the ECM of CRSsNP. However, there are some controversies regarding the TGF-β1 expression in CRS [17]. Cao et al. found that the TGF-β1 mRNA expression was downregulated in all types of CRS including CRSsNP, and eosinophilic and non-eosinophilic CRSwNP in Chinese patients [11]. However, Li et al. and Van Bruaene et al. found that TGF-β1 protein levels were significantly increased in CRSsNP but decreased in CRSwNP of Chinese and Caucasians [3, 13]. The factors contributing to these discrepancies are not very clear. Nevertheless, it is well known that the regulation of TGF-β1 mainly occurs at the posttranscriptional level [16]. TGF-β1 is mainly expressed by infiltrating inflammatory cells and ciliary cells in epithelium of CRSsNP and CRSwNP [18]. The dominant inflammatory cells producing TGF-β1are granulocytes [18].

TGF-β1 is an important cytokine to induce EMT, and cause local aggregation of interstitial fibroblasts which derive from epithelial cells [12, 19]. EMT is a cellular process whereby epithelial cells acquire mesenchymal properties, and lose cell–cell interactions and apico-basal polarity, eventually contributing to the local fibroblast pool [20]. The features of EMT include decreased expression of epithelial markers, such as E-cadherin, β-catenin, and cytokeratin, and increased expression of mesenchymal markers, including α-smooth muscle actin (α-SMA), vimentin, and fibronectin. TGF-β/Smad is the main pathway that is activated in EMT, nevertheless, TGF-β can also promote EMT through non-Smad signaling pathways, including mitogen activated protein kinase (MAPK) pathway, Rho-like GTPase signaling pathway, and phosphatidylinositol 3-kinase/Akt pathways, etc. [21]. Although nasal polyps are characterized by significant edema formation, EMT has also been found involved in tissue remodeling in CRSwNP by some studies. It has been reported that EMT was initiated by TGF-β1-induced MAPK and Snail/Slug signaling pathways in CRSwNP [22]. TGF-β1 can also induce EMT through microRNA-21 and via activation of histone deacetylase 2 (HDAC2) and HDAC4 in CRSwNP [23, 24]. In addition, hypoxia is considered a critical factor of initiating EMT in CRSwNP via hypoxia-inducible factor (HIF)-1α [25]. In addition to hypoxia, IFN-γ is able to induce EMT of nasal epithelial cells through the p38 and extracellular signal-regulated kinase (ERK) pathways, distinct from HIF-1α and Smad signaling pathways in CRSwNP [26]. However, generally, EMT is associated with ECM production and tissue fibrosis. Therefore, the role of EMT in nasal polyps, where the edema is the predominant tissue remodeling type with low levels of TGF-β pathway activation, requires further investigation. On the other hand, although CRSsNP is characterized by tissue fibrosis, the contribution of EMT to tissue remodeling in CRSsNP remain poorly studied.

Except for TGF-β1, TGF-β2 has been reported to be the predominant isoform expressed in severe asthma and associated with local fibrosis [27]. Van Bruaene found that TGF-β2 protein levels increased comparably in CRSsNP and CRSwNP compared to controls in Caucasians [17]. However, Shi LL et al. found that TGF-β2 protein level was significantly upregulated in CRSsNP in comparison with CRSwNP and controls in Chinese [10]. Notably, TGF-β2 levels were positively correlated with the number of myofibroblasts and the expression of fibronectin in CRS, underscoring the potential importance of the TGF-β2 in local fibrosis formation in CRS [28]. Importantly, neutrophils have been found as the main sources of TGF-β2 in CRS [10].

Other cytokines have also been reported involved in fibrosis in CRS. Platelet-derived growth factor (PDGF) is indicated to be an important cytokine in the pathogenesis of rhinosinusitis by promoting tissue fibrosis [29]. PDGF can be produced by gland cells, vascular endothelial cells, inflammatory cells, and epithelial cells in CRSwNP with asthma, which acts on epithelial cells and fibroblasts and may play a role in polyp formation [29]. In addition, periostin, a tissue remodeling molecule secreted by epithelial cells in type 2 inflammation, is associated with basement membrane thickening, tissue eosinophilia, and fibrosis in CRS [28].

Edema is the featured tissue remodeling in CRSwNP, especially in eosinophilic type. Imbalance of MMPs and TIMPs is critical for the edema formation in CRSwNP [3, 30, 31]. Reduced TIMP-1 and -4 expression lead to the disinhibition of MMP-1, 2, 7, 9, resulting in ECM degradation and edema formation in CRSwNP [3, 10, 32]. Of note, the expression of MMPs has been found to be regulated by damage-associated molecular pattern molecules (DAMPs) [33]. It is well known that chronic inflammation can be triggered and sustained not only by exogenous pathogen-associated molecular pattern molecules that are expressed on invading microorganisms, but also the endogenous DAMPs released from host cells under pathological stress [33]. DAMPs have been indicated to participate in tissue remodeling process of CRSwNP [33, 34]. Cold-inducible RNA-binding protein (CIRP) is a newly identified DAMP. Shi et al. found that CIRP expressed in nasal epithelial cells and $CD68^+$ macrophages in sinonasal tissues. The upregulated production and release of CIRP from nasal epithelial cells and macrophages may contribute to the edema formation in both eosinophilic and non-eosinophilic CRSwNP by inducing MMPs (MMP2, MMP7, MMP9, and MMP12) and VEGF-A production from epithelial cells and macrophages [33].

Recently, dysregulation of the coagulation cascade has been reported to play an important role in CRSwNP, associating with excessive deposition of fibrin and edema formation [35]. Extravascular fibrin can be degraded to fibrin degradation products (FDPs) by plasmin, thereby preventing excessive fibrin deposition [36]. Plasmin is generated through cleavage of plasminogen by t-PA [37]. The downregulated t-PA production in airway epithelial cells may contribute to the excessive fibrin deposition and edema formation in CRSwNP [38]. t-PA level is reduced in the presence of type-1 and type-2 cytokines, which facilitates dysregulated fibrin deposition and then promotes water retaining and edema formation in nasal polyps [15, 39]. Although IL-17A upregulates the production of t-PA at both mRNA and protein levels, the combination of IFN-γ and IL-13 significantly reduces t-PA level even in the presence of IL-17A [15]. In CRSwNP, type-2 inflammation can lead to the recruitment of M2 macrophages and the subsequent production of FXIII-A, which induces excessive fibrin deposition by cross-linking fibrin directly and blocking the action of plasmin through the cross-link of α2-plasmin inhibitor (α2PI) with fibrin [38]. Additionally, the role of the complement system in CRSwNP has been studied [39]. The levels of C3a and C5a are significantly increased in nasal secretions from CRSwNP patients compared to controls [39]. Both C3a and C5a can increase vascular permeability and lead to plasma exudation and albumin accumulation as a consequence.

10.4 Correlation Between Tissue Remodeling and Inflammation Patterns in CRS

Different types of CRS show distinct remodeling patterns. Tissue remodeling is demonstrated to be associated with inflammation patterns in CRS of Chinese patients. It has been showed that eosinophilic and neutrophilic inflammation is positively correlated with the severity of edema and fibrosis in CRS, respectively. The eosinophil cationic protein (ECP) levels are positively correlated with edema but negatively correlated with the expression of profibrotic factors. Eosinophil-derived neurotoxin (EDN) is an eosinophil granule protein that induces production of MMP-9 by the nasal epithelium [40]. Therefore, eosinophilic inflammation may contribute to the remarkable edema in eosinophilic CRSwNP [10]. As mentioned above, TGF-β2 mainly derived from neutrophils is upregulated in CRSsNP and non-eosinophilic CRSwNP compared with control and eosinophilic CRSwNP [10]. The number of TGF-β2-positive cells is positively correlated with the number of myofibroblasts and the expression level of fibronectin. In the context of CRS, both epithelial shedding and BM thickness are strongly correlated with the number of infiltrating eosinophils and IL-17A-positive cells [41, 42]. $CD8^+$ cytotoxic T lymphocytes (Tc) are the main IL-17A production cells in the polyp tissues of CRSwNP patients [43]. IL-17A promotes the expression of MMP-9 in human primary nasal epithelial cells by activating the NF-κB signal pathway, revealing the crucial role of IL-17A and Tc in the tissue remodeling of CRSwNP [43]. In addition, $V\gamma 1^+$ γδT cells can induce eosinophilic inflammation, which promotes the formation of edema [44]. In Caucasian patients, IL-5 levels correlate with TIMP-1 levels in CRSwNP, while multiple correlations are found between ECP, MMP-9, MMP-2, TGF-β1, and tryptase [45].

On the other hand, tissue remodeling may promote inflammation. There are significant correlations between the levels of tryptase, MMP-2, MMP-9, and TGF-β1. MMP-2, MMP-9, and TGF-β1 facilitate the migration of eosinophil and mast cell to nasal polyps [46]. Thrombin is regarded as a regulator of tissue remodeling with the ability to promote inflammatory responses, which affects airway permeability and eosinophil migration by elevating the production of inflammatory cytokines in airway epithelial cells, including IL-6, IL-8, prostaglandin E2 (PGE2), chemokine (C-C motif) ligand 2 (CCL2), PDGF, and the mucin MUC5AC [35].

Airway remodeling in asthma could occur in early life, probably on the basis of specific genetic background or epigenetic phenomena [4], challenging the paradigm that remodeling depends on the prior development of inflammation. Based on the study of "early stage" CRSsNP, Van Bruaene et al. found that TGF-β1 and collagen production could be upregulated in sinonasal mucosa before the advent of obvious inflammation [47], indicating that remodeling might be independent from the prior inflammation. Meng J et al. demonstrated that the epithelial loss was more prominent in the early stage polypoid tissues in the middle turbinate of CRSwNP patients, coupled with increased M2 type macrophages and markedly high expression of fibronectin. Remodeling appeared to occur in parallel with, rather than subsequent to, inflammation [2].

10.5 Conclusion

In brief, eosinophilic inflammation, type-2 inflammation, increased vascular permeability as well as deposition of fibrin may contribute to the remarkable edema in eosinophilic CRSwNP, whereas neutrophilic inflammation with the overproduction of TGF-β2 may closely relate to fibrosis in CRSsNP and non-eosinophilic CRSwNP.

References

1. Thiele A, Holzhausen HJ, Riederer A, Knipping S. Mucosal remodeling in chronic rhinosinusitis without nasal polyposis - an ultrastructural evaluation. Laryngorhinootologie. 2010;89(6):352–7. https://doi.org/10.1055/s-0030-1249022.
2. Meng J, Zhou P, Liu Y, Liu F, Yi X, Liu S, et al. The development of nasal polyp disease involves early nasal mucosal inflammation and remodelling. PLoS One. 2013;8(12):e82373. https://doi.org/10.1371/journal.pone.0082373.
3. Li X, Meng J, Qiao X, Liu Y, Liu F, Zhang N, et al. Expression of TGF, matrix metalloproteinases, and tissue inhibitors in Chinese chronic rhinosinusitis. J Allergy Clin Immunol. 2010;125(5):1061–8. https://doi.org/10.1016/j.jaci.2010.02.023.
4. Bousquet J, Jacot W, Vignola AM, Bachert C, Van Cauwenberge P. Allergic rhinitis: a disease remodeling the upper airways? J Allergy Clin Immunol. 2004;113(1):43–9. https://doi.org/10.1016/j.jaci.2003.09.047.
5. Fokkens WJ, Lund VJ, Mullol J, Bachert C, Alobid I, Baroody F, et al. European position paper on rhinosinusitis and nasal polyps 2012. Rhinol Suppl. 2012;23:3 p preceding table of contents, 1–298.
6. Watelet JB, Dogne JM, Mullier F. Remodeling and repair in rhinosinusitis. Curr Allergy Asthma Rep. 2015;15(6):34. https://doi.org/10.1007/s11882-015-0531-3.
7. Hellquist HB. Nasal polyps update. Histopathology. Allergy Asthma Proc. 1996;17(5):237–42.
8. Van Crombruggen K, Zhang N, Gevaert P, Tomassen P, Bachert C. Pathogenesis of chronic rhinosinusitis: inflammation. J Allergy Clin Immunol. 2011;128(4):728–32. https://doi.org/10.1016/j.jaci.2011.07.049.
9. Wang X, Zhang N, Bo M, Holtappels G, Zheng M, Lou H, et al. Diversity of T(H) cytokine profiles in patients with chronic rhinosinusitis: a multicenter study in Europe, Asia, and Oceania. J Allergy Clin Immunol. 2016;138(5):1344–53. https://doi.org/10.1016/j.jaci.2016.05.041.
10. Shi LL, Xiong P, Zhang L, Cao PP, Liao B, Lu X, et al. Features of airway remodeling in different types of Chinese chronic rhinosinusitis are associated with inflammation patterns. Allergy. 2013;68(1):101–9. https://doi.org/10.1111/all.12064.
11. Cao PP, Li HB, Wang BF, Wang SB, You XJ, Cui YH, et al. Distinct immunopathologic characteristics of various types of chronic rhinosinusitis in adult Chinese. J Allergy Clin Immunol. 2009;124(3):478–84, 84.e1–2. https://doi.org/10.1016/j.jaci.2009.05.017.
12. Hackett TL, Warner SM, Stefanowicz D, Shaheen F, Pechkovsky DV, Murray LA, et al. Induction of epithelial-mesenchymal transition in primary airway epithelial cells from patients with asthma by transforming growth factor-beta1. Am J Respir Crit Care Med. 2009;180(2):122–33. https://doi.org/10.1164/rccm.200811-1730OC.
13. Van Bruaene N, Derycke L, Perez-Novo CA, Gevaert P, Holtappels G, De Ruyck N, et al. TGF-beta signaling and collagen deposition in chronic rhinosinusitis. J Allergy Clin Immunol. 2009;124(2):253–9, 9.e1–2. https://doi.org/10.1016/j.jaci.2009.04.013.
14. Takabayashi T, Schleimer RP. Formation of nasal polyps: the roles of innate type 2 inflammation and deposition of fibrin. J Allergy Clin Immunol.

2020;145(3):740–50. https://doi.org/10.1016/j.jaci.2020.01.027.
15. Chen CL, Yao Y, Pan L, Hu ST, Ma J, Wang ZC, et al. Common fibrin deposition and tissue plasminogen activator downregulation in nasal polyps with distinct inflammatory endotypes. J Allergy Clin Immunol. 2020; https://doi.org/10.1016/j.jaci.2020.02.010.
16. Li YC, An YS, Wang T, Zang HR. Analysis of transforming growth factor β signaling in chronic rhinosinusitis. Chin Med J. 2013;126(17):3340–3.
17. Watelet JB, Claeys C, Perez-Novo C, Gevaert P, Van Cauwenberge P, Bachert C. Transforming growth factor beta1 in nasal remodeling: differences between chronic rhinosinusitis and nasal polyposis. Am J Rhinol. 2004;18(5):267–72.
18. Liu Z, Lu X, Wang H, Gao Q, Cui Y. The up-regulated expression of tenascin C in human nasal polyp tissues is related to eosinophil-derived transforming growth factor beta1. Am J Rhinol. 2006;20(6):629–33. https://doi.org/10.2500/ajr.2006.20.2918.
19. Iwano M, Plieth D, Danoff TM, Xue C, Okada H, Neilson EG. Evidence that fibroblasts derive from epithelium during tissue fibrosis. J Clin Invest. 2002;110(3):341–50. https://doi.org/10.1172/jci15518.
20. Thiery JP, Sleeman JP. Complex networks orchestrate epithelial-mesenchymal transitions. Nat Rev Mol Cell Biol. 2006;7(2):131–42. https://doi.org/10.1038/nrm1835.
21. Zhang YE. Non-Smad pathways in TGF-beta signaling. Cell Res. 2009;19(1):128–39. https://doi.org/10.1038/cr.2008.328.
22. Yang HW, Lee SA, Shin JM, Park IH, Lee HM. Glucocorticoids ameliorate TGF-β1-mediated epithelial-to-mesenchymal transition of airway epithelium through MAPK and Snail/Slug signaling pathways. Sci Rep. 2017;7(1):3486. https://doi.org/10.1038/s41598-017-02358-z.
23. Li X, Li C, Zhu G, Yuan W, Xiao ZA. TGF-β1 induces epithelial-mesenchymal transition of chronic sinusitis with nasal polyps through microRNA-21. Int Arch Allergy Immunol. 2019;179(4):304–19. https://doi.org/10.1159/000497829.
24. Park IH, Kang JH, Shin JM, Lee HM. Trichostatin a inhibits epithelial mesenchymal transition induced by TGF-β1 in airway epithelium. PLoS One. 2016;11(8):e0162058. https://doi.org/10.1371/journal.pone.0162058.
25. Shin HW, Cho K, Kim DW, Han DH, Khalmuratova R, Kim SW, et al. Hypoxia-inducible factor 1 mediates nasal polypogenesis by inducing epithelial-to-mesenchymal transition. Am J Respir Crit Care Med. 2012;185(9):944–54. https://doi.org/10.1164/rccm.201109-1706OC.
26. Lee M, Kim DW, Khalmuratova R, Shin SH, Kim YM, Han DH, et al. The IFN-γ-p38, ERK kinase axis exacerbates neutrophilic chronic rhinosinusitis by inducing the epithelial-to-mesenchymal transition. Mucosal Immunol. 2019;12(3):601–11. https://doi.org/10.1038/s41385-019-0149-1.
27. Balzar S, Chu HW, Silkoff P, Cundall M, Trudeau JB, Strand M, et al. Increased TGF-beta2 in severe asthma with eosinophilia. J Allergy Clin Immunol. 2005;115(1):110–7. https://doi.org/10.1016/j.jaci.2004.09.034.
28. Ebenezer JA, Christensen JM, Oliver BG, Oliver RA, Tjin G, Ho J, et al. Periostin as a marker of mucosal remodelling in chronic rhinosinusitis. Rhinology. 2017;55(3):234–41. https://doi.org/10.4193/Rhin16.215.
29. Kouzaki H, Seno S, Fukui J, Owaki S, Shimizu T. Role of platelet-derived growth factor in airway remodeling in rhinosinusitis. Am J Rhinol Allergy. 2009;23(3):273–80. https://doi.org/10.2500/ajra.2009.23.3310.
30. Bhandari A, Takeuchi K, Suzuki S, Harada T, Hayashi S, Imanaka-Yoshida K, et al. Increased expression of matrix metalloproteinase-2 in nasal polyps. Acta Otolaryngol. 2004;124(10):1165–70. https://doi.org/10.1080/00016480410017152.
31. Kahveci OK, Derekoy FS, Yilmaz M, Serteser M, Altuntas A. The role of MMP-9 and TIMP-1 in nasal polyp formation. Swiss Med Wkly. 2008;138(45–46):684–8.
32. Malinsky RR, Valera FC, Cavallari FE, Küpper DS, Milaneze C, Silva JS, et al. Matrix metalloproteinases and their impact on sinusal extension in chronic rhinosinusitis with nasal polyps. Eur Archiv Otorhinolaryngol. 2013;270(4):1345–8. https://doi.org/10.1007/s00405-012-2219-9.
33. Shi LL, Ma J, Deng YK, Chen CL, Wang H, Cao PP, et al. Cold-inducible RNA-binding protein contributes to tissue remodeling in chronic rhinosinusitis with nasal polyps. Allergy. 2020; https://doi.org/10.1111/all.14287.
34. Van Crombruggen K, Jacob F, Zhang N, Bachert C. Damage-associated molecular patterns and their receptors in upper airway pathologies. Cell Mol Life Sci. 2013;70(22):4307–21. https://doi.org/10.1007/s00018-013-1356-7.
35. Kim DY, Cho SH, Takabayashi T, Schleimer RP. Chronic rhinosinusitis and the coagulation system. Allergy, Asthma Immunol Res. 2015;7(5):421–30. https://doi.org/10.4168/aair.2015.7.5.421.
36. Idell S. Coagulation, fibrinolysis, and fibrin deposition in acute lung injury. Crit Care Med. 2003;31(4 Suppl):S213–20. https://doi.org/10.1097/01.Ccm.0000057846.21303.Ab.
37. Del Rosso M, Fibbi G, Pucci M, Margheri F, Serrati S. The plasminogen activation system in inflammation. Front Biosci. 2008;13:4667–86. https://doi.org/10.2741/3032.
38. Takabayashi T, Kato A, Peters AT, Hulse KE, Suh LA, Carter R, et al. Increased expression of factor XIII-A in patients with chronic rhinosinusitis with nasal polyps. J Allergy Clin Immunol. 2013;132(3):584–92.e4. https://doi.org/10.1016/j.jaci.2013.02.003.
39. Van Zele T, Coppieters F, Gevaert P, Holtappels G, Van Cauwenberge P, Bachert C. Local complement activation in nasal polyposis. Laryngoscope.

2009;119(9):1753–8. https://doi.org/10.1002/lary.20484.
40. Tsuda T, Maeda Y, Nishide M, Koyama S, Hayama Y, Nojima S, et al. Eosinophil-derived neurotoxin enhances airway remodeling in eosinophilic chronic rhinosinusitis and correlates with disease severity. Int Immunol. 2019;31(1):33–40. https://doi.org/10.1093/intimm/dxy061.
41. Saitoh T, Kusunoli T, Yao T, Kawano K, Kojima Y, Miyahara K, et al. Relationship between epithelial damage or basement membrane thickness and eosinophilic infiltration in nasal polyps with chronic rhinosinusitis. Rhinology. 2009;47(3):275–9. https://doi.org/10.4193/Rhin08.109.
42. Saitoh T, Kusunoki T, Yao T, Kawano K, Kojima Y, Miyahara K, et al. Role of interleukin-17A in the eosinophil accumulation and mucosal remodeling in chronic rhinosinusitis with nasal polyps associated with asthma. Int Arch Allergy Immunol. 2010;151(1):8–16. https://doi.org/10.1159/000232566.
43. Chen X, Chang L, Li X, Huang J, Yang L, Lai X, et al. Tc17/IL-17A up-regulated the expression of MMP-9 via NF-κB pathway in nasal epithelial cells of patients with chronic rhinosinusitis. Front Immunol. 2018;9:2121. https://doi.org/10.3389/fimmu.2018.02121.
44. Yang LY, Li X, Li WT, Huang JC, Wang ZY, Huang ZZ, et al. Vγ1$^+$ γδT cells are correlated with increasing expression of eosinophil cationic protein and metalloproteinase-7 in chronic rhinosinusitis with nasal polyps inducing the formation of edema. Allergy, Asthma Immunol Res. 2017;9(2):142–51. https://doi.org/10.4168/aair.2017.9.2.142.
45. Chen YS, Langhammer T, Westhofen M, Lorenzen J. Relationship between matrix metalloproteinases MMP-2, MMP-9, tissue inhibitor of matrix metalloproteinases-1 and IL-5, IL-8 in nasal polyps. Allergy. 2007;62(1):66–72. https://doi.org/10.1111/j.1398-9995.2006.01255.x.
46. Lee YM, Kim SS, Kim HA, Suh YJ, Lee SK, Nahm DH, et al. Eosinophil inflammation of nasal polyp tissue: relationships with matrix metalloproteinases, tissue inhibitor of metalloproteinase-1, and transforming growth factor-beta1. J Korean Med Sci. 2003;18(1):97–102. https://doi.org/10.3346/jkms.2003.18.1.97.
47. Van Bruaene N, C PN, Van Crombruggen K, De Ruyck N, Holtappels G, Van Cauwenberge P, et al. Inflammation and remodelling patterns in early stage chronic rhinosinusitis. Clin Exp Allergy. 2012;42(6):883–90. https://doi.org/10.1111/j.1365-2222.2011.03898.x.

Nasal Mucociliary Clearance

11

Jian Jiao and Luo Zhang

Key Points

- Mucociliary clearance is a key first-line defense of the respiratory tract.
- Mucus and cilia are two principal components of the mucociliary clearance apparatus.
- Several approaches and techniques have been used to assess mucociliary clearance and ciliary function.
- Impairment of nasal mucociliary clearance has commonly been reported in CRS and plays an important role in disease progression.
- Common microbial pathogens, environmental toxins, and inflammatory cytokines play important roles in mucociliary dysfunction in CRS.

J. Jiao
Department of Otolaryngology, Head and Neck Surgery, Beijing Tongren Hospital, Capital Medical University, Beijing, China

Beijing Key Laboratory of Nasal Diseases, Beijing Institute of Otolaryngology, Beijing, China

L. Zhang (✉)
Department of Otolaryngology, Head and Neck Surgery, Beijing Tongren Hospital, Capital Medical University, Beijing, China

Beijing Key Laboratory of Nasal Diseases, Beijing Institute of Otolaryngology, Beijing, China

Department of Allergy, Beijing Tongren Hospital, Capital Medical University, Beijing, China

11.1 Introduction

The sinonasal cavity is constantly exposed to environmental irritants such as particulate matter, allergens, microbes, and toxins [1]. Mucociliary clearance is a key first-line defense of the respiratory tract that clears the upper airways of inhaled pathogens and debris. This defense mechanism is dependent on appropriate mucus production and coordinated ciliary activity. Coordinated and directional ciliary beating enables transport of the overlying debris-laden mucus to the oropharynx, where it is swallowed or expectorated. Patients with chronic rhinosinusitis (CRS) have been reported to have impaired mucociliary clearance, which might lead to chronic exposure of the airways to inflammatory or environmental stimuli, contributing to the development and progression of this disease. In this regard, while common microbial pathogens, allergens and irritants of the respiratory mucosa have been reported to interrupt normal mucociliary function [1–4]; inflammatory factors present in patients with CRS may also play a role in impaired mucociliary clearance [5, 6]. Several approaches and techniques have been used to assess mucociliary clearance and ciliary function.

L. Zhang, C. Bachert (eds.), *Chronic Rhinosinusitis*, https://doi.org/10.1007/978-981-16-0784-4_11

11.2 Components of Mucociliary Clearance

The sinonasal epithelium provides an interface between the body and the external environment, and serves as the first-line defense barrier against inhaled particulate matter, allergens, microbes, and toxins. The majority of the epithelium in nasal cavity is pseudostratified columnar ciliated epithelium consisting of ciliated columnar epithelial cells (75%), goblet cells (20%), and a small number of progenitor basal cells (less than 5%) [7]. The ciliated cells are lined with multiple motile cilia that are composed of unique structural proteins and motor proteins that drive the coordinated directional ciliary beating critical for mucociliary clearance [8]. The goblet cells contribute to mucociliary clearance by producing mucus, which contains mucin, the principal component generating viscosity, and elasticity of mucus. Basal cells reside on the basement membrane and function as progenitor cells for other cell types during natural turnover and repair after injury.

Mucus and cilia are two principal components of the mucociliary clearance apparatus. The mucus covering the nasal epithelium traps and transports the inhaled particles and pathogens out of the airway by means of ciliary beating. The dysfunction of either mucus or cilia impairs the mucociliary clearance and contributes to the pathogenesis of multiple airway diseases, such as primary ciliary dyskinesia (PCD), cystic fibrosis (CF), chronic obstructive pulmonary disease (COPD), asthma, and chronic rhinosinusitis (CRS).

The airway surface is covered with a two-layered mucus layer, which consists of the mucus gel layer and the less viscous periciliary layer (PCL). The overlying mucus layer is a gel with properties of both a soft, elastic solid and a viscous fluid, and consists of 97% water and 3% solids (mucins, non-mucin proteins, salts, lipids, and cellular debris) [6]. The viscous properties of mucus depend on the high molecular weight glycoproteins known as mucins, which are the major protein components of the gel layer. To date, 21 human MUC genes have been identified, of which 13 are found in the airway [9]. Among these 13 mucins, 7 mucins predominate in airway protein expression: MUC1, MUC4, MUC16, MUC20, MUC5AC, MUC5B, and MUC7 [9]. MUC5AC and MUC5B are the principal gel-forming mucins in airway. In normal human airway, MUC5AC is produced primarily in proximal airways by goblet cells, whereas MUC5B is produced throughout the airways by secretory cells and by submucosal glands. The production of MUC5AC and MUC5B changes in patients with airway diseases and inflammation, for example, upregulation of MUC5AC is implicated in the pathogenesis of asthma, CF, COPD, and MUC5B is elevated in the airway of smokers [6, 9].

The production of airway mucins is regulated at transcriptional, posttranscriptional, and epigenetic level. Different stimuli, such as respiratory virus, bacterial enterotoxins, allergens, air pollutants, tobacco smoke, and cytokines (e.g. IL-4, IL-9, IL-13 IL-17, IL-23, IL-25), have been shown to increase mucin production in the airways [5, 6, 9]. Mucin production can also be regulated at posttranscriptional level and by epigenetic mechanisms, including DNA methylation and histone modification, and regulation of distant repressors via interaction with the trans factor, the CCCTC-binding factor (CTCF) [9].

The periciliary sol layer lies below the mucus gel layer and surrounds the cilia, allowing them to beat in concert to propel mucus out of the airway. It has a height of approximately 7 μm, which is equal to the height of the extended cilium, and maintenance of the depth of this layer is critically important for mucociliary clearance. Furthermore, the periciliary sol layer can prevent compression of the cilia from the overlying gel layer, and provide a water reservoir to control water distribution [10].

Each airway ciliated epithelial cell has approximately 50 to 200 cilia, measuring 5 ~ 7 μm in length and 0.2 ~ 0.3 μm in diameter [7]. The cilium is composed of the highly conserved 9 + 2 axoneme that extends from the basal body and has an overlying membrane, which is a continuous part of the cell plasma membrane. The axoneme of motile cilia consists of nine outer doublet microtubules surrounding two central singlet microtubules, surrounded by an inner sheath. Each outer doublet consists of a complete tubule (the A tubule) containing 13 tubulin subunits, and a partial tubule (the B tubule) containing 11 tubulin subunits. The doublets are connected to each other by a large protein complex, the nexin-dynein regulatory complex (N-DRC). The two central microtubules are attached to each other by paired bridges and to the outer doublets by radial spokes. Furthermore, the A tubule is attached to inner dynein arm (IDA) and outer dynein arm (ODA), which are multi-subunit protein complexes composed of one or more dynein heavy chain (DHC) proteins, dynein intermediate chain proteins, and dynein light chain proteins [11]. For ciliary motility, the DHC is activated by ATP, leading the doublet microtubules to slide relative to one another. The presence of N-DRC and radial spokes-central pair interactions generate a controlled bending, yielding a ciliary beat with an effective stroke and a recovery stroke within the same plane [11].

Physiologically, the airway cilia beat in a coordinated manner known as metachronal wave to clear the mucus containing pathogens and debris out of the nasal sinuses and airways. The basal ciliary beat frequency (CBF) ranges from 10 to 20 Hz, yielding a mucociliary clearance velocity of approximately 5.5 mm/min. The coordination of ciliary beating is achieved through multistep events occurring both at submicrometer scale and at the entire organ scale [12]. Studies in different types of multiciliated cells have shown that basal bodies of a given cell are oriented in the same direction, which is necessary for coordinated beating of cilia within individual multiciliated cells [12]. The distribution and orientation of basal bodies rely on their interaction with the cytoskeletal elements. In this regard the actin network is necessary for docking basal bodies to the cell membrane and connecting basal bodies for their correct spacing, while microtubules connecting basal bodies are required for their alignment and orientation [12]. In order to establish a coordinated ciliary beat pattern, ciliary beating needs to be coordinated at the tissue-level. This is achieved by a planar cell polarity driven multistep process [12].

Ciliary beating can be increased by purinergic, adrenergic, cholinergic, and adenosine-receptor agonists, as well as various mechanical, chemical, hormonal stimuli [6, 13]. Intracellular second messengers including cyclic adenosine monophosphate (cAMP), cyclic guanosine monophosphate (cGMP), and calcium play important roles in CBF regulation [14]. CBF can additionally be affected by changes in temperature and pH [13].

11.3 Measurement of Mucociliary Clearance

The saccharin test is the easiest and most widely applied test to assess nasal mucociliary clearance. This involves the placement of 5 mg of saccharin particles on the inferior turbinate, 1 cm behind the mucocutaneous junction, and the patient is asked to sit quietly with the head tilted forward. The time taken from the placement of the particle to the first perception of a sweet taste is reported as the saccharin clearance time. Normal saccharin clearance time varies between 7 and 15 min, and patients with saccharin clearance times greater than 20 min are regarded as having abnormal nasal mucociliary clearance. In case the patient has not been able to perceive a sweet taste after 30 min, another saccharin particle is placed on the tongue to confirm the ability to taste saccharin.

A more objective and least invasive method for measuring mucociliary transport rates in vivo requires the inhalation of a radiolabeled marker that deposits on the airway surface. The short half-life isotope technetium-99 is used to label the inhaled marker, and the movement of the radioactivity is recorded using a gamma camera over periods of 1–24 h. This technique has been used in different animal models and in humans [11]. An alternative method to measure mucociliary clearance in vivo is to record the movement of individual radiopaque disks [15]. However, these methods employing radiolabeled markers are labor-intensive and expensive, and therefore not suitable for routine use. Some investigators measured mucociliary transport by recording the movement of fluorescent particles along the trachea or nasopharynx in mouse models, while others have used ex vivo preparations of trachea or bronchi to study mucociliary transport [11]. Although these studies provide valuable information, these procedures are more invasive and not easy to manipulate.

A method to measure mucociliary clearance in vitro has been established with the development of well-differentiated human airway epithelial air–liquid interface cultures. By adding fluorescence beads to the apical surfaces of these cultures, the mucociliary transport can be assessed by tracking movement of the beads appearing as swirls or hurricanes [16]. However, this method is limited because the speed of mucociliary transport and the height of mucus layer, as well as the location and size of transport area are variable in these cultures. To avoid these limitations, investigators have developed a modified mucociliary transport device (MCTD) that allows human airway epithelial cells to differentiate into a mucociliary epithelium that transports mucus in a continuous circular track. This device allows the measurement and manipulation of all features of mucociliary transport in a controlled in vitro system [17].

11.4 Assessment of Ciliary Structure and Function

The assessment of cilia includes static structure and dynamic function assessment. This involves sampling the nasal epithelium and assessing the structure of cilia, CBF, and ciliary beat pattern (CBP). Nasal ciliated epithelium can be obtained by nasal brushing, swab, and curettage; of which brushing is the most efficient method for sampling the ciliated epithelium and suitable for the evaluation of both ciliary structure and function. Nasal brushing technique usually involves brushing the inferior nasal turbinate with a cytology brush to obtain samples of the nasal epithelium [18].

The structure of ciliated epithelium and ultrastructure of cilia are commonly evaluated by transmission electron microscopy. The ciliated epithelium can be evaluated by analysis of the number of ciliated cells, mucous cells, and dead cells, as well as by analysis of damaged epithelium with incorporated ciliary loss, cellular projection, cytoplasmic bleeding, and mitochondrial damage. The assessment of ciliary structure also includes the incidence of compound cilia, central and peripheral microtubule defects, and defects in the inner and outer dynein arms. The alignment of individual cilia within the cell can be assessed by measuring the ciliary orientation [19, 20].

The CBF can be measured by video-coupled photomultiplier and photodiode techniques. These techniques capture the light intensity fluctuations from beating cilia and convert them into voltage changes, which are transferred to an oscilloscope and analyzed by special software to calculate the CBF [21]. However, these techniques are limited due to their slow sampling rate (about 30 frames per second). The development of digital imaging techniques has made it possible to perform high-speed imaging (as high as 400 frames per second) with multiple analyses for measuring CBF. Moreover, by using digital high-speed video microscopy (DHSV), investigators can perform real-time visualization of the ciliary waveform and assess complete ciliary function, including CBF and CBP [18]. Using this technology, it is recommended that CBF is be determined manually by measuring the time required for a group of cilia to complete a minimum of five ciliary beat cycles. In addition to manual evaluation, CBF can also be calculated using computer algorithms developed based on the variations in light intensity in the pixels of the recorded video images over time. Computer-assisted calculation of CBF can be either semi-automated or fully automated. Semi-automated programing requires the operator to select the specific regions of interest (ROIs) in a captured image before the CBF is calculated by the software, while fully automated whole field analysis (WFA) automatically analyzes the entire captured image without the need for selection of ROIs. Although computer-assisted CBF analysis is time-saving and ensures a certain degree of reproducibility, there are also some limitations of the technique; in particular the manual selection of ROIs might introduce a selection bias in semi-automated methods, whereas the setting of CBF ranges in some automated programs miss ciliary beating outside these ranges [18, 22].

11.5 Mucociliary Clearance in Chronic Rhinosinusitis

An impairment of mucociliary clearance has commonly been reported in CRS, and the degree of impairment correlated with the severity of CRS [4, 23, 24]. Multiple studies have reported decreased ciliation, increased cilia loss, abnormal ciliary structure or inactivity of cilia in CRS sinonasal mucosa compared with control mucosa [25–27]. Li and colleagues [28] showed an increase in the number of cilia per ciliated cell and abnormal cilia architecture, as well as a decreased CBF in CRS patients compared with healthy controls. These authors further showed that the expression of three important ciliogenesis-related genes; CP110, Foxj1, and TAp73; was elevated in CRS and correlated with ciliary length, indicating that both ciliary injury and an abnormal upregulation of ciliogenesis led to impairment of ciliary architecture and function in CRS. By using whole-transcriptome sequencing, Peng and colleagues [29] revealed that defective host defences including cilia dysfunction are involved in CRSwNP. However, there are conflicting findings with regard to the changes of CBF in CRS; with some studies indicating a decrease of basal beat frequency whereas some studies demonstrating no alterations in baseline CBF between CRS patients and controls [4, 28, 30]. Moreover, a blunted ciliary response to environmental stimuli has also been reported in a subset of CRS patients. For example, Chen and colleagues [23] have reported a marked decrease of ciliary adaptation to exogenously applied adenosine triphosphate in CRS patients compared to controls.

Mucus hypersecretion is another common characteristic feature of CRS [31]. Increased expression of several mucins including MUC1, 2, 4, 5AC, 5B, 7, and 8, were reported in CRS tissues [32]. MUC5AC and MUC5B are the most important secreted mucins and both are upregulated in both CRSwNP and CRSsNP patients [33]. Zhang and colleagues [34] divided CRSwNP samples into IL-5(+) CRSwNP and IL-5(−) CRSwNP endotypes, and found that IL-5(+) CRSwNP samples had significantly increased expression of both MUC5AC and MUC5B compared with IL-5(−) CRSwNP samples and control samples. Seshadri and colleagues [35] showed that the elevation of MUC5AC in nasal polyps correlated with increased expression of pendrin, which might lead to increased inflammation, mucus production, and decreased mucociliary clearance. Indeed, the numbers of mucus secretory elements, including goblet cells and submucosal glands have also been shown to be increased in sinus mucosa of CRS patients [36].

Defects in mucociliary clearance in CRS occur directly as a consequence of exposure to environmental or microbial toxins and/or as a secondary consequence of exposure to inflammatory stimuli. In this regard several common respiratory bacteria associated with CRS; including *Pseudomonas aeruginosa*, *Haemophilus influenzae*, and *Streptococcus pneumoniae*; can produce specific toxins that impair ciliary function. Similarly, viruses, allergens, and irritants of respiratory mucosa can interrupt normal mucociliary clearance by disrupting the ciliary function [4, 37], and inflammatory mediators such as TNF-α, IFN-γ, IL-6, IL-8, and IL-13 present in patients with CRS have been reported to play an important role in modulating ciliary function or ciliogenesis [26, 30, 38, 39].

Increased mucin production in nasal mucosa has also been shown to be induced by different stimuli. Respiratory pathogens such as rhinovirus, influenza virus, fungi, and *Pseudomonas aeruginosa* have been reported to increase different mucins such as MUC1, 2, 4, 5AC, 5B, and 8 [32]. Multiple inflammatory cytokines such as IL-4, IL-9, IL-13, IL-17, IL-19, IL-33, TNF-α, IFN-γ, and IL-1β have also been shown to be involved in the upregulation of mucins or goblet cell hyperplasia in sinonasal epithelial cells, thus contributing to mucociliary dysfunction in CRS [5, 6, 32]. In addition, the hypoxic condition occurring in the sinus is associated with MUC5AC overproduction via the HIF-1α-mediated mechanism in the sinonasal epithelium of CRS [40].

Cigarette smoking and passive smoke exposure have been demonstrated to be involved in mucociliary dysfunction in CRS [41]. Cigarette smoke challenge to sinonasal epithelial cells leads to altered ciliary motility, with conflicting results showing no change, an increase, or a decrease in CBF [41]. Histologic changes of goblet cell hyperplasia were reported in sinus mucosa of smokers [41]. In a pediatric population exposed to passive smoking, the ultrastructural changes of nasal mucosa including patchy loss of cilia, generalized loss of cilia, and hyperplasia of goblet cells were observed, suggesting passive cigarette smoke may have negative effects on ciliary activity and mucociliary function [42].

11.6 Summary

Mucociliary clearance is a primary defense mechanism of the respiratory tract. The impairment of nasal mucociliary clearance has commonly been reported in CRS and plays an important role in disease progression. Cilia and mucus are principle components of mucociliary clearance, and dysfunction of either component results in the impairment of mucociliary function. The impairment of mucociliary clearance may lead to microbial colonization and nasal inflammation contributing to CRS. Consequently, approaches designed to improve mucociliary clearance remain attractive strategies for the treatment of CRS.

References

1. Schleimer RP, Lane AP, Kim J. Innate and acquired immunity and epithelial cell function in chronic rhinosinusitis. Clin Allergy Immunol. 2007;20:51–78.
2. Stevens WW, Lee RJ, Schleimer RP, Cohen NA. Chronic rhinosinusitis pathogenesis. J Allergy Clin Immunol. 2015;136(6):1442–53. https://doi.org/10.1016/j.jaci.2015.10.009.
3. Navarrette CR, Sisson JH, Nance E, Allen-Gipson D, Hanes J, Wyatt TA. Particulate matter in cigarette smoke increases ciliary axoneme beating through mechanical stimulation. J Aerosol Med Pulm Drug Deliv. 2012;25(3):159–68. https://doi.org/10.1089/jamp.2011.0890.
4. London NR Jr, Lane AP. Innate immunity and chronic rhinosinusitis: What we have learned from animal models. Laryngoscope Investig Otolaryngol. 2016;1(3):49–56. https://doi.org/10.1002/lio2.21.
5. Zhang N, Van Crombruggen K, Gevaert E, Bachert C. Barrier function of the nasal mucosa in health and type-2 biased airway diseases. Allergy. 2016;71(3):295–307. https://doi.org/10.1111/all.12809.
6. Fahy JV, Dickey BF. Airway mucus function and dysfunction. N Engl J Med. 2010;363(23):2233–47. https://doi.org/10.1056/NEJMra0910061.
7. Antunes MB, Gudis DA, Cohen NA. Epithelium, cilia, and mucus: their importance in chronic rhinosinusitis. Immunol Allergy Clin N Am. 2009;29(4):631–43. https://doi.org/10.1016/j.iac.2009.07.004.
8. Whitsett JA. Airway epithelial differentiation and mucociliary clearance. Ann Am Thorac Soc. 2018;15(Suppl 3):S143–s8. https://doi.org/10.1513/AnnalsATS.201802-128AW.
9. Ma J, Rubin BK, Voynow JA. Mucins, mucus, and goblet cells. Chest. 2018;154(1):169–76. https://doi.org/10.1016/j.chest.2017.11.008.
10. Bonser LR, Erle DJ. Airway mucus and asthma: the role of MUC5AC and MUC5B. J Clin Med. 2017;6(12):112. https://doi.org/10.3390/jcm6120112.
11. Bustamante-Marin XM, Ostrowski LE. Cilia and mucociliary clearance. Cold Spring Harbor Perspect Biol. 2017;9(4):a028241. https://doi.org/10.1101/cshperspect.a028241.
12. Boutin C, Kodjabachian L. Biology of multiciliated cells. Curr Opin Genet Dev. 2019;56:1–7. https://doi.org/10.1016/j.gde.2019.04.006.
13. Gudis DA, Cohen NA. Cilia dysfunction. Otolaryngol Clin N Am. 2010;43(3):461–72, vii. https://doi.org/10.1016/j.otc.2010.02.007.
14. Salathe M. Regulation of mammalian ciliary beating. Annu Rev Physiol. 2007;69:401–22. https://doi.org/10.1146/annurev.physiol.69.040705.141253.
15. Hoegger MJ, Awadalla M, Namati E, Itani OA, Fischer AJ, Tucker AJ, et al. Assessing mucociliary transport of single particles in vivo shows variable speed and preference for the ventral trachea in newborn pigs. Proc Natl Acad Sci U S A. 2014;111(6):2355–60. https://doi.org/10.1073/pnas.1323633111.
16. Matsui H, Randell SH, Peretti SW, Davis CW, Boucher RC. Coordinated clearance of periciliary liquid and mucus from airway surfaces. J Clin Invest. 1998;102(6):1125–31. https://doi.org/10.1172/jci2687.
17. Sears PR, Yin WN, Ostrowski LE. Continuous mucociliary transport by primary human airway epithelial cells in vitro. Am J Physiol Lung Cell Mol Physiol.

2015;309(2):L99–108. https://doi.org/10.1152/ajplung.00024.2015.
18. Kempeneers C, Seaton C, Garcia Espinosa B, Chilvers MA. Ciliary functional analysis: beating a path towards standardization. Pediatr Pulmonol. 2019;54(10):1627–38. https://doi.org/10.1002/ppul.24439.
19. Chilvers MA, Rutman A, O'Callaghan C. Functional analysis of cilia and ciliated epithelial ultrastructure in healthy children and young adults. Thorax. 2003;58(4):333–8. https://doi.org/10.1136/thorax.58.4.333.
20. Rayner CF, Rutman A, Dewar A, Greenstone MA, Cole PJ, Wilson R. Ciliary disorientation alone as a cause of primary ciliary dyskinesia syndrome. Am J Respir Crit Care Med. 1996;153(3):1123–9. https://doi.org/10.1164/ajrccm.153.3.8630555.
21. Antunes MB, Cohen NA. Mucociliary clearance--a critical upper airway host defense mechanism and methods of assessment. Curr Opin Allergy Clin Immunol. 2007;7(1):5–10. https://doi.org/10.1097/ACI.0b013e3280114eef.
22. Raidt J, Wallmeier J, Hjeij R, Onnebrink JG, Pennekamp P, Loges NT, et al. Ciliary beat pattern and frequency in genetic variants of primary ciliary dyskinesia. Eur Respir J. 2014;44(6):1579–88. https://doi.org/10.1183/09031936.00052014.
23. Chen B, Shaari J, Claire SE, Palmer JN, Chiu AG, Kennedy DW, et al. Altered sinonasal ciliary dynamics in chronic rhinosinusitis. Am J Rhinol. 2006;20(3):325–9. https://doi.org/10.2500/ajr.2006.20.2870.
24. Orlandi RR, Kingdom TT, Hwang PH, Smith TL, Alt JA, Baroody FM, et al. International consensus statement on allergy and rhinology: rhinosinusitis. Int Forum Allergy Rhinol. 2016;6(Suppl 1):S22–209. https://doi.org/10.1002/alr.21695.
25. Schleimer RP. Immunopathogenesis of chronic rhinosinusitis and nasal polyposis. Annu Rev Pathol. 2017;12:331–57. https://doi.org/10.1146/annurev-pathol-052016-100401.
26. Lai Y, Chen B, Shi J, Palmer JN, Kennedy DW, Cohen NA. Inflammation-mediated upregulation of centrosomal protein 110, a negative modulator of ciliogenesis, in patients with chronic rhinosinusitis. J Allergy Clin Immunol. 2011;128(6):1207–15.e1. https://doi.org/10.1016/j.jaci.2011.09.001.
27. Demarco RC, Tamashiro E, Rossato M, Ferreira MD, Valera FC, Anselmo-Lima WT. Ciliary ultrastructure in patients with chronic rhinosinusitis and primary ciliary dyskinesia. Eur Archiv Otorhinolaryngol. 2013;270(7):2065–70. https://doi.org/10.1007/s00405-012-2342-7.
28. Li YY, Li CW, Chao SS, Yu FG, Yu XM, Liu J, et al. Impairment of cilia architecture and ciliogenesis in hyperplastic nasal epithelium from nasal polyps. J Allergy Clin Immunol. 2014;134(6):1282–92. https://doi.org/10.1016/j.jaci.2014.07.038.
29. Peng Y, Zi XX, Tian TF, Lee B, Lum J, Tang SA, et al. Whole-transcriptome sequencing reveals heightened inflammation and defective host defence responses in chronic rhinosinusitis with nasal polyps. Eur Respir J. 2019;54(5):1900732. https://doi.org/10.1183/13993003.00732-2019.
30. Jiao J, Duan S, Meng N, Li Y, Fan E, Zhang L. Role of IFN-γ, IL-13, and IL-17 on mucociliary differentiation of nasal epithelial cells in chronic rhinosinusitis with nasal polyps. Clin Exp Allergy. 2016;46(3):449–60. https://doi.org/10.1111/cea.12644.
31. Burgel PR, Escudier E, Coste A, Dao-Pick T, Ueki IF, Takeyama K, et al. Relation of epidermal growth factor receptor expression to goblet cell hyperplasia in nasal polyps. J Allergy Clin Immunol. 2000;106(4):705–12. https://doi.org/10.1067/mai.2000.109823.
32. Kato K, Song BH, Howe CL, Chang EH. A comprehensive systematic review of the association between airway mucins and chronic rhinosinusitis. Am J Rhinol Allergy. 2019;33(4):433–48. https://doi.org/10.1177/1945892419837042.
33. Luo Q, Zhang J, Wang H, Chen F, Luo X, Miao B, et al. Expression and regulation of transcription factor FoxA2 in chronic rhinosinusitis with and without nasal polyps. Allergy, Asthma Immunol Res. 2015;7(5):458–66. https://doi.org/10.4168/aair.2015.7.5.458.
34. Zhang Y, Derycke L, Holtappels G, Wang XD, Zhang L, Bachert C, et al. Th2 cytokines orchestrate the secretion of MUC5AC and MUC5B in IL-5-positive chronic rhinosinusitis with nasal polyps. Allergy. 2019;74(1):131–40. https://doi.org/10.1111/all.13489.
35. Seshadri S, Lu X, Purkey MR, Homma T, Choi AW, Carter R, et al. Increased expression of the epithelial anion transporter pendrin/SLC26A4 in nasal polyps of patients with chronic rhinosinusitis. J Allergy Clin Immunol. 2015;136(6):1548–58.e7. https://doi.org/10.1016/j.jaci.2015.05.024.
36. Luo Q, Zhang Z, Liu D, Feng K, Jin X, Zhang J. Human neutrophil elastase induces MUC5AC overexpression in chronic rhinosinusitis through tumour necrosis factor-α converting enzyme. Acta Otolaryngol. 2016;136(6):641–8. https://doi.org/10.3109/00016489.2016.1144145.
37. Ahmadzada S, Ende JA, Alvarado R, Christensen JM, Kim JH, Rimmer J, et al. Responses of well-differentiated human sinonasal epithelial cells to allergen exposure and environmental pollution in chronic rhinosinusitis. Am J Rhinol Allergy. 2019;33(6):624–33. https://doi.org/10.1177/1945892419853103.
38. Gudis D, Zhao KQ, Cohen NA. Acquired cilia dysfunction in chronic rhinosinusitis. Am J Rhinol Allergy. 2012;26(1):1–6. https://doi.org/10.2500/ajra.2012.26.3716.
39. Ma Y, Sun Y, Jiang L, Zuo K, Chen H, Guo J, et al. WDPCP regulates the ciliogenesis of human sinonasal epithelial cells in chronic rhinosinusitis. Cytoskeleton (Hoboken, NJ). 2017;74(2):82–90. https://doi.org/10.1002/cm.21351.
40. Cho HJ, Kim CH. Oxygen matters: hypoxia as a pathogenic mechanism in rhinosinusitis. BMB

Rep. 2018;51(2):59–64. https://doi.org/10.5483/bmbrep.2018.51.2.014.
41. Christensen DN, Franks ZG, McCrary HC, Saleh AA, Chang EH. A systematic review of the association between cigarette smoke exposure and chronic rhinosinusitis. Otolaryngol Head Neck Surg. 2018;158(5):801–16. https://doi.org/10.1177/0194599818757697.
42. Elwany S, Ibrahim AA, Mandour Z, Talaat I. Effect of passive smoking on the ultrastructure of the nasal mucosa in children. Laryngoscope. 2012;122(5):965–9. https://doi.org/10.1002/lary.23246.

Sinonasal Epithelium

12

Michael Soyka and Cezmi A. Akdis

Key Points

- Different layers of the epithelium contribute to the barrier function.
- The barrier is composed of a supraepithelial mucus layer, the epithelial cilia, the epithelium itself and the junctions between the cells.
- Different aspects of the epithelial barrier are impaired in CRS.
- Epithelial barrier dysfunction may explain different aspects of CRS pathophysiology.

12.1 Introduction

Chronic Rhinosinusitis is a disorder of the sinonasal mucosal surfaces and underlying submucosal tissues. The nose and its inner surfaces are among the first and most exposed parts of the human body to airborne pollutants. Its pathophysiology is only partly understood and affection of the general population is high, with one in ten of affected patients additionally suffering from NSAID exacerbated respiratory disease [1–4]. Daily, more than 10,000 liters of air pass through the nose. Thereby the mucosa is facing the stress of drying, attack by viruses and bacteria as well as harm from environmental pollutants and other molecules including allergens. Although fully covered by pseudostratified columnar epithelium, research has mainly focused on the subepithelial compartment and immunologic processes rather than on the epithelium itself. Only in cystic fibrosis (CF) and primary ciliary dyskinesia the dysfunction of the epithelium, either by thick tenacious secretions or the inadequate mucocilliary clearance, have been identified and directly linked to its pathophysiology. It is not intended to describe these well-known genetic pathologies in this chapter.

The epithelial barrier is the first site of contact to the outer world and also first line of defense. An intact and functioning barrier is the prerequisite for a functioning organ and entire body homeostasis. Not only is it of utmost importance to keep foreign particles out, it is just as important to keep moisture, tissue water and proteins confined to inner compartments. It is in close contact with resident cells of the tissues, such as mast cells, macrophages, resident T cells, and mucosal associated T (MAIT) cells. Furthermore, the epithelium itself is capable of interacting with non-resident immunological cells by antigen

M. Soyka
Department of Otorhinolaryngology, Head and Neck Surgery, University Hospital Zurich, Zurich, Switzerland
e-mail: michael.soyka@usz.ch

C. A. Akdis (✉)
Swiss Institute of Allergy and Asthma Research (SIAF), University Zurich, Davos, Switzerland

Christine Kühne Center for Allergy Research and Education, Davos, Switzerland
e-mail: akdisac@siaf.uzh.ch

L. Zhang, C. Bachert (eds.), *Chronic Rhinosinusitis*, https://doi.org/10.1007/978-981-16-0784-4_12

presentation and the release of various cytokines and other intercellular mediators.

Different inflammatory patterns are found in subgroups of CRS referred to as endotypes. Depending on the basic pathophysiology of the barrier dysfunction and its consequence on inflammatory cells, the difference in endotypes could also be explained [5, 6]. A good example again is mucostasis in CF and ciliary dyskinesia leading to a more TH1/TH17 skewed inflammatory pattern, while type 2 inflammatory processes are more likely to be found in "idiopathic" polyps in Western countries.

12.2 Multiple Epithelial Barrier Layers and Their Functions

The mucosal barrier is composed of different parts, where the epithelium itself plays a major, but not the only, role. Therefore, we need to define distinct layers that contribute to this function. It would be wrong to look at layers as separate players since they highly interact with each other. Their contribution, however, to defense and homeostasis is best understood when they are looked at separately.

Four layers of epithelial barrier have been identified (Fig. 12.1). The first layer comprises the supraepithelial barrier that is mainly created by secreted proteins including mucins, other peptides, and water. Second layer is the epithelial cilia. Third layer of the barrier is constituted by the junctions between those cells and the last layer is formed by the epithelial cells themselves as an immune organ. A healthy and diverse microbiome and factors that keep the microbiome healthy such as prebiotics, vitamins, and cellulose are also thought to be part of the mucosal barrier. In the next sections, we will focus on each segment separately and then try to show the links in between.

12.2.1 The Supraepithelial Barrier

The very first contact with the environment is made by a viscous layer above the cells that is composed of antimicrobial proteins and peptides. Cathelicidins, defensins, lysozyme, and lactoferrin are good examples [7, 8]. In addition, the S-100 protein family contributes to the defense by activating toll-like receptors [9]. The just-mentioned proteins are secreted by epithelial cells. It is a normal and adequate reaction of the body to increase expression of these proteins upon exogenic stimulation. In CRS, however, some of those defense mechanisms seem to be downregulated: Lactoferrin and psoriasin as well as calprotectin (from the S-100 Family) are expressed less [10]. This seems to lead to an imbalance of the innate epithelial immunity and a functionally intact supraepithelial barrier cannot be built. As a consequence, the patient gets prone to bacterial or fungal colonization. This in turn may lead to an activation of the adaptive immune system and to secretion of cytokines, which can contribute to the vicious cycle of inflammation in CRS [11, 12]. Taste receptors like T2Rs were identified on cilia of the sinonasal epithelium. Physiologic reactions to bacteria include activation by bacterial quorum-sensing molecules that leads to stimulation of nitiric oxide production, increasing ciliary beat frequency and improves direct killing of bacteria [13]. This is a good example of the communication between the different parts of the epithelial barrier and its interaction. Dysfunctions of the bitter taste receptor have been suggested to impact on the pathophysiology in CRS.

The nasal microbiome has both a positive and negative impact on the epithelium of the nose and sinuses. This section will not focus on the diverse effects but stresses the interaction of bacteria and the epithelial barrier. Very recently microbial-derived butyrate, a short chain fatty acid, has been shown to promote barrier integrity as described below. Chemical and natural histone deacetylase (HDAC) inhibitors—sodium butyrate as a natural inhibitor—have been shown to be therapeutic in allergic rhinitis, while blocking HDAC activity leads to promotion of TJ integrity both in vivo and in vitro [14]. Similarly in allergic rhinitis general HDAC activity was higher in nasal epithelial cells and correlated inversely with epithelial integrity. Treatment of nasal epi-

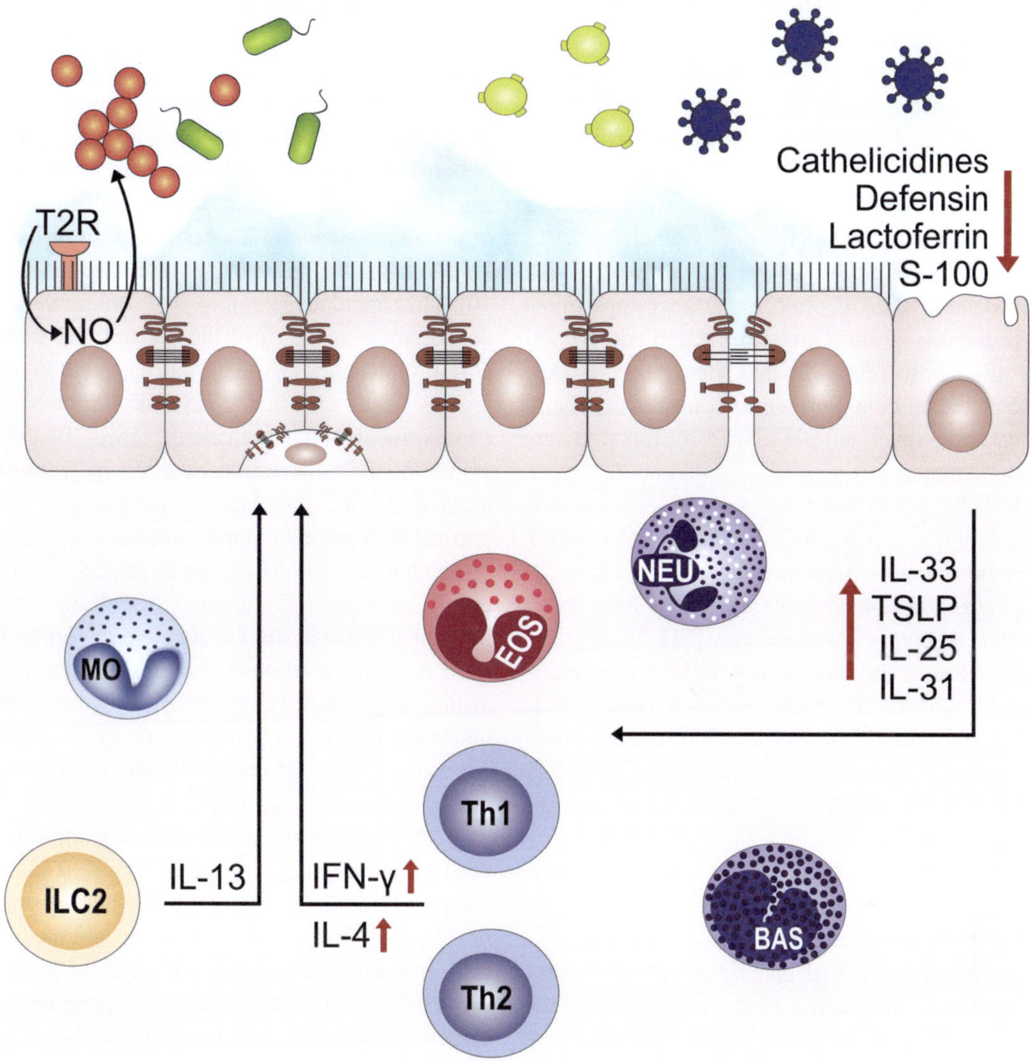

Fig. 12.1 The sinonasal epithelium is under constant strain caused by pollutants, allergens, viruses, and bacteria. An intact barrier is a prerequisite to sustain homeostasis. Different cytokines may directly or indirectly influence this barrier. Epithelial-derived alarmins such as IL-33 may increase Th2 inflammation and lead to the release of pro-inflammatory cytokines increasing leakiness of the epithelium. *EOS* eosinophil, *NEU* neutrophil, *BAS* basophil, *Th* T helper cell, *MO* macrophage, *ILC* innate lymphoid cell, *IFN* interferon, *TSLP* thymic stromal lymphopoietin, *T2R* bitter taste receptor type 2, *NO* nitrogen oxide

thelial cells with a synthetic HDAC inhibitor, JNJ-26481585, restored epithelial integrity by promoting tight junction expression. To demonstrate the in vivo role of HDACs, house dust mite-sensitized mice were treated with JNJ-26481585 in a prevention model and these mice did not develop allergic airway inflammation and had no bronchial hyperreactivity [15]. Similarly the same HDAC inhibitor was previously shown to treat asthmatic epithelial barrier defect [16].

12.2.2 The Epithelial Cilia

Mucocilliary clearance is of utmost importance for a well-functioning nose. When the nasal vibrissae have not withheld particles from entering the nostrils, these foreign bodies will, under physiological circumstances, be transported by coordinated mucocilliary movement towards the pharynx and then expectorated or swallowed [17]. While the supraepithelial mucus barrier influences directly the potential of the movement of cilia, they may be affected by other factors as well. In genetic disorders, such as primary ciliary dyskinesia and CF, direct or indirect impairment of the cilia causes chronic infection and inflammation, with reversible and irreversible damage to epithelial cilia. Furthermore, mechanic, chemical, hormonal, and pH-related dysfunctions are well known, just as well as temperature dependent changes in beat frequency [18–20]. Bacteria including Pseudomonas aeruginosa, Streptococcus pneumoniae, Staphylococcus aureus, and Haemophilus influenzae have direct effect on ciliary beat frequency [21]. Their toxins and biofilm formations may reduce movement, and coordination of cilia or even destroy cilia bearing cells, disrupting the physiologic clearance [22]. Different cytokines including TNF-alpha, IL-13, and IL-6 play a relevant role in the pathogenesis of CRS [20, 23, 24]. Even after surgery, where mucosa has been stripped of the bone completely, regeneration of cilia bearing cells may take several months before a fully functional epithelium is restored, one of the reasons why the functional endoscopic sinus surgery technique was introduced. At the same time, they exert negative effects on ciliary activity. These effects all lead to mucostasis that again promotes the growth of bacteria and contribute to the vicious cycle of chronic inflammation [20, 25]. Biofilm formation may be promoted and is thought to contribute to CRS, especially in recalcitrant cases [26].

12.2.3 Junctional Proteins and the Tightness of the Epithelial Cells

Different cell–cell junctions are found in the mucosa of healthy noses and paranasal sinuses. A tight epithelium forms a mechanical barrier to separate the apical from the basolateral side. TJs form a part of the functional complex of desmosomes, gap junctions, and adherens junctions in epithelial cell connections (Fig. 12.2) [27]. TJs are the most apical, intercellular components of polarized epithelium and the main determinants of barrier function responsible for the integrity of a cell layer. These proteins have a multifold way of action consisting of a barrier function, a fence function and also influence on transcription [28–30]. They regulate signaling, cell differentiation, proliferation and control the paracellular transport of molecules. While the barrier function represents the classical separation of two compartments, the so-called fence function maintains the polarization of a cell by avoiding movement of membrane components. TJs encompass transmembrane molecules, scaffold- and signal proteins. They consist of occludin, the family of claudins, angulines, tricellulins, and junctional adhesion molecules. Neighboring TJ form homo/heterodimers enabling a tight connection between cells. On the cytosolic side, they bind through adaptor proteins such as the zonula occludens (ZO1–3) to the cytoskeleton [31]. The cell connections prevent the intrusion of bacteria and other pathogens, while avoiding unwanted fluid loss. Recently, a disrupted TJ pattern and an increased leakiness of the epithelial barrier could be found in lower airway biopsies affected by bronchial asthma. An intact barrier is the prerequisite for a functioning and healthy epithelium. A defective epithelium could promote the uptake of pathogens, such as Staphylococcus aureus, an endotoxin secreting bacterium with a potentially central role in the development of CRSwNP. A common pathophysiological pathway for both upper and lower airway disorders has been propagated. CRSwNP is directly associated with non-atopic bronchial asthma. Different studies could so far identify defects in TJ in asthma.

In the late nineties Bernstein et al. performed first functional analyses of nasal epithelial cells to investigate the tightness of the layer [32]. This was followed by a second study, where no difference in the transepithelial resistance (TER is an indicator of epithelial integrity and correlates nicely with the condition of TJs) was found between CRS- and control epithelium. However,

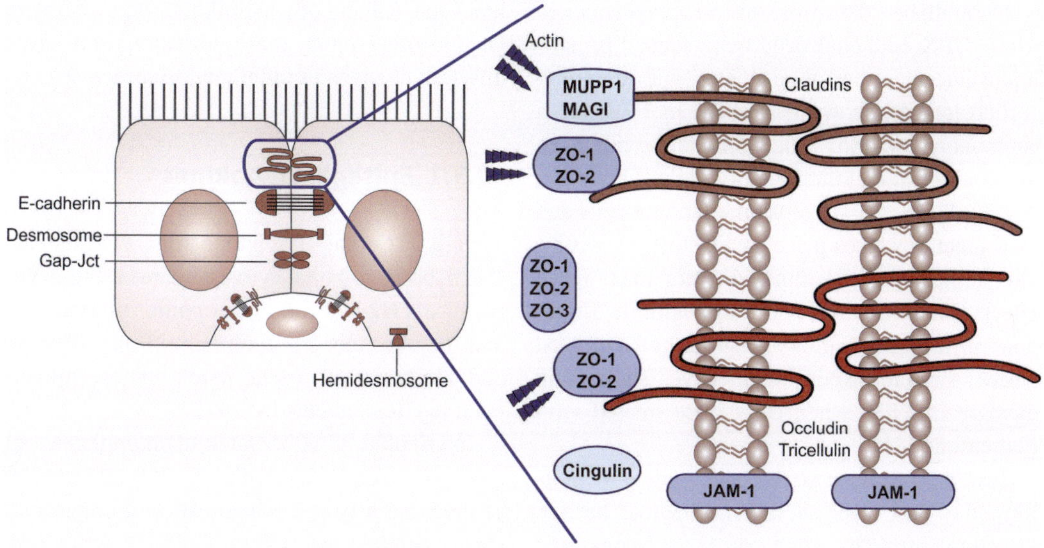

Fig. 12.2 The epithelial barrier consists of different components including desmosomes, hemidesmosomes, adherens junctions, and tight junctions (TJ). TJ-proteins like Claudins, Occludin and Tricellulin bind to the cytoskeleton through adaptor proteins like zonula occludens (ZO), MUPP (multi-PDZ domain protein), and MAGI (membrane-associated guanylate kinases with inverted domain structure)

no distinction between CRSwNP and CRSsNP was made [33]. The TJ associated protein ZO-1 was found to be downregulated in CRSwNP, particularly in dedifferentiated epithelium [34]. Interestingly no differences in TJ expression could be found in biopsies of CRSwNP/CRSsNP compared to controls, when patients were pretreated with corticosteroids. Rhinovirus is directly capable of destroying TJs in cases of acute rhinosinusitis [35]. Junctional adhesion molecules are involved in the attachment of adenovirus to the cell membrane and RSV is even capable of downregulating occludin expression [36, 37]. A direct disruption of TJs by pollen was shown in vitro, while their effects on TJs in CRS have not been investigated yet. The pollen peptidases lead to a loosening of the mechanical barrier [38].

Our own studies showed a downregulation of the proteins occludin, claudin-4 and ZO-1 both on mRNA and protein levels in diseased CRS biopsies [39]. The expression of occludin mRNA correlated negatively with the mRNA of ECP (eosinophil cationic protein), a marker of eosinophilic inflammation in CRS. Ex vivo, a lowered trans-tissue-resistance (TTR) in CRSwNP was demonstrated. In vitro results also show a lower trans-epithelial-resistance (TER or TEER) in air–liquid interface (ALI) cultured epithelia from CRSwNP patients. Paracellular flux can be measured by evaluating FITC-labeled 4000 kDa molecular weight dextran diffusion across the barrier. TER nicely correlates with FITC-dextran permeability in air–liquid interface cultures. The influence of different cytokines like IL-4 (a typical T helper 2 cytokine), IFN-gamma (a typical T helper 1 cytokine), IL-17 (T helper 17 cytokine), and IL-35 (Treg cytokine) on the TER was also tested. While IL-17 does not exert any effect on the epithelial integrity, the integrity of the cell layer is reduced through stimulations with IL-4 and IFN-gamma. Similar results have been shown in allergic rhinitis [15, 40, 41]. As described above histone deacetylase (HDAC) has been identified as a crucial driver of allergic inflammation and tight junction dysfunction. HDAC activity is negatively correlated with epithelial integrity in allergic rhinitis. The use of HDAC inhibitor JNJ-26481585 in vivo experiments with HDM-sensitized mice showed alleviation of the allergic reaction and restoration of tight junction function [15].

Unpublished data from in vitro experiments, where CRS epithelial cells were seeded on air–liquid interfaces and then treated with common corticosteroids, show an increase in TER and a potential restoration of the epithelial barrier, even in the absence of inflammatory cells. Therefore, direct influence of steroids on epithelial cells and their junctions takes place. Azelastine, as a common topical antihistamine, did not exert these effects. These findings are in line with investigations in allergic rhinitis epithelial cell cultures, where similar experiments have shown an increase in TER, when cells were treated with Fluticasone [41].

Just below the TJs, the adherens junctions form the next layer of the mechanical barrier. Structural proteins such as E-cadherins and anchor proteins like catenins again connect the actin-filaments of the cytoskeleton and the cell membrane. In contrast to the defective TJs in CRS, E-cadherin seem to be increased in strength in nasal polyps, possibly as a counter-regulatory mechanism to overcome the lack in TJs. Cadherin-related family member 3 is a receptor for rhinovirus-C and a missense variant seems to be associated with childhood asthma and exacerbations [42].

Desmosomes are the anchoring proteins for the intermediate filaments and thereby also connect the cytoskeleton and the cell membrane, specifically to stabilize the cells against pulling and shearing forces [43]. Desmoglein 2 & 3 expression in CRSwNP is low, which is common both in Th1 and Th2 inflammatory processes [44]. This again contributes to an insufficient barrier in CRS.

12.3 Interaction of the Epithelium and the Adaptive Immune System

As discussed in the appropriate sections of this book the immune system is highly active in CRS. Different inflammatory endotypes can be found presenting as similar phenotypes. As described above the epithelial barrier is actively influenced by inflammatory cells and their cytokines in CRS and other similar chronic disorders. On the other hand, the epithelium itself exerts different changes in inflammatory processes.

12.3.1 Epithelial Cytokines

Thymic stromal lymphopoietin (TSLP) and IL-25, both epithelial cytokines, are strong inducers of a TH2 skewed eosinophilic inflammation and may be released upon stimuli like allergens and viruses. Both tissue cytokines are upregulated in CRS patients [45–47].

Interleukin 33 is liberated upon epithelial cell death [48]. Acting as an alarmin it is also capable of inducing a type 2 inflammation. Furthermore, these cytokines are able to bind to dendritic cells that themselves support Th2 cell development through IL-6 and IL-4 [12]. They are capable of activating innate lymphoid cells (ILCs), where type II ILCs (ILC2) support the skew towards a Th2 inflammation [49]. ILCs seem to play an important role in type 2 inflammatory processes of CRS. Even in NERD ILC2s are increased in nasal scrapings, when stimulated with COX1 inhibitors, while peripheral ILC2s decrease as an effect of migration [49]. While ILC2s contribute to inflammation, retinoic acid is capable of converting these into IL-10-producing ILC regulatory cells that express CTLA-4. These cells also occur in inflamed CRSwNP tissue most likely as a counter-regulatory effect, while they are rarely found in healthy individuals' noses [50]. Furthermore, ILC2s interact with the epithelial barrier, where a tight junctional disruption through IL-13 was seen in asthmatic patients [51].

Interleukin 32 is expressed in pure epithelial cell cultures from CRS patients, especially when stimulated with IFN-gamma, TNF-alpha or in the presence of TH1 cells. This cytokine is found to be elevated in CRS, especially in polyps [52]. While its functional role in CRS is unclear it has been shown to enhance inflammation in different diseases including atopic dermatitis. Zink depletion was observed in CRS patients' mucosa especially in polyposis. The same group could demonstrate a negative effect on the barrier function through interference with ZO-1 [53].

The epithelial cell, in particular basal cells, which are considered to be part of the stem cells, seem to play a role in CRS pathogenesis. Growth and proliferation of epithelial progenitor cells of nasal polyp patients were found to be reduced. Mesenchymal progenitor cells can have immunoregulatory effects in nasal polyps and may contribute to control of inflammation [54].

Antiviral mediators like interferons (IFN) are also part of the barrier and are produced by human nasal epithelial cells directly. Human Rhinovirus induced cytokine release seems to be impaired in CRS, suggesting a deficiency in virus clearance of affected patients [55]. IFN-beta on the other hand seems to contribute to the eosinophilic inflammation by CCL11 production in a mouse model of CRS [56].

12.3.2 The Link Between Layers of Epithelial Barrier

Chronic rhinosinusitis in both phenotypic forms is a complex disease with unknown pathophysiology. The concept of a defective epithelial barrier is not new, but different aspects of its origin have only lately been described. In general, different parts of current knowledge can be explained by using this theory: An insufficiently functioning supraepithelial barrier will allow colonization with potentially pathogenic proteins, cells, and viruses, while impaired cilia will lead to mucostasis and prolonged elimination of intruders. In a defective epithelium and barrier, pathogens such as *Staphylococcus aureus* may penetrate easier and perpetuate inflammation by superantigen release, as has been shown in different studies that could augment the type 2 inflammation in polyps, which again contributes to the vicious cycle of CRS inflammation (Fig. 12.1).

12.3.3 Translation of the Mechanistic Knowledge into Daily Practice

It is still unclear if barrier dysfunction is the cause or consequence of inflammation in chronic inflammatory disorders. It, however, has been impressively shown to be part of the pathophysiology in CRS. Restoring the epithelial function and the barrier in CRS should be one of the central aims when targeting this disease. This translates directly into daily clinical practice: Novel treatments including biologics have proven to play a relevant role in CRS therapy. Monoclonal antibodies directed against IL-5 or its receptor, as well as IL-4/13 antibodies could bring the epithelium back to a less inflamed state and indirectly improve the barrier function. Probiotics may also play a crucial role in restoring epithelial integrity. Short-chain fatty acids along with topical steroids are promising candidates to directly "heal" the damaged barrier. This could potentially interrupt the vicious cycle of pathogen intrusion, fluid loss and perpetuation of inflammation.

References

1. Kowalski ML, Agache I, Bavbek S, Bakirtas A, Blanca M, Bochenek G, et al. Diagnosis and management of NSAID-Exacerbated Respiratory Disease (N-ERD)-a EAACI position paper. Allergy. 2019;74(1):28–39. https://doi.org/10.1111/all.13599.
2. Samitas K, Carter A, Kariyawasam HH, Xanthou G. Upper and lower airway remodelling mechanisms in asthma, allergic rhinitis and chronic rhinosinusitis: the one airway concept revisited. Allergy. 2018;73(5):993–1002. https://doi.org/10.1111/all.13373.
3. Breiteneder H, Diamant Z, Eiwegger T, Fokkens WJ, Traidl-Hoffmann C, Nadeau K, et al. Future research trends in understanding the mechanisms underlying allergic diseases for improved patient care. Allergy. 2019; https://doi.org/10.1111/all.13851.
4. Fokkens WJ, Lund V, Bachert C, Mullol J, Bjermer L, Bousquet J, et al. EUFOREA consensus on biologics for CRSwNP with or without asthma. Allergy. 2019; https://doi.org/10.1111/all.13875.
5. Akdis CA, Bachert C, Cingi C, Dykewicz MS, Hellings PW, Naclerio RM, et al. Endotypes and phenotypes of chronic rhinosinusitis: a PRACTALL document of the European Academy of Allergy and Clinical Immunology and the American Academy of Allergy, Asthma & Immunology. J Allergy Clin Immunol. 2013;131(6):1479–90. https://doi.org/10.1016/j.jaci.2013.02.036.
6. Bachert C, Akdis CA. Phenotypes and emerging endotypes of chronic rhinosinusitis. J Allergy Clin Immunol Pract. 2016;4(4):621–8. https://doi.org/10.1016/j.jaip.2016.05.004.

7. Travis SM, Conway BA, Zabner J, Smith JJ, Anderson NN, Singh PK, et al. Activity of abundant antimicrobials of the human airway. Am J Respir Cell Mol Biol. 1999;20(5):872–9. https://doi.org/10.1165/ajrcmb.20.5.3572.
8. Bals R. Epithelial antimicrobial peptides in host defense against infection. Respir Res. 2000;1(3):141–50. https://doi.org/10.1186/rr25.
9. Donato R, Cannon BR, Sorci G, Riuzzi F, Hsu K, Weber DJ, et al. Functions of S100 proteins. Curr Mol Med. 2013;13(1):24–57.
10. Tieu DD, Peters AT, Carter RG, Suh L, Conley DB, Chandra R, et al. Evidence for diminished levels of epithelial psoriasin and calprotectin in chronic rhinosinusitis. J Allergy Clin Immunol. 2010;125(3):667–75. https://doi.org/10.1016/j.jaci.2009.11.045.
11. Seshadri S, Lin DC, Rosati M, Carter RG, Norton JE, Suh L, et al. Reduced expression of antimicrobial PLUNC proteins in nasal polyp tissues of patients with chronic rhinosinusitis. Allergy. 2012;67(7):920–8. https://doi.org/10.1111/j.1398-9995.2012.02848.x.
12. Lam K, Schleimer R, Kern RC. The etiology and pathogenesis of chronic rhinosinusitis: a review of current hypotheses. Curr Allergy Asthma Rep. 2015;15(7):41. https://doi.org/10.1007/s11882-015-0540-2.
13. Lee RJ, Cohen NA. Role of the bitter taste receptor T2R38 in upper respiratory infection and chronic rhinosinusitis. Curr Opin Allergy Clin Immunol. 2015;15(1):14–20. https://doi.org/10.1097/ACI.0000000000000120.
14. Wang J, Wen L, Wang Y, Chen F. Therapeutic effect of histone deacetylase inhibitor, sodium butyrate, on allergic rhinitis in vivo. DNA Cell Biol. 2016;35(4):203–8. https://doi.org/10.1089/dna.2015.3037.
15. Steelant B, Wawrzyniak P, Martens K, Jonckheere AC, Pugin B, Schrijvers R, et al. Blocking histone deacetylase activity as a novel target for epithelial barrier defects in patients with allergic rhinitis. J Allergy Clin Immunol. 2019; https://doi.org/10.1016/j.jaci.2019.04.027.
16. Wawrzyniak P, Wawrzyniak M, Wanke K, Sokolowska M, Bendelja K, Ruckert B, et al. Regulation of bronchial epithelial barrier integrity by type 2 cytokines and histone deacetylases in asthmatic patients. J Allergy Clin Immunol. 2017;139(1):93–103. https://doi.org/10.1016/j.jaci.2016.03.050.
17. Houtmeyers E, Gosselink R, Gayan-Ramirez G, Decramer M. Regulation of mucociliary clearance in health and disease. Eur Respir J. 1999;13(5):1177–88.
18. Sutto Z, Conner GE, Salathe M. Regulation of human airway ciliary beat frequency by intracellular pH. J Physiol. 2004;560(Pt 2):519–32. https://doi.org/10.1113/jphysiol.2004.068171.
19. Winters SL, Davis CW, Boucher RC. Mechanosensitivity of mouse tracheal ciliary beat frequency: roles for Ca2+, purinergic signaling, tonicity, and viscosity. Am J Physiol Lung Cell Mol Physiol. 2007;292(3):L614–24. https://doi.org/10.1152/ajplung.00288.2005.
20. Gudis D, Zhao KQ, Cohen NA. Acquired cilia dysfunction in chronic rhinosinusitis. Am J Rhinol Allergy. 2012;26(1):1–6. https://doi.org/10.2500/ajra.2012.26.3716.
21. Ferguson JL, McCaffrey TV, Kern EB, Martin WJ II. The effects of sinus bacteria on human ciliated nasal epithelium in vitro. Otolaryngol Head Neck Surg. 1988;98(4):299–304. https://doi.org/10.1177/019459988809800405.
22. Palmer J. Bacterial biofilms in chronic rhinosinusitis. Ann Otol Rhinol Laryngol Suppl. 2006;196:35–9.
23. Laoukili J, Perret E, Willems T, Minty A, Parthoens E, Houcine O, et al. IL-13 alters mucociliary differentiation and ciliary beating of human respiratory epithelial cells. J Clin Invest. 2001;108(12):1817–24. https://doi.org/10.1172/JCI13557.
24. Papathanasiou A, Djahanbakhch O, Saridogan E, Lyons RA. The effect of interleukin-6 on ciliary beat frequency in the human fallopian tube. Fertil Steril. 2008;90(2):391–4. https://doi.org/10.1016/j.fertnstert.2007.07.1379.
25. Al-Rawi MM, Edelstein DR, Erlandson RA. Changes in nasal epithelium in patients with severe chronic sinusitis: a clinicopathologic and electron microscopic study. Laryngoscope. 1998;108(12):1816–23.
26. Tajudeen BA, Schwartz JS, Palmer JN. Understanding biofilms in chronic sinusitis. Curr Allergy Asthma Rep. 2016;16(2):10. https://doi.org/10.1007/s11882-015-0591-4.
27. Denker BM, Nigam SK. Molecular structure and assembly of the tight junction. Am J Phys. 1998;274(1 Pt 2):F1–9.
28. Chiba H, Osanai M, Murata M, Kojima T, Sawada N. Transmembrane proteins of tight junctions. Biochim Biophys Acta. 2008;1778(3):588–600. https://doi.org/10.1016/j.bbamem.2007.08.017.
29. Tsukita S, Furuse M, Itoh M. Multifunctional strands in tight junctions. Nat Rev Mol Cell Biol. 2001;2(4):285–93. https://doi.org/10.1038/35067088.
30. Kohler K, Zahraoui A. Tight junction: a co-ordinator of cell signalling and membrane trafficking. Biol Cell. 2005;97(8):659–65. https://doi.org/10.1042/BC20040147.
31. Hartsock A, Nelson WJ. Adherens and tight junctions: structure, function and connections to the actin cytoskeleton. Biochim Biophys Acta. 2008;1778(3):660–9. https://doi.org/10.1016/j.bbamem.2007.07.012.
32. Bernstein JM, Gorfien J, Noble B, Yankaskas JR. Nasal polyposis: immunohistochemistry and bioelectrical findings (a hypothesis for the development of nasal polyps). J Allergy Clin Immunol. 1997;99(2):165–75.
33. Dejima K, Randell SH, Stutts MJ, Senior BA, Boucher RC. Potential role of abnormal ion transport in the pathogenesis of chronic sinusitis. Arch Otolaryngol Head Neck Surg. 2006;132(12):1352–62. https://doi.org/10.1001/archotol.132.12.1352.

34. Jang YJ, Kim HG, Koo TW, Chung PS. Localization of ZO-1 and E-cadherin in the nasal polyp epithelium. Eur Arch Otorhinolaryngol. 2002;259(9):465–9. https://doi.org/10.1007/s00405-002-0500-z.
35. Sajjan U, Wang Q, Zhao Y, Gruenert DC, Hershenson MB. Rhinovirus disrupts the barrier function of polarized airway epithelial cells. Am J Respir Crit Care Med. 2008;178(12):1271–81. https://doi.org/10.1164/rccm.200801-136OC.
36. Guttman JA, Finlay BB. Tight junctions as targets of infectious agents. Biochim Biophys Acta. 2009;1788(4):832–41. https://doi.org/10.1016/j.bbamem.2008.10.028.
37. Kast JI, McFarlane AJ, Globinska A, Sokolowska M, Wawrzyniak P, Sanak M, et al. Respiratory syncytial virus infection influences tight junction integrity. Clin Exp Immunol. 2017;190(3):351–9. https://doi.org/10.1111/cei.13042.
38. Runswick S, Mitchell T, Davies P, Robinson C, Garrod DR. Pollen proteolytic enzymes degrade tight junctions. Respirology. 2007;12(6):834–42. https://doi.org/RES1175 [pii]. https://doi.org/10.1111/j.1440-1843.2007.01175.x.
39. Soyka MB, Wawrzyniak P, Eiwegger T, Holzmann D, Treis A, Wanke K, et al. Defective epithelial barrier in chronic rhinosinusitis: the regulation of tight junctions by IFN-gamma and IL-4. J Allergy Clin Immunol. 2012;130(5):1087–96. e10. https://doi.org/10.1016/j.jaci.2012.05.052.
40. Steelant B, Seys SF, Van Gerven L, Van Woensel M, Farre R, Wawrzyniak P, et al. Histamine and T helper cytokine-driven epithelial barrier dysfunction in allergic rhinitis. J Allergy Clin Immunol. 2018;141(3):951–63. e8. https://doi.org/10.1016/j.jaci.2017.08.039.
41. Steelant B, Farre R, Wawrzyniak P, Belmans J, Dekimpe E, Vanheel H, et al. Impaired barrier function in patients with house dust mite-induced allergic rhinitis is accompanied by decreased occludin and zonula occludens-1 expression. J Allergy Clin Immunol. 2016;137(4):1043–53 e1–5. https://doi.org/10.1016/j.jaci.2015.10.050.
42. Bonnelykke K, Coleman AT, Evans MD, Thorsen J, Waage J, Vissing NH, et al. Cadherin-related family member 3 genetics and rhinovirus c respiratory illnesses. Am J Respir Crit Care Med. 2018;197(5):589–94. https://doi.org/10.1164/rccm.201705-1021OC.
43. Huber O. Structure and function of desmosomal proteins and their role in development and disease. Cell Mol Life Sci. 2003;60(9):1872–90. https://doi.org/10.1007/s00018-003-3050-7.
44. Zuckerman JD, Lee WY, DelGaudio JM, Moore CE, Nava P, Nusrat A, et al. Pathophysiology of nasal polyposis: the role of desmosomal junctions. Am J Rhinol. 2008;22(6):589–97. https://doi.org/10.2500/ajr.2008.22.3235.
45. Liu T, Li TL, Zhao F, Xie C, Liu AM, Chen X, et al. Role of thymic stromal lymphopoietin in the pathogenesis of nasal polyposis. Am J Med Sci. 2011;341(1):40–7. https://doi.org/10.1097/MAJ.0b013e3181f20489.
46. Boita M, Bucca C, Riva G, Heffler E, Rolla G. Release of type 2 cytokines by epithelial cells of nasal polyps. J Immunol Res. 2016;2016:2643297. https://doi.org/10.1155/2016/2643297.
47. Lam M, Hull L, Imrie A, Snidvongs K, Chin D, Pratt E, et al. Interleukin-25 and interleukin-33 as mediators of eosinophilic inflammation in chronic rhinosinusitis. Am J Rhinol Allergy. 2015;29(3):175–81. https://doi.org/10.2500/ajra.2015.29.4176.
48. Soyka MB, Holzmann D, Basinski TM, Wawrzyniak M, Bannert C, Burgler S, et al. The induction of IL-33 in the sinus epithelium and its influence on T-helper cell responses. PLoS One. 2015;10(5):e0123163. https://doi.org/10.1371/journal.pone.0123163.
49. Kortekaas Krohn I, Shikhagaie MM, Golebski K, Bernink JH, Breynaert C, Creyns B, et al. Emerging roles of innate lymphoid cells in inflammatory diseases: clinical implications. Allergy. 2018;73(4):837–50. https://doi.org/10.1111/all.13340.
50. Morita H, Kubo T, Ruckert B, Ravindran A, Soyka MB, Rinaldi AO, et al. Induction of human regulatory innate lymphoid cells from group 2 innate lymphoid cells by retinoic acid. J Allergy Clin Immunol. 2019;143(6):2190–201. e9. https://doi.org/10.1016/j.jaci.2018.12.1018.
51. Sugita K, Steer CA, Martinez-Gonzalez I, Altunbulakli C, Morita H, Castro-Giner F, et al. Type 2 innate lymphoid cells disrupt bronchial epithelial barrier integrity by targeting tight junctions through IL-13 in asthmatic patients. J Allergy Clin Immunol. 2018;141(1):300–10 e11. https://doi.org/10.1016/j.jaci.2017.02.038.
52. Soyka MB, Treis A, Eiwegger T, Menz G, Zhang S, Holzmann D, et al. Regulation and expression of IL-32 in chronic rhinosinusitis. Allergy. 2012;67(6):790–8. https://doi.org/10.1111/j.1398-9995.2012.02820.x.
53. Murphy J, Ramezanpour M, Roscioli E, Psaltis AJ, Wormald PJ, Vreugde S. Mucosal zinc deficiency in chronic rhinosinusitis with nasal polyposis contributes to barrier disruption and decreases ZO-1. Allergy. 2018;73(10):2095–7. https://doi.org/10.1111/all.13532.
54. Klimek L, Koennecke M, Mullol J, Hellings PW, Wang DY, Fokkens W, et al. A possible role of stem cells in nasal polyposis. Allergy. 2017;72(12):1868–73. https://doi.org/10.1111/all.13221.
55. Kim JH, Kim YS, Cho GS, Kim NH, Gong CH, Lee BJ, et al. Human Rhinovirus-induced Proinflammatory Cytokine and Interferon-beta Responses in Nasal Epithelial Cells From Chronic Rhinosinusitis Patients. Allergy Asthma Immunol Res. 2015;7(5):489–96. https://doi.org/10.4168/aair.2015.7.5.489.
56. Jang YJ, Lim JY, Kim S, Lee Y, Kweon MN, Kim JH. Enhanced interferon-beta response contributes to eosinophilic chronic rhinosinusitis. Front Immunol. 2018;9:2330. https://doi.org/10.3389/fimmu.2018.02330.

Microbiology

13

Mahboobeh Mahdavinia and Robert P. Schleimer

Key Points

- The human respiratory tract is home to a large community of microorganisms, which are found throughout the system; from the small airways in the lung to the sinonasal cavity.
- Both healthy and diseased sinuses are inhabited by bacteria, fungi, and viruses. An imbalance of these microbes (i.e. dysbiosis) has the potential to cause sinonasal inflammation, which in a susceptible host can result in chronic rhinosinusitis (CRS).
- An increased presence and diversity of the so-called gatekeeping microbes keeps the respiratory tract healthy by limiting inflammation and controlling infections.
- Studying the composition of nasal microbiota in patients with CRS is important because of its potential therapeutic implications.

13.1 Introduction

Microorganisms are found throughout the human respiratory tract [1]. Commensal microorganisms—the beneficial microbes that make up the vast majority of the microbiome of the respiratory tract—and their metabolites are essential to maintaining the stability and health of mucosal membranes. At the molecular signaling level, crosstalk between microbes and immune system elements in the sinonasal cavity maintains a crucial equilibrium which, when disrupted, can lead to an increase in pathogenic species and ultimately the initiation and progression of inflammatory processes [2].

We now understand that chronic rhinosinusitis (CRS) is an inflammatory condition typically not caused by infection. Indeed, CRS has a complex pathophysiology linked to multiple contributing factors, including environmental exposures, host physiology, and host microbiome. Multiple studies have demonstrated changes in both commensal microbes and pathogens in CRS [2–6]. The microorganisms associated with CRS include bacteria [2, 6], fungi [7, 8], and viruses [9], all of which have the capacity to interact in ways that change the overall composition of the nasal microbiome and/or activate the immune system [9, 10]. An imbalance within the nasal microbiome (i.e. dysbiosis) is associated with various allergic and inflammatory diseases of the airways, such as allergic rhinitis (AR) [11–13] and

M. Mahdavinia
Division of Allergy-Immunology, Internal Medicine Department, Rush University Medical Center, Chicago, IL, USA
e-mail: mahboobeh_mahdavinia@rush.edu

R. P. Schleimer (✉)
Division of Allergy and Immunology, Department of Medicine, Northwestern University Feinberg School of Medicine, Chicago, IL, USA
e-mail: rpschleimer@northwestern.edu

L. Zhang, C. Bachert (eds.), *Chronic Rhinosinusitis*, https://doi.org/10.1007/978-981-16-0784-4_13

asthma [14]. Dysbiosis can also trigger sinonasal inflammation which, in a susceptible host, can lead to CRS [15].

It is not possible to fully understand whether changes in microbiota are a cause or an effect of inflammatory diseases. Imbalances in the microbial communities can be a trigger for initiation of immune response as evidenced by the impacts of gut microbiome in infancy on development of allergic diseases later on in life [16–18]. On the other hand, an unregulated immune response, especially in the setting of dysfunctional immune barrier due to inflamed mucosal epithelium [19], can present a suitable environment for growth of pathogenic microorganisms and further dysbiosis.

13.2 Bacterial Microbiota in CRS

The most common bacteria in the nasal cavity are of the phyla *Firmicutes*, *Actinobacteria*, *Proteobacteria*, *Bacteroidetes*, and *Fusobacteria*. Together, these bacteria account for 95–99% of phylum-level assigned sequences in both healthy subjects and CRS patients [2–4, 6, 11, 15]. At the genus-level, the most abundant bacteria in the nose of healthy patients are *Staphylococcus*, *Propionibacterium*, *Corynebacterium*, and *Streptococcus* [2–4, 6, 11, 15]. Microbiome composition can be highly variable among individuals with CRS, reflecting dysbiosis across multiple taxonomic levels, with most reported changes at the genus level (The results of supporting studies are summarized in Table 13.1).

We now know that greater biodiversity and abundance of the so-called gatekeeping or keystone bacteria are key to a healthy respiratory tract. These bacteria help limit inflammation and control infections [1]. Underrepresentation of these bacteria results in an environment that may support expansion of more potentially pathogenic species, such as *Staphylococcus* spp. or *Streptococcus pneumoniae*. One example of an important "keystone" bacterial genus in the nose is *Corynebacterium* [3, 5, 28, 29]. *Corynebacterium* is one of the main bacterial genera dominating the upper respiratory tract in healthy children [29] and healthy adults [3, 5]. These organisms may operate actively within the nasal passages to keep pathogenic bacteria at bay. For example, one common *Corynebacterium* species, *C. accolens*, can modify its local habitat to inhibit the growth of pathogens by releasing antibacterial fatty acids [28]. Another common member of this group, *C. pseudodiphtheriticum*, exerts strong contact-independent antibacterial activity against *Staphylococcus aureus* (*S. aureus*) [30], which can play a key role in airway disease [31]. Perhaps not surprisingly, *Corynebacerium* species are significantly underrepresented within the context of CRS [3, 5], and the relative abundance (RA) of *S. aureus* in CRS patients, especially those with nasal polyps (CRSwNP), is higher than in control subjects [6, 8, 20, 24, 32].

It may not be simply the size of the population of pathogenic bacteria that determines pathogenicity in CRS-related inflammation. Because of the link between *S. aureus* and CRS, one might expect asthmatic patients with CRS to have an even greater abundance of *S. aureus*. However, one study [6] found that it was not the overall population of *S. aureus* that was larger in affected asthmatic CRSwNP patients compared to non-asthmatic subjects, but the abundance of IgE specific to staphylococcal enterotoxins (SE-IgE). This result suggests that it may be, at least in part, the virulence of *S. aureus* strain that drives CRS-related inflammation and disease [31, 33]. Consistent with this idea, one study of microbial interactions demonstrates that *Corynebacterium* species impact *S. aureus* by increasing the transcription of genes linked to human nasal colonization and decreasing the transcription of virulence genes [34], thus effectively shifting the population of *S. aureus* from virulence towards a more commensal state [34]. Certain intra-species interactions may also serve to reinforce this shift. For instance, certain non-pathogenic strains of *S. aureus* may interfere with the establishment of pathogenic strains. This is similar to the protective effect of *Staphylococcus epidemisdis* against colonization with skin pathogens [35]. Thus, the RA of specific strains of *S. aureus* may effectively control the pathogenicity of a host's nasal microbiome.

Table 13.1 Results of studies on Nasal microbiome in CRS

Authors, year	Number of sample	Sampling method	Analysis method	Microbial diversity	Differences at phylum level	Differences at genus level	Differences at species level
Bacterial microbiome studies							
Stephenson et al. 2010 [20]	18 CRS 9 controls	Anterior ethmoid mucosal biopsy	Bacterial tag-encoded FLX amplicon pyrosequencing (bTEFAP)	–	–	*Propionibacterium* found in 83% of CRS vs. 67% of controls (no statistics available) *Diaphorobacter* spp. and *Peptoniphilus* only reported in CRS (78% and 72% respectively)	*Staphylococcus aureus* found in 50% of CRS vs 100% of controls (no statistics available)
Stressmann et al. 2011 [21]	70 samples from 43 CRS No control	Mucosal biopsy	16S-rDNA sequencing and terminal restriction fragment length polymorphism (T-RFLP)	No control	–	Most abundant: *Pseudomonas, Citrobacter, Haemophilus, Propionibacterium, Staphylococcus and Streptococcus*	–
Abreu et al. 2012 [22]	7 CRS 7 control	Endoscopically guided maxillary sinus brushing	16S rRNA PhyloChip Phylogenetic microarray approach	Decreased in CRS	–	Decreased: order *Lactobacillales*	Increased: *Corynebacterium tuberculostearicum* Decreased: *Lactobacillus Sakai, Carnobacterium alterfunditum, Enterococcus mundtii,* and *Pediococcus pentosaceus*
Feazel et al. 2012 [23]	15 CRS (2 wNP and 13sNP) 5 controls	Middle meatus swabs	16-rDNA pyrosequencing and comparison with Silva version 104	Diversity was not different A trend towards lower evenness in CRS	–	–	Increased: a trend towards increase for *Staphylococcus aureus*

(continued)

Table 13.1 (continued)

Authors, year	Number of sample	Sampling method	Analysis method	Microbial diversity	Differences at phylum level	Differences at genus level	Differences at species level
Aurora et al. 2013 [8]	30 CRS 12 control	Lavage of the middle meatus	16S rRNA sequenced and submitted to NCBI; analyzed using scripts in the QIIME (Quantitative Insights into Microbial Ecology)	Increased diversity in CRS: 2333 in controls vs 3780 in CRS	No difference at phylum level	–	Increased *Corynebacterium accolens*, *Curtobacterium* species S22, *Pseudomonas* DT3–61, *Staphylococcus aureus* *Pseudomonas aeruginosa* *Decreased: Alicycliphilus* and *Cloacibacterium*
Boase et al. 2013 [24]	38 CRS and 6 controls	Ethmoid sinus mucosal tissue	Ibis T5000 analysis PCR coupled with electrospray ionization mass spectrometry	Trends towards increased diversity; mean isolates per patient in controls was 2, in CRSsNP was 2.5 and in CRSwNP was 3.2	–	–	Increased: *Staphylococcus aureus* in abundance and frequency Less frequently: *Propionibacterium acnes*
Choi et al. 2014 [25]	8 CRS (5wNP and 3sNP) 3 controls	Nasal lavage (NAL) fluid	16S-rDNA high-throughput pyrosequencing followed by identification using ExTaxon database.	Decreased diversity in CRS	Increased: Proteobacteria Decreased: Bacteroidetes decreased, from 25.42% to 7.37%	Increased: *Staphylococcus, Corynebacterium,* and *Propionibacterium* Decreased: *Prevotella, Streptococcus,* and *Veillonella* **Pseudomonas* increased in CRSwNP compared with CRSsNP	Increased: *Staphylococcus epidermidis*, *Pseudomonas monteilii* Decreased: *Prevotella melaninogenica* *Staphylococcus aureus* increased in CRSwNP compared to CRSsNP

Ramakrishnan et al. 2015 [4]	56 CRS and 26 controls	Swabs from Ethmoid region obtained during surgery	16-rRNA	Not reported between CRS and Controls, Diversity was associated with optimal surgical outcome in CRS	No difference	Decreased: *Propionibacterium* and *Peptoniphilus* at genum level	Not reported between CRS and controls
Lal et al. (2017) [11]	46 CRS 8 controls 11 Allergic rhinitis	Middle and inferior meatus swabs under guide	16S rRNA	Decreased diversity in CRSsNP compared with CRSwNP and controls (in middle meatus samples)	–	Increased • (only in CRSsNP): Streptococcus compared with controls • (only in CRSsNP): Haemophilus, and Fusobacterium compared with CRSwNP and controls • (only in CRSwNP): Alloiococcus compared with CRSsNP	–
Mahdavinia et al. 2018 [3]	111 CRS and 21 controls	Middle meatus swabs under guide	16S rRNA	No difference	Decreased: Actinobacteria	Decreased: Corynebacterium, peptiniphilus at genum level	–

(continued)

Table 13.1 (continued)

Authors, year	Number of sample	Sampling method	Analysis method	Microbial diversity	Differences at phylum level	Differences at genus level	Differences at species level
Chalermwatanachai et al. 2018 [6]	21 CRSwNP patients without asthma (CRSwNP-A) 20 CRSwNP patients with comorbid asthma (CRSwNP+A) 0.17 controls	Nasal swab	16S rRNA	Significantly decreased bacterial diversity (Shannon H index) and evenness (Pielou's evenness index),	Phylum Proteobacteria was more abundance in CRSwNP than control, phylum Actinobacteria and Bacteroidetes, were dominant in healthy control	Increased: Haemophilus was more abundance in CRSwNP Decreased: Bacteroides was dominant in healthy control	Increased: Haemophilus influenzae was significantly enriched in CRSwNP patients, Staphylococcus aureus was abundant in the CRSwNP-A group Decreased: Propionibacterium acnes in the healthy group

Authors, year	Number of sample	Sampling method	Analysis method	Microbial Diversity	Differences at Phylum level	Differences at order, family or genus level	Differences at Species level
Fungal microbiome studies							
Aurora et al. 2013 [8]	30 CRS 12 controls	Lavage of the middle meatus	18S rRNA deep sequencing	Increased diversity in CRS	Increased: Ascomycota Decreased: Basidiomycota	–	Increased: Cryptococcus neofromans, Rhodosporidium diabovatum, Davadiella Tassaiana Decreased: Malassezia-uncultured stramenopile
Boase et al. 2013 [24]	38 CRS and 6 controls	Ethmoid sinus mucosal tissue	Ibis T5000 analysis PCR coupled with electrospray ionization mass spectrometry	Fungi were only detected in 3 CRSwNP cases and in none of the control or CRSsNP	–	–	Only 3 positive samples; 2 CRSwNP cases had Aspergillus Fumigatus and 1 CRSwNP case had Penicilium Chrysogenum
Cleland et al. 2014 [7]	23 CRS 11 controls	Middle meatus or anterior ethmoid swabs	18S rDNA tag-encoded FLX amplicon pyrosequencing	Not different	–	Increased: *Scutellospora* 33 genera had differential abundance in CRS vs. Controls	–
Zhao, et al. 2018 [26]	63 CRS 27 controls	Middle meatus Swabs	Internal transcribed spacer (ITS) region.	Not different	–	Increased: Aspergillus only in culture positive CRSwNP cases	–
Gerber et al. 2016 [27]	15 CRSwNP 3 fungus ball 3 AFRS 7 controls	Brush samples of ethmoid or maxillary sinuses		Not different	–	Aspergillus only in AFRS and fungus ball patients	–

Other potential gatekeeping bacteria are *Propionobacterium acnes* [6, 15, 24] and *Peptoniphilus* genus [3] which has been shown to decrease in the setting of CRS.

Prediction of functional pathways in microbiota using PICRUSt analysis has shown that lipopolysaccharide (LPS) biosynthetic proteins and bacterial invasion of epithelial cell pathways were significantly higher in CRS patients compared to controls [3]. However, in that study, the analysis could not identify a single LPS producing bacterium which was increased and could explain the results. This suggests that there may be different groups of LPS producers that are increased in different CRS patients. This capacity has enabled these different bacteria to overcome the community in CRS.

13.3 Virome

The community of viruses, i.e., the virome, present in the nose may also play a role in CRS pathology. Healthy adults carry a large number of viruses including DNA viruses, single-stranded RNA viruses, and bacteriophages [36]. A few studies have examined the abundance of viruses in CRS [37–40]. Although the exact role of viruses in CRS is still unknown, the majority of CRS patients present with an initial viral upper respiratory tract infection prior to developing CRS or prior to a period of exacerbated CRS symptoms. Indeed, one recent study of a large population of patients showed that common respiratory viruses are more common in CRSsNP patients compared to healthy controls [37]. However, although the virome of patients with CRS appears to be relatively rich in rhinovirus and coronavirus [37–40], CRSwNP patients do not have an overall greater total population of viruses compared to controls. This study also found a significant association between presence of viruses in nasal cavity with radiological and endoscopic severity of CRS disease in CRSwNP patients [40].

An imbalance in the total abundance and/or types of viruses present in the nasal passages may contribute to CRS pathology. For instance, human rhinovirus infection can have multiple different impacts on the nasal epithelium. It can damage the mucosal lining by disrupting tight junction proteins [41, 42], thus priming the epithelium for bacterial invasion and infection [42]. It can also induce secondary bacterial invasion by significantly increasing the adherence of potentially harmful bacteria, such as *S. aureus*, to the respiratory mucosa [43]. Finally, some strains of human rhinovirus upregulate surface molecules, e.g., fibronectin, platelet-activating factor receptor, and carcinoembryonic antigen-related cell adhesion molecule, within primary human nasal epithelial cells [43]. These data support the notion that viral-bacterial interplay may contribute to the development of CRS, as viruses can facilitate bacterial binding and translocation by disrupting airway epithelial barrier function. This principle is particularly well established with influenza infections, where mortality is more often due to bacterial superinfections after the flu virus has run its course.

13.4 Mycobiome

The fungal microbiota (mycobiome) of the human respiratory tract is not well characterized. Findings from the few molecular-based studies that analyzed the mycobiome of the sinonasal cavity show evidence of fungal microorganisms in both healthy and CRS subjects [7, 8, 26]. The most commonly detected fungus in the nasal cavity of non-CRS individuals is *Malassezia* genus [7, 27, 44]. Aspergillus is abundant in sinus cavities as well, and is the most common fungus found in patients with CRS [26]. As with bacterial populations, fungal populations can go out of balance (i.e. fungal dysbiosis), with potentially deleterious effects on host health. However, one recent study, which used the internal transcribed spacer (ITS) region specific to only fungi to track balance within the mycobiome, found that fungal dysbiosis only occurs in a subset of CRS patients [26]. The same study showed that a large percentage of healthy and CRS cases have no evidence of fungal DNA [26]. Interestingly, another study focused on analyzing fungal microbiota in CRS, found evidence for the presence of *Aspergillus* only in CRS patients with known fungal subtypes of CRS including those with fungus ball and allergic fungal rhinosinusitis (AFRS) [27]. *Aspergillus fumigatus* is the primary fungus involved in the development of AFRS, which is a specific subtype of CRS accounting for 6–9% of all patients needing surgery [45]. AFRS is characterized by chronic eosinophilic-lymphocytic inflammation and nasal polyps. Similar to Allergic bronchopulmonary aspergillosis (ABPA), AFRS patients have elevated levels of serum IgE in response to fungus [45].

Not surprisingly, bacteria and fungi that co-inhabit the nasal cavity can sometimes interact with one another. Bacterial co-colonizers can affect fungal morphology, survival, and growth [46]. For example, the bacterium *S. aureus* penetrates the hyphae of the *Candida albicans* (*C. albicans*) fungus during mixed biofilm growth [46–48]. In an ex vivo experiment on mouse tongue epithelium, *S. aureus* only penetrated within the epithelial tissue when invasive *C. albicans* hyphae were present in the culture [47].

13.5 Interplay Between the Immune System and Microbes

The innate immune system is responsible for mounting the first line of defense and establishing a barrier to protect the airways. Toward this end, sinonasal epithelium and mucosal cells produce a large group of antimicrobial molecules, and epithelial cells also possess multiple pattern recognition receptors, such as Toll-like receptors (TLRs) and bitter taste receptors [49], that recognize potentially hazardous microbes and/or microbial products. In some cases, activating innate defense mechanisms may actually lead to some of the inflammatory symptoms associated with CRS. For instance, certain pattern recognition receptors are found on inflammatory granulocytes like basophils and eosinophils, which are commonly detected in inflamed sinonasal tissue of CRS patients [50]. Activated granulocytes recruit other inflammatory cells involved in the T helper 2 type (Th2) response, thus driving inflammation. Th2 inflammation can in turn downregulate multiple elements of innate immunity, such as production of antimicrobial and anti-inflammatory agents including human beta-defensin 2(hBD-2), antileukoproteinase, Immunoglobulin J chain and surfactant protein-A (SP-A) [19, 49, 51]. This can result in a weakened innate immune response, which in turn further exposes the individual to the risks of microbes and their pathogenic products.

There are a few examples of microbial and fungal products that interact with the immune system, as described above, with particular implications for CRS. Enterotoxins produced by *S. aureus* can act as superantigens and promote Th2 inflammation in CRS [52]. Increased Th2 inflammation include production of IL-13, IL-4, and IL-5 cytokines which recruit and activate multiple inflammatory cells such as eosinophils, basophils, mast cells, and alternatively activated macrophages [49]. As discussed above, these cells recognize and respond to multiple microbial products through their pattern recognition receptors and create a feed forward loop of inflammation. Other examples of pro-inflammatory microbial products are bacterial and fungal proteases, which can induce epithelial production of Thymic Stromal Lymphopoietin (TSLP) by activating Protease-Activated Receptor-2 (PAR-2) [10]. TSLP can subsequently activated dendritic cells to promote Th2 responses and activate innate lymphoid type 2 cells (ILC-2), which are potent inflammatory cells found in CRS [53]. It is worth mentioning that many of the discoveries discussed above were made by studying the interplay of the immune system with microbes.

Specific to the mycobiome, there are some pattern recognition receptors, such as C-type lectins, that recognize the fungal polysaccharide β-1,3 glucan motif found on fungal cell walls. Absence of such receptors may have pathological consequences, as mice lacking dectin-1 (a type of C-type lectin) were susceptible to more severe epithelial inflammation compared to wild-type mice [54]. Other C-type lectins, namely Clec4e and Clecsf9, specifically recognize the fungi of the genus *Malassezia* [55]. When these receptors sense *Malassezia*, they signal the activation of macrophages, which in turn promotes pro-inflammatory responses [55]. Interestingly, these receptors have also been implicated in Th2 inflammation [56]. Thus, as is also true with bacteria, we see that interactions among commensal fungi and the mucosal immune system are important in maintaining host and microbial homeostasis, and that disequilibrium has the potential to drive chronic inflammation.

13.6 Conclusions

Findings of studies of the nasal microbiome and its impact on CRS pathology have been inconsistent and highly variable, making it difficult to draw actionable conclusions. The variations in findings may be caused by differences in methods of collection or analysis or may reflect underlying complexity that is not yet appreciated. Despite these challenges, our understanding of the role of microbes in CRS pathology has evolved from a narrow focus on a single pathogenic organism to a more holistic view that considers the entire microbiome residing in the sinonasal cavity. We also now appreciate that interactions among microbes, microbial products, the environment, and the host immune system could all contribute to dysbiosis, chronic inflammation and, ultimately, the development of disease. Whereas bacteria had been the focus of research in past, we now understand that fungal and viral populations must also be considered for their role in CRS pathology. Though it is clear that the nasal cavity microbiome differs in CRS patients compared to their healthy counterparts, one key challenge that remains is dissecting whether these observed variations are the cause or the effect of chronic inflammation/disease. Thus, the relationship between sinonasal microbiota and CRS must remain at the forefront of study in the field. The findings of such studies have and will continue to guide future endeavors to find new therapeutic or preventive modalities in CRS.

13.7 Implications of Microbiome Equilibrium for Medical Practice

The composition, distribution, and overall abundance of microbiota have an impact on mucosal health by influencing the growth and function of pathogenic microbes and production of inflammatory microbial products. This suggests that any therapeutic approach based on use of broad spectrum antimicrobial agents has the potential to cause harm by triggering disequilibrium. There is a critical need to understand the mechanistic details underlying host–microbiome relationships so as to better inform the use of antimicrobial treatments and/or develop new treatments that leverage such relationships to strengthen innate defenses and minimize inflammation. This is relevant to the treatment of CRS, known to be the result of rampant inflammation, and is likely to be particularly relevant to treating patients with CRS-related asthma, in whom nasal microbiome dysbiosis may underlie their severe atopic endotype.

References

1. Man WH, de Steenhuijsen Piters WA, Bogaert D. The microbiota of the respiratory tract: gatekeeper to respiratory health. Nat Rev Microbiol. 2017;15(5):259–70. https://doi.org/10.1038/nrmicro.2017.14.
2. Mahdavinia M, Keshavarzian A, Tobin MC, Landay AL, Schleimer RP. A comprehensive review of the nasal microbiome in chronic rhinosinusitis (CRS). Clin Exp Allergy. 2016;46(1):21–41. https://doi.org/10.1111/cea.12666.
3. Mahdavinia M, Engen PA, LoSavio PS, Naqib A, Khan RJ, Tobin MC, et al. The nasal microbiome in patients with chronic rhinosinusitis: analyzing the effects of atopy and bacterial functional pathways in 111 patients. J Allergy Clin Immunol. 2018;142(1):287–90 e4. https://doi.org/10.1016/j.jaci.2018.01.033.
4. Ramakrishnan VR, Hauser LJ, Feazel LM, Ir D, Robertson CE, Frank DN. Sinus microbiota varies among chronic rhinosinusitis phenotypes and predicts surgical outcome. J Allergy Clin Immunol. 2015;136(2):334–42.e1. https://doi.org/10.1016/j.jaci.2015.02.008.
5. Hoggard M, Biswas K, Zoing M, Wagner Mackenzie B, Taylor MW, Douglas RG. Evidence of microbiota dysbiosis in chronic rhinosinusitis. Int Forum Allergy

Rhinol. 2017;7(3):230–9. https://doi.org/10.1002/alr.21871.

6. Chalermwatanachai T, Vilchez-Vargas R, Holtappels G, Lacoere T, Jauregui R, Kerckhof FM, et al. Chronic rhinosinusitis with nasal polyps is characterized by dysbacteriosis of the nasal microbiota. Sci Rep. 2018;8(1):7926. https://doi.org/10.1038/s41598-018-26327-2.
7. Cleland EJ, Bassioni A, Boase S, Dowd S, Vreugde S, Wormald PJ. The fungal microbiome in chronic rhinosinusitis: richness, diversity, postoperative changes and patient outcomes. Int Forum Allergy Rhinol. 2014;4(4):259–65. https://doi.org/10.1002/alr.21297.
8. Aurora R, Chatterjee D, Hentzleman J, Prasad G, Sindwani R, Sanford T. Contrasting the microbiomes from healthy volunteers and patients with chronic rhinosinusitis. JAMA Otolaryngol Head Neck Surg. 2013;139(12):1328–38. https://doi.org/10.1001/jamaoto.2013.5465.
9. van den Bergh MR, Biesbroek G, Rossen JW, de Steenhuijsen Piters WA, Bosch AA, van Gils EJ, et al. Associations between pathogens in the upper respiratory tract of young children: interplay between viruses and bacteria. PLoS One. 2012;7(10):e47711. https://doi.org/10.1371/journal.pone.0047711.
10. Kouzaki H, O'Grady SM, Lawrence CB, Kita H. Proteases induce production of thymic stromal lymphopoietin by airway epithelial cells through protease-activated receptor-2. J Immunol. 2009;183(2):1427–34. https://doi.org/10.4049/jimmunol.0900904.
11. Lal D, Keim P, Delisle J, Barker B, Rank MA, Chia N, et al. Mapping and comparing bacterial microbiota in the sinonasal cavity of healthy, allergic rhinitis, and chronic rhinosinusitis subjects. Int Forum Allergy Rhinol. 2017;7(6):561–9. https://doi.org/10.1002/alr.21934.
12. Choi CH, Poroyko V, Watanabe S, Jiang D, Lane J, de Tineo M, et al. Seasonal allergic rhinitis affects sinonasal microbiota. Am J Rhinol Allergy. 2014;28(4):281–6. https://doi.org/10.2500/ajra.2014.28.4050.
13. Wise SK, Lin SY, Toskala E, Orlandi RR, Akdis CA, Alt JA, et al. International consensus statement on allergy and rhinology: allergic rhinitis. Int Forum Allergy Rhinol. 2018;8(2):108–352. https://doi.org/10.1002/alr.22073.
14. Fazlollahi M, Lee TD, Andrade J, Oguntuyo K, Chun Y, Grishina G, et al. The nasal microbiome in asthma. J Allergy Clin Immunol. 2018;142(3):834–843.e2. https://doi.org/10.1016/j.jaci.2018.02.020.
15. Wagner Mackenzie B, Waite DW, Hoggard M, Douglas RG, Taylor MW, Biswas K. Bacterial community collapse: a meta-analysis of the sinonasal microbiota in chronic rhinosinusitis. Environ Microbiol. 2017;19(1):381–92. https://doi.org/10.1111/1462-2920.13632.
16. Teo SM, Mok D, Pham K, Kusel M, Serralha M, Troy N, et al. The infant nasopharyngeal microbiome impacts severity of lower respiratory infection and risk of asthma development. Cell Host Microbe. 2015;17(5):704–15. https://doi.org/10.1016/j.chom.2015.03.008.
17. Cardenas PA, Cooper PJ, Cox MJ, Chico M, Arias C, Moffatt MF, et al. Upper airways microbiota in antibiotic-naive wheezing and healthy infants from the tropics of rural Ecuador. PLoS One. 2012;7(10):e46803. https://doi.org/10.1371/journal.pone.0046803.
18. Bisgaard H, Hermansen MN, Buchvald F, Loland L, Halkjaer LB, Bonnelykke K, et al. Childhood asthma after bacterial colonization of the airway in neonates. N Engl J Med. 2007;357(15):1487–95. https://doi.org/10.1056/NEJMoa052632.
19. Tomazic PV, Birner-Gruenberger R, Leitner A, Obrist B, Spoerk S, Lang-Loidolt D. Nasal mucus proteomic changes reflect altered immune responses and epithelial permeability in patients with allergic rhinitis. J Allergy Clin Immunol. 2014;133(3):741–50. https://doi.org/10.1016/j.jaci.2013.09.040.
20. Stephenson MF, Mfuna L, Dowd SE, Wolcott RD, Barbeau J, Poisson M, et al. Molecular characterization of the polymicrobial flora in chronic rhinosinusitis. J Otolaryngol Head Neck Surg. 2010;39(2):182–7.
21. Stressmann FA, Rogers GB, Chan SW, Howarth PH, Harries PG, Bruce KD, et al. Characterization of bacterial community diversity in chronic rhinosinusitis infections using novel culture-independent techniques. Am J Rhinol Allergy. 2011;25(4):e133–40. https://doi.org/10.2500/ajra.2011.25.3628.
22. Abreu NA, Nagalingam NA, Song Y, Roediger FC, Pletcher SD, Goldberg AN, et al. Sinus microbiome diversity depletion and Corynebacterium tuberculostearicum enrichment mediates rhinosinusitis. Sci Transl Med. 2012;4(151):151ra24. https://doi.org/10.1126/scitranslmed.3003783.
23. Feazel LM, Robertson CE, Ramakrishnan VR, Frank DN. Microbiome complexity and Staphylococcus aureus in chronic rhinosinusitis. Laryngoscope. 2012;122(2):467–72. https://doi.org/10.1002/lary.22398.
24. Boase S, Foreman A, Cleland E, Tan L, Melton-Kreft R, Pant H, et al. The microbiome of chronic rhinosinusitis: culture, molecular diagnostics and biofilm detection. BMC Infect Dis. 2013;13:210. https://doi.org/10.1186/1471-2334-13-210.
25. Choi EB, Hong SW, Kim DK, Jeon SG, Kim KR, Cho SH, et al. Decreased diversity of nasal microbiota and their secreted extracellular vesicles in patients with chronic rhinosinusitis based on a metagenomic analysis. Allergy. 2014;69(4):517–26. https://doi.org/10.1111/all.12374.
26. Zhao YC, Bassiouni A, Tanjararak K, Vreugde S, Wormald PJ, Psaltis AJ. Role of fungi in chronic rhinosinusitis through ITS sequencing. Laryngoscope. 2018;128(1):16–22. https://doi.org/10.1002/lary.26702.
27. Gelber JT, Cope EK, Goldberg AN, Pletcher SD. Evaluation of malassezia and common fungal pathogens in subtypes of chronic rhinosinusitis. Int

Forum Allergy Rhinol. 2016;6(9):950–5. https://doi.org/10.1002/alr.21777.
28. Bomar L, Brugger SD, Yost BH, Davies SS, Lemon KP. Corynebacterium accolens releases antipneumococcal free fatty acids from human nostril and skin surface triacylglycerols. MBio. 2016;7(1):e01725–15. https://doi.org/10.1128/mBio.01725-15.
29. Biesbroek G, Tsivtsivadze E, Sanders EA, Montijn R, Veenhoven RH, Keijser BJ, et al. Early respiratory microbiota composition determines bacterial succession patterns and respiratory health in children. Am J Respir Crit Care Med. 2014;190(11):1283–92. https://doi.org/10.1164/rccm.201407-1240OC.
30. Hardy BL, Dickey SW, Plaut RD, Riggins DP, Stibitz S, Otto M, et al. Corynebacterium pseudodiphtheriticum exploits Staphylococcus aureus virulence components in a novel polymicrobial defense strategy. MBio. 2019;10(1):e02491–18. https://doi.org/10.1128/mBio.02491-18.
31. Bachert C, van Steen K, Zhang N, Holtappels G, Cattaert T, Maus B, et al. Specific IgE against Staphylococcus aureus enterotoxins: an independent risk factor for asthma. J Allergy Clin Immunol. 2012;130(2):376–81 e8. https://doi.org/10.1016/j.jaci.2012.05.012.
32. Bachert C, Zhang N, van Zele T, Gevaert P, Patou J, van Cauwenberge P. Staphylococcus aureus enterotoxins as immune stimulants in chronic rhinosinusitis. Clin Allergy Immunol. 2007;20:163–75.
33. Bachert C, Zhang N. Chronic rhinosinusitis and asthma: novel understanding of the role of IgE 'above atopy'. J Intern Med. 2012;272(2):133–43. https://doi.org/10.1111/j.1365-2796.2012.02559.x.
34. Ramsey MM, Freire MO, Gabrilska RA, Rumbaugh KP, Lemon KP. Staphylococcus aureus shifts toward commensalism in response to corynebacterium species. Front Microbiol. 2016;7:1230. https://doi.org/10.3389/fmicb.2016.01230.
35. Lai Y, Cogen AL, Radek KA, Park HJ, Macleod DT, Leichtle A, et al. Activation of TLR2 by a small molecule produced by Staphylococcus epidermidis increases antimicrobial defense against bacterial skin infections. J Invest Dermatol. 2010;130(9):2211–21. https://doi.org/10.1038/jid.2010.123.
36. Wylie KM, Mihindukulasuriya KA, Zhou Y, Sodergren E, Storch GA, Weinstock GM. Metagenomic analysis of double-stranded DNA viruses in healthy adults. BMC Biol. 2014;12:71. https://doi.org/10.1186/s12915-014-0071-7.
37. Rowan NR, Lee S, Sahu N, Kanaan A, Cox S, Phillips CD, et al. The role of viruses in the clinical presentation of chronic rhinosinusitis. Am J Rhinol Allergy. 2015;29(6):e197–200. https://doi.org/10.2500/ajra.2015.29.4242.
38. Cho GS, Moon BJ, Lee BJ, Gong CH, Kim NH, Kim YS, et al. High rates of detection of respiratory viruses in the nasal washes and mucosae of patients with chronic rhinosinusitis. J Clin Microbiol. 2013;51(3):979–84. https://doi.org/10.1128/JCM.02806-12.
39. Wood AJ, Antoszewska H, Fraser J, Douglas RG. Is chronic rhinosinusitis caused by persistent respiratory virus infection? Int Forum Allergy Rhinol. 2012;1(2):95–100. https://doi.org/10.1002/alr.20030.
40. Goggin RK, Bennett CA, Bialasiewicz S, Vediappan RS, Vreugde S, Wormald PJ, et al. The presence of virus significantly associates with chronic rhinosinusitis disease severity. Allergy. 2019;74(8):1569–72. https://doi.org/10.1111/all.13772.
41. Sajjan U, Wang Q, Zhao Y, Gruenert DC, Hershenson MB. Rhinovirus disrupts the barrier function of polarized airway epithelial cells. Am J Respir Crit Care Med. 2008;178(12):1271–81. https://doi.org/10.1164/rccm.200801-136OC.
42. Kim KA, Jung JH, Kang IG, Choi YS, Kim ST. ROS is involved in disruption of tight junctions of human nasal epithelial cells induced by HRV16. Laryngoscope. 2018;128(12):E393–401. https://doi.org/10.1002/lary.27510.
43. Wang JH, Kwon HJ, Jang YJ. Rhinovirus enhances various bacterial adhesions to nasal epithelial cells simultaneously. Laryngoscope. 2009;119(7):1406–11. https://doi.org/10.1002/lary.20498.
44. Jung WH, Croll D, Cho JH, Kim YR, Lee YW. Analysis of the nasal vestibule mycobiome in patients with allergic rhinitis. Mycoses. 2015;58(3):167–72. https://doi.org/10.1111/myc.12296.
45. Ryan MW, Clark CM. Allergic fungal rhinosinusitis and the unified airway: the role of antifungal therapy in AFRS. Curr Allergy Asthma Rep. 2015;15(12):75. https://doi.org/10.1007/s11882-015-0573-6.
46. Zhang I, Pletcher SD, Goldberg AN, Barker BM, Cope EK. Fungal microbiota in chronic airway inflammatory disease and emerging relationships with the host immune response. Front Microbiol. 2017;8:2477. https://doi.org/10.3389/fmicb.2017.02477.
47. Peters BM, Ovchinnikova ES, Krom BP, Schlecht LM, Zhou H, Hoyer LL, et al. Staphylococcus aureus adherence to Candida albicans hyphae is mediated by the hyphal adhesin Als3p. Microbiology. 2012;158(Pt 12):2975–86. https://doi.org/10.1099/mic.0.062109-0.
48. Peters BM, Jabra-Rizk MA, Scheper MA, Leid JG, Costerton JW, Shirtliff ME. Microbial interactions and differential protein expression in Staphylococcus aureus -Candida albicans dual-species biofilms. FEMS Immunol Med Microbiol. 2010;59(3):493–503. https://doi.org/10.1111/j.1574-695X.2010.00710.x.
49. Hulse KE, Stevens WW, Tan BK, Schleimer RP. Pathogenesis of nasal polyposis. Clin Exp Allergy. 2015;45(2):328–46. https://doi.org/10.1111/cea.12472.
50. Mahdavinia M, Carter RG, Ocampo CJ, Stevens W, Kato A, Tan BK, et al. Basophils are elevated in nasal polyps of patients with chronic rhinosinusitis without aspirin sensitivity. J Allergy Clin Immunol. 2014;133(6):1759–63. https://doi.org/10.1016/j.jaci.2013.12.1092.
51. Tesse R, Pandey RC, Kabesch M. Genetic variations in toll-like receptor pathway genes influence asthma

and atopy. Allergy. 2011;66(3):307–16. https://doi.org/10.1111/j.1398-9995.2010.02489.x.
52. Van Zele T, Gevaert P, Watelet J-B, Claeys G, Holtappels G, Claeys C, et al. Staphylococcus aureus colonization and IgE antibody formation to enterotoxins is increased in nasal polyposis. J Allergy Clin Immunol. 2004;114(4):981. https://doi.org/10.1016/j.jaci.2004.07.013.
53. Poposki JA, Klingler AI, Tan BK, Soroosh P, Banie H, Lewis G, et al. Group 2 innate lymphoid cells are elevated and activated in chronic rhinosinusitis with nasal polyps. Immun Inflamm Dis. 2017;5(3):233–43. https://doi.org/10.1002/iid3.161.
54. Iliev ID, Funari VA, Taylor KD, Nguyen Q, Reyes CN, Strom SP, et al. Interactions between commensal fungi and the C-type lectin receptor Dectin-1 influence colitis. Science. 2012;336(6086):1314–7. https://doi.org/10.1126/science.1221789.
55. Yamasaki S, Matsumoto M, Takeuchi O, Matsuzawa T, Ishikawa E, Sakuma M, et al. C-type lectin Mincle is an activating receptor for pathogenic fungus, Malassezia. Proc Natl Acad Sci U S A. 2009;106(6):1897–902. https://doi.org/10.1073/pnas.0805177106.
56. Geijtenbeek TB, Gringhuis SI. C-type lectin receptors in the control of T helper cell differentiation. Nat Rev Immunol. 2016;16(7):433–48. https://doi.org/10.1038/nri.2016.55.

14 *Staphylococcus aureus* and Its Proteins

Goran Abdurrahman and Barbara M. Bröker

Key Points

- *Staphylococcus aureus* is an opportunistic pathogen that can cause a wide range of infections.
- The bacterium can develop a long-lasting relationship with human and asymptomatically colonizes up to 20% of general populations, while this rate can be significantly higher in patients with allergic conditions such as chronic rhinosinusitis (CRS).
- Colonization with *S. aureus* is considered as a risk factor for the development of both infections and allergic reactions.
- *S. aureus* promotes type 2 (allergic) immune responses through the release of a number of different virulence factors, namely superantigens and staphylococcal serine protease-like proteins.
- Driving an allergic response is an immune evasion mechanism employed by *S. aureus* that is increasing the bacterial survival chances because allergic inflammation is less active at killing the pathogen than a type 1 immune response.

Staphylococcus aureus is a Gram-positive bacterium that can persist in nature under hostile environmental conditions and interacts with humans as both commensal and pathogen. It is responsible for a multitude of hospital- and community-acquired infections. The bacterium is often found on the skin of the axilla, chest/abdomen, groin, and perineum as well as on the mucosa of pharynx and intestine [1, 2], but the main site of colonization in humans is the *vestibulum nasi* (anterior nares) [3, 4]. With regard to *S. aureus* colonization, humans are grouped into three categories: non-carriers, intermittent carriers, and persistent carriers [2]. Around 20% of human population are persistently colonized with *S. aureus* [5]. Nasal colonization depends on both host and microbial factors that will be described below. The differential rates of colonization among individuals are linked to their immune status, gene polymorphisms, and competition of *S. aureus* with other microorganisms [2]. Patients with airway diseases, such as asthma or chronic rhinosinusitis with nasal polyps (CRSwNP), show significantly higher rates of *S. aureus* colonization than healthy adults [6]. It has long been recognized that nasal carriage of *S. aureus* is a major risk factor for infections, which are mostly caused by the colonizing strain [7].

In this chapter we will discuss the influence of *S. aureus* on CRS with the focus on its involve-

The original version of this chapter was revised. The correction to this chapter can be found at https://doi.org/10.1007/978-981-16-0784-4_55

G. Abdurrahman · B. M. Bröker (✉)
Institute of Immunology, University Medicine Greifswald, Greifswald, Germany
e-mail: goran.abdurrahman@uni-greifswald.de; broeker@uni-greifswald.de

L. Zhang, C. Bachert (eds.), *Chronic Rhinosinusitis*, https://doi.org/10.1007/978-981-16-0784-4_14

ment in the development of an allergic inflammation. First, we will show how *S. aureus* colonizes the host and the obstacles it has to overcome in order to do so. Later, we will shed light on the components of *S. aureus* that have allergenic properties and illustrate how these can be involved in driving allergic reactions and, therefore, contribute to the symptoms in CRS. Finally, we will argue that *S. aureus* may benefit from stimulating allergic inflammation.

14.1 Interaction Between *S. aureus* and the Host

The species *S. aureus* has a diverse range of virulence factors that, due to genetic variability, are not equally expressed among different clinical strains. The degree of conservation within the species *S. aureus* determines the classification of genes into the core genome, the core variable genome, and the variable genome [8]. About 75% of the bacterial genome belongs to the core genome which is highly conserved among different isolates. It encodes genes associated with central metabolism and other housekeeping functions. The core variable genome comprises about 10% of the pathogen's genome and includes regulators of virulence gene expression, e.g., the accessory gene regulator (*agr*), and surface proteins [9]. Fifteen percent of the total genome, the variable genome, is encoded on mobile genetic elements such as plasmids, bacteriophages, pathogenicity islands, and transposons [10, 11]. Many of the bacterial virulence factors are encoded on such genetic elements. For example, bacteriophages contribute to the virulence of *S. aureus* by carrying accessory virulence genes, encoding for example, Panton–Valentine leukocidin (PVL), staphylokinase, enterotoxins, and exfoliative toxin A [12, 13].

The plethora of virulence factors are crucial to the success of *S. aureus* as a commensal bacterium and as a pathogen. As an example, the bacterium expresses a range of cell wall-anchored (CWA) proteins. The most predominant group of the CWA is the family of microbial surface components recognizing adhesive matrix molecules (MSCRAMMs). These surface proteins are defined by the presence of two adjacent IgG-like folded subdomains that mediate the binding to their ligands on host cells. Examples of MSCRAMMs include, but are not limited to, clumping factor A (ClfA), ClfB, fibronectin binding protein A (FnBPA), FnBPB, serine-aspartate repeat proteins C-E (Sdr C-E), and collagen adhesin (Cna) [14]. These MSCRAMMs have many functions, including adhesion to and invasion of host cells and tissues, evasion of the immune response and biofilm formation [15]. Additionally, the bacterium secretes a number of pore-forming beta-barrel toxins, the most prominent member being alpha (α)-toxin. The toxin was initially named as α-hemolysin due to its ability to cause red blood cell lysis. However, based on its broad range of virulence functions, α-toxin is an important cause of injury in skin and soft tissue necrosis as well as necrotizing pneumonia, which is often lethal [16].

S. aureus can interfere with the host's immune system through factors that block complement activation, phagocyte chemotaxis, phagocytic uptake, and oxidative killing [17–19]. Conversely, the bacterium can exploit host defense mechanisms such as neutrophil extracellular traps (NET) or fibrin formation to favor its own replication and survival. *S. aureus* is also known for the manipulation of the adaptive immune response, such as disruption of the proliferative response of B- and T cells, which prevents these cells from mounting a protective immune response [20].

14.2 Colonization

S. aureus has evolved a complex relationship with the human host and its colonization is a multifactorial process that is yet to be fully understood. Persistent colonization requires the bacterium to establish a stable interaction with the epithelium through various cell surface components and the release of virulence factors. Also, in order for the bacterium to survive in the nasal niche, it has to compete with the local microbiome and avoid or misdirect recognition and elimination by the immune system. Hence, the process of colonization is the result of complex interplay between a multitude of host and bacterial factors that ends up in a tight and, sometimes, long-lasting relationship between the two parties [21]. In a study, it was shown that persistent *S. aureus* carriers will eventually re-obtain their own strain after they have been de-colonized and then artificially re-colonized with a mixed *S. aureus* culture [22]. The composition of the nasal microbiome is not entirely fixed by host genetics and is therefore susceptible to environmental conditions [23]. Moreover, certain bacterial species interfere with the *S. aureus* colonization in the nose. For example, some *Staphylococcus epidermidis* strains secrete a serine protease (Esp) that inhibits *S. aureus* biofilm formation and nasal colonization. The epidemiological data from healthy subjects show that the presence of Esp-secreting *Staphylococcus epidermidis* in the nose correlates with the absence of *S. aureus* [24]. Also, *Bacillus subtilis* [25] and *Staphylococcus lugdunensis* [26] have been shown to abolish *S. aureus* colonization.

The anterior nares of humans, where *S. aureus* mostly colonizes, is lined by skin. Its uppermost layer is keratinized squamous epithelium that contains proteins such as loricrin, cytokeratin 10, involucrin, and filaggrin [27]. The bacterium efficiently adheres to these proteins through surface factors including ClfB [21, 28], and iron-regulated surface determinant A (IsdA) [28]. Other *S. aureus* surface proteins, such as surface protein G (SasG), SasX [2] as well as SdrC and SdrD [29] may also serve as ligands for host proteins on the epithelial cells. Additionally, staphylococcal cell wall teichoic acids (WTAs), non-protein adhesins, are vital for the colonization process [30]. The bacterium can bind to the ciliated epithelium in the posterior nasal cavity through WTAs [31]. Once colonization is established, *S. aureus* grows exponentially in nasal cavity to avoid elimination by epithelial cell shedding and mucous release [15]. Besides, *S. aureus* can survive intracellularly in different cell types including epithelial cells, endothelial cells, inflammatory cells, and mast cells [2]. The bacterium invades these cells, adapts to the intracellular environment, and exerts its toxic effects while hiding from immune recognition [15] and antibiotic killing [2, 32]. Intracellular persistence might explain the recurrence of infections and failure of decolonization observed in patients with CRS [33]. In the upper airway mucosa of patients with CSRwNP, more than 600 proteins released by *S. aureus* were identified with high resolution mass spectrometry; among these were staphylococcal enterotoxins (SEs) and serine protease-like proteins (Spls) [34] which are going to be discussed further in this chapter.

Successful colonization requires *S. aureus* to overcome the challenges imposed by the host's immune system. With regard to this, the bacterium has evolved a broad range of mechanisms to escape the immune system such as avoiding, inhibiting and misdirecting the host's immune system [35]. As an example, *S. aureus* releases protein A that inhibits phagocytosis. Opsonization for phagocytosis requires IgG antibody to bind to the antigens on the surface of the bacterial cells followed by activation of complement and enhanced recognition by phagocytes via IgG-Fc receptors and complement receptors. *S. aureus*-produced protein A binds to the Fc part of the IgG, such that the antibodies bind to the bacterial cells in the wrong orientation preventing antibody- and complement enhanced phagocytosis [20, 36]. Additionally, ClfA has been shown to mediate complement protein C3b inhibition by recruiting host complement regulators [37]. Also, staphylokinase, an exoprotein produced by *S. aureus*, was shown to resist the antimicrobial activity of α-defensin which is secreted by neutrophils to disrupt the integrity of bacterial cell walls (Fig. 14.1) [35].

There is increasing evidence that colonization by *S. aureus* is associated with the development of allergic inflammation. The bacteria can release some components with documented allergenic properties [38–41]. In T helper 2 (Th2) cells, these proteins will induce the release of interleukin (IL)-4 and IL-13, which are known to promote immunoglobulin class switching to IgE and IgE formation. We propose that driving an allergic immune response is an immune evasion

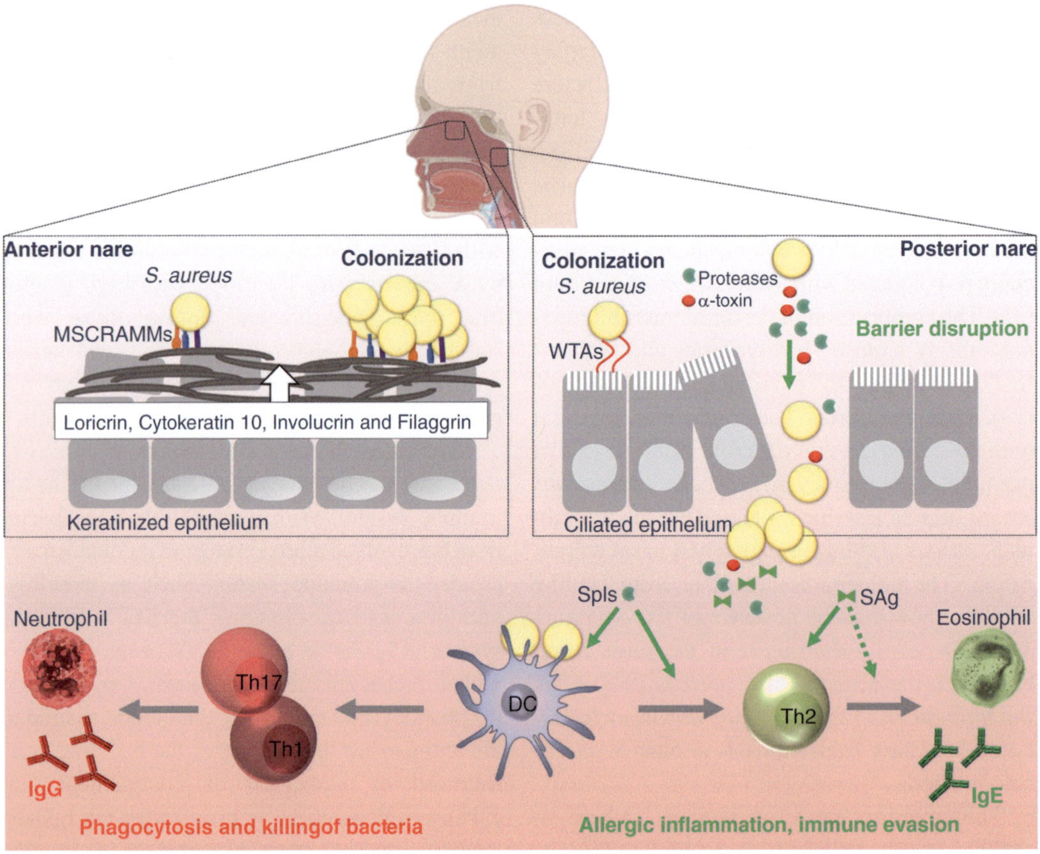

Fig. 14.1 *S. aureus* colonization, invasion and induction of an adaptive immune response. *S. aureus* uses MSCRAMMs to bind to loricrin, cytokeratin 10, involucrin and filaggrin which are abundunt in the keratinized epithelium in the anterior nares (left panel). However, in the posterior nares (right panel), the bacterium binds to the ciliated cells through its WTAs. Proteases and α-toxin can disrupt the epithelial barrier, facilitating the entry of *S. aureus* and its components. Moreover, secreted allergens, namely Spls and SAgs trigger allergic inflammation and elicit an IgE-biased specific antibody response. As a result of this concerted action, *S. aureus* is able to shift the host immune response away from a Th1/Th17 profile, which would be required for efficient clearance of the bacteria, towards type 2 inflammation, which is less harmful to this microorganism. *DC* dendritic cell, *MSCRAMM* microbial surface components recognizing adhesive matrix molecule, *SAg* superantigen, *Spl* staphylococcal serine protease-like protein, *Th* T helper cell, *WTA* wall-teichoic acid

mechanism employed by *S. aureus* to increase its survival chances within the host because an allergic immune profile (type 2) is less effective at killing the bacterium than the more typical antibacterial immune response that is dominated by IFN-γ- and IL-17 (type 1). Due to the increasing evidence for involvement of *S. aureus* in allergic diseases, there is a growing interest in the allergome, i.e., all the IgE binding proteins of *S. aureus* [6, 42]. So far, the proteins of *S. aureus* with documented allergenic properties include some members of the superantigen family (enterotoxins A-E and toxic shock syndrome toxin-1) and Spls.

14.3 Superantigens

Superantigens (SAgs) are a family of potent toxins that have a very strong immunomodulatory effects. SAgs are mitogens for T cells and cause aberrant activation of large proportions of this cell population that is usually subject to stringent regulation. The toxins crosslink major histocompatibility complex-II on an antigen presenting cell with the T cell receptor, independent of its antigen specificity. Thus they bypass the normal antigen processing and presentation and activate a large proportion of T cells. The massive synchronous T cell activation results in the release of high amounts of cytokines, a cytokine storm. The staphylococcal SAg family is composed of at least 26 different toxins with the protein size ranging between 19 kDa to 27 kD [43]. It encompasses staphylococcal enterotoxins (SEs), staphylococcal enterotoxin-like molecules (SEls), and the toxic shock syndrome toxin-1 (TSST-1). Two SAgs, SElX, and the putative SElW [43] are universally present, and around 80% of clinical *S. aureus* isolates harbor additional SAg genes [44] that are encoded on mobile genetic elements [43].

After more than 30 years of research, the advantage gained by *S. aureus* from SAgs is still under discussion. SAgs are thought to create an immunological "smokescreen" [34] in which *S. aureus* hides itself from specific immune recognition through stimulating the release of a storm of cytokines that makes T cells refractory to specific activation [36, 45, 46]. Also, T cells exposed to the cytokine storm become anergic and many of them ultimately die [45, 46]. Another concept suggests that SAgs aid *S. aureus* in the process of colonizing the host. Antibodies directed against SAgs have been found in persistent carriers [47, 48]. Also, SAg transcripts have been detected in the nose of carriers [47]. These indicate that SAgs are expressed during colonization. In a mouse infection model, deletion of *seb* increased the bacterial burden. The authors propose that SAgs act as a checkpoint through promoting an inflammatory response that keeps the bacterial number below pathogenic densities, therefore, fostering asymptomatic carriage, while preventing complete elimination by the immune system [43].

However, SAgs are known to cause a number of different diseases ranging from self-limiting episodes of food poisoning to multi-organ dysfunction. First and foremost, SEs are potent gastrointestinal toxins causing vomiting and diarrhea. A rare but well-known condition triggered by SAgs is the toxic shock syndrome (TSS) which is caused by the storm of pro-inflammatory cytokines released by non-specifically-activated T cells. TSS is a life-threatening condition manifested by sudden fever, hypotension and potential progression to multi-organ failure [49]. Moreover, SAgs are associated with pneumonia, endocarditis, and autoimmune disorders [43, 50]. Being dangerous virulence factors, SAgs are interesting vaccine targets. Vaccination protocols using genetically modified inactive SAg toxoids of TSST-1 and SEB, respectively, have been successful in phase I clinical trials, proving safety and immunogenicity [51, 52]. Of particular relevance to this review, there is increasing evidence that *S. aureus* is involved in the severity, exacerbation, and recurrence of CRS, especially CRSwNP. It has been shown that the presence of *S. aureus* in the local tissue of the patients undergoing sinus surgery was associated with the recurrence of CRS [53]. The allergenic properties of the SAgs are evident because they induce specific IgE formation in susceptible individuals. SAg-specific IgE (SE-IgE) has been detected in the sera of patients with different allergic disorders, including CRS.

In CRS, these toxins may have multiple pathophysiologic functions: (i) Superantigen: stimulation of local T cells independent of their antigen specificity and function; (ii) "superallergen": stimulation of Th2 cells independent of their antigen specificity; (iii) superantigen: Stimulation of local B cells by recruiting T cell help, independent of the immune cells' antigen specificity and function; (iv) "superallergen" stimulation of IgE-positive B cells by recruiting help from Th2 cells, independent of the immune cells' antigen specificity; (v) antigen:—SAgs are dominant staphylococcal antigens, shown only for the B cell and antibody response; (vi) allergen:—SAgs elicit a specific IgE response (SE-IgE). The frequently observed anti-SAg IgG- and IgE responses (v, vi) point to a large pool of SAg-specific T cells, including Th2 cells. These T cells, however, have not yet been demonstrated.

Many CRSwNP patients exhibit high concentrations of polyclonal IgE, which may be significantly higher locally in the nasal polyp tissue than the circulation. This increase of polyclonal IgE in the nasal fluids has been linked to the SAgs of *S. aureus*. These may polyclonally activate Th2 cells to induce Ig class switching in B cells, resulting in the release of polyclonal IgE [39]. In line with the higher rate of colonization by *S. aureus*, the formation of serum SE-IgE is also increased in patients with chronic airway diseases compared with healthy individuals. It has been demonstrated that SE-IgE levels in CRSwNP correlate with disease severity and asthma comorbidity, showing their role as an important cofactor in chronic inflammatory airway diseases [40, 54]. In another study screening more than 2900 individuals in 19 different centers in Europe, it was found that SE-IgE was significantly associated with asthma severity. It was shown that 59.6% of severe asthma patients have SE-IgE, whereas only 13% of healthy control subjects were SE-IgE positive [55]. Currently, there is a commercial kit available to measure IgE against 5 different SEs (SE A-E) and TSST-1, the question of whether there are IgEs against the other 21 SAgs cannot be answered at the moment. The specific IgE antibodies against SAgs detected in the nasal polyps from CRS are functional. They bind to the surfaces of mast cells and basophils via Fcε receptors and trigger degranulation upon ligation by their antigen, i.e., SAgs of *S. aureus* [56–58], thereby promoting an allergic inflammation in CRS.

14.4 *S. aureus* Proteases

Proteases are enzymes that break down polypeptides or proteins by cleaving peptide bonds. Proteases comprise a large functional group of proteins in living systems, with thousands being described in different organisms [59]. Due to their importance in bacterial fitness and virulence, bacterial proteases are interesting candidates for both therapeutic and diagnostic purposes. Moreover, studying the bacterial proteases and their substrates could reveal means of inhibiting their destructive effects during infections [60]. In bacteria proteases are involved in proliferation and virulence and can serve the microorganisms in a number of ways. Firstly, proteases hydrolyze proteins into short chains of amino acids that can be used by bacteria as energy supply and for biosynthesis. Secondly, proteases help the bacteria to penetrate host barriers, invade the host tissues and even gain access to the intracellular niche where they can hide from detection by the immune system. Moreover, these enzymes may have a direct effect on a broad range of host immune functions, including the inhibition of immune cell activation, the prevention of opsonophagocytosis, and the blockade of classical and alternative complement pathways. Besides, proteases can degrade the tight junctions between the epithelial cells, paving the way for the bacteria to the underlying connective tissue where they will induce a strong innate immune response. Last not least, recent reports show that some of these proteases are able to deviate the immune response in the direction of a type 2 profile, promoting an allergic inflammation. Some proteases can activate protease-activated receptors (PAR) that are widely expressed in human airway epithelium. PAR activation has been linked to initiation of allergic immune response [61].

To date, 10 major extracellular proteases are known in *S. aureus*, including the serine protease V8, 6 serine protease-like proteins Spl (A-F), the metalloprotease aureolysin and two cysteine proteases, staphopain A and B [62]. Previously, it was thought that these proteases are only important for nutrient acquisition, but recent findings suggest that they also interact with the host immune system, weakening or misdirecting the immune response in a way that favors the bacterial survival [63].

The V8 and staphopain proteases were shown to disrupt tight junctions of the airway epithelium, modulate cytokine production [64], and activate nuclear factor kappa light-chain enhancer of activated B cells (NF-κB) in the airway epithelial cells [65]. These findings suggest an involvement of V8 and staphopain proteases in the pathophysiology of CRS. Barrier disruption further predisposes for allergic sensitization.

Serine protease-like proteins (Spls), a group of six proteins, Spls A-F, encoded on a single operon, can be released by the majority of *S. aureus* clinical isolates. Spls have recently been identified as triggering allergens stimulating allergic airway inflammation in mice [66]. Interestingly, human T cells exposed to Spls in vitro released typical Th2 cytokines including: IL-4, IL-5, and IL-13. Meanwhile, IFN-γ- and IL-17 production was shown to be very low. This tends to be opposite in the case of other *S. aureus* antigens which typically stimulate a Th1/Th17 profile with increased IFN-γ- and IL-17 production. The nasal polyp tissues from patients colonized with *S. aureus* contain detectable amounts of IgG binding to SplA, SplB, and SplD/F. Moreover, specific IgE against different Spls has been detected in the sera of asthma patients at higher concentrations than in control subjects [66].

In a mouse model, repeated endotracheal applications of SplD induced typical features of allergic asthma such as SplD-specific IgE formation, Th2 cytokine production in the local draining lymph nodes, and eosinophilic infiltration of the airways [67]. This allergic inflammation was dependent on IL-33 as the administration of a soluble IL-33 receptor as a decoy resulted in a significant reduction of symptoms. IL-33 is an alarmin that activates type 2 innate lymphoid cells (ILC2), which in return secrete IL-4. The IL-4 released by ILC2s acts on B cells nonspecifically and leads to antibody class switching and polyclonal IgE formation [42]. ILC2s can be found in significantly increased numbers in the nasal polyps from CRS patients with comorbid asthma [68]. The IL-33 released upon exposure to SplD in mice could exacerbate characteristic features of allergic asthma and even break immune tolerance to other antigens/allergens [62]. Of note, Spls have been detected in nasal polyp tissues [69] confirming their presence in the local tissue where they may trigger a type 2 immune response in CRS.

These results show that *S aureus* Spls act as novel allergens that induce a specific Th2/IgE response in mice. They give rise to the hypothesis that *S. aureus* Spls can cause allergies in humans. Further understanding of interactions and the mechanisms through which *S. aureus* secreted factors induce a Th2 biased immune response will help to develop means of preventing or mitigating the pathogenic potential of *S. aureus* in CRS.

14.5 δ-Toxin

There are other components of *S. aureus* that are believed to contribute to allergic airway inflammation. As an example, *S. aureus* delta-toxin (δ-toxin) has been shown to directly activate mast cells in the absence of antigens [1]. *In vitro*, human mast cells are triggered to produce tryptase which is the most abundant protease in mast cell granules and a biomarker for mast cell activation. The bacterial toxin belongs to the hemolysin family, which is composed of four quite different toxins, known as α-, β-, γ-, and δ-toxins. Δ-toxin degrades host cell membranes upon contact, causing pore formation and subsequent cell lysis. Furthermore, δ-toxin helps *S. aureus* to evade phagosomes and enter the host cell cytoplasm, supporting the bacterial persistence in the nasal polyp tissues. There is a tight link between *agr*, a global regulator system in *S. aureus*, which controls the expression of numerous virulence factors, and δ-toxin. Activation of the *agr* system induces RNAIII, one of the main intracellular effectors of the *agr* quorum-sensing system of *S. aureus*. As a second function, RNAIII encodes δ-toxin [70]. Δ-toxin-producing *S. aureus* strains are more abundant in patients with atopic skin diseases than in healthy controls and colonization with δ-toxin-producing *S. aureus* in mice induces IgE and IL-4 production [1], creating an allergenic microenvironment within the host. Therefore, *S. aureus* benefits twice from δ-toxin: by evading immune system and, at the same time, promoting allergic inflammation.

14.6 Why Does *S. aureus* Drive Allergy?

In summary, results obtained by numerous research groups agree that *S. aureus*, through its secreted proteins, including—but not limited to—SAgs, Spls, and δ-toxin, contributes to the development of type 2 immune responses. Deviation of the immune response towards a type 2 profile and development of an allergic response in the host probably benefits *S. aureus* during colonization and infection because this immune response module counteracts the Th1/Th17 profile which is efficient at neutrophil recruitment and pathogen clearance. Therefore, it is plausible that the type 2 modulation of the immune system functions as a staphylococcal immune evasion mechanism [6]. This idea is supported by the high colonization rates of *S. aureus* among allergic patients, especially in CRSwNP, which are significantly higher than healthy individuals. As a "side effect," type 2 immune responses against pathogens requiring Th1/Th17 cells for clearance increase the risk of life-threatening infections [71, 72].

14.7 Translation into Future Daily Practice

The evidence for a crucial involvement of *S. aureus* and its components in CRSwNP is based on clinical association, cell culture experiments, and animal models, which in sum are very compelling. Nevertheless, to demonstrate causation, provocation tests, e.g., skin prick tests, are needed. A prerequisite for the application of the putative allergens, SAgs and Spls, in this diagnostic procedure is the elimination of their toxic potential. Diagnostics of therapy-refractory CRS should include the measurement of *S. aureus*-specific IgE.

To eliminate *S. aureus* as a driver of CRS, the application of proven decolonization procedures is an obvious consideration. However, permanent decolonization is difficult to achieve, especially in the highly inflamed and swollen nasal tissue in florid CRS. Prior treatment of the allergic inflammation using anti-allergic regimens, such as anti-IgE monoclonal antibodies, may facilitate bacterial decolonization. Taking into account the increasing problem of antibiotic resistance, promising alternative anti-*S. aureus* strategies could be bacteriophages or bacterial interference using harmless microorganisms.

To prevent infection with the dangerous pathogen *S. aureus* or provide clinical protection, effective vaccines are urgently needed and their development is actively pursued by the *S. aureus* research community. As a "side effect," anti-*S. aureus* vaccination could also reduce the risk of developing allergic reactions to *S. aureus*. Finally, allergen-specific immunotherapy (AIT) using detoxified *S. aureus* allergens could be a future strategy for alleviating CRSwNP.

References

1. Nakamura Y, Oscherwitz J, Cease KB, Chan SM, Muñoz-Planillo R, Hasegawa M, et al. Staphylococcus δ-toxin induces allergic skin disease by activating mast cells. Nature. 2013;503(7476):397–401.
2. Sakr A, Brégeon F, Mège J-L, Rolain J-M, Blin O. *Staphylococcus aureus* nasal colonization: an update on mechanisms, epidemiology, risk factors, and subsequent infections. Front Microbiol. 2018;9:2419.
3. Sollid JUE, Furberg AS, Hanssen AM, Johannessen M. *Staphylococcus aureus*: determinants of human carriage. Infect Genet Evol. 2014;21:531–41.
4. de Benito S, Alou L, Becerro-de-Bengoa-Vallejo R, Losa-Iglesias ME, Gómez-Lus ML, Collado L, et al. Prevalence of Staphylococcus spp. nasal colonization among doctors of podiatric medicine and associated risk factors in Spain. Antimicrob Resist Infect Control. 2018;7:24.
5. van Belkum A, Verkaik NJ, de Vogel CP, Boelens HA, Verveer J, Nouwen JL, et al. Reclassification of *Staphylococcus aureus* nasal carriage types. J Infect Dis. 2009;199(12):1820–6.
6. Nordengrün M, Michalik S, Völker U, Bröker BM, Gómez-Gascón L. The quest for bacterial allergens. Int J Med Microbiol. 2018;308(6):738–50.
7. von Eiff C, Becker K, Machka K, Stammer H, Peters G. Nasal carriage as a source of *Staphylococcus aureus* bacteremia. Study Group. N Engl J Med. 2001;344(1):11–6.
8. Lindsay JA, Holden MTG. Understanding the rise of the superbug: investigation of the evolution and genomic variation of *Staphylococcus aureus*. Funct Integr Genomics. 2006;6(3):186–201.
9. Lindsay JA, Moore CE, Day NP, Peacock SJ, Witney AA, Stabler RA, et al. Microarrays reveal that each of the ten dominant lineages of *Staphylococcus aureus* has a unique combination of surface-associated and regulatory genes. J Bacteriol. 2006;188(2):669–76.
10. Kuroda M, Ohta T, Uchiyama I, Baba T, Yuzawa H, Kobayashi I, et al. Whole genome sequencing of

meticillin-resistant *Staphylococcus aureus*. Lancet. 2001;357(9264):1225–40.

11. Lindsay JA, Holden MTG. *Staphylococcus aureus*: superbug, super genome? Trends Microbiol. 2004;12(8):378–85.
12. Holtfreter S, Grumann D, Balau V, Barwich A, Kolata J, Goehler A, et al. Molecular epidemiology of *Staphylococcus aureus* in the general population in northeast Germany: results of the study of health in Pomerania (SHIP-TREND-0). J Clin Microbiol. 2016;54(11):2774–85.
13. Goerke C, Pantucek R, Holtfreter S, Schulte B, Zink M, Grumann D, et al. Diversity of prophages in dominant *Staphylococcus aureus* clonal lineages. J Bacteriol. 2009;191(11):3462–8.
14. Foster TJ. The MSCRAMM family of cell-wall-anchored surface proteins of gram-positive cocci. Trends Microbiol. 2019;
15. Foster TJ, Geoghegan JA, Ganesh VK, Höök M. Adhesion, invasion and evasion: the many functions of the surface proteins of *Staphylococcus aureus*. Nat Rev Microbiol. 2014;12(1):49–62.
16. Berube B, Wardenburg J. *Staphylococcus aureus* α-toxin: nearly a century of intrigue. Toxins. 2013;5(6):1140–66.
17. Spaan AN, Surewaard BGJ, Nijland R, van Strijp JAG. Neutrophils versus *Staphylococcus aureus*: a biological tug of war. Annu Rev Microbiol. 2013;67:629–50.
18. de Jong NWM, van Kessel KPM, van Strijp JAG. Immune evasion by *Staphylococcus aureus*. Microbiol Spectr. 2019;7(2)
19. van Kessel KPM, Bestebroer J, van Strijp JAG. Neutrophil-mediated phagocytosis of *Staphylococcus aureus*. Front Immunol. 2014;5:467.
20. Thammavongsa V, Kim HK, Missiakas D, Schneewind O. Staphylococcal manipulation of host immune responses. Nat Rev Microbiol. 2015;13(9):529–43.
21. Mulcahy ME, Geoghegan JA, Monk IR, O'Keeffe KM, Walsh EJ, Foster TJ, et al. Nasal colonisation by *Staphylococcus aureus* depends upon clumping factor B binding to the squamous epithelial cell envelope protein loricrin. PLoS Pathog. 2012;8(12):e1003092.
22. Nouwen J, Boelens H, van Belkum A, Verbrugh H. Human factor in *Staphylococcus aureus* nasal carriage. Infect Immun. 2004;72(11):6685–8.
23. Liu CM, Price LB, Hungate BA, Abraham AG, Larsen LA, Christensen K, et al. *Staphylococcus aureus* and the ecology of the nasal microbiome. Sci Adv. 2015;1(5):e1400216.
24. Iwase T, Uehara Y, Shinji H, Tajima A, Seo H, Takada K, et al. *Staphylococcus epidermidis* Esp inhibits *Staphylococcus aureus* biofilm formation and nasal colonization. Nature. 2010;465(7296):346–9.
25. Piewngam P, Zheng Y, Nguyen TH, Dickey SW, Joo H-S, Villaruz AE, et al. Pathogen elimination by probiotic *Bacillus* via signalling interference. Nature. 2018;562(7728):532–7.
26. Zipperer A, Konnerth MC, Laux C, Berscheid A, Janek D, Weidenmaier C, et al. Human commensals producing a novel antibiotic impair pathogen colonization. Nature. 2016;535(7613):511–6.
27. Eckhart L, Lippens S, Tschachler E, Declercq W. Cell death by cornification. Biochim Biophys Acta. 2013;1833(12):3471–80.
28. Clarke SR, Andre G, Walsh EJ, Dufrêne YF, Foster TJ, Foster SJ. Iron-regulated surface determinant protein A mediates adhesion of *Staphylococcus aureus* to human corneocyte envelope proteins. Infect Immun. 2009;77(6):2408–16.
29. Corrigan RM, Miajlovic H, Foster TJ. Surface proteins that promote adherence of *Staphylococcus aureus* to human desquamated nasal epithelial cells. BMC Microbiol. 2009;9:22.
30. Weidenmaier C, Kokai-Kun JF, Kristian SA, Chanturiya T, Kalbacher H, Gross M, et al. Role of teichoic acids in *Staphylococcus aureus* nasal colonization, a major risk factor in nosocomial infections. Nat Med. 2004;10(3):243–5.
31. Krismer B, Weidenmaier C, Zipperer A, Peschel A. The commensal lifestyle of *Staphylococcus aureus* and its interactions with the nasal microbiota. Nat Rev Microbiol. 2017;15(11):675–87.
32. Tuchscherr L, Kreis CA, Hoerr V, Flint L, Hachmeister M, Geraci J, et al. *Staphylococcus aureus* develops increased resistance to antibiotics by forming dynamic small colony variants during chronic osteomyelitis. J Antimicrob Chemother. 2016;71(2):438–48.
33. Ou J, Bassiouni A, Drilling A, Psaltis AJ, Vreugde S, Wormald PJ. The persistence of intracellular *Staphylococcus aureus* in the sinuses: a longitudinal study. Rhinology. 2017;55(4):305–11.
34. Schmidt F, Meyer T, Sundaramoorthy N, Michalik S, Surmann K, Depke M, et al. Characterization of human and *Staphylococcus aureus* proteins in respiratory mucosa by in vivo- and immunoproteomics. J Proteome. 2017;155:31–9.
35. Jin T, Bokarewa M, Foster T, Mitchell J, Higgins J, Tarkowski A. *Staphylococcus aureus* resists human defensins by production of staphylokinase, a novel bacterial evasion mechanism. J Immunol. 2004;172(2):1169–76.
36. Bröker BM, Holtfreter S, Bekeredjian-Ding I. Immune control of *Staphylococcus aureus* - regulation and counter-regulation of the adaptive immune response. Int J Med Microbiol. 2014;304(2):204–14.
37. Hair PS, Ward MD, Semmes OJ, Foster TJ, Cunnion KM. *Staphylococcus aureus* clumping factor A binds to complement regulator factor I and increases factor I cleavage of C3b. J Infect Dis. 2008;198(1):125–33.
38. Kim Y-C, Won H-K, Lee JW, Sohn K-H, Kim M-H, Kim T-B, et al. *Staphylococcus aureus* nasal colonization and asthma in adults: systematic review and meta-analysis. J Allergy Clin Immunol Pract. 2019;7(2):606–615.e9.
39. Bachert C, Gevaert P, Holtappels G, Johansson SG, van Cauwenberge P. Total and specific IgE in nasal polyps is related to local eosinophilic inflammation. J

Allergy Clin Immunol. 2001;107(4):607. https://doi.org/10.1067/mai.2001.112374.
40. Bachert C, Gevaert P, Howarth P, Holtappels G, van Cauwenberge P, Johansson SGO. IgE to *Staphylococcus aureus* enterotoxins in serum is related to severity of asthma. J Allergy Clin Immunol. 2003;111(5):1131–2.
41. Bachert C, van Steen K, Zhang N, Holtappels G, Cattaert T, Maus B, et al. Specific IgE against *Staphylococcus aureus* enterotoxins: an independent risk factor for asthma. J Allergy Clin Immunol. 2012;130(2):376–81 e8. https://doi.org/10.1016/j.jaci.2012.05.012.
42. Teufelberger AR, Bröker BM, Krysko DV, Bachert C, Krysko O. *Staphylococcus aureus* orchestrates type 2 airway diseases. Trends Mol Med. 2019;25(8):696–707.
43. Tuffs SW, Haeryfar SMM, McCormick JK. Manipulation of innate and adaptive immunity by Staphylococcal superantigens. Pathogens. 2018;7(2)
44. Holtfreter S, Grumann D, Schmudde M, Nguyen HTT, Eichler P, Strommenger B, et al. Clonal distribution of superantigen genes in clinical *Staphylococcus aureus* isolates. J Clin Microbiol. 2007;45(8):2669–80.
45. Watson ARO, Janik DK, Lee WT. Superantigen-induced CD4 memory T cell anergy. I. Staphylococcal enterotoxin B induces Fyn-mediated negative signaling. Cell Immunol. 2012;276(1–2):16–25.
46. Janik DK, Lee WT. Staphylococcal enterotoxin B (SEB) induces memory CD4 T cell anergy in vivo and impairs recall immunity to unrelated antigens. J Clin Cell Immunol. 2015;6(4):1–8.
47. Burian M, Grumann D, Holtfreter S, Wolz C, Goerke C, Bröker BM. Expression of staphylococcal superantigens during nasal colonization is not sufficient to induce a systemic neutralizing antibody response in humans. Eur J Clin Microbiol Infect Dis. 2012;31(3):251–6.
48. Verkaik NJ, de Vogel CP, Boelens HA, Grumann D, Hoogenboezem T, Vink C, et al. Anti-staphylococcal humoral immune response in persistent nasal carriers and noncarriers of *Staphylococcus aureus*. J Infect Dis. 2009;199(5):625–32.
49. Lappin E, Ferguson AJ. Gram-positive toxic shock syndromes. Lancet Infect Dis. 2009;9(5):281–90.
50. Proft T, Fraser JD. Bacterial superantigens. Clin Exp Immunol. 2003;133(3):299–306.
51. Schwameis M, Roppenser B, Firbas C, Gruener CS, Model N, Stich N, et al. Safety, tolerability, and immunogenicity of a recombinant toxic shock syndrome toxin (rTSST)-1 variant vaccine: a randomised, double-blind, adjuvant-controlled, dose escalation first-in-man trial. Lancet Infect Dis. 2016;16(9):1036–44.
52. Chen WH, Pasetti MF, Adhikari RP, Baughman H, Douglas R, El-Khorazaty J, et al. Safety and immunogenicity of a parenterally administered, structure-based rationally modified recombinant staphylococcal enterotoxin B protein vaccine, STEBVax. Clin Vaccine Immunol. 2016;23(12):918–25.
53. Maniakas A, Asmar M-H, Renteria Flores AE, Nayan S, Alromaih S, Mfuna Endam L, et al. *Staphylococcus aureus* on sinus culture is associated with recurrence of chronic rhinosinusitis after endoscopic sinus surgery. Front Cell Infect Microbiol. 2018;8:150.
54. Bachert C, Claeys SEM, Tomassen P, van Zele T, Zhang N. Rhinosinusitis and asthma: a link for asthma severity. Curr Allergy Asthma Rep. 2010;10(3):194–201.
55. Tomassen P, Jarvis D, Newson R, van Ree R, Forsberg B, Howarth P, et al. *Staphylococcus aureus* enterotoxin-specific IgE is associated with asthma in the general population: a GA(2)LEN study. Allergy. 2013;68(10):1289–97.
56. Shamji MH, Thomsen I, Layhadi JA, Kappen J, Holtappels G, Sahiner U, et al. Broad IgG repertoire in patients with chronic rhinosinusitis with nasal polyps regulates proinflammatory IgE responses. J Allergy Clin Immunol. 2019;143(6):2086–2094.e2.
57. Ono HK, Nishizawa M, Yamamoto Y, Hu D-L, Nakane A, Shinagawa K, et al. Submucosal mast cells in the gastrointestinal tract are a target of staphylococcal enterotoxin type A. FEMS Immunol Med Microbiol. 2012;64(3):392–402.
58. Ono HK, Hirose S, Narita K, Sugiyama M, Asano K, Hu D-L, et al. Histamine release from intestinal mast cells induced by staphylococcal enterotoxin A (SEA) evokes vomiting reflex in common marmoset. PLoS Pathog. 2019;15(5):e1007803.
59. Bond JS. Proteases: history, discovery, and roles in health and disease. J Biol Chem. 2019;294(5):1643–51.
60. Kaman WE, Hays JP, Endtz HP, Bikker FJ. Bacterial proteases: targets for diagnostics and therapy. Eur J Clin Microbiol Infect Dis. 2014;33(7):1081–7.
61. Wu D, Wei Y, Bleier BS. Emerging role of proteases in the pathogenesis of chronic rhinosinusitis with nasal polyps. Front Cell Infect Microbiol. 2017;7:538.
62. Krysko O, Teufelberger A, van Nevel S, Krysko DV, Bachert C. Protease/antiprotease network in allergy: the role of *Staphylococcus aureus* protease-like proteins. Allergy. 2019;
63. Pietrocola G, Nobile G, Rindi S, Speziale P. *Staphylococcus aureus* manipulates innate immunity through own and host-expressed proteases. Front Cell Infect Microbiol. 2017;7:166.
64. Murphy J, Ramezanpour M, Stach N, Dubin G, Psaltis AJ, Wormald P-J, et al. *Staphylococcus aureus* V8 protease disrupts the integrity of the airway epithelial barrier and impairs IL-6 production in vitro. Laryngoscope. 2018;128(1):E8–E15.
65. Rudack C, Sachse F, Albert N, Becker K, von Eiff C. Immunomodulation of nasal epithelial cells by *Staphylococcus aureus*-derived serine proteases. J Immunol. 2009;183(11):7592–601.
66. Stentzel S, Teufelberger A, Nordengrün M, Kolata J, Schmidt F, van Crombruggen K, et al. Staphylococcal serine protease-like proteins are pacemakers of aller-

gic airway reactions to *Staphylococcus aureus*. J Allergy Clin Immunol. 2017;139(2):492–500.e8.
67. Teufelberger AR, Nordengrün M, Braun H, Maes T, de Grove K, Holtappels G, et al. The IL-33/ST2 axis is crucial in type 2 airway responses induced by *Staphylococcus aureus* –derived serine protease–like protein D. J Allergy Clin Immunol. 2018;141(2):549–559.e7.
68. van Crombruggen K, Taveirne S, Holtappels G, Leclercq G, Bachert C. Innate lymphoid cells in the upper airways: importance of CD117 and IL-1RI expression. Eur Respir J. 2018;52(6):1800742.
69. Bachert C, Holtappels G, Merabishvili M, Meyer T, Murr A, Zhang N, et al. *Staphylococcus aureus* controls interleukin-5 release in upper airway inflammation. J Proteome. 2018;180:53–60.
70. Tan L, Li SR, Jiang B, Hu XM, Li S. Therapeutic targeting of the *Staphylococcus aureus* accessory gene regulator (agr) system. Front Microbiol. 2018;9:55.
71. Joshi A, Pancari G, Cope L, Bowman EP, Cua D, Proctor RA, et al. Immunization with *Staphylococcus aureus* iron regulated surface determinant B (IsdB) confers protection via Th17/IL17 pathway in a murine sepsis model. Hum Vaccin Immunother. 2012;8(3):336–46.
72. Milner JD, Brenchley JM, Laurence A, Freeman AF, Hill BJ, Elias KM, et al. Impaired T(H)17 cell differentiation in subjects with autosomal dominant hyper-IgE syndrome. Nature. 2008;452(7188):773–6.

15 Viruses

Feng Lan and Luo Zhang

Key Points

Chronic rhinosinusitis (CRS) has a high detection rate for viruses. Viruses play an important role in persistent inflammation in CRS patients by enhancement of bacterial adhesion and exacerbation of local inflammation, which may contribute to longer duration of CRS symptoms during acute viral infection.

15.1 Introduction

The nasopharynx is regarded as a considerable reservoir for microbiomes in humans. Multiple viruses have been detected in the upper airways; with a higher rate of respiratory viruses observed in the nasal washes and mucosa of chronic rhinosinusitis (CRS) patients compared to control subjects [1]. Although viral activity influences the pathogenesis of CRS, limited research to date and contradictory findings have led to a poor understanding of the role of viruses in CRS.

15.1.1 Epidemiology

Human rhinovirus (HRV), respiratory syncytial virus (RSV), influenza virus (IFV), and coronavirus (CorV) have been considered as the frequent viruses detected in CRS patients (Table 15.1) [4]. In particular, HRV has been detected more frequently in both lavage fluids and scrapings of turbinate epithelial cells from CRS patients (26.1%) than from control subjects [1, 5]. One recent study from China, employing the polymerase chain reaction (PCR) technique to detect viral DNA and RNA, demonstrated that HRV could be detected all year round, peaking between July and September [6]. However, undetectable HRV in lavage fluids samples from both CRS and control groups in summer time from March to July may lead to a false-negative result [7]. Similarly, RSV can also be found significantly more frequently in nasal lavage fluid and scrapings of epithelial cells from CRS patients (11–12%) than from control subjects [1, 8]. RSV leads to severe illness in infants and older adults especially in winter, and false-negative results for RSV may occur particularly in summer.

A culture-based method, which is regarded as a reliable method for virus isolation, has also been utilized to determine the presence of viruses

F. Lan
Beijing Key Laboratory of Nasal Diseases, Beijing Institute of Otolaryngology, Beijing, China

L. Zhang (✉)
Beijing Key Laboratory of Nasal Diseases, Beijing Institute of Otolaryngology, Beijing, China

Department of Otolaryngology, Head and Neck Surgery, Beijing Tongren Hospital, Capital Medical University, Beijing, China

Department of Allergy, Beijing Tongren Hospital, Capital Medical University, Beijing, China

L. Zhang, C. Bachert (eds.), *Chronic Rhinosinusitis*, https://doi.org/10.1007/978-981-16-0784-4_15

Table 15.1 The prevalence of viruses in airways

Characteristic of subjects	Sample source	Identification technique	The common viruses	Refs.
Chronic rhinosinusitis patients	Nasal lavage/scraping epithelial cells	RT-PCR	Rhinovirus (26.1/31.4%); Parainfluenza (23.4/21.6%); IFV (13.5/12.6%); RSV (10.8%);	[1]
Chronic rhinosinusitis patients	Turbinate epithelial cells	RT-PCR	Picornavirus (21%)	[2]
Chronic rhinosinusitis patients	Sinus mucosa	RT-PCR	Rhinovirus (26.1%); RSV (11.8%)	[3]

RSV human respiratory syncytial virus, *IFV* influenza viruses, *RT-PCR* reverse transcription polymerase chain reaction

in the airways. Exceptionally, although it has not been possible to successfully propagate the more virulent HRV-C species in any cell type using the traditional 2D cellular culture technique [9], a recently developed 3D cellular culture, which mimics the physiological complexity of in vivo microenvironments, has made it possible to propagate HRV-C in vitro [10]. Based on the knowledge of viruses, PCR can unveil selected DNA and RNA viruses in nasal mucosa using specific primers [11]. A new next-generation sequencing (NGS)-based method efficiently can also uncover potentially pathogenic viruses in CRS without the prior knowledge of virus genomic sequences, thus making this technique more convenient than the PCR for detection of viruses [12]. Respiratory viruses can be detected in several types of tissues; including nasopharynx secretion, nasal swab, nasal lavage, nasal tissue or epithelial cell scrapings from inferior turbinate [2]. Although nasopharynx secretion is regarded as the sample with highest sensitivity for detection of IFV, nasal and oropharyngeal swab samples are less-invasive compared to nasopharynx secretion [13]. Thus, sampling from different sites, the type of specimen and the timing of sampling in the nasal cavity can contribute to variation in viral detection rates in CRS patients [3]. Besides the effect of differences in sampling, the CRS subtype of the patient may also be an important factor; particularly as chronic rhinosinusitis with nasal polyps (CRSwNP) is mainly characterized by Th2-biased inflammation, whereas chronic rhinosinusitis without nasal polyps (CRSsNP) often exhibits a Th1-cell associated inflammation. Thus, owing to the different inflammatory patterns and disease severity, it is necessary to characterize the prevalence of viruses in CRSsNP and CRSwNP according to inflammatory endotyping. Indeed, in this regard most of the studies investigating the role of viruses in CRS to date are limited by the observation that CRSwNP or CRSsNP subgroups were not distinguished, and thus detection of a particular virus cannot be attributed to a specific subgroup.

15.2 Mechanisms

Viruses may affect the pathogenesis of CRS via two aspects: (i) impairing epithelial barrier integrity; (ii) enhancing bacterial attachment to the nasal epithelial cells, indirectly inducing an inflammatory response (Fig. 15.1). It has been reported that HRV or RSV infections decrease the expression of tight junction and adhesion junction proteins such as zona occludens-1 (ZO-1), occludin, claudin-1, and E-cadherin in healthy human nasal epithelial cells (NECs), and upregulate pro-inflammatory cytokines such as TNF-α and IL-8 [14–16]. The epithelial barrier acts as the first-line defense against viral infection, which disrupts the integrity of the epithelial barrier and lays the foundation for viral invasion of the lamina propria. RSV infection has additionally been shown to enhance the adhesion of Haemophilus influenzae and Streptococcus pneumonia to respiratory epithelial cells by upregulat-

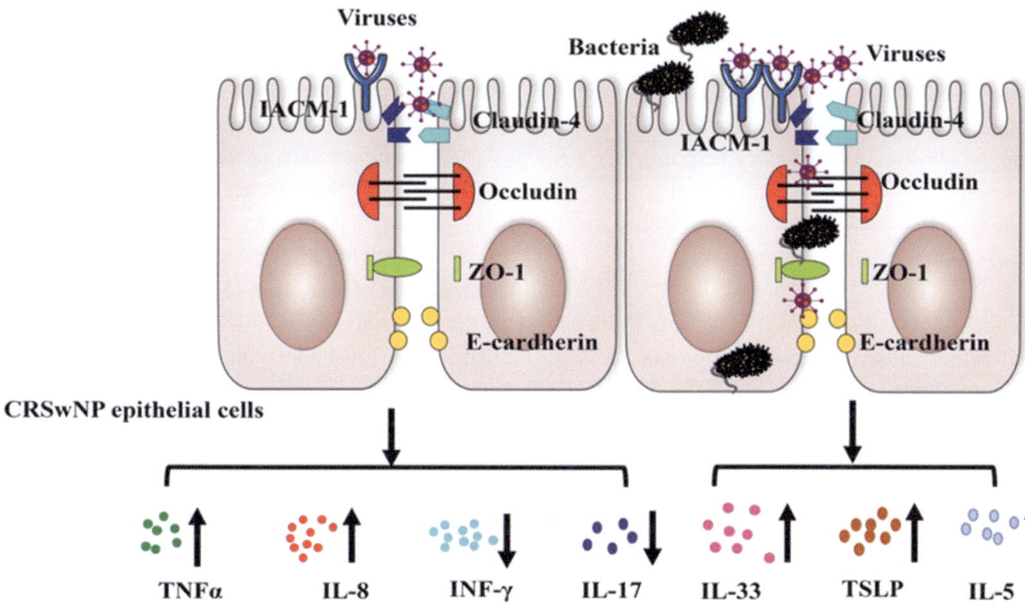

Fig. 15.1 Interaction between viruses and bacteria induces persistent inflammation in chronic rhinosinusitis with nasal polyps (CRSwNP). The integrity of epithelial layer in CRSwNP is compromised as a result of decreased expression of tight junction proteins such as claudin-4, occluding, E-cadherin, and zona occludens-1 (ZO-1). Viral infection further decreases the expression of tight junction proteins leading to disruption of the epithelial barrier. Concurrently, virus-induced expression of ICAM-1 on the epithelial cells leads to enhanced adhesion and invasion of bacteria; especially Staphylococcus aureus (*S. aureus*) and then *S. aureus*; which propagate type 2 responses in the CRSwNP mucosa via epithelial cell-derived cytokines such as IL-33 and thymic stromal lymphopoietin (TSLP). The release of pro-inflammatory cytokines such as TNF-α, IL-5, and IL-8 may also be increased, and cytokines such as IFN-γ and IL-17 decreased, in CRSwNP during viral infection

ing the expression of viral glycoproteins and bacterial receptors including ICAM-1, carcinoembryonic antigen-related cell adhesion molecule 1 (CEACAM1), and platelet-activating factor receptor (PAFr) [17]. However, all viruses do not have a similar effect as RSV, nor do all respiratory cell types respond similarly to viral infection.

While IFV-infected NECs from healthy donors with no concurrent history of viral infections induce a strong activation of type I immune responses against the viral infection [18], NECs from CRS patients demonstrate a mild impairment of IFN protein production [19]. In the event of significantly decreased release of interferon (IFN)-γ and IL-17, the CRSwNP mucosa has been shown to be more susceptible to herpes simplex virus type 1 (HSV1) invasion compared to healthy inferior turbinate mucosa; with the CRSwNP patients experiencing long-lasting symptoms upon acute infection [20]. Epithelial cell-derived cytokines IL-33 and thymic stromal lymphopoietin (TSLP) can initiate type 2 cytokine release from Th2 cells or group 2 innate lymphoid cells. While asthmatic patients exposed to HRV demonstrate induced levels of IL-33 [21] and elevated levels of TSLP in allergic asthma patients have been shown to be positively associated with the disease severity [22]; to date there is still no evidence that virus exposure directly triggers type 2 immune response in CRSwNP via epithelial cell-derived cytokines. We have recently demonstrated that HSV1 infection facilitated adhesion and invasion of *Staphylococcus aureus* (*S. aureus*) in the nasal mucosa and nasal polyp tissue from CRSwNP patients, and that *S. aureus* in the lamina propria further propagated Th2 response via induction of IL-33 and TSLP in CRSwNP tissue [23, 24]. Furthermore, bacterial superantigens staphylococcal enterotoxins A

(SEA) and SEB increased HRV replication in airway epithelial cells of CRS [25]. Collectively, these findings suggest that the interaction between viruses and bacteria in CRS may aggravate the chronic inflammatory response in CRS.

15.3 Antiviral Therapy

As mentioned above, viral infection influences the pathogenesis of and symptoms in CRS patients. Thus, treatment in CRSwNP patients infected by virus usually aims to target the virus itself or resolve and relieve the symptoms of CRSwNP. Saline irrigation and topical corticosteroids relieve nasal congestion and reduce nasal edema, and thus may lead to improvement in symptoms in CRSwNP patients [26]. In concert with the suggestion that specific anti-HRV molecules based on DNAzyme technology might be useful in preventing asthma exacerbations [27], it is possible that these molecules may also be effective for "viral silencing" in CRSwNP patients, by diminishing type 2 allergic immune responses. Although IFN-γ may act as first-line therapy against viral infection, the clinical usage of IFN-γ in CRSwNP patients is very limited considering the effective dosage and side effects [28]. It is noteworthy that commensal bacteria produce IFN-λ1 for protection against influenza virus infection [29] and IFN-λ1 favors the clearance of *S. aureus* by affecting the phagocytosis and endocytosis of macrophages in healthy nasal mucosa [30]. Herein, the use of IFN-λ1 for inhibiting viral and bacterial co-infection in CRSwNP patients may be a promising intervention strategy to diminish the post-infectious inflammation in CRSwNP. Currently a licensed vaccine is unavailable for the treatment of viral infection in CRS due to the vast numbers of virus serotypes, and thus the likelihood of a limited clinic effect.

15.4 Translation into Future Daily Practice

Owing to their different inflammatory patterns, it is necessary to characterize the prevalence of the virus in each subgroup of CRS according to inflammatory endotyping. The variability of virus prevalence in CRS may attribute to the specimen types used for viral detection and the time for specimen collection.

Viruses may interrupt the integrity of the epithelial barrier, which can further enhance the invasion of bacteria to exacerbate persistent upper airway inflammation. Although the direct contribution of the virus to Th2-biased response in the lower airway is at least partly understood, the mechanisms underlying virus-mediated propagation of type 2 responses in CRS await further investigations.

Using specific anti-virus molecules based on DNAzyme technology or IFN-λ1 might be promising interventions for viral infections in CRS patients in the future.

References

1. Cho GS, Moon BJ, Lee BJ, Gong CH, Kim NH, Kim YS, et al. High rates of detection of respiratory viruses in the nasal washes and mucosae of patients with chronic rhinosinusitis. J Clin Microbiol. 2013;51(3):979–84. https://doi.org/10.1128/JCM.02806-12.
2. Lan F, Zhang N, Gevaert E, Zhang L, Bachert C. Viruses and bacteria in Th2-biased allergic airway disease. Allergy. 2016;71(10):1381–92. https://doi.org/10.1111/all.12934.
3. Wood AJ, Antoszewska H, Fraser J, Douglas RG. Is chronic rhinosinusitis caused by persistent respiratory virus infection? Int Forum Allergy Rhinol. 2011;1(2):95–100. https://doi.org/10.1002/alr.20030.
4. Chonmaitree T, Revai K, Grady JJ, Clos A, Patel JA, Nair S, et al. Viral upper respiratory tract infection and otitis media complication in young children. Clin Infect Dis. 2008;46(6):815–23. https://doi.org/10.1086/528685.
5. Lee SB, Yi JS, Lee BJ, Gong CH, Kim NH, Joo CH, et al. Human rhinovirus serotypes in the nasal washes and mucosa of patients with chronic rhinosinusitis. Int Forum Allergy Rhinol. 2015;5(3):197–203. https://doi.org/10.1002/alr.21472.
6. Sun H, Sun Q, Jiang W, Chen Z, Huang L, Wang M, et al. Prevalence of rhinovirus in wheezing children: a comparison with respiratory syncytial virus wheezing. Br J Infect Dis. 2016;20(2):179–83. https://doi.org/10.1016/j.bjid.2015.12.005.
7. Jang YJ, Kwon HJ, Park HW, Lee BJ. Detection of rhinovirus in turbinate epithelial cells of chronic sinusitis. Am J Rhinol. 2006;20(6):634–6. https://doi.org/10.2500/ajr.2006.20.2899.
8. Abshirini H, Makvandi M, Seyyed Ashrafi M, Hamidifard M, Saki N. Prevalence of rhinovirus

and respiratory syncytial virus among patients with chronic rhinosinusitis. Jundishapur J Microbiol. 2015;8(3):e20068. https://doi.org/10.5812/jjm.20068.
9. Arden KE, Mackay IM. Newly identified human rhinoviruses: molecular methods heat up the cold viruses. Rev Med Virol. 2010;20(3):156–76. https://doi.org/10.1002/rmv.644.
10. Chen YX, Xie GC, Pan D, Du YR, Pang LL, Song JD, et al. Three-dimensional culture of human airway epithelium in matrigel for evaluation of human rhinovirus C and bocavirus infections. Biomed Environ Sci. 2018;31(2):136–45. https://doi.org/10.3967/bes2018.016.
11. Teo SM, Mok D, Pham K, Kusel M, Serralha M, Troy N, et al. The infant nasopharyngeal microbiome impacts severity of lower respiratory infection and risk of asthma development. Cell Host Microbe. 2015;17(5):704–15. https://doi.org/10.1016/j.chom.2015.03.008.
12. Kustin T, Ling G, Sharabi S, Ram D, Friedman N, Zuckerman N, et al. A method to identify respiratory virus infections in clinical samples using next-generation sequencing. Sci Rep. 2019;9(1):2606. https://doi.org/10.1038/s41598-018-37483-w.
13. Spencer S, Thompson MG, Flannery B, Fry A. Comparison of respiratory specimen collection methods for detection of influenza virus infection by reverse transcription-PCR: a literature review. J Clin Microbiol. 2019;57(9):e00027–19. https://doi.org/10.1128/jcm.00027-19.
14. Yeo NK, Jang YJ. Rhinovirus infection-induced alteration of tight junction and adherens junction components in human nasal epithelial cells. Laryngoscope. 2010;120(2):346–52. https://doi.org/10.1002/lary.20764.
15. Sajjan U, Wang Q, Zhao Y, Gruenert DC, Hershenson MB. Rhinovirus disrupts the barrier function of polarized airway epithelial cells. Am J Respir Crit Care Med. 2008;178(12):1271–81. https://doi.org/10.1164/rccm.200801-136OC.
16. Smallcombe CC, Linfield DT, Harford TJ, Bokun V, Ivanov AI, Piedimonte G, et al. Disruption of the airway epithelial barrier in a murine model of respiratory syncytial virus infection. Am J Physiol Lung Cell Mol Physiol. 2019;316(2):L358–l68. https://doi.org/10.1152/ajplung.00345.2018.
17. Avadhanula V, Rodriguez CA, Devincenzo JP, Wang Y, Webby RJ, Ulett GC, et al. Respiratory viruses augment the adhesion of bacterial pathogens to respiratory epithelium in a viral species- and cell type-dependent manner. J Virol. 2006;80(4):1629–36. https://doi.org/10.1128/jvi.80.4.1629-1636.2006.
18. Tan KS, Andiappan AK, Lee B, Yan Y, Liu J, Tang SA, et al. RNA sequencing of H3N2 influenza virus-infected human nasal epithelial cells from multiple subjects reveals molecular pathways associated with tissue injury and complications. Cells. 2019;8(9):986. https://doi.org/10.3390/cells8090986.
19. Kim JH, Kim YS, Cho GS, Kim NH, Gong CH, Lee BJ, et al. Human rhinovirus-induced proinflammatory cytokine and interferon-β responses in nasal epithelial cells from chronic rhinosinusitis patients. Allergy, Asthma Immunol Res. 2015;7(5):489–96. https://doi.org/10.4168/aair.2015.7.5.489.
20. Lan F, Wang XD, Nauwynck HJ, Holtappels G, Zhang L, Johnston SL, et al. Th2 biased upper airway inflammation is associated with an impaired response to viral infection with Herpes simplex virus 1. Rhinology. 2016;54(2):141–9. https://doi.org/10.4193/Rhin15.213.
21. Jackson DJ, Makrinioti H, Rana BM, Shamji BW, Trujillo-Torralbo MB, Footitt J, et al. IL-33-dependent type 2 inflammation during rhinovirus-induced asthma exacerbations in vivo. Am J Respir Crit Care Med. 2014;190(12):1373–82. https://doi.org/10.1164/rccm.201406-1039OC.
22. Shikotra A, Choy DF, Ohri CM, Doran E, Butler C, Hargadon B, et al. Increased expression of immunoreactive thymic stromal lymphopoietin in patients with severe asthma. J Allergy Clin Immunol. 2012;129(1):104–11.e1–9. https://doi.org/10.1016/j.jaci.2011.08.031.
23. Wang X, Zhang N, Glorieux S, Holtappels G, Vaneechoutte M, Krysko O, et al. Herpes simplex virus type 1 infection facilitates invasion of Staphylococcus aureus into the nasal mucosa and nasal polyp tissue. PLoS One. 2012;7(6):e39875. https://doi.org/10.1371/journal.pone.0039875.
24. Lan F, Zhang N, Holtappels G, De Ruyck N, Krysko O, Van Crombruggen K, et al. Staphylococcus aureus induces a mucosal type 2 immune response via epithelial cell-derived cytokines. Am J Respir Crit Care Med. 2018;198(4):452–63. https://doi.org/10.1164/rccm.201710-2112OC.
25. Wang JH, Kwon HJ, Lee BJ, Jang YJ. Staphylococcal enterotoxins A and B enhance rhinovirus replication in A549 cells. Am J Rhinol. 2007;21(6):670–4. https://doi.org/10.2500/ajr.2007.21.3101.
26. Li C, Shi L, Yan Y, Gordon BR, Gordon WM, Wang DY. Gene expression signatures: a new approach to understanding the pathophysiology of chronic rhinosinusitis. Curr Allergy Asthma Rep. 2013;13(2):209–17. https://doi.org/10.1007/s11882-012-0328-6.
27. Potaczek DP, Unger SD, Zhang N, Taka S, Michel S, Akdağ N, et al. Development and characterization of DNAzyme candidates demonstrating significant efficiency against human rhinoviruses. J Allergy Clin Immunol. 2019;143(4):1403–15. https://doi.org/10.1016/j.jaci.2018.07.026.
28. Basharat U, Aiche MM, Kim MM, Sohal M, Chang EH. Are rhinoviruses implicated in the pathogenesis of sinusitis and chronic rhinosinusitis exacerbations? A comprehensive review. Int Forum Allergy Rhinol. 2019;9(10):1159–88. https://doi.org/10.1002/alr.22403.
29. Kim HJ, Jo A, Jeon YJ, An S, Lee KM, Yoon SS, et al. Nasal commensal Staphylococcus epidermidis

enhances interferon-λ-dependent immunity against influenza virus. Microbiome. 2019;7(1):80. https://doi.org/10.1186/s40168-019-0691-9.

30. Lan F, Zhong H, Zhang N, Johnston SL, Wen W, Papadopoulos N, et al. IFN-λ1 enhances Staphylococcus aureus clearance in healthy nasal mucosa but not in nasal polyps. J Allergy Clin Immunol. 2019;143(4):1416–25.e4. https://doi.org/10.1016/j.jaci.2018.09.041.

Environmental and Allergic Triggers

16

Changyu Qiu and Lei Cheng

Key Points

- Correlation between CRS and microbes.
- Correlation between CRS and air pollutants.
- Correlation between CRS and allergy remains controversial; however, allergy does have a close relation to type 2 inflammation of CRS, which requires further validation.
- Asthma and airway hyperresponsiveness have a close association with CRS, but an unclear association with the phenotypes.

16.1 Introduction

Chronic rhinosinusitis (CRS) is a common chronic inflammation of the mucous membranes that line the sinuses. The pathophysiology of CRS may involve anatomical, genetic, and environmental factors. Very recently, great strides have been made on the research of CRS and its diverse classifications. The correlation between CRS and environmental and allergic triggers, currently, remains controversial. Potential factors triggering the pathogenesis of CRS require to be further analyzed. In the present study, we illustrate the correlation between environmental triggers and CRS, and that between allergic triggers and CRS phenotypes. This review aims to provide references for the clinical diagnosis and treatment of CRS.

C. Qiu
International Centre for Allergy Research, Nanjing Medical University, Nanjing, China

L. Cheng (✉)
Department of Otorhinolaryngology and Clinical Allergy Center, The First Affiliated Hospital, Nanjing Medical University, Nanjing, China

International Centre for Allergy Research, Nanjing Medical University, Nanjing, China
e-mail: chenglei@jsph.org.cn

16.2 Environmental Triggers of CRS

Environmental factors can trigger and exacerbate the development of CRS [1]. In the human airway, the nasal mucosa, as the first line of defense against harmful substances, is continuously exposed to infection sources, allergens, pollutants, and other environmental factors. CRS may be evoked by environmental factors, like microbes, contaminants and allergens, especially bacteria and fungi [2] (Fig. 16.1).

The airway microbial community is a dynamic system that responds to environmental, climate, and host factors. During CRS, symbiotic bacteria give way to pathogenic ones, thus resulting in CRS and sinus symptoms [3]. The microbial community in CRS is mainly composed of *Corynebacterium*, *Propionibacterium*, *Staphylococcus*, *Malassezia*, etc. [4]. The fol-

L. Zhang, C. Bachert (eds.), *Chronic Rhinosinusitis*, https://doi.org/10.1007/978-981-16-0784-4_16

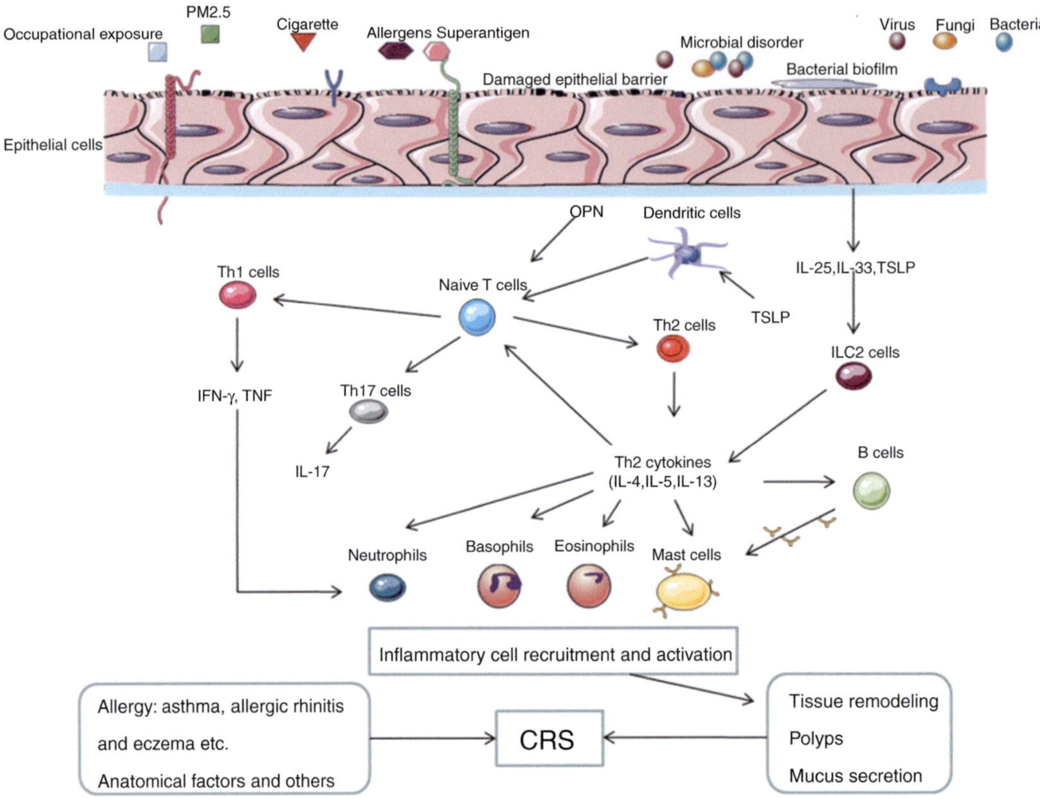

Fig. 16.1 Chronic rhinosinusitis triggered by environmental and allergic factors. *CRS* chronic rhinosinusitis, *INF* interferon, *IL* interleukin, *ILC2* group 2 innate lymphoid cell, *OPN* osteopontin, *PM2.5* fine particulate matter (particles smaller than 2.5 μm), *Th* T helper cell, *TNF* tumor necrosis factor, *TSLP* thymic stromal lymphopoietin

lowing three theories on CRS etiology and pathogenesis have been widely established: the superantigen hypothesis, the biofilm hypothesis and the microbiome hypothesis. *Staphylococcus aureus* (*S. aureus*) is the dominant microorganism in CRS [5]. *S. aureus* participates in the pathogenesis of CRS by destroying the epithelial barrier or triggering type 2 inflammation [6]. *S. aureus* has shown a considerable heterogeneity in chronic rhinosinusitis with nasal polyps (CRSwNP) and without nasal polyps (CRSsNP). For eosinophilic CRS (eCRS) patients, especially those with asthma, the superantigen exotoxins produced by *S. aureus* can amplify the local eosinophilic reaction, thus promoting the formation of nasal polyps, that is, the superantigen hypothesis. The superantigen exotoxins are believed as disease modifiers of nasal polyp formation [2, 7]. The specific role of biofilms in the etiology and pathogenesis of CRS remains largely unclear. Bacterial biofilms are highly organized complexes of protective extracellular matrix. As a vital characteristic of endogenous sinus bacteria, biofilms in CRSsNP and CRSwNP patients contain multiple species of microorganisms, including *S. aureus*, *Pseudomonas aeruginosa*, *Haemophilus influenzae,* and *Moraxella catarrhalis* [5]. The prevalence of biofilms in CRS ranges 29–72%, largely associated with severe preoperative condition, persistent postoperative symptoms, long-term infection in mucous membrane and inflammation [8]. Nevertheless, direct evidences are porous to support the biological role of bacteria biofilms in CRS [2]. Microbial disorders are associated with CRS. Following antibiotics intervention or virus infection, changes in the abundance and diversity of microbial community initiate the proliferation of pathogenic microorganisms of CRS. The colonization of pathogenic microorganisms and consequent microbial imbalance trigger chronic immune response of CRS [3]. *Citrobacter* and *S. aureus* are the main bacteria detected in CRSwNP and eCRS patients, respectively [5]. Taken together, the microbiome hypothesis of CRS requires to be further validated, and other possible reasons may contribute to type 2 inflammation of CRS [2].

Fungi are widespread in the upper respiratory tract. Abundant fungi can be found in the nasal mucus of CRS patients, including *Alternaria, Aspergillus, Candida, Cladosporium, Penicillium, Trichophyton*, etc. Although current evidences have proven that fungi infection is not causative of CRS, fungal aggregation still poses risk of CRS *via* mediating the immune system of the host and host microflora [9]. Allergic fungal rhinosinusitis (AFRS) and fungal balls are of significance in phenotypes of fungal CRS [2].

In addition, viral infection may worsen CRS. Viral-infection-caused CRS patients are often predisposed to factors like epithelial remodeling caused by long-term inflammation. Rhinovirus, respiratory syncytial virus, coronavirus, influenza virus, and parainfluenza virus are the most identified in CRS [10]. Experimental data support the fact that viral infection only exerts an initial role in inflammatory stimulation [11]. Besides, rhinovirus infection can cause eosinophilic inflammation and participate in the pathogenesis of CRS [5].

Sinus mucosa serves as the first buffer against inhaled environmental pollutants. Occupational, traffic-related air pollutants (e.g. $PM_{2.5}$, nitrogen dioxide, and diesel exhaust particles), as well as cigarette smoke are vital risk factors for CRS [1]. A latest study proposed that air pollutants are significantly correlated to the severity of CRS symptoms [12]. Occupational exposure to paper dust, cleaning agents, metal dust, animals, moisture/mold or toxic gases enhances the susceptibility to CRS [13, 14]. Moreover, exposure to abundant dusts, and living in poor, crowded or dilapidated houses are associated with an increase in the prevalence of CRS, and occupational dust has an important correlation with the formation of nasal polyps [15, 16]. Sufficient evidences have shown the relationship between $PM_{2.5}$ exposure and CRS. The proportion of CRSsNP needing surgery increases by 1.89 times as $PM_{2.5}$ exposure increases by one unit [1, 12]. Cigarette smoke disturbs the function of nasal cavity and paranasal sinuses relying on multiple mechanisms, including the destruction of ion transport, mucociliary clearance, vitamin D conversion and nasal epithelial barrier dysfunction, enhancement of oxidative stress, and production of inflammatory mediators. Both active and passive smoking have a strong correlation with CRS. Notably, exposure to second-hand smoke is found in 68% of children with CRS. The negative impact that cigarette smoke exerts on CRS worsens as inhaled amount and smoking duration increase, sometimes increasing the rate of endoscopic examination and reoperation after sinus surgery [17].

In CRS, inflammatory response comes as the result of epithelial barrier damage, immune response disorder, and infection or colonization of specific pathogens [6]. On the one hand, environmental factors can induce type 2 inflammation or other immune disorders through damaging the nasal mucosal epithelial barrier, weakening the ciliary function of nasal mucosa and promoting the oxidative stress cascade in the nasal mucosa, ultimately leading to CRS symptoms (e.g. nasal obstruction, increased nasal secretions, and dryness of nasal mucosa) [5, 6, 18]. On the other hand, environmental factors can directly alter key CRS-related genes by epigenetic modifications. Differing from genetic variations, epigenetic modifications trigger chronic inflammation through regulating the expressions of genes and proteins, a process that does not necessarily involve alterations in DNA sequences. DNA methylation decides gene activity. Kim et al. [19] reported abundant methylated genes in polyp tissues of CRSwNP patients. Regulatory roles of environmental factors in CRS, especially its different phenotypes, require to be explored in the future.

16.3 Allergic Triggers of CRS

Allergic or non-allergic reactions rise as a consequence of hypersensitivity to foreign antigens [20]. The relationship between allergies and CRS remains unclear. In 2014, Wilson et al. [21] retrospectively analyzed 18 studies on the relation between allergy and CRSwNP, and among them, the relation was confirmed in 10 studies, denied in 7 studies, and suspended in 1 study. Moreover, of the 9 studies, 4 studies reported a relation between allergy and CRSsNP, and the remaining showed no relation. Perennial exposure to inhaled allergens (e.g. molds, dust mites, and pollens) is associated with CRS and CRS progression [20]. A relevant study showed that the prevalence of inhaled allergy in control subjects, CRSsNP and CRSwNP patients is 13.1%, 20.3%, and 31.0%, respectively. Notably, a higher rate of allergy by *Dermatophagoides pteronyssinus* is detected in CRSwNP patients than in CRSsNP patients [22]. IgE-mediated allergic reactions are considered as precipitating factors or comorbidities of CRS. Mainly in the early phase of CRS, they trigger chronic inflammation through increasing tissue exudation, mucosal edema, and delaying mucociliary cleaning [23]. It is reported that allergic rhinitis (AR) is significantly linked to CRS, and the multimorbidity of CRS and AR is up to 60–80% [21]. Whether allergy affects the process of CRSwNP is controversial. Experimental data obtained a similar prevalence of nasal polyps between allergic patients and the normal population. However, another study showed that nasal polyps was more common in allergic patients, so was allergic reaction in patients with nasal polyps [20]. Taken together, the relationship between CRS (classified into CRSwNP, CRSsNP, and other broad phenotypes) and allergy is obscure.

The prevalence of allergy in CRS patients may vary in different phenotypes. Since allergic reaction is a type 2 inflammation, and CRS can be subtyped to different endotypes based on type 1 and type 2 inflammation, allergy and CRS may share inflammatory similarity. Primary CRS is dominated by endotypes, which are classified into type 2 and non-type 2, and the type 2 phenotypes are further divided into central compartment atopic disease (CCAD), AFRS, and CRSwNP/eCRS [5]. Previous evidences have demonstrated a stronger correlation between allergy and certain phenotypes of CRS. For example, AFRS and CCAD have a stronger association with CRS than CRSwNP and CRSsNP [5, 20]. CCAD is an allergic airway inflammation disease, which is highly prevalent in allergic patients. CCAD patients usually exhibit a history of atopic reactions, including AR, conjunctival symptoms and dermatitis. The prevalence of asthma in CCAD patients is low. As a common phenotype in clinically diagnosed CRSwNP, CCAD has been recently identified to have a close link to atopic reactions. In 2014, White et al. [24] for the first time discovered polypoid changes of turbinate and edema-like changes in patients tested positive to inhaled allergen. A central pattern of mucosal disease is highly correlated with allergy. Patients with an isolated middle turbinate lesion have a higher correlation with allergen sensitization than patients with diffuse polyposis [25]. As a non-invasive, recurrent subset of CRSwNP, AFRS is caused by non-invasive fungal hyphae, accounting for 5–10% of CRS cases. Typical allergic mucin causes nasal polyps, hyposmia/anosmia, and facial structural deformation. AFRS patients often show an atopic sensitivity to IgE in multiple air allergens, and presence of AR and/or asthma. In IgE-mediated AFRS, fungal allergens mainly include *Aspergillus*, *Bipolaris*, *Curvularis*, and *Alternaria* [26]. Currently, eosinophils, IgE and periostin are used as biomarkers for identifying type 2 inflammation in some more specialized centers. Mounting evidences have shown that eosinophils are a proper surrogate marker. Specifically, eosinophils/HPF $\geq$ 10 is used to predict CRS. Eosinophilic CRSwNP (eCRSwNP) is more detected in men who are prone to smoking, atopia, a higher absolute count of eosinophils in peripheral blood and IgE level. eCRSwNP features diffuse ethmoid sinus, olfactory involvement and high CT scores of ethmoid/maxillary sinus. eCRS is the only accurate predictor of CRS recurrence and is related to poor prognosis, high postoperative score, reduced life quality, and high recurrence rate of polyps [5, 27]. The EPOS 2020 guidelines propose that eosinophilic granulomatosis with polyangiitis (EGPA), also known as Churg-Strauss disease, causes bilateral sinusitis and inflammation in small- and medium-sized blood vessels. In a series of non-pulmonary symptoms, those in the nasal cavity and sinuses are common to EGPA that usually appears in asthma adults, manifested as chronic sinusitis and eosinophilic nasal polyps [5].

CRS is often accompanied with lower airway inflammation. Asthma and airway hyperresponsiveness are closely related to CRS. There is a tight correlation between CRS and asthma in all age groups [28, 29]. Typically, CRS is manifested as uncontrolled asthma and increases the risk of asthma exacerbation [5]. In 2012, a GA^{2}LEN survey conducted in 12 European countries found that the prevalence of asthma in CRS patients was more than twice of that in non-CRS patients [29]. Consistently, epidemiological investigations found 11.2% of CRS patients with concomitant asthma and 27.3% with co-existing airway hyperresponsiveness in China [28]. In a latest study, the prevalence of asthma in the normal, CRSsNP and CRSwNP group was 9.95%, 21.16%, and 46.9%, respectively [22]. Approximately, 9–10% of CRSwNP patients demonstrate aspirin intolerance syndrome and asthma [27]. In contrast, nasal polyps develop in 7% of asthma patients: 5% in atopic and 13% in non-atopic asthma patients. Asthma is an independent predictor of CRS, and each may precede the other [5, 30]. Interestingly, nasal colonization of *S. aureus* has a significant relationship with asthma prevalence in CRSwNP and CRSsNP patients, which may be explained by that *S. aureus* can induce type 2 inflammation [5]. In addition, eczema, food allergy, urticaria and chronic obstructive pulmonary disease (COPD) are also common comorbidities of CRS [31].

Mechanisms underlying the influences of allergy on CRS differ a lot. Severe CRS is generally not considered as an allergic disease, while comorbid allergies may aggravate type 2 inflammation in CRS. A recent study covering Chinese population has shown obvious mucosal immunopathological products in both atopic and non-atopic CRSsNP patients, indicating that Chinese CRSsNP patients with AR are predisposed to type 2 inflammation, and CRSsNP patients without AR to non-type 2 inflammation [32]. Local IgE production in patients with atopic nasal polyps may be induced by allergen stimulation. In patients with non-atopic nasal polyps, however, local hyperimmunoglobulinemia also arises, suggesting that IgE level may be maneuvered by other possible mechanisms [32]. Allergy may not be the primary cause of CRS, but can turn people susceptible to CRS through aggravating the inflammatory response of mucosa [28] (Fig. 16.1).

16.4 Conclusions

CRS is highly heterogeneous. Environmental and allergic factors trigger the onset of CRS and pose negative impacts on its prognosis. Among the environmental factors, microbes and air pollutants are culprits in the pathogenesis of CRS. Although the relationship between allergy and CRSwNP/CRSsNP remains controversial, allergy does have a close link with certain phenotypes of CRS (e.g. type 2 primary CRS, including CCAD and AFRS). Besides, eCRSwNP and EGPA are significantly correlated with allergy. Asthma and airway hyperresponsiveness are related to CRS, while their involvement in CRS phenotypes is unclear. Collectively, the roles of environmental and allergic factors in the processes of CRS, especially its phenotypes, require further study.

References

1. London NR Jr, Lina I, Ramanathan M Jr. Aeroallergens, air pollutants, and chronic rhinitis and rhinosinusitis. World J Otorhinolaryngol. 2018;4(3):209–15. https://doi.org/10.1016/j.wjorl.2018.08.006.
2. Lam K, Schleimer R, Kern RC. The etiology and pathogenesis of chronic rhinosinusitis: a review of current hypotheses. Curr Allergy Asthma Rep. 2015;15(7):41. https://doi.org/10.1007/s11882-015-0540-2.
3. Wang JC, Moore CA, Epperson MV, Sedaghat AR. Association of the sinonasal bacterial microbiome with clinical outcomes in chronic rhinosinusitis: a systematic review. Int Forum Allergy

Rhinol. 2020;10(4):433–43. https://doi.org/10.1002/alr.22524.
4. Wagner Mackenzie B, Chang K, Zoing M, Jain R, Hoggard M, Biswas K, et al. Longitudinal study of the bacterial and fungal microbiota in the human sinuses reveals seasonal and annual changes in diversity. Sci Rep. 2019;9(1):17416. https://doi.org/10.1038/s41598-019-53975-9.
5. Fokkens WJ, Lund VJ, Hopkins C, Hellings PW, Kern R, Reitsma S, et al. European position paper on rhinosinusitis and nasal polyps 2020. Rhinology. 2020;58(Suppl S29):1–464. https://doi.org/10.4193/Rhin20.600.
6. Staudacher AG, Stevens WW. Sinus infections, inflammation, and asthma. Immunol Allergy Clin N Am. 2019;39(3):403–15. https://doi.org/10.1016/j.iac.2019.03.008.
7. Kim Y-C, Won H-K, Lee JW, Sohn K-H, Kim M-H, Kim T-B, et al. *Staphylococcus aureus* nasal colonization and asthma in adults: systematic review and meta-analysis. J Allergy Clin Immunol Pract. 2019;7(2):606–615.e9. https://doi.org/10.1016/j.jaip.2018.08.020.
8. Singhal D, Psaltis AJ, Foreman A, Wormald PJ. The impact of biofilms on outcomes after endoscopic sinus surgery. Am J Rhinol Allergy. 2010;24(3):169–74. https://doi.org/10.2500/ajra.2010.24.3462.
9. Hoggard M, Zoing M, Biswas K, Taylor MW, Douglas RG. The sinonasal mycobiota in chronic rhinosinusitis and control patients. Rhinology. 2019;57(3):190–9. https://doi.org/10.4193/Rhin18.256.
10. Tan KS, Yan Y, Ong HH, Chow VTK, Shi L, Wang DY. Impact of respiratory virus infections in exacerbation of acute and chronic rhinosinusitis. Curr Allergy Asthma Rep. 2017;17(4):24. https://doi.org/10.1007/s11882-017-0693-2.
11. Brook I. Microbiology of chronic rhinosinusitis. Eur J Clin Microbiol Infect Dis. 2016;35(7):1059–68. https://doi.org/10.1007/s10096-016-2640-x.
12. Mady LJ, Schwarzbach HL, Moore JA, Boudreau RM, Tripathy S, Kinnee E, et al. Air pollutants may be environmental risk factors in chronic rhinosinusitis disease progression. Int Forum Allergy Rhinol. 2018;8(3):377–84. https://doi.org/10.1002/alr.22052.
13. Gao WX, Ou CQ, Fang SB, Sun YQ, Zhang H, Cheng L, et al. Occupational and environmental risk factors for chronic rhinosinusitis in China: a multicentre cross-sectional study. Respir Res. 2016;17(1):54. https://doi.org/10.1186/s12931-016-0366-z.
14. Clarhed UKE, Svendsen M, Schiöler L, Kongerud J, Torén K, Hellgren J, et al. Chronic rhinosinusitis related to occupational exposure: the telemark population study. J Occup Environ Med. 2018;60(7):656–60. https://doi.org/10.1097/jom.0000000000001312.
15. Weakley J, Hall CB, Liu X, Zeig-Owens R, Webber MP, Schwartz T, et al. The effect of World Trade Center exposure on the latency of chronic rhinosinusitis diagnoses in New York City firefighters: 2001-2011. Occup Environ Med. 2016;73(4):280–3. https://doi.org/10.1136/oemed-2015-103094.
16. Geramas I, Terzakis D, Hatzimanolis E, Georgalas C. Social factors in the development of chronic rhinosinusitis: a systematic review. Curr Allergy Asthma Rep. 2018;18(2):7. https://doi.org/10.1007/s11882-018-0763-0.
17. Christensen DN, Franks ZG, McCrary HC, Saleh AA, Chang EH. A systematic review of the association between cigarette smoke exposure and chronic rhinosinusitis. Otolaryngol Head Neck Surg. 2018;158(5):801–16. https://doi.org/10.1177/0194599818757697.
18. Ahmadzada S, Ende JA, Alvarado R, Christensen JM, Kim JH, Rimmer J, et al. Responses of well-differentiated human sinonasal epithelial cells to allergen exposure and environmental pollution in chronic rhinosinusitis. Am J Rhinol Allergy. 2019;33(6):624–33. https://doi.org/10.1177/1945892419853103.
19. Kim JY, Kim DK, Yu MS, Cha MJ, Yu SL, Kang J. Role of epigenetics in the pathogenesis of chronic rhinosinusitis with nasal polyps. Mol Med Rep. 2018;17(1):1219–27. https://doi.org/10.3892/mmr.2017.8001.
20. Marcus S, Roland LT, DelGaudio JM, Wise SK. The relationship between allergy and chronic rhinosinusitis. Laryngoscope Investig Otolaryngol. 2019;4(1):13–7. https://doi.org/10.1002/lio2.236.
21. Wilson KF, McMains KC, Orlandi RR. The association between allergy and chronic rhinosinusitis with and without nasal polyps: an evidence-based review with recommendations. Int Forum Allergy Rhinol. 2014;4(2):93–103. https://doi.org/10.1002/alr.21258.
22. Philpott CM, Erskine S, Hopkins C, Kumar N, Anari S, Kara N, et al. Prevalence of asthma, aspirin sensitivity and allergy in chronic rhinosinusitis: data from the UK National Chronic Rhinosinusitis Epidemiology Study. Respir Res. 2018;19(1):129. https://doi.org/10.1186/s12931-018-0823-y.
23. Marcus S, DelGaudio JM, Roland LT, Wise SK. Chronic rhinosinusitis: does allergy play a role? Med Sci (Basel). 2019;7(2):30. https://doi.org/10.3390/medsci7020030.
24. White LJ, Rotella MR, DelGaudio JM. Polypoid changes of the middle turbinate as an indicator of atopic disease. Int Forum Allergy Rhinol. 2014;4(5):376–80. https://doi.org/10.1002/alr.21290.
25. Hamizan AW, Loftus PA, Alvarado R, Ho J, Kalish L, Sacks R, et al. Allergic phenotype of chronic rhinosinusitis based on radiologic pattern of disease. Laryngoscope. 2018;128(9):2015–21. https://doi.org/10.1002/lary.27180.
26. Hoyt AE, Borish L, Gurrola J, Payne S. Allergic fungal rhinosinusitis. J Allergy Clin Immunol Pract. 2016;4(4):599–604. https://doi.org/10.1016/j.jaip.2016.03.010.
27. Liu Z, Chen J, Cheng L, Li H, Liu S, Lou H, et al. Chinese Society of Allergy and Chinese Society of Otorhinolaryngology-Head and Neck Surgery

guideline for chronic rhinosinusitis. Allergy, Asthma Immunol Res. 2020;12(2):176–237. https://doi.org/10.4168/aair.2020.12.2.176.
28. [Chinese guidelines for diagnosis and treatment of chronic rhinosinusitis (2018)]. Zhonghua Er Bi Yan Hou Tou Jing Wai Ke Za Zhi = Chinese J Otorhinolaryngol Head Neck Surg. 2019;54(2):81–100. https://doi.org/10.3760/cma.j.issn.1673-0860.2019.02.001.
29. Jarvis D, Newson R, Lotvall J, Hastan D, Tomassen P, Keil T, et al. Asthma in adults and its association with chronic rhinosinusitis: the GA2LEN survey in Europe. Allergy. 2012;67(1):91–8. https://doi.org/10.1111/j.1398-9995.2011.02709.x.
30. Tint D, Kubala S, Toskala E. Risk factors and comorbidities in chronic rhinosinusitis. Curr Allergy Asthma Rep. 2016;16(2):16. https://doi.org/10.1007/s11882-015-0589-y.
31. Khan A, Vandeplas G, Huynh TMT, Joish VN, Mannent L, Tomassen P, et al. The Global Allergy and Asthma European Network (GALEN) rhinosinusitis cohort: a large European cross-sectional study of chronic rhinosinusitis patients with and without nasal polyps. Rhinology. 2019;57(1):32–42. https://doi.org/10.4193/Rhin17.255.
32. Wang BF, Cao PP, Long XB, Zhang XH, Xu K, Cui YH, et al. Distinct mucosal immunopathologic profiles in atopic and nonatopic chronic rhinosinusitis without nasal polyps in Central China. Int Forum Allergy Rhinology. 2016;6(10):1013–9. https://doi.org/10.1002/alr.21799.

17 Dysfunctional Immune Regulatory System

Jinmei Xue, Pingchang Yang,
and Changqing Zhao

Key Points

- Nasal mucosa is an important part of the local mucosal immune system. The immune active components in the mucosa play an important role in the defense of upper respiratory mucosa. The acquired immunity and congenital immune system cooperate together in maintaining the immune balance of nasal mucosa.
- Innate and adaptive inflammatory responses are underlying the Pathogenesis of CRS. Effective barrier function is essential for survival, and chronic damage of the epithelial barrier is a characteristic feature of a number of significant diseases.
- The mechanism of Immune dysregulation in CRS is regulated by immunomodulators, antibacterial drugs, antihistamine and leukotriene receptor antagonism and saline irrigations.

J. Xue · C. Zhao (✉)
Department of Otolaryngology, Head and Neck Surgery, The Second Hospital, Shanxi Medical University, Taiyuan, China

P. Yang
Research Center of Allergy and Immunology, Shenzhen University School of Medicine, Shenzhen, China

17.1 Introduction

This part describes the mechanism of the dysfunction of the immune regulatory system of rhinosinusitis. The immune regulatory system is divided into acquired immune system and innate immune system. They jointly maintain the immune balance of the nasal mucosa, which is an important part of the local mucosal immune system, and plays an important role in defense through the immune active components. CRS is due to the effective barrier function of epithelium, through inflammation, cytokines, T and B lymphocytes, and congenital lymphocytes (ILCs) and other functions, resulting in the disorder of immune regulatory system. At present, it can be treated by immunomodulators, antibiotics, antihistamines and leukotrienes receptor antagonists and saline irrigation.

17.2 Immune Regulatory System

17.2.1 Congenital Immune System in Nasal Mucosa

Epithelial cells, submucosal glands (serous gland cells and mucous gland cells), and secretory cells (plasma cells) in the nasal mucosa not only produce secretions, but also make an permeation of blood plasma proteins from the blood vessels, or synthesize and secrete immune substances by

L. Zhang, C. Bachert (eds.), *Chronic Rhinosinusitis*, https://doi.org/10.1007/978-981-16-0784-4_17

these cells, which form the basis of nasal mucosal immune system [1, 2]. The nasal mucosa contains natural immune substances, mainly lysozyme and lactoferrin, the latter is stimulated by antigen to produce immunoglobulin A and G (IgA, IgG).

The term "innate" refers to the immune mechanisms that do not require prior exposure to specific antigens, such as pathogens. The congenital immunity consists of a series of components and induction processes, which can be either non-specific or pathogen-induced. Some innate immune pathways closely intertwine with tissue growth and repair. Persistent inflammation observed in chronic sinusitis may result from a pathologic imbalance of innate immune interactions between the host and the environment. Serious impairment of innate immune protection renders the sinonasal mucosal surface vulnerable to colonization and potential injury, which is characterized by chronic sinusitis, to stimulate a significant adaptive immune response.

The innate immune system is remarkably intricate. The continuously flowing mucus blanket is the main innate immune defense compartment in the nasal cavity. The nasal cavity can filter the inhaled air, trap particulates and potential pathogens in the mucus and propel them toward the pharynx through ciliary oscillation [3]. Mucus contains enzymes, immunoglobulins, opsonin, and antimicrobial peptides that restrict microorganism growth. Proteins in the mucus are derived from plasma exudates, mucus, and serous cells in submucosal glands, goblet cells, Clara cells, epithelial cells, and other cells in the mucosa (plasma cells, mast cells, phagocytes, and fibroblasts). The quantity and viscoelastic properties of the mucus and pulsation frequency of cilia determine the effectiveness of mucociliary clearance. Antimicrobial proteins and peptides secreted from mucus, as well as immunoglobulins, contribute to mucosal defense on the airway surface. Sinonasal epithelial cells are involved in this process, secreting proteins into the mucus and propelling the mucus blanket out of the nose with coordinated ciliary movement. In mucosal homeostasis, local stimulants and pathogens can be eliminated rapidly and effectively through the innate immune response of nasal mucosa without wider stimulation of the adaptive immune system.

Additionally, innate immune responses can identify pathogen-related molecular patterns in parasites, viruses, bacteria, yeasts, and mycobacteria by membrane binding and cytoplasmic antigen immune responses. Patterns-recognition receptors (PRRs) may be more exposed to epithelial damage than pathogen-associated molecular patterns (PAMPs) and amplify the immune response; if PAMP is strong enough, acquired immune response can be triggered. The two most distinctive membrane receptors are Toll-like receptors (TLR) and NOD (nucleotide-binding oligomerization domain)-like receptors (NLR) [4]. The TLR family contains 10 receptors, which have specific recognition for different ligands. Important factors in TLRs signal transduction pathway include myeloid differential protein-88, interleukin-1 receptor-associated kinase, tumor necrosis factor receptor-associated factor, mitogen-activated protein kinases (MPKs), and nuclear factor (NF)- Kappa B. TLR is a transmembrane receptor, which is expressed in most cells including respiratory epithelial cells. Studies have shown that TLRs and their transduction pathways are abnormally expressed in chronic sinusitis and nasal polyps, suggesting that innate immunity plays a role in the pathogenesis of CRS [5]. NOD-like receptor families include NODl and NOD2, which play an important role in the identification of bacterial cell wall products.

17.2.2 Acquired Immune System in Nasal Mucosa

It has become increasingly appreciated that adaptive immune response likely plays a primary role in the pathogenesis of CRS. CRS is a chronic inflammatory disease of respiratory mucosa. Its pathological characteristics are a large number of activated lymphocyte infiltration, and lymphocyte activation constantly initiates inflammatory response, which makes the inflammatory response persistent [6–9].

In nasal adaptive immune response, dendritic cells act as initial antigen presenting cells, presenting antigens to primitive T lymphocytes in draining lymph nodes or local lymphoid aggregation. In addition, basophilic granulocytes in circulating blood can also enter tissues together with dendritic cells in local tissues or even replace dendritic cells as antigen presenting cells to perform antigen presenting function.

CRS is considered an inflammatory disease that is regulated by T cell subsets. After antigen presentation, CD4+ primitive T lymphocytes will differentiate into one of several T cell lines to determine the nature of adaptive immune response. T lymphocyte subsets involved in the response included Th1, Th2, Th17, and regulatory T lymphocyte. Each cell has unique molecular, cellular, and functional properties. Helper T cells (Th) are key cells in the adaptive immune system and have recently been found to be related to many chronic diseases [8, 9]. In a non-disease state, the cells in the adaptive immune system and the cells in the innate immune system work together to form an effective immune response. Disorders of this response can lead to immune dysfunction and prevent the clearance of invading pathogens, leading to a continuous state of inflammation [10].

Once Th cells are stimulated, they have the ability to differentiate into Th1, Th2, Th17, follicular helper T cells and Treg, each of which has a specific immune regulatory function. Typical effector cells of Th1 cells are macrophages. Their response to viral and intracellular bacterial infections is particularly effective. Interferon (IFN-γ), as a recognized cytokine, can enhance the immune response of cell antigens. The key transcription factor of Th2 cells is GATA-3 and the related cytokines are IL-4, IL-5, and IL-13 [11]. Effective cells of Th2 are eosinophils, which play an important role in parasite immunity, especially those too large to be removed by phagocytosis. The key transcription factor of Th17 cells is RORc, and the related cytokine is IL-17A. The typical effector cells involved in the response are neutrophils. Extracellular bacteria, especially Staphylococcus aureus, are the main targets of attack. Treg cells characterized by CD4 + CD25 + CD127 low surface marker expression have a suppressor function, downregulating downstream T cell effector immune responses. Treg cell transcription factor (TRF) is FOXP3 and its main function is to restrict overreaction through other subpopulations. They mediate their activity by direct cell-to-cell contact and through the production of transforming growth factor (TGF)-B and interleukin (IL)-10 cytokines, which downgrade immune responses and contribute to self-tolerance [12].

17.3 Dysfunctional Immune Regulation in Rhinosinusitis

17.3.1 Epithelial Dysfunction in CRS

Effective barrier function is essential for survival, and chronic damage of the epithelial barrier is a characteristic feature of a number of significant diseases. Together, the physical barrier, local innate antimicrobial responses and mucociliary escalator compose what is called the immune barrier at times. Several studies have revealed a physical or functional defect in the barrier in patients with CRS [6, 13]. Many studies also have identified the loss of epithelial markers and gain of mesenchymal markers in CRS. Loss of barrier can result from genetic defects or decreased expression of barrier structural proteins resulting from infection, injury, or inflammation.

Proper mucociliary function is essential in nasal physiology and immunity. Ciliary motion through the sol phase of the mucus blanket propels mucus and the intercepted microbes and particulates out of the sinuses and nasal airways. The majority of early studies found that mucociliary function is impaired and that the degree of impairment of clearance is mutually related with the severity of CRS. Many studies have reported inactivity or loss of cilia in CRS tissue due to ciliary injury. Defects in mucociliary function promote bacterial growth and formation of biofilms, creating a vicious cycle.

More than 100 molecules are involved in pathogen recognition and killing, most of which are expressed by the epithelium in the upper airways and sinuses. No surprise, many of these molecules are highly induced in CRS. Although not all have been evaluated, some have been reported to be dysfunctional or reduced at the mucosal surface in CRS, including Toll-like receptors, Bitter taste receptors, Endotoxin-binding molecules, Antimicrobial peptides, Enzymatic mediators, etc.

17.3.2 Innate and Adaptive Inflammatory Responses Underlying the Pathogenesis of CRS

CRS pathogenesis has been focused on inflammation, cytokines, T and B lymphocytes, and innate lymphoid cells (ILCs) [14, 15]. When rapid local innate immune responses are inadequate to prevent growth or entry of pathogens, adaptive immune T cells and B cells are activated and converged to reinforce the response. Although the injured epithelium makes at least three T helper cell type 2 (Th2)-promoting cytokines, IL-25, IL-33, and TSLP, among these three TSLP is most highly produced in the CRS tissue [16–18]. In the presence of TSLP, ILC2s and mast cells express considerable amounts of type 2 cytokines, especially IL-5 and IL-13, and relatively little IL-4 [19]. This is the same event as seen in nasal polyps, suggesting a role of ILC2s in the type 2 cytokine production in CRSwNP. Unlike T cells, ILC2s do not depend on antigen for activation, and they rapidly activate these cytokines.

Type 2 cytokines from ILC2 are significant in recruitment of adaptive immune cells by induction of production of chemokines, activation of endothelial adhesion molecules, and provision of cytokines that shape T cell differentiation. The nature of the ILC that is activated shapes the T cell response; In this case, ILC2s promote Th2 responses. Eosinophilic polyps include type 2 cytokines, whereas non-eosinophilic polyps generally do not. Whether type 2 cytokines are derived from Th2 cells, ILC2, or mast cells and basophils, the importance of IL-5 and IL-13 in the formation of polyps is persuasive. IL-5 and IL-13 drive many features of the inflammation and the effector cell recruitment that is characteristic of the disease. In unison with an expansion of T cells in CRSwNP, there is an impressive expansion of plasmablasts, plasma cells and B cells. Local activation, proliferation, production of antibodies and class switch recombination take place within polyps [20–22]. Whether there are defects in regulatory T cells in CRS is controversial.

17.3.3 Eosinophilia and CRS

Eosinophils and their products are of great significance in airway barrier dysfunction, injury, and induction of epithelial mesenchymal transition (EMT). Eosinophil was recognized in the CRS tissues soon after Ehrlich recognizes the dyes that bind to eosinophil granules, and eosinophil granule proteins were related to pathology [23]. Eosinophils have inflammatory and tissue remodeling effects, and their derivative mediators can damage epithelial cells, stimulate EMT, activate or inhibit sensory nerves, regulate the activity of stem cells and plasma cells, and change the mechanical responses of the airway [24–26]. The correlations between disease severity and eosinophils detected in the blood or nasal tissues are well certificated. Eosinophilia is closely related to type 2 immune and inflammatory responses. Patients with eosinophilic polyp usually have higher levels of IgE, higher prevalence of allergies, and higher prevalence and severity of asthma [27]. Environmental factors that may affect eosinophilia include breastfeeding, the birth season, and the use of antibiotic during infancy; these are considered to be risk factors that may change the microbiome [28–30].

17.4 Restoration of Immune Regulation in Rhinosinusitis

17.4.1 The Regulatory Mechanism of Immune Dysregulation of CRS by Immunomodulators

Th2 response is characterized by the production of IL-4, IL-5 and IL-13, followed by eosinophilia, mast cell and basophilia. Asian CRSwNP showed neutrophil inflammation and Th1/Th17/Th22 mixed inflammatory reactions. IL-4 and IL-13 responsible for isotype conversion and upregulation of sIgE receptors on eosinophils, mast cells, monocytes and basophils. The other role of IL-4 is chemotaxis in inflammatory cells and upregulates vascular cell adhesion molecule-1 (VCAM-1). IL-5 mainly promotes the maturation, differentiation and activation of eosinophils, involved in innate immune epithelial responses with IL-13. The type 2 innate lymphoid cells (ILC2s), which are early responders within the sinonasal mucosa and activated by epithelial cell, amplify the Th2 inflammatory response in CRSwNP [17, 31–33].

- **Anti-IgE Monoclonal Antibody**
- The regulatory mechanism of immune dysregulation of CRS by anti-IgE monoclonal antibody is that anti-IgE binds free circulating IgE molecules, inhibiting its interaction with receptors on mast cells and basophils. It results in a reduction of the allergen-induced mast cell degranulation and release of inflammatory mediators. Omalizumab (Xolair) is a human anti-IgE monoclonal antibody [34].
- **Anti-IL-5 Monoclonal Antibody**
- IL-5 is a key cytokine in the activation, chemotaxis and survival of eosinophils. The anti-IL-5 acts by binding free IL-5 or inhibiting the IL-5 receptor (IL-5Rα) on the surface of eosinophils. Mepolizumab and reslizumab are anti-IL-5 monoclonal antibodies, which bind free IL-5 while benrazilumab inhibits the IL-5 receptor [35].
- **Anti-IL-4/IL-13 Monoclonal Antibody**
- Although IL-4 and IL-13 do not have high sequence homology, they share the IL-4 α receptor and signaling pathways. IL-4 and IL-13 are involved in the synthesis of IgE, activation of eosinophilic cells, mucus secretion and airway remodeling. Dupilumab is a fully humanized monoclonal antibody that effectively blocks the signaling pathways mediated by the cytokines IL-4 and IL-13 [36].
- **Siglec-8 Monoclonal Antibody**
- The receptor of sialic acid-binding immunoglobulin-type lectin (siglec)-8 is found on the surface of mast cells, eosinophils, and basophils. Siglec-8 monoclonal antibody binds the receptor to lead to selective apoptosis of cytokine-primed cells. In mast cells, engagement of siglec-8 inhibits the activity of FcεR I, down regulating the release of inflammatory mediators such as histamine and prostaglandin D2. AK001 is an IgG4 monoclonal antibody against siglec-8 [37].
- **Anti-TSLP Monoclonal Antibody**
- TSLP is an IL-7 cytokine that is mainly expressed in the lungs, skin and intestines. Under external stimulation, TSLP promotes primitive T cells differentiation to Th2 cell and increases the release of IL-4, IL-5 and IL-13. Tezepelumab, the first new potential drug to target TSLP, is a human monoclonal antibody against TSLP. It can bind to free TSLP receptors, and prevent TSLP attacking immune cells and releasing pro-inflammatory cytokines, thus preventing asthma from worsening and controlling asthma [33].

17.4.2 The Regulatory Mechanism of Immune Dysregulation of CRS by Antibacterial Drugs

Whether bacteria are the initial cause of CRS is still unclear, and the imbalance of bacterial flora may be related to the pathogenesis, inflammatory state and treatment effect of CRS. Bacterial biofilms can play a pathogenic role as infectious pathogens. *S. aureus* enterotoxins increase the Th2 cytokines IL-2, IL-4, IL-5 greater than two fold as superantigens, but not the T-regcytokines IL-10 and TGF-β1. Furthermore, The enterotoxins influence local immunoglobulin synthesis and induce polyclonal IgE production, which may contribute to severe inflammation via activation of mast cells [38].

In addition, bacterial biofilms can be used as antigens, superantigens and inflammatory factors to promote the occurrence and development of CRS [39].

Macrolides are a class of antibiotics produced by streptomycin, which are widely used in the clinical treatment of chronic rhinosinusitis due to their anti-inflammatory and immunomodulatory effects. Macrolides inhibit the production of

IL-1, IL-5, IL-6, IL-8, granulocyte macrophage colony–stimulating factor and tumor necrosis factor-α.

Macrolides also inhibit formation of leukotriene B4, which attracts neutrophils, and inhibit the release of superoxide anion by neutrophils. Macrolides can downregulate the expression of cell surface adhesion molecules on neutrophils, which is necessary for neutrophil migration. Both erythromycin and roxithromycin can accelerate apoptosis in vitro in human neutrophils. Braga and colleagues demonstrated that rokitamycin could restrain the oxidative burst of neutrophils in vitro and that after removing the macrolide, the oxidative burst ability was recovered.

Macrolides directly inhibit secretion of mucus by preventing the release of glycoproteins. Hirakata and colleagues showed that erythromycin inhibits the release of elastase, protease, phospholipase C, and eotaxin A by P aeruginosa. Besides, macrolides change the structure and architecture of bacterial biofilm, which play a role in epithelial adhesion and antimicrobial resistance. Macrolide antibiotic clarithromycin can reduce the cellular expression of TGF-β and NF-κB in nasal biopsies in vitro. Nakano and colleagues show that roxithromycin treatment in rabbits speeds the tracheal mucociliary transport. Clarithromycin decreases lipopolysaccharide-induced goblet cell hypersecretion in the guinea-pig trachea [40–42].

17.4.3 The Regulatory Mechanism of Antihistamine and Leukotriene Receptor Antagonism on Immune Dysregulation of CRS

CRSwNP is one of the most refractory forms of CRS to treat, which characterized by T helper 2 (Th2)-skewed eosinophilic inflammation with massive tissue edema. These immunopathologic features are well recognized to be mediated by numerous inflammatory mediators, such as Th2 cytokines (IL-4, IL-5 and IL-13), cysteinyl leukotriene (LT), etc. In addition to mediating robust and sustained vascular permeability, they also contribute to eosinophil recruitment and activation, mucus secretion, and tissue edema.

Studies have shown increased levels of leukotrienes (LTs) and the mRNA and protein expression of CysLT1R and CysLT2R are localized to nasal polyps. Furthermore, the upregulation of CysLT receptors and overproduction of CysLTs have been demonstrated in patients with allergic rhinitis, asthma, and CRS.

Leukotrienes promote bronchoconstriction, mucus production, edema, and chemotaxis of neutrophils and eosinophils. This process can be inhibited by blocking the receptor with an LT receptor antagonist, such as montelukast [26, 43].

Recent evidence indicates that histamine H1 receptors modulate immune responses to antigens. Treatment with desloratadine did not impair IgE production. OVA-responsive T cells from desloratadine-treated mice exhibited decreased production of IL-4, IL-5 and IL-13 and normal amounts of IFN-c. Desloratadine, administered at the time of exposure to the allergen, inhibits Th2 responses.

It was found that combining azelastine a second-generation antihistamine with budesonide (a corticosteroid) in vitro was able to upregulate expression of mitogen-activated protein kinase phosphatase-1 (MKP-1), an anti-inflammatory gene induced by corticosteroids, more than with budesonide alone. MKP-1 expression decreases intercellular adhesion molecule-1 (ICAM-1) expression, a molecule required for the extravasation of inflammatory cells from the bloodstream [44].

17.4.4 The Regulatory Mechanism of Saline Irrigations on Immune Dysregulation of CRS

Saline irrigation mechanically removes secretions, pathogens, mucus, crusts, debris, and allergens from the sinonasal cavity, and potentially has the additional benefit of improving mucociliary clearance, ciliary beat frequency, and protecting the sinonasal mucosa [45, 46].

17.5 Conclusion

This part deals with dysfunctional immune regulatory system in rhinosinusitis from the following three aspects.

First, it introduces that the acquired immunity and congenital immune system cooperate together to maintain the immune balance of nasal mucosa. The nasal mucosa contains natural immune substances, in which lysozyme and lactoferrin dominate. It has become increasingly appreciated that adaptive immune response is likely to play a primary role in the pathogenesis of CRS.

Second, it explains the dysfunctional immune regulation in rhinosinusitis. Several studies have revealed a physical and functional defect in the immune barrier in patients with CRS. When rapid local innate immune responses are inadequate to prevent growth or entry of pathogens, adaptive immune T cells and B cells are activated and converged to reinforce the response. Eosinophils have both inflammatory and tissue remodeling effects, modulate the activity of plasma cells and stem cells, and alter mechanical responses of the airways.

Then, it discusses the restoration of immune regulation in rhinosinusitis, and further introduces the regulatory mechanism of immune dysregulation of CRS by immunomodulators, antibacterial drugs, antihistamine as well as leukotriene receptor antagonism and saline irrigations.

References

1. Polito AJ, Proud D. Epithelia cells as regulators of airway inflammation. J Allergy Clin Immunol. 1998;102(5):714–8. https://doi.org/10.1016/s0091-6749(98)70008-9.
2. Takizawa H. Airway epithelial cells as regulators of airway inflammation (Review). Int J Mol Med. 1998;1(2):367–78. https://doi.org/10.3892/ijmm.1.2.367.
3. Knowles MR, Boucher RC. Mucus clearance as a primary innate defense mechanism for mammalian airways. J Clin Invest. 2002;109(5):571–7. https://doi.org/10.1172/jci15217.
4. Vasselon T, Detmers PA. Toll receptors: a central element in innate immune responses. Infect Immun. 2002;70(3):1033–41. https://doi.org/10.1128/iai.70.3.1033-1041.2002.
5. Ramanathan M Jr, Lee WK, Dubin MG, Lin S, Spannhake EW, Lane AP. Sinonasal epithelial cell expression of toll-like receptor 9 is decreased in chronic rhinosinusitis with polyps. Am J Rhinol. 2007;21(1):110–6. https://doi.org/10.2500/ajr.2007.21.2997.
6. Dejima K, Randell SH, Stutts MJ, Senior BA, Boucher RC. Potential role of abnormal ion transport in the pathogenesis of chronic sinusitis. Archiv Otolaryngol Head Neck Surg. 2006;132(12):1352–62. https://doi.org/10.1001/archotol.132.12.1352.
7. Kern RC, Conley DB, Walsh W, Chandra R, Kato A, Tripathi-Peters A, et al. Perspectives on the etiology of chronic rhinosinusitis: an immune barrier hypothesis. Am J Rhinol. 2008;22(6):549–59. https://doi.org/10.2500/ajr.2008.22.3228.
8. Zhang N, Van Zele T, Perez-Novo C, Van Bruaene N, Holtappels G, DeRuyck N, et al. Different types of T-effector cells orchestrate mucosal inflammation in chronic sinus disease. J Allergy Clin Immunol. 2008;122(5):961–8. https://doi.org/10.1016/j.jaci.2008.07.008.
9. Shen Y, Tang XY, Yang YC, Ke X, Kou W, Pan CK, et al. Impaired balance of Th17/Treg in patients with nasal polyposis. Scand J Immunol. 2011;74(2):176–85. https://doi.org/10.1111/j.1365-3083.2011.02546.x.
10. Shi LL, Song J, Xiong P, Cao PP, Liao B, Ma J, et al. Disease-specific T-helper cell polarizing function of lesional dendritic cells in different types of chronic rhinosinusitis with nasal polyps. Am J Respir Crit Care Med. 2014;190(6):628–38. https://doi.org/10.1164/rccm.201402-0234OC.
11. Sokol CL, Chu NQ, Yu S, Nish SA, Laufer TM, Medzhitov R. Basophils function as antigen-presenting cells for an allergen-induced T helper type 2 response. Nat Immunol. 2009;10(7):713–20. https://doi.org/10.1038/ni.1738.
12. Zhu J, Yamane H, Paul WE. Differentiation of effector CD4 T cell populations (*). Annu Rev Immunol. 2010;28:445–89. https://doi.org/10.1146/annurev-immunol-030409-101212.
13. Bernstein JM, Gorfien J, Noble B, Yankaskas JR. Nasal polyposis: immunohistochemistry and bioelectrical findings (a hypothesis for the development of nasal polyps). J Allergy Clin Immunol. 1997;99(2):165–75.
14. Akdis CA, Bachert C, Cingi C, Dykewicz MS, Hellings PW, Naclerio RM, et al. Endotypes and phenotypes of chronic rhinosinusitis: a PRACTALL document of the European Academy of Allergy and Clinical Immunology and the American Academy of Allergy, Asthma & Immunology. J Allergy Clin Immunol. 2013;131(6):1479–90. https://doi.org/10.1016/j.jaci.2013.02.036.
15. Hulse KE, Stevens WW, Tan BK, Schleimer RP. Pathogenesis of nasal polyposis. Clin Exp Allergy. 2015;45(2):328–46. https://doi.org/10.1111/cea.12472.

16. Liu T, Li TL, Zhao F, Xie C, Liu AM, Chen X, et al. Role of thymic stromal lymphopoietin in the pathogenesis of nasal polyposis. Am J Med Sci. 2011;341(1):40–7. https://doi.org/10.1097/MAJ.0b013e3181f20489.
17. Nagarkar DR, Poposki JA, Tan BK, Comeau MR, Peters AT, Hulse KE, et al. Thymic stromal lymphopoietin activity is increased in nasal polyps of patients with chronic rhinosinusitis. J Allergy Clin Immunol. 2013;132(3):593–600.e12. https://doi.org/10.1016/j.jaci.2013.04.005.
18. Miljkovic D, Bassiouni A, Cooksley C, Ou J, Hauben E, Wormald PJ, et al. Association between group 2 innate lymphoid cells enrichment, nasal polyps and allergy in chronic rhinosinusitis. Allergy. 2014;69(9):1154–61. https://doi.org/10.1111/all.12440.
19. McKenzie ANJ, Spits H, Eberl G. Innate lymphoid cells in inflammation and immunity. Immunity. 2014;41(3):366–74. https://doi.org/10.1016/j.immuni.2014.09.006.
20. Gevaert P, Holtappels G, Johansson SG, Cuvelier C, Cauwenberge P, Bachert C. Organization of secondary lymphoid tissue and local IgE formation to Staphylococcus aureus enterotoxins in nasal polyp tissue. Allergy. 2005;60(1):71–9. https://doi.org/10.1111/j.1398-9995.2004.00621.x.
21. Mechtcheriakova D, Sobanov Y, Holtappels G, Bajna E, Svoboda M, Jaritz M, et al. Activation-induced cytidine deaminase (AID)-associated multigene signature to assess impact of AID in etiology of diseases with inflammatory component. PLoS One. 2011;6(10):e25611. https://doi.org/10.1371/journal.pone.0025611.
22. Hulse KE, Norton JE, Suh L, Zhong Q, Mahdavinia M, Simon P, et al. Chronic rhinosinusitis with nasal polyps is characterized by B-cell inflammation and EBV-induced protein 2 expression. J Allergy Clin Immunol. 2013;131(4):1075–83.e1–7. https://doi.org/10.1016/j.jaci.2013.01.043.
23. Mygind N, Dahl R, Bachert C. Nasal polyposis, eosinophil dominated inflammation, and allergy. Thorax. 2000;55(Suppl 2):S79–83. https://doi.org/10.1136/thorax.55.suppl_2.s79.
24. Lee JJ, Jacobsen EA, McGarry MP, Schleimer RP, Lee NA. Eosinophils in health and disease: the LIAR hypothesis. Clin Exp Allergy. 2010;40(4):563–75. https://doi.org/10.1111/j.1365-2222.2010.03484.x.
25. Postma DS, Rabe KF. The asthma-COPD overlap syndrome. N Engl J Med. 2015;373(13):1241–9. https://doi.org/10.1056/NEJMra1411863.
26. George L, Brightling CE. Eosinophilic airway inflammation: role in asthma and chronic obstructive pulmonary disease. Ther Adv Chronic Dis. 2016;7(1):34–51. https://doi.org/10.1177/2040622315609251.
27. Wang ET, Zheng Y, Liu PF, Guo LJ. Eosinophilic chronic rhinosinusitis in East Asians. World J Clin Cases. 2014;2(12):873–82. https://doi.org/10.12998/wjcc.v2.i12.873
28. Rothenberg ME. Biology and treatment of eosinophilic esophagitis. Gastroenterology. 2009;137(4):1238–49. https://doi.org/10.1053/j.gastro.2009.07.007.
29. Alexander ES, Martin LJ, Collins MH, Kottyan LC, Sucharew H, He H, et al. Twin and family studies reveal strong environmental and weaker genetic cues explaining heritability of eosinophilic esophagitis. J Allergy Clin Immunol. 2014;134(5):1084–92.e1. https://doi.org/10.1016/j.jaci.2014.07.021.
30. Schleimer RP. Immunopathogenesis of chronic rhinosinusitis and nasal polyposis. Annu Rev Pathol. 2017;12:331–57. https://doi.org/10.1146/annurev-pathol-052016-100401.
31. Mjösberg JM, Trifari S, Crellin NK, Peters CP, van Drunen CM, Piet B, et al. Human IL-25- and IL-33-responsive type 2 innate lymphoid cells are defined by expression of CRTH2 and CD161. Nat Immunol. 2011;12(11):1055–62. https://doi.org/10.1038/ni.2104.
32. Shaw JL, Fakhri S, Citardi MJ, Porter PC, Corry DB, Kheradmand F, et al. IL-33-responsive innate lymphoid cells are an important source of IL-13 in chronic rhinosinusitis with nasal polyps. Am J Respir Crit Care Med. 2013;188(4):432–9. https://doi.org/10.1164/rccm.201212-2227OC.
33. Lavigne P, Lee SE. Immunomodulators in chronic rhinosinusitis. World J Otorhinolaryngol Head Neck Surg. 2018;4(3):186–92. https://doi.org/10.1016/j.wjorl.2018.09.002.
34. Baroody FM, Suh SH, Naclerio RM. Total IgE serum levels correlate with sinus mucosal thickness on computerized tomography scans. J Allergy Clin Immunol. 1997;100(4):563–8. https://doi.org/10.1016/s0091-6749(97)70151-9.
35. Bachert C, Sousa AR, Lund VJ, Scadding GK, Gevaert P, Nasser S, et al. Reduced need for surgery in severe nasal polyposis with mepolizumab: randomized trial. J Allergy Clin Immunol. 2017;140(4):1024–31.e14. https://doi.org/10.1016/j.jaci.2017.05.044.
36. Castro M, Corren J, Pavord ID, Maspero J, Wenzel S, Rabe KF, et al. Dupilumab efficacy and safety in moderate-to-severe uncontrolled asthma. N Engl J Med. 2018;378(26):2486–96. https://doi.org/10.1056/NEJMoa1804092.
37. Schleimer RP, Schnaar RL, Bochner BS. Regulation of airway inflammation by Siglec-8 and Siglec-9 sialoglycan ligand expression. Curr Opin Allergy Clin Immunol. 2016;16(1):24–30. https://doi.org/10.1097/aci.0000000000000234.
38. Bachert C, Zhang N, Patou J, van Zele T, Gevaert P. Role of staphylococcal superantigens in upper airway disease. Curr Opin Allergy Clin Immunol. 2008;8(1):34–8. https://doi.org/10.1097/ACI.0b013e3282f4178f.
39. Pinto JM, Mehta N, DiTineo M, Wang J, Baroody FM, Naclerio RM. A randomized, double-blind, placebo-controlled trial of anti-IgE for chronic rhinosinusitis. Rhinology. 2010;48(3):318–24. https://doi.org/10.4193/Rhin09.144.

40. Tamaoki J, Kadota J, Takizawa H. Clinical implications of the immunomodulatory effects of macrolides. Am J Med. 2004;117(Suppl 9A):5s–11s. https://doi.org/10.1016/j.amjmed.2004.07.023.
41. Wallwork B, Coman W, Mackay-Sim A, Cervin A. Effect of clarithromycin on nuclear factor-kappa B and transforming growth factor-beta in chronic rhinosinusitis. Laryngoscope. 2004;114(2):286–90. https://doi.org/10.1097/00005537-200402000-00019.
42. Cervin A, Wallwork B. Anti-inflammatory effects of macrolide antibiotics in the treatment of chronic rhinosinusitis. Otolaryngol Clin N Am. 2005;38(6):1339–50. https://doi.org/10.1016/j.otc.2005.08.002.
43. Wu X, Hong H, Zuo K, Han M, Li J, Wen W, et al. Expression of leukotriene and its receptors in eosinophilic chronic rhinosinusitis with nasal polyps. Int Forum Allergy Rhinol. 2016;6(1):75–81. https://doi.org/10.1002/alr.21625.
44. Dutta R, Dubal PM, Eloy JA. The connection between seasonal allergies, food allergies, and rhinosinusitis: what is the evidence? Curr Opin Otolaryngol Head Neck Surg. 2015;23(1):2–7. https://doi.org/10.1097/moo.0000000000000123.
45. Sanan A, Rabinowitz M, Rosen M, Nyquist G. Topical therapies for refractory chronic rhinosinusitis. Otolaryngol Clin N Am. 2017;50(1):129–41. https://doi.org/10.1016/j.otc.2016.08.011.
46. Brietzke SE, Shin JJ, Choi S, Lee JT, Parikh SR, Pena M, et al. Clinical consensus statement: pediatric chronic rhinosinusitis. Otolaryngol Head Neck Surg. 2014;151(4):542–53. https://doi.org/10.1177/0194599814549302.

18 Chronic Rhinosinusitis with and Without Nasal Polyps

Bradley F. Marple

Key Points

- Chronic rhinosinusitis represents an inflammatory disorder involving the mucosa of the nasal cavity and sinuses persisting for a period of at least 12 weeks.
- Diagnosis requires objective findings of inflammation within the paranasal sinuses.
- Phenotypic subtypes of chronic rhinosinusitis (Chronic Rhinosinusitis with Nasal Polyps, Chronic Rhinosinusitis without Nasal Polyps) are based upon differences in physical characteristics of disease expression, and served as a preliminary step toward a directing treatment strategy.

18.1 Introduction

Consensus definitions for chronic rhinosinusitis (CRS) began to emerge in 2003 in order to address the need for uniformity within clinical research trials, to target various potential causes of the disease, and to better elucidate effective prevention and treatment plans [1]. At this point in time, two clinically distinct patterns of disease had been recognized. The first pattern was of CRS that occurred in patients who concomitantly suffered asthma. This was thought to be supportive of the "one-airway disease" hypothesis and implicated a more systemic inflammatory process broadly involving airway respiratory epithelium [2]. This population of patients was also more likely to manifest allergies, bilateral sinus involvement, and nasal polyposis. The second pattern of disease differed from the first, most significantly in that patients suffered no other evidence of airway disease. The pattern of sinus involvement could be asymmetric, and an association with dental disease or anatomic variants was noted. The lack of consensus around a single definition at the time highlighted the difficulty in consolidating these observations of CRS as a single disease entity, and supported the concept that CRS may exist more as a syndrome of several underlying etiologies [2].

In order to address the need for a common set of definitions that would provide a foundation for future evidence-based guidance for the treatment of CRS, a panel of international experts and representatives of five major professional societies representing was convened the summer of 2003 [3]. During the course of the 2-day meeting, the panel discussed the need for a series of definitions that would account for the potential that multiple mechanisms may contribute to the phenotypic expression of CRS within a given patient.

B. F. Marple (✉)
Department of Otolaryngology, Head and Neck Surgery, University of Texas, Southwestern Medical Center, Dallas, TX, USA
e-mail: bradley.marple@utsouthwestern.edu

L. Zhang, C. Bachert (eds.), *Chronic Rhinosinusitis*, https://doi.org/10.1007/978-981-16-0784-4_18

The correlation between specific phenotypic expressions of CRS and clusters of inflammatory mediators within the respiratory epithelium had been recently described and seemed to be an obvious strategy for classification [4]. Unfortunately, the lack of clinically available methods to assess these mediators precluded its use at the time. A strategy based upon clinically available disease characteristics was adopted. Polyps, and their correlation with the histologic presence of eosinophils, were proposed as a clinical surrogate for eosinophilic inflammation. The panel reached consensus around the following definitions for rhinosinusitis [3]:

1. Acute presumed bacterial rhinosinusitis.
2. CRS without polyps.
3. CRS with polyps.
4. Classic Allergic Fungal Rhinosinusitis.

The development of a standard series of definitions for CRS paved the way for our current understanding of the disease, its pathogenesis, and novel approaches for its treatment.

Table 18.1 Diagnostic criteria for chronic rhinosinusitis [7]

Diagnostic criteria	CRS phenotype	
	CRSsNP	CRSwNP
Duration	Symptoms present ≥12 weeks	Symptoms present ≥12 weeks
Symptoms of Disease	Requires ≥2 of the following symptoms • Mucopurulent drainage. • Nasal obstruction. • Facial pressure, fullness, or pain.	Requires ≥2 of the following symptoms • Mucopurulent drainage. • Nasal obstruction. • Hyposmia.
Objective Findings (Requires both endoscopic AND CT findings required)	Endoscopic evidence of inflammation as demonstrated by: • Discolored mucus, or. • Middle meatus mucosal edema, or. • Ethmoid mucosal edema.	Endoscopic evidence of inflammation as demonstrated by: • Presence of nasal polyps.
	CT evidence of rhinosinusitis	CT evidence of rhinosinusitis

18.2 Definition and Epidemiology

Chronic rhinosinusitis (CRS) is defined as an inflammatory process involving the mucosa of the nasal cavity and paranasal sinuses that persists for greater than 12 weeks. It also requires the presence of at least two or more recognized symptoms, as well as evidence of inflammation as demonstrated by radiologic or endoscopic exam [1, 3, 5, 6] (Table 18.1). The inflammation that underlies CRS involves the respiratory epithelium of the upper airway in much the same way that the respiratory mucosa is involved in diseases of the lower respiratory track such as asthma and chronic obstructive pulmonary disease, where medical management strategies have enjoyed success. Better use of the phenotypes (and subsequent endotypes) of CRS holds the promise of better selection of medical and surgical management [8].

CRS ranks as one of the most prevalent chronic diseases [9–12], affecting 10.9% of European, 13.4% of American, and 8% of the Chinese populations [13–15]. Given the worldwide prevalence of CRS, the disease is commonly encountered within the practice of many medical specialties [16]. Estimates from 2011 suggest CRS is responsible for a cost of $8 billion to the United States health care system annually [17]. The overall cost of CRS on society, however, is likely far greater when quality of life and function are taken into account. Gliklich and Metson measured CRS burden in 158 patients using a validated questionnaire and found the impact of CRS in the domains of societal functioning and bodily pain to be greater than other chronic diseases such as back pain, chronic obstructive pulmonary disease, and angina [18].

18.3 History and Physical Examination

18.3.1 History

Elucidating an accurate diagnosis of CRS can be challenging. Evaluation of the patient with CRS begins with a detailed history and physical examination. This provides the necessary data critical to better classify an individual patient's disease. Primary complaints may include facial pain or discomfort, congestion, nasal airway obstruction, discolored nasal drainage from the nares or into the posterior pharynx, foul smell or taste, hyposmia, lethargy, fatigue, etc. In most cases, patients will describe ≥2 of these symptoms, but in some cases symptoms are absent despite objective evidence of sinus pathology [19]. Co-morbid conditions such as asthma, allergic rhinitis, sensitivity to non-steroidal anti-inflammatory medications, recurrent infections, primary or secondary immune-deficiency, cystic fibrosis, mucociliary dysfunction, etc. serve as important factors that further help in the process of understanding the patient [8].

In many cases, a patient may present with a chief complaint of "chronic sinusitis." Given the lack of specificity of many of the individual symptoms in isolation, care should be taken to ensure correct attribution of the patient's complaints. As an example, a patient may assume facial pain or headache is a manifestation of an underlying sinonasal disorder: the so-called sinus headache. In many cases, such a headache may be caused by temporomandibular joint disorders, vascular headaches, neurogenic headaches, or muscle tension. Likewise, post-nasal drainage from laryngopharyngeal reflux can be confused with primary CRS [8].

A comprehensive physical examination is performed in the course of evaluation of all patients under evaluation for CRS. Emphasis should be placed on any indication of any signs suggestive of suppurative complications of rhinosinusitis or the presence of neoplastic disease. Particular interest should be placed in a comprehensive nasal examination including nasal endoscopy [19].

18.3.2 Nasal Endoscopy

Anterior rhinoscopy, while a standard component of a head and neck examination, is inadequate due to limited visualization of the middle meatus and surrounding structures, and is therefore of limited value for CRS [16].

Nasal endoscopy provides improved visual access to the areas within the nasal cavity, and is used to evaluate the inflammatory status of the sinonasal mucosa. The middle meatus, superior meatus, and nasopharynx are easily accessible for visual inspection, culture, or biopsy when needed. Several studies have demonstrated a correlation between normal endoscopic examination and normal CT scan [20], suggesting that in many clinical scenarios nasal endoscopy can result in more judicious use of CT scans.

18.3.3 Imaging

Although readily available, the utility of plain sinus x-rays compared to that of computed tomography (CT) limits its utility [19].

Magnetic resonance imaging (MRI) scanning is extremely sensitive to soft tissue changes, poorly suited to demonstrate bony anatomy, and costly. Its use is therefore not recommended for the routine evaluation of CRS, and is limited to assessment of neoplasms or invasive soft tissue disease (invasive fungal sinusitis) [19].

Computed tomography has been the modality of choice for evaluation of the paranasal sinuses for the past several decades. This modality offers high resolution, multiplanar imaging of bony structures and soft tissue [19, 21], which provides both an overall assessment of paranasal sinus status (obstruction, bony changes, structural abnormalities, etc.) and an ability to provide semi-quantitative analysis of inflammatory mucosal disease. Several CT staging systems have been described, but the Lund-MacKay system remains validated rating system that is most commonly used and referenced. The Lund-MacKay system relies upon sinus location and degree of opacification: 0 = normal, 1 = partial opacification, 2 = total opacification. These ratings are then applied to separately to the frontal, anterior ethmoid, posterior ethmoid, maxillary, and sphenoid sinuses. The infundibulum is graded as either a score of 0 (no involvement) or 2 (involved). A maximum score of 12 per side can be achieved [22, 23].

Computed tomography correlates poorly with symptoms, a fact that is particularly true when CT scans are obtained prior to assessment and treatment [20]. Therefore, it is not considered as a primary step in the assessment of CRS, except in the case of unilateral findings or suspicion of suppurative complications of rhinosinusitis [16]. Given the potential reversibility of many inflammatory findings on CT, it is common in most cases to perform the study following an appropriate course of medical management in order to differentiate medical from surgical disease [19].

18.4 Phenotypes of CRS

Information collected from a thorough clinical evaluation enables a phenotypic description of CRS (Table 18.2) from which assumptions related to the underlying cause and reasonable treatment options can be made. CRS phenotypes are primarily based upon the presence (CRSwNP) or absence (CRSsNP) of nasal polyposis, which serves as a general surrogate for the type of underlying inflammation [24]. In many cases there is a reasonably high correlation of TH2-mediated eosinophilic (elevated IL-4, IL-5, and IL-13) inflammation with CRSwNP, whereas CRSsNP is more likely to represent non-eosinophilic forms of inflammation [25]. This association of nasal polyps with eosinophilic inflammation, however, is not absolute. Nasal polyps associated with underlying neutrophilic inflammation and high tissue Th17 levels are recognized in Asian countries [26], demonstrating the potential shortcomings of over-reliance upon CRS phenotypes for therapeutic direction.

Further refinement of CRS phenotypes can be accomplished through consideration of other co-morbid conditions within an individual patient [27]. Asthma co-morbidity and CRS recurrence, for example, appear to be predictive of the presence of *Staphylococcus aureus* enterotoxin-specific IgE and high levels of tis-

Table 18.2 Phenotypes of CRS [8]

CRS Phenotypes	CRSsNP		
	CRSwNP		
	Allergic fungal sinusitis		
	CRS with aspirin-exacerbated respiratory disease		
	Infectious CRS		
	CRS with cystic fibrosis		
	Other CRS phenotypes	CRS with immune deficiencies such as common variable immunodeficiency and specific antibody deficiency	
		CRS with immotile cilia syndrome	
		CRS with anatomical abnormalities	
		Biomarker based (endotypes)	Eosinophilic CRS vs non-eosinophilic CRS
			Allergic CRS vs non-allergic CRS
			Type 2 high vs Type 2 low
			High IgE vs normal IgE

sue IL-5. Another example of this type of refinement is the co-existence of aspirin-exacerbated respiratory disease (AERD) and CRS, which is highly associated with underlying tissue eosinophilia [28]. A variety of laboratory assessments can provide additional information helpful in the process of phenotyping CRS. In vivo and in vitro IgE tests, aspirin challenge, immunologic evaluation, and tissue biopsy may be indicated in selected cases [8].

Tomassen et al. acknowledging that reliance upon clinically determined phenotypes may not adequately reflect the pathophysiologic diversity of the disease, performed a multicenter, case-control study of CRS. 173 patients undergoing surgery had tissue analyzed for IL-5, IFN-gamma, IL-17A, TNF-alpha, IL-22, IL-1beta, IL-6, IL-8, eosinophilic cationic protein (ECP), myeloperoxidase, TGF-beta1, IgE, *Staphylococcus aureus* enterotoxin-specific IgE, and albumin. Partition-based clustering revealed 10 clusters. Six of these clusters demonstrated high levels of IL-5, ECP, and albumin, while the remaining four had low or undetectable levels of the same markers. Three of the four IL-5-negative clusters were phenotypically classified as CRSsNP without asthma, while remaining cluster demonstrated a TH17 inflammatory profile and had a mixed CRScNP/CRSsNP phenotype. Those IL-5 positive clusters could be phenotypically stratified based upon IL-5 levels. High levels of tissue IL-5 were associated with CRSwNP and greatly increased prevalence of asthma. Moderate levels of IL-5 demonstrated a mixed CRScNP/CRSsNP phenotype and some increase in asthma prevalence. Of note, the two clusters with the highest IL-5 concentrations also expressed *Staphylococcus aureus* enterotoxin-specific IgE. The overall conclusion was that while phenotypes were largely correlated with specific inflammatory patterns, it was the discreet inflammatory patterns within each cluster that provided a more accurate description of the disease, supporting the concept of targeted therapy within CRS endotypes [13, 29] (see Chap. 20).

18.5 CRS Without Nasal Polyposis (CRSsNP)

CRS is divided into two phenotypes based upon the presence or absence of polyps on examination, as supported by histologic and inflammatory cytokine findings [3, 29]. Use of nasal polyps as a clinical surrogate for the inflammatory response underlying the disease is supported reasonably well when applied to populations within the Western hemisphere. This clinical categorization of CRS is also supported by differences in treatment responses and recurrence rates [30]. CRSsNP enjoys lower recurrence rates and better response to standard therapies than CRSwNP. Because of the overlap of many of the symptoms of CRSsNP and other common maladies (e.g. headache, allergic rhinitis, rhinitis medicamentosa, etc.), it can be difficult to differentiate from other diseases. Appropriate use of nasal endoscopy, allergy evaluation, and radiologic examination are employed to ensure an appropriate diagnosis [20, 31].

18.6 CRS with Nasal Polyposis (CRSwNP)

The etiology and underlying pathogenesis of CRSwNP remain controversial. Initial hypotheses broadly focused upon either the role of exogenous factors or that of the host response to the environment as potential explanations for CRSwNP with and without polyps.

18.7 Exogenous Factors in CRSwNP

Allergens, viruses, fungi, bacterial biofilms, and *Staphylococcus aureus* endotoxins have been suggested as such potential exogenous factors are capable of initiating inflammation within the respiratory epithelium in affected individuals. While some objective evidence supports a potential role for each of these as a contributor to the pathogenesis of CRS, no single "pathogen" has proven to be universally causative.

18.7.1 Fungus

The "fungal hypothesis of CRS" is perhaps the best example of the frailty that underlies the concept of external pathogens serving a sole causative role in CRS. A group of researchers during the late 1990s made use of sensitive detection techniques to identify the presence of fungi within the nose in almost 100% of patients with CRS and controls. Those patients with CRS, however, differed from controls by demonstrating eosinophilic inflammation within the nasal epithelium and absence of corresponding systemic IgE-mediated sensitivity to fungi [32]. Subsequent ex-vivo studies showed that peripheral blood monocytes from patients with CRS elicited high levels of IL-5 in response to exposure to *Alternaria alternata* extract [33]. This was interpreted as a unique, non-IgE mediated immune response to *Alternaria alternata* suggesting a potential universal cause for CRS [34]. Initial enthusiasm for this proposed explanation for CRS began to wane when results could not be duplicated at other institutions [35]. In the end, a large multi-institutional, blinded, randomized, controlled trial using intranasal amphotericin failed to show any evidence of efficacy.

18.7.2 Bacteria and the Microbiome

Bacteria have long been speculated to contribute to the development of CRS. Cultures obtained from the nasal vestibule yield several bacterial species, out of which Staphylococcus sp. and Corynebacterium constitute the majority [36]. Active bacterial antagonism along the nasal mucosa, otherwise known as "bacterial interference," contributes to the complexity of the nasal microbiome [37, 38]. As an example of this phenomenon, *S. epidermidis* appears to compete at the mucosal surface with S. *aureus* [39]. Commensal bacteria colonizing the sinonasal mucosa may serve to both interfere with growth of bacterial pathogens, while also modulating the host innate immune response [40]. So, while the role of bacteria in initiating CRS remains unclear, it appears that the presence and interaction of bacteria along the surface of the mucosa possess the ability to impact disease.

18.7.3 *Staphylococcus aureus* Enterotoxin

Staphylococcus aureus warrants some unique consideration as a disease modifier in CRS. *S aureus* has been observed at higher rates in CRS when compared to controls [41], but rather than focusing upon its role a pathogen, researchers have studied its potential to interact in concert with local innate and specific immune mechanisms to contribute to the recruitment of a Type 2 inflammatory response (e.g. mediated by IL-4, IL-5, and IL-13). Evidence supportive of this concept is provided by studies demonstrating concordance between nasal polyposis and the presence of *S. aureus* [42, 43]. More importantly, enterotoxin produced by *S. aureus* has been isolated within polyp homogenates, but not from tissue obtained patients with CRSsNP [44]. These enterotoxins possess the ability to upregulate polyclonal production of local IgE independent of the normally required antigen [45]. The "Superantigen Hypothesis" proposes that Staphylococcal aureus enterotoxin produced locally serves to amplify local eosinophilic responses, thereby acting as a disease modifier in the development of nasal polyps [46].

18.7.4 Biofilms

Biofilms, existing as a protective bacterial adaptation against host defenses and antibiotics, have been observed in CRS and associated with poorer outcomes following surgery [47]. This argues a potential role in perpetuation of disease in some cases, but no clear evidence exists proving that the presence of biofilms contributes to the initiation of, or causes, CRS [48].

18.7.5 Host Factors in CRSwNP

Fungi, commensal bacteria and pathogens, bacterial biofilms, and *S. aureus* are present in a large percentage of the population, yet the reason why polyps develop in some patients and not in others remain unknown. Recent studies have demonstrated significant differences in inflammatory patterns amongst separate populations suffering from CRSwNP. Histological examination of respiratory epithelium from American or European patients with CRSwNP demonstrates both high levels of eosinophils and type 2 cytokines (e.g. IL-4, IL-5, IL-13) [49]. Chinese patients with CRSwNP, however, are more likely to express a neutrophilic inflammatory response, demonstrating that hosts responses may be influenced by genetic factors [50]. Further study of the Chinese population since 2006 has demonstrated a significant shift toward an increase in the proportion of this population expressing eosinophilic polyps [26]. The precise reason for this increase in eosinophilic inflammation is not yet known, but this shift appears to temporally coincide with an era of increased "westernization" of Asia and may represent indirect evidence that environmental factors may impact the host response.

18.7.6 Immune Barrier Function

The "immune barrier hypothesis" proposed that defects in the barrier function of the respiratory epithelium have been implicated in pathogenesis of CRSwNP [16]. Increasing evidence, however, suggests innate interactions between the host and its environment may play a critical part in the initiation of mucosal inflammation. The potential for an exogenous trigger of inflammation to interact with a host occurs at an epithelial surface, which functions as an innate immune barrier through a combination of mucociliary clearance, innate local immunity, and epithelial-derived inflammatory responses [51]. Epithelial cells have the ability to interact with surface microbes leading to the release of IL-25, IL-33 and thymic stromal lymphopoietin. Innate lymphoid cells (ILC2) activate and recruit T- and B-lymphocytes, as well as producing local type 2 cytokines [27]. Type-2 cytokines (i.e. IL-4, IL-5, IL-13, etc.), specifically IL-4, and IFN-γ have further been implicated in attenuation of tight junctions between epithelial cells [52]. Additionally, mucus production is increased in the presence of IL-4 and IL-13, and serves to decrease mucociliary function [53].

18.7.7 Eicosanoid Hypothesis

Eicosanoids are signaling molecules generated through the metabolism of arachidonic acid present within the cell membranes of a wide range of cells. This class of inflammatory mediators has immunologic properties critical to local regulation of inflammation [49]. Several families of eicosanoids with differing properties exist. Leukotrienes exhibit pro-inflammatory properties and are generated by lipoxygenase (5-LO). Prostaglandins and prostacyclins, both generally anti-inflammatory in function, are generated by the cyclooxygenase enzyme (Cox-1, Cox-2). Defects within the eicosanoid pathway are associated with aspirin intolerance, asthma, and CRSwNP [54]. Alterations in this pathway have been identified specifically within the CRSwNP population, specifically noting an up-regulation of the leukotriene pathway and a down-regulation of the prostaglandin pathway. Some evidence suggests feedback loop interplay between the presence of *S. aureus* enterotoxin B (SEB) and prostaglandin E2 (PGE2), whereby SEB can regulate PGE2 synthesis, while PGE2 has the ability to suppress SEB-induced eosinophilia [55, 56]. The impact of *S. aureus* colonization upon the pro-inflammatory environment that occurs in the setting of defects in the eicosanoid pathway has been suggested as central to the etiology of nasal polyposis [49].

18.8 Comprehensive Overview of CRSwNP

A single comprehensive theory addressing the etiology and pathogenesis remains unclear, and in many cases individually proposed lines of research may appear to compete or conflict with one another. This leaves us to ask the question, which hypothesis is correct? The answer may be both "neither and all."

Chronic rhinosinusitis with nasal polyps (CRSwNP) among western populations is generally characterized by type 2 inflammation (e.g. mediated by IL-4, IL-5, and IL-13) and manifests as eosinophilic mucosal infiltration [49]. The phenotypic expression of CRSwNP results from the recruitment of several immunological processes occurring in concert with one another, ultimately contributing to the onset and the perpetuation of tissue changes and leading to polyp formation [57]. The role of the airway epithelium and its interaction with surface antigens, bacteria environmental toxins, and viruses may lead to: (1) increased epithelial permeability though loosening of tight junctions [52], (2) activation of epithelial cells leading to production of epithelial-derived cytokines (i.e. TSLP, IL-25, IL-33) [58], (3) recruitment of Th2 and ILC2 cells [59], and (4) direct production of prostaglandins (PGE2) [56], especially in patients with AERD. Epithelial activation and the downstream immunologic response may be further modified by the presence of *S. aureus* enterotoxin leading to polyclonal expansion of local IgE, amplification of the type 2 response, and impairment of regulatory T-cells [60].

18.9 Summary

As more light is shed upon the many differing triggers, modifiers, and common inflammatory mediators that contribute to ultimate phenotypic expression of CRS with or without polyposis, targets for more specific therapeutic interventions become apparent.

References

1. Meltzer EO, Hamilos DL, Hadley JA, Lanza DC, Marple BF, Nicklas RA, et al. Rhinosinusitis: developing guidance for clinical trials. J Allergy Clin Immunol. 2006;118:S17–61. https://doi.org/10.1016/j.jaci.2006.09.005.
2. Benninger MS, Ferguson BJ, Hadley JA, Hamilos DL, Jacobs M, Kennedy DW, et al. Adult chronic rhinosinusitis: definitions, diagnosis, epidemiology, and pathophysiology. Otolaryngol Head Neck Surg. 2003;129:S1–32. https://doi.org/10.1016/s0194-5998(03)01397-4.
3. Meltzer EO, Hamilos DL, Hadley JA, Lanza DC, Marple BF, Nicklas RA, et al. Rhinosinusitis: establishing definitions for clinical research and patient care. Otolaryngol Head Neck Surg. 2004;114:155–212. https://doi.org/10.1016/j.jaci.2004.09.029.
4. Hamilos DL, Leung DY, Wood R, Cunningham L, Bean DK, Yasruel Z, et al. Evidence for distinct cytokine expression in allergic versus nonallergic chronic sinusitis. J Allergy Clin Immunol. 1995;96(4):537–44. https://doi.org/10.1016/s0091-6749(95)70298-9.
5. Kern RC, Conley DB, Walsh W, Chandra R, Kato A, Tripathi-Peters A, et al. Perspectives on the etiology of chronic rhinosinusitis: an immune barrier hypothesis. Am J Rhinol. 2008;22(6):549–59. https://doi.org/10.2500/ajr.2008.22.3228.
6. Fokkens WJ, Lund VJ, Mullol J, Bachert C, Alobid I, Baroody F, et al. EPOS 2012: European position paper on rhinosinusitis and nasal polyps 2012. A summary for otorhinolaryngologists. Rhinology. 2012;50(1):1–12. https://doi.org/10.4193/Rhino50E2.
7. Meltzer EOHD, Hadley JA, et al. Rhinosinusitis: developing guidance for clinical trials. J Allergy Clin Immunol Pract. 2006;118:S17–61.
8. Cho SH, Bachert C, Lockey RF. Chronic rhinosinusitis phenotypes: an approach to better medical care for chronic rhinosinusitis. J Allergy Clin Immunol Pract. 2016;4(4):639–42. https://doi.org/10.1016/j.jaip.2016.05.007.
9. Smith TL, Kern RC, Palmer JN, Schlosser RJ, Chandra RK, Chiu AG, et al. Medical therapy vs surgery for chronic rhinosinusitis: a prospective, multi-institutional study. Int Forum Allergy Rhinol. 2011;1(4):235–41. https://doi.org/10.1002/alr.20063.
10. Smith TL, Kern R, Palmer JN, Schlosser R, Chandra RK, Chiu AG, et al. Medical therapy vs surgery for chronic rhinosinusitis: a prospective, multi-institutional study with 1-year follow-up. Int Forum Allergy Rhinol. 2013;3(1):4–9. https://doi.org/10.1002/alr.21065.
11. Smith KA, Smith TL, Mace JC, Rudmik L. Endoscopic sinus surgery compared to continued medical therapy for patients with refractory chronic rhinosinusitis. Int Forum Allergy Rhinol. 2014;4(10):823–7. https://doi.org/10.1002/alr.21366.
12. Soler ZM, Hyer JM, Rudmik L, Ramakrishnan V, Smith TL, Schlosser RJ. Cluster analysis and predic-

tion of treatment outcomes for chronic rhinosinusitis. J Allergy Clin Immunol. 2016;137(4):1054–62. https://doi.org/10.1016/j.jaci.2015.11.019.
13. Tomassen P, Vandeplas G, Van Zele T, Cardell LO, Arebro J, Olze H, et al. Inflammatory endotypes of chronic rhinosinusitis based on cluster analysis of biomarkers. J Allergy Clin Immunol. 2016;137(5):1449–56.e4. https://doi.org/10.1016/j.jaci.2015.12.1324.
14. Hastan D, Fokkens WJ, Bachert C, Newson RB, Bislimovska J, Bockelbrink A, et al. Chronic rhinosinusitis in Europe – an underestimated disease. A GA²LEN study. Allergy. 2011;66(9):1216–23. https://doi.org/10.1111/j.1398-9995.2011.02646.x.
15. Shi JB, Fu QL, Zhang H, Cheng L, Wang YJ, Zhu DD, et al. Epidemiology of chronic rhinosinusitis: results from a cross-sectional survey in seven Chinese cities. Allergy. 2015;70(5):533–9. https://doi.org/10.1111/all.12577.
16. Fokkens WJ, Lund VJ, Mullol J, Bachert C, Alobid I, Baroody F, et al. European position paper on rhinosinusitis and nasal polyps 2012. Rhinol Suppl. 2012;23:3 p preceding table of contents, 1–298.
17. DeMarcantonio MA, Han JK. Nasal polyps: pathogenesis and treatment implications. Otolaryngol Clin N Am. 2011;44(3):685–95., ix. https://doi.org/10.1016/j.otc.2011.03.005.
18. Gliklich RE, Metson R. The health impact of chronic sinusitis in patients seeking otolaryngologic care. Otolaryngol Head Neck Surg. 1995;113(1):104–9. https://doi.org/10.1016/s0194-5998(95)70152-4.
19. Marple BF, Stankiewicz JA, Baroody FM, Chow JM, Conley DB, Corey JP, et al. Diagnosis and management of chronic rhinosinusitis in adults. Postgrad Med. 2009;121(6):121–39. https://doi.org/10.3810/pgm.2009.11.2081.
20. Stankiewicz JA, Chow JM. Nasal endoscopy and the definition and diagnosis of chronic rhinosinusitis. Otolaryngol Head Neck Surg. 2002;126(6):623–7. https://doi.org/10.1067/mhn.2002.125602.
21. Rosenfeld RM, Andes D, Bhattacharyya N, Cheung D, Eisenberg S, Ganiats TG, et al. Clinical practice guideline: adult sinusitis. Otolaryngol Head Neck Surg. 2007;137(3 Suppl):S1–31. https://doi.org/10.1016/j.otohns.2007.06.726.
22. Lund VJ, Mackay IS. Staging in rhinosinusitis. Rhinology. 1993;31(4):183–4.
23. Metson R, Gliklich RE, Stankiewicz JA, Kennedy DW, Duncavage JA, Hoffman SR, et al. Comparison of sinus computed tomography staging systems. Otolaryngol Head Neck Surg. 1997;117(4):372–9. https://doi.org/10.1016/s0194-5998(97)70129-3.
24. Bayar Muluk N, Cingi C, Scadding GK, Scadding G. Chronic rhinosinusitis-could phenotyping or endotyping aid therapy? Am J Rhinol Allergy. 2019;33(1):83–93. https://doi.org/10.1177/1945892418807590.
25. Wang X, Zhang N, Bo M, Holtappels G, Zheng M, Lou H, et al. Diversity of T(H) cytokine profiles in patients with chronic rhinosinusitis: a multicenter study in Europe, Asia, and Oceania. J Allergy Clin Immunol. 2016;138(5):1344–53. https://doi.org/10.1016/j.jaci.2016.05.041.
26. Zhang Y, Gevaert E, Lou H, Wang X, Zhang L, Bachert C, et al. Chronic rhinosinusitis in Asia. J Allergy Clin Immunol. 2017;140(5):1230–9. https://doi.org/10.1016/j.jaci.2017.09.009.
27. Bachert C, Akdis CA. Phenotypes and emerging endotypes of chronic rhinosinusitis. J Allergy Clin Immunol Pract. 2016;4(4):621–8. https://doi.org/10.1016/j.jaip.2016.05.004.
28. Dennis SK, Lam K, Luong A. A review of classification schemes for chronic rhinosinusitis with nasal polyposis endotypes. Laryngoscope Investig Otolaryngol. 2016;1(5):130–4. https://doi.org/10.1002/lio2.32.
29. Malekzadeh S, Hamburger MD, Whelan PJ, Biedlingmaier JF, Baraniuk JN. Density of middle turbinate subepithelial mucous glands in patients with chronic rhinosinusitis. Otolaryngol Head Neck Surg. 2002;127(3):190–5. https://doi.org/10.1067/mhn.2002.126800.
30. Kennedy DW, Wright ED, Goldberg AN. Objective and subjective outcomes in surgery for chronic sinusitis. Laryngoscope. 2000;110(3 Pt 3):29–31. https://doi.org/10.1097/00005537-200003002-00008.
31. Bhattacharyya N. Clinical and symptom criteria for the accurate diagnosis of chronic rhinosinusitis. Laryngoscope. 2006;116(7 Pt 2 Suppl 110):1–22. https://doi.org/10.1097/01.mlg.0000224508.59725.19.
32. Ponikau JU, Sherris DA, Kern EB, Homburger HA, Frigas E, Gaffey TA, et al. The diagnosis and incidence of allergic fungal sinusitis. Mayo Clin Proc. 1999;74(9):877–84. https://doi.org/10.4065/74.9.877.
33. Shin SH, Ponikau JU, Sherris DA, Congdon D, Frigas E, Homburger HA, et al. Chronic rhinosinusitis: an enhanced immune response to ubiquitous airborne fungi. J Allergy Clin Immunol. 2004;114(6):1369–75. https://doi.org/10.1016/j.jaci.2004.08.012.
34. Sasama J, Sherris DA, Shin SH, Kephart GM, Kern EB, Ponikau JU. New paradigm for the roles of fungi and eosinophils in chronic rhinosinusitis. Curr Opin Otolaryngol Head Neck Surg. 2005;13(1):2–8. https://doi.org/10.1097/00020840-200502000-00003.
35. Orlandi RR, Marple BF. Fungus and chronic rhinosinusitis: weighing the evidence. Otolaryngol Head Neck Surg. 2010;143(5):611–3. https://doi.org/10.1016/j.otohns.2010.07.002.
36. Hilty M, Burke C, Pedro H, Cardenas P, Bush A, Bossley C, et al. Disordered microbial communities in asthmatic airways. PLoS One. 2010;5(1):e8578. https://doi.org/10.1371/journal.pone.0008578.
37. Lemon KP, Klepac-Ceraj V, Schiffer HK, Brodie EL, Lynch SV, Kolter R. Comparative analyses of the bacterial microbiota of the human nostril and oropharynx. mBio. 2010;1(3). https://doi.org/10.1128/mBio.00129-10.
38. Benninger M, Brook I, Bernstein JM, Casey JR, Roos K, Marple B, et al. Bacterial interference in upper respiratory tract infections: a systematic review.

Am J Rhinol Allergy. 2011;25(2):82–8. https://doi.org/10.2500/ajra.2011.25.3594.
39. Frank DN, Feazel LM, Bessesen MT, Price CS, Janoff EN, Pace NR. The human nasal microbiota and *Staphylococcus aureus* carriage. PLoS One. 2010;5(5):e10598. https://doi.org/10.1371/journal.pone.0010598.
40. Cernadas M. It takes a microbiome: commensals, immune regulation, and allergy. Am J Respir Crit Care Med. 2011;184(2):149–50. https://doi.org/10.1164/rccm.201105-0828ED.
41. Larson DA, Han JK. Microbiology of sinusitis: does allergy or endoscopic sinus surgery affect the microbiologic flora? Curr Opin Otolaryngol Head Neck Surg. 2011;19(3):199–203. https://doi.org/10.1097/MOO.0b013e328344f67a.
42. Van Zele T, Gevaert P, Watelet JB, Claeys G, Holtappels G, Claeys C, et al. *Staphylococcus aureus* colonization and IgE antibody formation to enterotoxins is increased in nasal polyposis. J Allergy Clin Immunol. 2004;114(4):981–3. https://doi.org/10.1016/j.jaci.2004.07.013.
43. Ramakrishnan VR, Feazel LM, Abrass LJ, Frank DN. Prevalence and abundance of *Staphylococcus aureus* in the middle meatus of patients with chronic rhinosinusitis, nasal polyps, and asthma. Int Forum Allergy Rhinol. 2013;3(4):267–71. https://doi.org/10.1002/alr.21101.
44. Seiberling KA, Conley DB, Tripathi A, Grammer LC, Shuh L, Haines GK III, et al. Superantigens and chronic rhinosinusitis: detection of staphylococcal exotoxins in nasal polyps. Laryngoscope. 2005;115(9):1580–5. https://doi.org/10.1097/01.mlg.0000168111.11802.9c.
45. Seiberling KA, Grammer L, Kern RC. Chronic rhinosinusitis and superantigens. Otolaryngol Clin N Am. 2005;38(6):1215–36., ix. https://doi.org/10.1016/j.otc.2005.08.006.
46. Bachert C, Gevaert P, Holtappels G, Johansson SG, van Cauwenberge P. Total and specific IgE in nasal polyps is related to local eosinophilic inflammation. J Allergy Clin Immunol. 2001;107(4):607–14. https://doi.org/10.1067/mai.2001.112374.
47. Psaltis AJ, Weitzel EK, Ha KR, Wormald PJ. The effect of bacterial biofilms on post-sinus surgical outcomes. Am J Rhinol. 2008;22(1):1–6. https://doi.org/10.2500/ajr.2008.22.3119.
48. Foreman A, Jervis-Bardy J, Wormald PJ. Do biofilms contribute to the initiation and recalcitrance of chronic rhinosinusitis? Laryngoscope. 2011;121(5):1085–91. https://doi.org/10.1002/lary.21438.
49. Van Crombruggen K, Zhang N, Gevaert P, Tomassen P, Bachert C. Pathogenesis of chronic rhinosinusitis: inflammation. J Allergy Clin Immunol. 2011;128(4):728–32. https://doi.org/10.1016/j.jaci.2011.07.049.
50. Zhang N, Holtappels G, Claeys C, Huang G, van Cauwenberge P, Bachert C. Pattern of inflammation and impact of *Staphylococcus aureus* enterotoxins in nasal polyps from southern China. Am J Rhinol. 2006;20(4):445–50. https://doi.org/10.2500/ajr.2006.20.2887.
51. Tam A, Wadsworth S, Dorscheid D, Man SF, Sin DD. The airway epithelium: more than just a structural barrier. Ther Adv Respir Dis. 2011;5(4):255–73. https://doi.org/10.1177/1753465810396539.
52. Soyka MB, Wawrzyniak P, Eiwegger T, Holzmann D, Treis A, Wanke K, et al. Defective epithelial barrier in chronic rhinosinusitis: the regulation of tight junctions by IFN-γ and IL-4. J Allergy Clin Immunol. 2012;130(5):1087–96.e10. https://doi.org/10.1016/j.jaci.2012.05.052.
53. Seshadri S, Lu X, Purkey MR, Homma T, Choi AW, Carter R, et al. Increased expression of the epithelial anion transporter pendrin/SLC26A4 in nasal polyps of patients with chronic rhinosinusitis. J Allergy Clin Immunol. 2015;136(6):1548–58.e7. https://doi.org/10.1016/j.jaci.2015.05.024.
54. Roca-Ferrer J, Garcia-Garcia FJ, Pereda J, Perez-Gonzalez M, Pujols L, Alobid I, et al. Reduced expression of COXs and production of prostaglandin E(2) in patients with nasal polyps with or without aspirin-intolerant asthma. J Allergy Clin Immunol. 2011;128(1):66–72.e1. https://doi.org/10.1016/j.jaci.2011.01.065.
55. Pérez-Novo CA, Waeytens A, Claeys C, Cauwenberge PV, Bachert C. *Staphylococcus aureus* enterotoxin B regulates prostaglandin E2 synthesis, growth, and migration in nasal tissue fibroblasts. J Infect Dis. 2008;197(7):1036–43. https://doi.org/10.1086/528989.
56. Okano M, Fujiwara T, Haruna T, Kariya S, Makihara S, Higaki T, et al. Prostaglandin E(2) suppresses staphylococcal enterotoxin-induced eosinophilia-associated cellular responses dominantly through an E-prostanoid 2-mediated pathway in nasal polyps. J Allergy Clin Immunol. 2009;123(4):868–74.e13. https://doi.org/10.1016/j.jaci.2009.01.047.
57. Heffler E, Malvezzi L, Boita M, Brussino L, De Virgilio A, Ferrando M, et al. Immunological mechanisms underlying chronic rhinosinusitis with nasal polyps. Expert Rev Clin Immunol. 2018;14(9):731–7. https://doi.org/10.1080/1744666x.2018.1512407.
58. Mitchell PD, O'Byrne PM. Biologics and the lung: TSLP and other epithelial cell-derived cytokines in asthma. Pharmacol Ther. 2017;169:104–12. https://doi.org/10.1016/j.pharmthera.2016.06.009.
59. Ho J, Bailey M, Zaunders J, Mrad N, Sacks R, Sewell W, et al. Group 2 innate lymphoid cells (ILC2s) are increased in chronic rhinosinusitis with nasal polyps or eosinophilia. Clin Exp Allergy. 2015;45(2):394–403. https://doi.org/10.1111/cea.12462.
60. Patou J, Gevaert P, Van Zele T, Holtappels G, van Cauwenberge P, Bachert C. *Staphylococcus aureus* enterotoxin B, protein A, and lipoteichoic acid stimulations in nasal polyps. J Allergy Clin Immunol. 2008;121(1):110–5. https://doi.org/10.1016/j.jaci.2007.08.059.

Allergic Fungal Sinusitis

19

Fenghong Chen, Matthew W. Ryan, and Bradley F. Marple

Key Points

- Allergic fungal sinusitis is a distinct phenotype of eosinophilic chronic rhinosinusitis with nasal polyposis.
- Unlike other forms of CRS with polyps, AFS has the potential to cause facial disfigurement and orbital complications such as diplopia and vision loss.
- Allergy, fungal hypersensitivity, and *Staphylococcus aureus* colonization are implicated in the pathogenesis of the disease.
- Current medical and surgical treatments for AFS are similar to that employed for other forms of type 2 CRS with polyps.
- New targeted molecular therapies (Biologics) should be specifically evaluated in the treatment of AFS.

F. Chen
Otorhinolaryngology Hospital, First Affiliated Hospital, Sun Yat-sen University, Guangzhou, Guangdong, China

M. W. Ryan (✉)
Department of Otolaryngology, The University of Texas Southwestern Medical Center, Dallas, TX, USA
e-mail: Matthew.Ryan@utsouthwestern.edu

B. F. Marple
Department of Otolaryngology, Head and Neck Surgery, University of Texas, Southwestern Medical Center, Dallas, TX, USA
e-mail: bradley.marple@utsouthwestern.edu

19.1 Introduction

Allergic fungal sinusitis is a distinct phenotype of chronic rhinosinusitis (CRS) with nasal polyposis that was first described in the 1980s. Since its description AFS has garnered considerable interest because of its tendency to recur and be difficult to control, patients may suffer facial deformity or orbital complications, and the precise pathophysiology of the condition remains elusive.

Allergic fungal sinusitis (AFS) was first recognized by pathologists who noted that sinus contents in these patients resemble that seen in the bronchial passages of patients with allergic bronchopulmonary aspergillosis (ABPA) [1–3]. The "Allergic mucin" (now more appropriately termed "eosinophilic mucin") containing clumps and clusters of eosinophils and non-invasive fungal hyphae that accumulates in patients' sinuses was once considered to be pathognomonic for the disease. However, many cases of CRS with polyps are associated with eosinophilic mucin accumulation [4, 5], and some cases with eosinophilic mucin without detectable fungus have different clinical features [6]. On the other hand, with sophisticated sampling and detection techniques, almost all CRS cases can be associated with the presence of fungus [7]. Therefore, the utility of relying on solely on detection of fungus or identification of eosinophilic mucin to differentiate AFS is limited.

L. Zhang, C. Bachert (eds.), *Chronic Rhinosinusitis*, https://doi.org/10.1007/978-981-16-0784-4_19

19.2 Pathophysiology

A hypersensitivity to fungus is believed to underlie the pathogenesis of AFS, but the nature of this hypersensitivity is unclear. Both "allergic" and "non-allergic" fungal hypersensitivity may be important components of the underlying pathophysiology of AFS. It appears that AFS develops in susceptible patients with a convergence of local anatomic as well as environmental factors [8]. The inflammatory response is usually limited to particular sinuses and may be unilateral. This inflammation induces polyp formation and the accumulation of eosinophilic mucin. Trapped fungi and other co-pathogens continue to stimulate the immune system in a vicious cycle. Over time, polyposis develops and fungal mucoceles distort the sinonasal anatomy.

For many years, the pathogenesis of AFS was assumed to be the same as ABPA [8]: a combination of Gell and Coombs Type 1 and Type 3 hypersensitivity to fungal allergens causes inflammation [9]. And indeed, AFS was clearly associated with allergy and the detection of elevated serum levels of total and fungal antigen-specific IgE and IgG [10, 11]. Most patients with AFS also have detectable fungal-specific IgE in their allergic mucin [12, 13]. Elevated levels of fungal-specific IgG3 are a consistent finding in patients with AFS and AFS-like disease [13]. Type 1 hypersensitivity to fungal antigens thus helps to distinguish AFS from other forms of CRS with polyps and eosinophilic mucin. Additionally, total serum IgE levels are often markedly elevated in AFS. One hypothesis is that *Staphylococcus aureus* is a microbiologic co-factor in the disease and high IgE levels are related to *Staphylococcus aureus* superantigens [14].

Allergy is clearly not the only cause of AFS, and other immunologic mechanisms, anatomic, and physical factors are required in explaining the clinical observations in AFS [8].

19.3 Epidemiology and Microbiology

Allergic fungal sinusitis is a common subtype of CRS with polyps in particular regions of the world. Perhaps because climate determines exposure to fungi, the highest incidence in the USA is in the southern states and along the Mississippi basin [15]. The disease has a worldwide distribution, though certain regions such as the middle east and India appear to have a high prevalence. AFS typically develops in young adults and adolescents [8] with a history of atopy [16, 17]. However, the prevalence of co-morbid asthma appears to be lower than other CRS with polyps [18]. By definition, AFS patients have allergy that should be evident by skin or in vitro testing.

Aspergillus species were once deemed to be the causative pathogen in this disease, but further experience with cases in the USA showed that the dematiaceous fungi were most commonly found in AFS mucus [16, 19], The terminology for this condition subsequently changed from "allergic *Aspergillus* sinusitis" to "allergic fungal sinusitis." In series of AFS from other parts of the world, *Aspergillus* is still found to be a common isolate [20–22]. However, the specific fungal organism does not appear to be clinically important. Nevertheless, the identification of fungus in eosinophilic mucin either via histopathology or culture is still considered to be important to make the diagnosis of AFS.

19.4 Clinical Presentation

Symptoms of AFS are usually insidious in onset and the symptom burden is often disproportionately mild compared to the extent of disease. Common signs and symptoms include nasal obstruction, hyposmia, headaches, thick dark sinus drainage, visual disturbance, or facial dysmorphia. Symptoms are frequently unilateral. Proptosis or telecanthus is not infrequently seen at presentation, especially in younger patients [8, 20, 23, 24]. Disease is often well advanced before a diagnosis is made.

The physical exam findings in AFS often reflect the advanced nature of disease at presentation. Proptosis/exophthalmos or other globe displacement is common. Intranasal examination will reveal bulky polyps that are asymmetric, often involving the more patent nasal cavity with an associated deviated septum. With nasal endoscopy dense yellow to brown mucus may be visualized among the polyps.

Testing is important to establish evidence of atopy, as demonstration of Type 1 hypersensitivity is required for diagnosis. This may be accomplished with skin testing or in vitro testing for antigen-specific IgE. Possible laboratory abnormalities in AFS patients include peripheral eosinophilia and markedly elevated total serum IgE levels. Skin testing or in vitro testing will usually demonstrate IgE-mediated hypersensitivity to multiple fungal and non-fungal antigens [8].

19.5 Diagnostic Criteria

The diagnosis of AFS requires a combination of clinical, radiographic, microbiologic, and histopathologic information. Therefore, the diagnosis of AFS requires surgical specimens, sinus imaging, and allergy testing. The classic and still widely accepted diagnostic criteria for AFS were described by Bent and Kuhn, who proposed the following: type 1 hypersensitivity; nasal polyposis; characteristic CT scan findings; eosinophilic mucus without fungal invasion into sinus tissue; and a positive fungal stain of sinus contents removed at surgery [25]. However, it has become clear that the only truly distinct features of the diagnostic criteria for AFS (i.e. not shared with other CRS with polyps) are Type 1 hypersensitivity and characteristic imaging findings [26].

19.5.1 Eosinophilic Mucin

Grossly, eosinophilic mucin is thick, tenacious, and darkly colored (Fig. 19.1). Microscopically, eosinophilic mucin consists of clusters and laminations of necrotic and degranulating eosinophils in a background of mucin with occasional Charcot–Leyden crystals (Fig. 19.2). Fungal hyphae are present in variable abundance, and special fungal stains may be needed for identification (Fig. 19.3). Adjacent mucosa and polyps demonstrate a prominent eosinophilic inflammatory infiltrate.

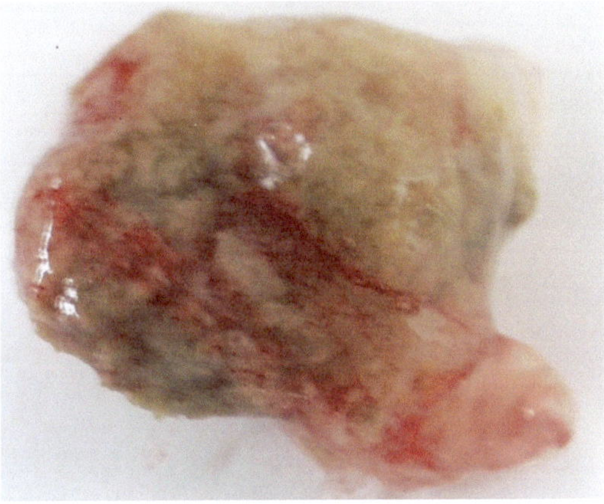

Fig. 19.1 Gross photo of eosinophilic mucin

19.6 Radiologic Features

AFS has characteristic features on computed tomography (CT) or magnetic resonance (MR) imaging. CT imaging shows multiple opacified sinuses with central hyperattenuation, sinus mucocele formation, and erosion of the lamina papyracea or skull base with a pushing border (Figs. 19.4 and 19.5) in a pattern that is rarely seen with other forms for CRS with polyps [21, 23, 27].

Magnetic resonance imaging is not usually clinically necessary, but may be employed in children to limit radiation exposure or in cases with central nervous system or orbital complications. On MR imaging, the sinuses have a central isointense or low signal on T1 and low signal on T2 imaging, corresponding to areas of eosinophilic mucin, with peripheral high signal intensity corresponding to inflamed mucosa [28–30].

19.7 Treatment

Treatment for AFS aims to prevent complications from sinus expansion (such as facial dysmorphia, diplopia, and vision loss) and reduce patient symptom burden. This is an important difference compared to other forms of CRS with polyps: AFS has the potential to cause permanent vision loss. Successful treatment of AFS usually requires a combination of surgery and medical therapy

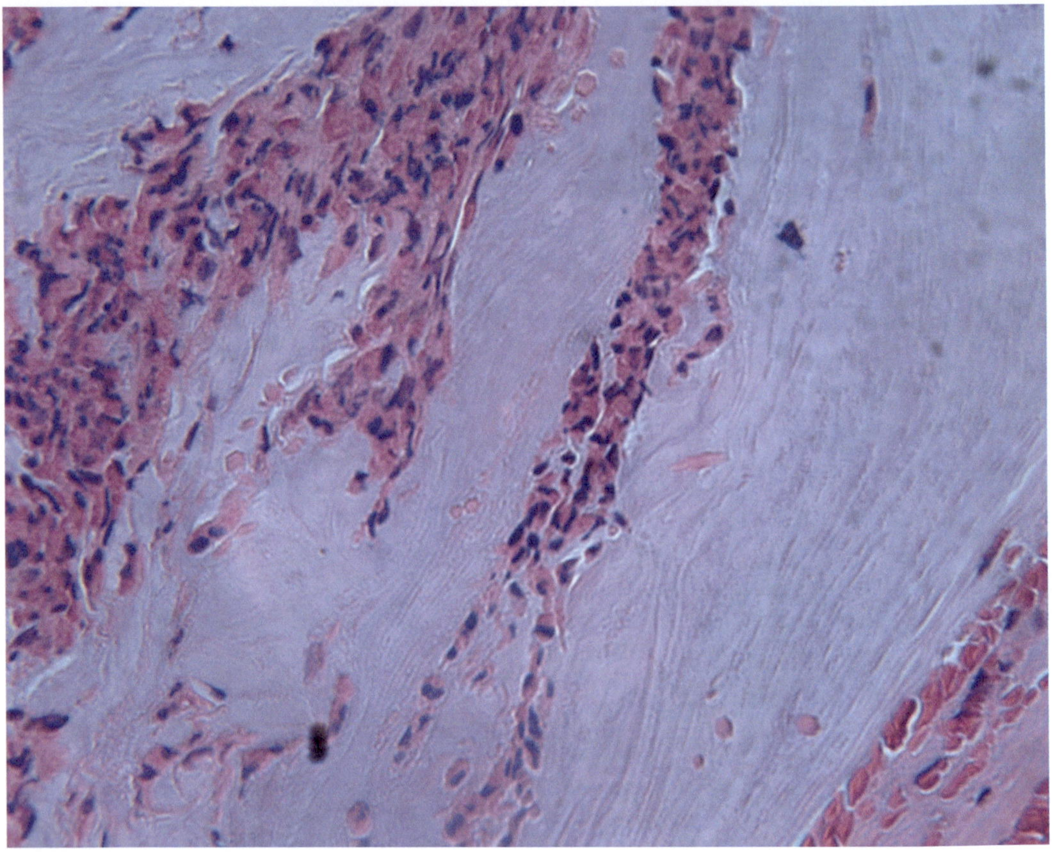

Fig. 19.2 Photomicrograph of an H&E stained section of eosinophilic mucin from a patient with AFS. There are layers of eosinophils in a background of mucin with many Charcot–Leyden crystals

directed at suppressing inflammation, reducing microbial stimuli that promote that inflammation, and supporting normal mucociliary clearance.

Surgery is required in almost all newly diagnosed cases of AFS. An aggressive surgical approach utilizing external approaches, stripping of sinus mucosa, or sinus obliteration is not appropriate. Contemporary surgical management relies on endoscopic tissue approaches to remove obstructing polyps and polypoid mucosa, resect sinus dividing walls and partitions, and evacuate sinus contents [8]. External surgeries are only necessary in rare circumstances. Often surgical access is improved by massive polyposis and mucocele formation that widens the surgical spaces. However, expansile disease may distort the normal intranasal landmarks and erode the important bony barriers to the orbit or brain, potentially increasing the risk and difficulty of surgery. Image guidance is therefore extremely helpful for orientation and to facilitate more complete surgery. Incomplete surgery, with retention of cells filled with eosinophilic mucin appears to be a risk factor for early recurrence [31] and may limit the effectiveness of anti-inflammatory therapies. Revision surgical treatment for polyp recurrences is indicated when intensive medical management fails to clear an exacerbation.

Medical treatment for AFS is essential to prevent or delay recurrence of polyps. Systemic anti-inflammatory agents are usually required in the treatment of AFS. Systemic corticosteroids have the best substantiation in the literature [17, 32]. A brief course of pre-operative systemic corticosteroids will shrink polyps and decrease bleeding during surgery [8]. Systemic corticosteroids given in the immediate post-op period will prevent early recurrence of polypoid

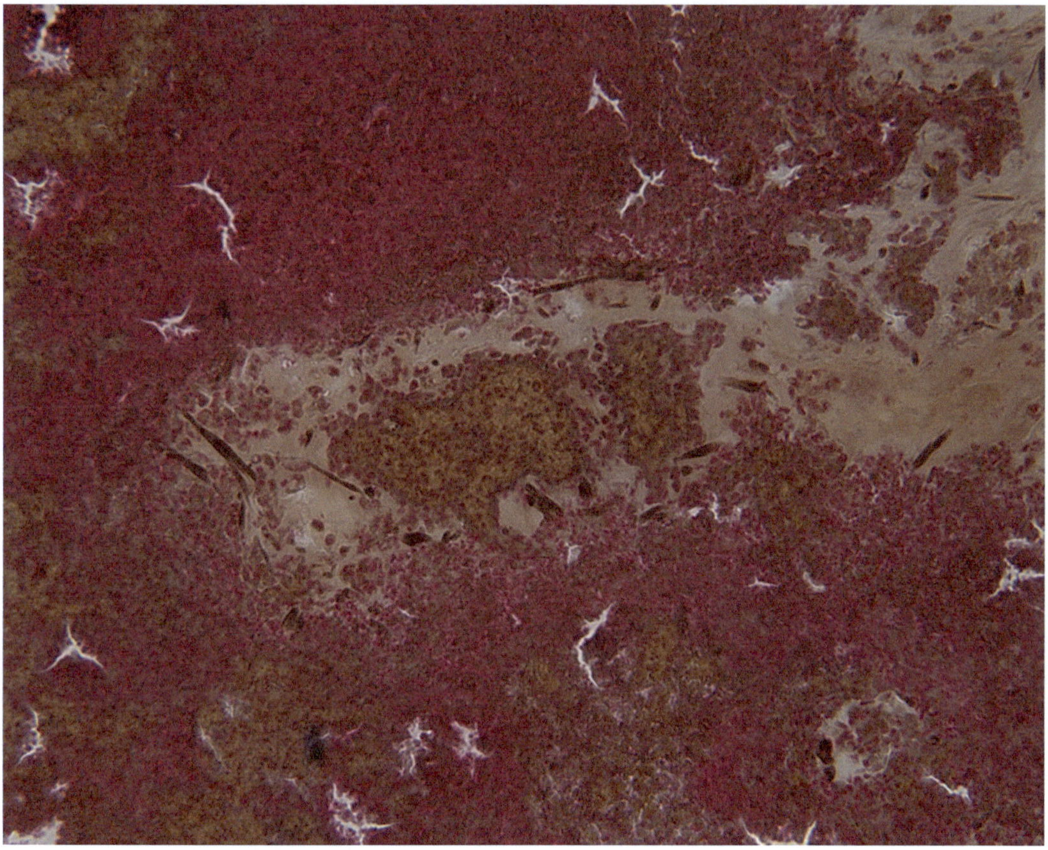

Fig. 19.3 Fontana-Masson stain that shows the melanin pigment of dematiaceous fungi. In this image, clusters of eosinophils are interspersed with a few scattered, dark brown fungal hyphae

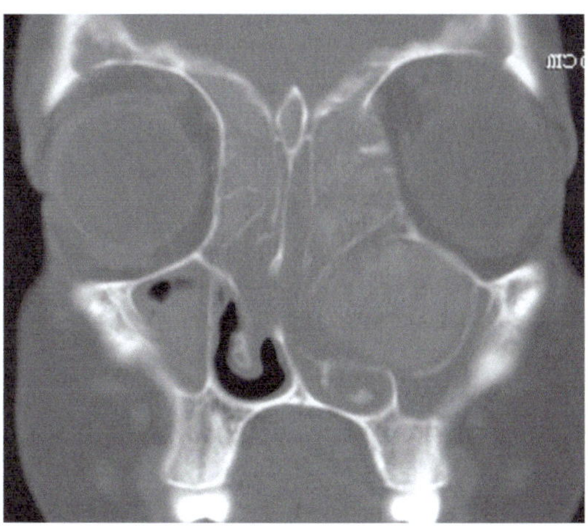

Fig. 19.4 Coronal non-contrasted CT image with bone windowing from a patient with AFS. Faint hyperattenuation of sinus contents is seen with left ethmoid expansion and mucocele impinging on the left maxillary sinus

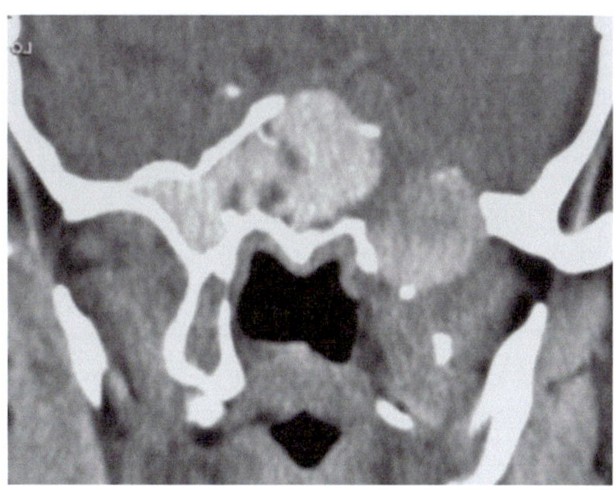

Fig. 19.5 Coronal non-contrasted CT image of the sphenoid region in soft tissue windows. There has been expansion of bilateral sphenoid sinuses with hyperdense contents and pronounced bone erosion

inflammation [33]. Long-term treatment with systemic corticosteroids entails considerable risk; therefore, short courses of oral corticosteroids (1–3 weeks duration) are usually employed to gain control over sinonasal inflammation, and topical intranasal steroids are utilized for long-term control. Leukotriene receptor antagonists are sometimes employed, though strong evidence for efficacy is lacking. Anti-leukotriene agents are attractive because of their safety and possible steroid-sparing effect [34]. Other anti-inflammatory agents such as itraconazole, macrolide antibiotics, or doxycycline may have an ancillary steroid-sparing role [32, 34–36].

In addition to systemic treatment, topical treatments are important medical adjuncts. Topical nasal corticosteroids and saline irrigations are mainstays of treatment. Nasal steroids have a minimal side effect profile, and are effective at decreasing sinonasal inflammation or shrinking nasal polyps. Local treatments are unfortunately often not sufficient to dampen the brisk inflammatory reaction of AFS and prevent recurrence, however.

Immunotherapy (IT) is another treatment modality that has been proposed to decrease the reliance on systemic steroids in the treatment of AFS. The rationale for immunotherapy presupposes that AFS is an IgE-mediated process. Folker, et al. reported their experience with IT in AFS patients and made a comparison to non-immunotherapy treated historical controls. After an average 33 months of follow-up, they showed that immunotherapy treated patients had better endoscopic mucosal appearance, lower chronic rhinosinusitis survey scores, required fewer courses of oral steroids (2 vs. 0), and showed less reliance on nasal steroids (73% vs. 27%) [37]. While this was not a randomized double blind study, these results suggest a potential role for immunotherapy in the management of AFS.

19.8 Prognosis

Like other forms of CRS with polyps, AFS is best considered to be an incurable chronic disease. While the long-term clinical course varies, and many patients do indeed "outgrow" their disease, a long-term disease management approach is warranted. After initiation of treatment, patients should be followed at intervals with endoscopic monitoring to guide titration of medical therapies. Surgical treatment without subsequent medical management is usually met with failure [38]. In AFS, significant recurrence of polyps or inflammation after initial treatment has been reported to range from 10% to 100% [8]. There are few longitudinal studies of the natural history of AFS, but most patients require multiple surgeries and continue to require repeated treatment with systemic steroids [31]. So while the disease may become quiescent over a period of years, a significant number of patients will have persistent sinonasal inflammation that requires ongoing treatment.

19.9 Unanswered Questions About AFS

While AFS is now recognized as a distinct phenotype of CRS with polyps, it is unclear if this phenotype is due to a distinct *endotype* of eosinophilic inflammation, and whether this distinction has relevance to treatment. To date, the roles of allergy, fungal entrapment, and *Staphylococcus aureus* colonization in driving the robust eosinophilic inflammation seen in these patients are unclear. Current treatment approaches for AFS are generally similar to those employed for other manifestations of CRS with polyps; aside from the urgency of treatment to prevent complications, we do not know if AFS should be treated any differently. Targeted molecular therapies (Biologics) are now available to treat CRS with nasal polyps; specific investigation will be required to determine their effectiveness and role in managing AFS.

References

1. Katzenstein AL, Sale SR, Greenberger PA. Allergic Aspergillus sinusitis: a newly recognized form of sinusitis. J Allergy Clin Immunol. 1983;72(1):89–93. https://doi.org/10.1016/0091-6749(83)90057-x.

2. Millar JW, Johnston A, Lamb D. Allergic aspergillosis of the maxillary sinuses. Thorax. 1981;36:710.
3. Safirstein BH. Allergic bronchopulmonary aspergillosis with obstruction of the upper respiratory tract. Chest. 1976;70(6):788–90. https://doi.org/10.1378/chest.70.6.788.
4. Allphin AL, Strauss M, Abdul-Karim FW. Allergic fungal sinusitis: problems in diagnosis and treatment. Laryngoscope. 1991;101(8):815–20. https://doi.org/10.1288/00005537-199108000-00003.
5. Cody DT II, Neel HB III, Ferreiro JA, Roberts GD. Allergic fungal sinusitis: the Mayo Clinic experience. Laryngoscope. 1994;104(9):1074–9. https://doi.org/10.1288/00005537-199409000-00005.
6. Ferguson BJ. Eosinophilic mucin rhinosinusitis: a distinct clinicopathological entity. Laryngoscope. 2000;110(5 Pt 1):799–813. https://doi.org/10.1097/00005537-200005000-00010.
7. Ponikau JU, Sherris DA, Kern EB, Homburger HA, Frigas E, Gaffey TA, et al. The diagnosis and incidence of allergic fungal sinusitis. Mayo Clin Proc. 1999;74(9):877–84. https://doi.org/10.4065/74.9.877.
8. Marple BF. Allergic fungal rhinosinusitis: current theories and management strategies. Laryngoscope. 2001;111(6):1006–19. https://doi.org/10.1097/00005537-200106000-00015.
9. Schubert MS, Goetz DW. Evaluation and treatment of allergic fungal sinusitis. I. Demographics and diagnosis. J Allergy Clin Immunol. 1998;102(3):387–94. https://doi.org/10.1016/s0091-6749(98)70125-3.
10. Manning SC, Holman M. Further evidence for allergic pathophysiology in allergic fungal sinusitis. Laryngoscope. 1998;108(10):1485–96. https://doi.org/10.1097/00005537-199810000-00012.
11. Stewart AE, Hunsaker DH. Fungus-specific IgG and IgE in allergic fungal rhinosinusitis. Otolaryngol Head Neck Surg. 2002;127(4):324–32. https://doi.org/10.1067/mhn.2002.126801.
12. Collins M, Nair S, Smith W, Kette F, Gillis D, Wormald PJ. Role of local immunoglobulin E production in the pathophysiology of noninvasive fungal sinusitis. Laryngoscope. 2004;114(7):1242–6. https://doi.org/10.1097/00005537-200407000-00019.
13. Pant H, Kette FE, Smith WB, Wormald PJ, Macardle PJ. Fungal-specific humoral response in eosinophilic mucus chronic rhinosinusitis. Laryngoscope. 2005;115(4):601–6. https://doi.org/10.1097/01.mlg.0000161341.00258.54.
14. Dutre T, Al Dousary S, Zhang N, Bachert C. Allergic fungal rhinosinusitis-more than a fungal disease? J Allergy Clin Immunol. 2013;132(2):487–9.e1. https://doi.org/10.1016/j.jaci.2013.02.040.
15. Ferguson BJ, Barnes L, Bernstein JM, Brown D, Clark CE III, Cook PR, et al. Geographic variation in allergic fungal rhinosinusitis. Otolaryngol Clin N Am. 2000;33(2):441–9. https://doi.org/10.1016/s0030-6665(00)80018-3.
16. Ence BK, Gourley DS, Jorgensen NL, Shagets FW, Parsons DS. Allergic fungal sinusitis. Am J Rhinol. 1990;4(5):169–78.
17. Schubert MS, Goetz DW. Evaluation and treatment of allergic fungal sinusitis. II. Treatment and follow-up. J Allergy Clin Immunol. 1998;102(3):395–402. https://doi.org/10.1016/s0091-6749(98)70126-5.
18. Promsopa C, Kansara S, Citardi MJ, Fakhri S, Porter P, Luong A. Prevalence of confirmed asthma varies in chronic rhinosinusitis subtypes. Int Forum Allergy Rhinol. 2016;6(4):373–7. https://doi.org/10.1002/alr.21674.
19. Manning SC, Schaefer SD, Close LG, Vuitch F. Culture-positive allergic fungal sinusitis. Arch Otolaryngol Head Neck Surg. 1991;117(2):174–8. https://doi.org/10.1001/archotol.1991.01870140062007.
20. Gupta AK, Bansal S, Gupta A, Mathur N. Is fungal infestation of paranasal sinuses more aggressive in pediatric population? Int J Pediatr Otorhinolaryngol. 2006;70(4):603–8. https://doi.org/10.1016/j.ijporl.2005.08.014.
21. Saravanan K, Panda NK, Chakrabarti A, Das A, Bapuraj RJ. Allergic fungal rhinosinusitis: an attempt to resolve the diagnostic dilemma. Arch Otolaryngol Head Neck Surg. 2006;132(2):173–8. https://doi.org/10.1001/archotol.132.2.173.
22. Singh N, Bhalodiya NH. Allergic fungal sinusitis (AFS) – earlier diagnosis and management. J Laryngol Otol. 2005;119(11):875–81. https://doi.org/10.1258/002221505774783412.
23. McClay JE, Marple B, Kapadia L, Biavati MJ, Nussenbaum B, Newcomer M, et al. Clinical presentation of allergic fungal sinusitis in children. Laryngoscope. 2002;112(3):565–9. https://doi.org/10.1097/00005537-200203000-00028.
24. Manning SC, Vuitch F, Weinberg AG, Brown OE. Allergic aspergillosis: a newly recognized form of sinusitis in the pediatric population. Laryngoscope. 1989;99(7 Pt 1):681–5. https://doi.org/10.1288/00005537-198907000-00003.
25. Bent JP III, Kuhn FA. Diagnosis of allergic fungal sinusitis. Otolaryngol Head Neck Surg. 1994;111(5):580–8. https://doi.org/10.1177/019459989411100508.
26. Fokkens WJ, Lund VJ, Mullol J, Bachert C, Alobid I, Baroody F, et al. EPOS 2012: European position paper on rhinosinusitis and nasal polyps 2012. A summary for otorhinolaryngologists. Rhinology. 2012;50(1):1–12. https://doi.org/10.4193/Rhino50E2.
27. Ghegan MD, Lee FS, Schlosser RJ. Incidence of skull base and orbital erosion in allergic fungal rhinosinusitis (AFRS) and non-AFRS. Otolaryngol Head Neck Surg. 2006;134(4):592–5. https://doi.org/10.1016/j.otohns.2005.11.025.
28. Aribandi M, McCoy VA, Bazan C III. Imaging features of invasive and noninvasive fungal sinusitis: a review. Radiographics. 2007;27(5):1283–96. https://doi.org/10.1148/rg.275065189.
29. Manning SC, Merkel M, Kriesel K, Vuitch F, Marple B. Computed tomography and magnetic resonance diagnosis of allergic fungal sinusitis. Laryngoscope. 1997;107(2):170–6. https://doi.org/10.1097/00005537-199702000-00007.

30. Zinreich SJ, Kennedy DW, Malat J, Curtin HD, Epstein JI, Huff LC, et al. Fungal sinusitis: diagnosis with CT and MR imaging. Radiology. 1988;169(2):439–44. https://doi.org/10.1148/radiology.169.2.3174990.
31. Marple B, Newcomer M, Schwade N, Mabry R. Natural history of allergic fungal rhinosinusitis: a 4- to 10-year follow-up. Otolaryngol Head Neck Surg. 2002;127(5):361–6. https://doi.org/10.1067/mhn.2002.129806.
32. Kuhn FA, Javer AR. Allergic fungal sinusitis: a four-year follow-up. Am J Rhinol. 2000;14(3):149–56. https://doi.org/10.2500/105065800782102780.
33. Sohail MA, Al Khabori MJ, Hyder J, Verma A. Allergic fungal sinusitis: can we predict the recurrence? Otolaryngol Head Neck Surg. 2004;131(5):704–10. https://doi.org/10.1016/j.otohns.2004.04.004.
34. Schubert MS. Antileukotriene therapy for allergic fungal sinusitis. J Allergy Clin Immunol. 2001;108(3):466–7. https://doi.org/10.1067/mai.2001.117592.
35. Erwin GE, Fitzgerald JE. Case report: allergic bronchopulmonary aspergillosis and allergic fungal sinusitis successfully treated with voriconazole. J Asthma. 2007;44(10):891–5. https://doi.org/10.1080/02770900701750197.
36. Rains BM III, Mineck CW. Treatment of allergic fungal sinusitis with high-dose itraconazole. Am J Rhinol. 2003;17(1):1–8.
37. Folker RJ, Marple BF, Mabry RL, Mabry CS. Treatment of allergic fungal sinusitis: a comparison trial of postoperative immunotherapy with specific fungal antigens. Laryngoscope. 1998;108(11 Pt 1):1623–7. https://doi.org/10.1097/00005537-199811000-00007.
38. Kupferberg SB, Bent JP III, Kuhn FA. Prognosis for allergic fungal sinusitis. Otolaryngol Head Neck Surg. 1997;117(1):35–41. https://doi.org/10.1016/s0194-5998(97)70203-1.

Type 2 Immune Reactions and Consequences

20

Claus Bachert

Key Points

- Understanding of the role of type 2 immune reaction is central to a better management of CRSwNP patients.
- Type 2 immune reactions are characterized by tissue eosinophilia, increase in IgE producing B-cells, and increased concentrations of type 2 cytokines IL-4, IL-5, and IL-13.
- Patients with type 2 CRSwNP have comorbid asthma in up to 70%, and are more likely to develop recurrence after surgery or pharmacotherapy.
- Biologics currently developed for CRSwNP all target type 2 immune reactions.

The immune mechanisms prominent in type 2 immune reactions are described in Chaps. 5–17. These pathomechanisms translate into biomarkers, such as local eosinophilia in the mucosal tissue and nasal secretions, and the expression of high concentrations of total and allergen-specific IgE within the tissue and secretions; the pathomechanisms also induce the typical symptoms, such as nasal obstruction by growing masses of polyps in CRSwNP due to fibrin deposition, but also swelling of nasal and sinus mucosa at areas without polyp growth. Type 2 cytokines orchestrate the production of typical viscous secretions, which are getting even more sticky and glue-like by the type 2 induced formations of eosinophil extracellular traps (EETs) and Charcot–Leyden crystals (CLCs) [1]. Type 2 cytokines also impact the olfactory nerve, inducing malfunction even without complete obstruction; the fast onset of Dupilumab, a potent IL4 receptor antagonist, even before the involution of the polyp mass, argues in that direction [2].

Clinicians are used to focus on eosinophils in tissues or peripheral blood; it is clinical routine to measure this parameter in blood and to ask the pathologist for a statement on the presence of tissue eosinophilia in the tissue harvested during surgery [3–5]. CRSwNP is usually "eosinophilic", depending on the threshold for eosinophils per vision field chosen and the region in the world in which the patient lives. In cases with low numbers of tissue eosinophils, the clinicians called it "neutrophilic". This way, already some distinction was possible, and even predictions for recurrence after surgery could be made based on eosinophil and neutrophil counts [3]. However, this dichotomy is an important misconception; in every eosinophilic polyp, neutrophils also are present and activated, reflected by increased concentrations of neutrophilic biomarkers [6, 7].

C. Bachert (✉)
Upper Airways Research Laboratory and Department of Oto-Rhino-Laryngology, Ghent University, Ghent, Belgium

Division of ENT Diseases, CLINTEC, Karolinska Institute, University of Stockholm, Stockholm, Sweden
e-mail: claus.bachert@ugent.be

L. Zhang, C. Bachert (eds.), *Chronic Rhinosinusitis*, https://doi.org/10.1007/978-981-16-0784-4_20

Cells are unevenly distributed throughout the tissue, and numbers may vary according to the region within the polyp. It is also clear that eosinophils do not reflect all aspects of type 2 immune reactions, as they do not mirror IgE production (not equivalent to allergy, again something different)!

To better reflect the inflammatory processes within a mucosal tissue, endotyping should employ quantifiable inflammatory mediators and cytokines. Tomassen et al. [6] succeeded to cluster subjects with CRS solely based on a variety of immune markers, independent of clinical phenotypic segregation; only secondarily, the authors matched the defined clusters with the clinical information or phenotypes. In a multicentre case–control study, 173 CRS cases and 89 controls undergoing surgery were included, and tissues were analysed for various T-cell cytokines including IL-5, IFN-γ, IL-17A, TNF-α, IL-22; pro-inflammatory cytokines IL-1β, IL-6, IL-8; granulocyte activation markers eosinophil cationic protein and myeloperoxidase; remodelling factors such as TGF-β1 and albumin; and finally total IgE and SE-IgE to reflect adaptive immune responses (Fig. 20.1). Clustering of the CRS cases resulted in four clusters with low or undetectable IL-5, ECP, IgE, and albumin concentrations, and six clusters having high concentrations of those markers. Three of four IL-5-low clusters showed limited inflammation, a type 1, type 17, or a type 22 profile; these cases clinically resembled predominantly the CRSsNP phenotype without increased asthma prevalence. The IL-5-high clusters were divided into a group of three clusters with moderate IL-5 levels and moderately increased asthma prevalence, and a group with high IL-5 concentrations, almost exclusively representing the NP phenotype with strongly increased asthma prevalence. In the latter, two clusters demonstrated highest concentrations of IgE and other type 2 markers and asthma prevalence, with all samples expressing SE-IgE. In summary, distinct CRS clusters with diverse inflammatory mechanisms may result in the same clinical phenotype, but endotypes provided a more accurate description of the inflammatory mechanisms involved than phenotype information only.

Analysing biomarkers in an unbiased way, we have thus described the first cluster-based endotype differentiation in CRS [6], which turned out to be of clinical relevance; risks for asthma comorbidity as well as local recurrences can be

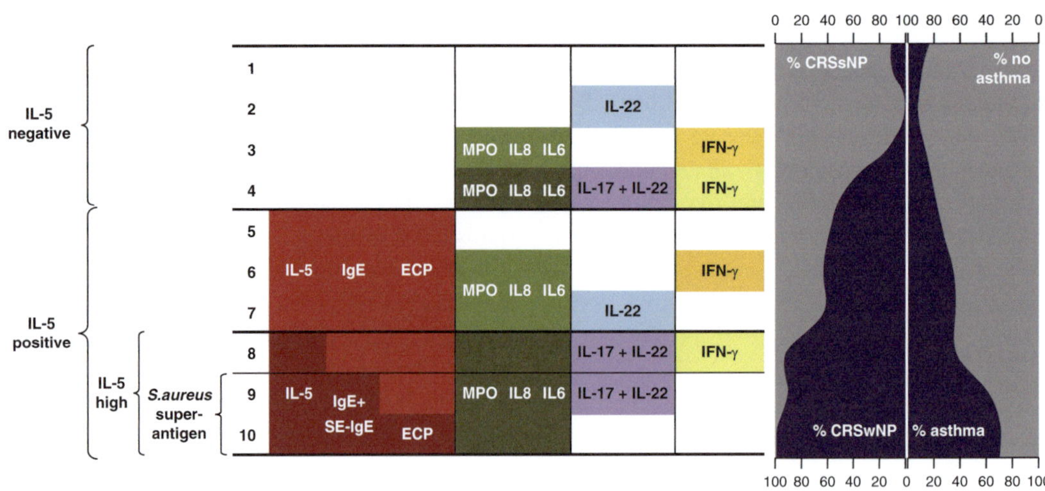

Fig. 20.1 Simplified graphic depiction of the clusters and their characteristic cytokines, as well as the distribution of CRSsNP versus CRSwNP and asthma. For cytokines, white indicates no increased concentration, light colours indicate moderately increased concentrations, and dark colours indicate strongly increased concentrations. Horizontal lines indicate groups of clusters, as determined by IL-5, SE-IgE, and CRSwNP and asthma characteristics (Source from P Tomassen et al. J Allergy Clin Immunol 2016)

deduced from the endotypes, with moderate and severe type 2 endotypes in contrast to the non-type 2 endotype, which turns the approach into a clinically usable and relevant tool. This is the condition sine qua non, e.g. only if endotyping supports treatment decisions and prediction of the course of disease, it contributes to a superior management with advantages for the patients, but also for the adequate usage of resources. Endotyping gains additional importance with the differentiation of surgical approaches and the advent of biologics into treatment algorisms; it is evident that monoclonal antibodies are highly targeted approaches and only should be given to severe patients, but specifically to matching patients in terms of molecules perpetuating the disease. It is clear that an expensive anti-type 2 cytokine antibody should not be indicated in a patient not suffering from a type 2 disease! In the future, this selection may even gain more momentum, as it might be possible to tailor the treatment to specific cytokines within the type 2 immune reaction (Fig. 20.2).

The immune reactions within the nasal cavities and the lungs can often also be read in the peripheral blood in terms of increased eosinophil numbers, or increased serum IgE concentrations mostly with a specific polyclonal character, e.g. the presence of small entities of allergen-specific IgEs to inhalant allergens, but also staphylococcal antigens, in great numbers. This polyclonality can be extreme, resulting in specific IgE idiotypes below detection limit, but high total serum IgE concentrations far above normal. Blood eosinophilia and high serum total IgE are both indicators for type 2 immune reactions.

A consequence of type 2 immune reactions also is disease recurrence, which is considerably higher in type 2 nasal polyposis compared to non-type 2 polyps, but also to CRS without polyps (CRSsNP) with or without type 2 disease [6, 7]. Factors such as eosinophils, IL-5, ECP, total IgE, and SE-IgE have been demonstrated to be associated with disease recurrence [8, 9]. The increased risk for recurrence persists over more than a decade [10], and multiple surgeries may be necessary over a life time. The likelihood of recurrence within the sinuses may of course very much depend on the surgical approach, which may be mucosa-sparing or complete (also referred to as "reboot approach" [11], see Chaps. 46–51). It is now evident that the severe mucosal type 2 inflammation is present in all sinuses, in polyps as well as in thickened or even normal looking sinus mucosa [12], and that an incomplete removal of the inflamed mucosa may result in rapid and severe recur-

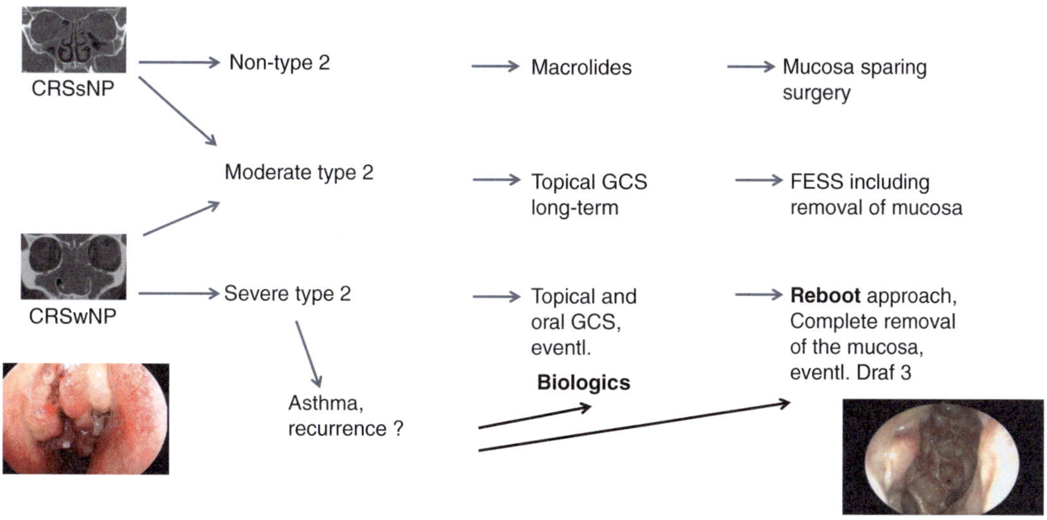

Fig. 20.2 Endotypes and consequences

rence. Also the nasal turbinates are part of the inflammation, but do only rarely form polyps (see Chaps. 46–51 for more detail).

However, type 2 immune reactions do not only have local disease consequences. There is a whole range of comorbidities linked to upper airway type 2 immune reactions, including early-onset diseases such as allergic rhinitis and late-onset nasal polyps [13]. Allergic rhinitis typically is characterized by comorbid atopic skin disease, by food allergy and allergic asthma [14]. CRSwNP is prominently associated with late-onset asthma [15], which may be diagnosed before or after nasal polyposis, or develop within a decade after the diagnosis of CRSwNP.

Typically, the comorbid asthma is mild to moderate, but may develop into severe disease [16] over time, and the type 2 immune reaction to staphylococcal superantigens (serum SE-IgEs) is predictive, whereas inhalant allergen-specific IgEs are not. However, there also is a group of severe asthma patients suffering from nasal polyps and impacting on the asthma severity [17]. Those polyps are often not diagnosed, as no referral to a rhinologist was done, and therefore not properly treated. In the area of biologics, however, they may also be controlled together with the treatment of asthma complaints, as the same biologics also may reduce burden of nasal polyp disease. In fact, type 2 comorbidities should be considered an important factor for the indication of biologics in either CRSwNP or asthma, and possibly atopic dermatitis.

Thus, type 2 immune reactions in CRSwNP result in local recurrence and asthma comorbidity as well as increased eosinophils in the peripheral blood and an increase in serum IgE with polyclonality. This fact can be used also in the diagnostic management, as e.g. a CRSwNP patient with late-onset asthma is highly likely to suffer from a type 2 disease; blood or serum biomarkers may confirm this. Repeated surgery in the past may also indicate type 2 immune reactions, but of course are dependent from the completeness of mucosal removal. The environment of disease expression may always be considered; in Europe, with more than 80% of polyps characterized by type 2 immune disease and frequent asthma comorbidity in up to 70%, the need for biomarkers additional to the clinical traits may be low, whereas in China, with less frequent and severe type 2 immune reactions and less asthma comorbidity (see Chap. 21), the need for biomarkers may be significantly higher.

It is evident that several clinical phenotypes share characteristic pathways and should be summarized as one common endotype: type 2 CRSwNP, AERD [18, 19], and AFRS [20] are all type 2 inflammatory responses, and may therefore be "clinical relatives"; in fact, they all are characterized by polyp formation in the sinuses, asthma comorbidity, and recurrence after sinus surgery. In contrast, immune deficits, cilia motility defects, CF, and infectious sinus diseases are characterized by type 1 and/or type 17 "neutrophilic" immune responses of the mucosa. Thus, a clinical phenotype such as CRSwNP may be characterized by different endotypes, and an endotype such as a type 2 immune reaction may form the background for several phenotypes. The understanding of endotyping rather than phenotyping, however, will guide progress in setting up diagnostic measures, understanding the natural course of disease, estimating prognosis and risk, and finally the determination of innovative therapeutic perspectives specifically for patients suffering from severe disease (Table 20.1).

Table 20.1 Clinical traits and Indicators for type 2 CRS

Strong indicator	Moderate indicators
Comorbid late-onset asthma	Other type 2 comorbidities, allergy
Former surgery with tissue eosinophilia in histology	One or more surgeries for CRSwNP
Non-steroidal anti-inflammatory drugs (NSAIDs)-exacerbated disease (N-ERD)	One or more oral GCS course in last 2 years for CRS
Blood eosinophils >300 cell/mm^3	Blood eosinophils 150 cell/mm^3
Serum IgE > 150 kU/L, polyclonality	Serum IgE >100 kU/L
SE-IgE positivity	

References

1. Gevaert E, Delemarre T, De Volder J, Zhang N, Holtappels G, De Ruyck N, et al. Charcot-Leyden crystals promote neutrophilic inflammation in patients with nasal polyposis. J Allergy Clin Immunol. 2020;145(1):427–30.e4. https://doi.org/10.1016/j.jaci.2019.08.027.
2. Bachert C, Han JK, Desrosiers M, Hellings PW, Amin N, Lee SE, et al. Efficacy and safety of dupilumab in patients with severe chronic rhinosinusitis with nasal polyps (LIBERTY NP SINUS-24 and LIBERTY NP SINUS-52): results from two multicentre, randomised, double-blind, placebo-controlled, parallel-group phase 3 trials. Lancet (London, England). 2019;394(10209):1638–50. https://doi.org/10.1016/s0140-6736(19)31881-1.
3. Vlaminck S, Vauterin T, Hellings PW, Jorissen M, Acke F, Van Cauwenberge P, et al. The importance of local eosinophilia in the surgical outcome of chronic rhinosinusitis: a 3-year prospective observational study. Am J Rhinol Allergy. 2014;28(3):260–4. https://doi.org/10.2500/ajra.2014.28.4024.
4. Hu Y, Cao PP, Liang GT, Cui YH, Liu Z. Diagnostic significance of blood eosinophil count in eosinophilic chronic rhinosinusitis with nasal polyps in Chinese adults. Laryngoscope. 2012;122(3):498–503. https://doi.org/10.1002/lary.22507.
5. Lou H, Meng Y, Piao Y, Zhang N, Bachert C, Wang C, et al. Cellular phenotyping of chronic rhinosinusitis with nasal polyps. Rhinology. 2016;54(2):150–9. https://doi.org/10.4193/Rhin15.271.
6. Tomassen P, Vandeplas G, Van Zele T, Cardell LO, Arebro J, Olze H, et al. Inflammatory endotypes of chronic rhinosinusitis based on cluster analysis of biomarkers. J Allergy Clin Immunol. 2016;137(5):1449–56.e4. https://doi.org/10.1016/j.jaci.2015.12.1324.
7. Stevens WW, Peters AT, Tan BK, Klingler AI, Poposki JA, Hulse KE, et al. Associations between inflammatory endotypes and clinical presentations in chronic rhinosinusitis. J Allergy Clin Immunol Pract. 2019;7(8):2812–20.e3. https://doi.org/10.1016/j.jaip.2019.05.009.
8. Zhang N, Van Zele T, Perez-Novo C, Van Bruaene N, Holtappels G, DeRuyck N, et al. Different types of T-effector cells orchestrate mucosal inflammation in chronic sinus disease. J Allergy Clin Immunol. 2008;122(5):961–8. https://doi.org/10.1016/j.jaci.2008.07.008.
9. Van Zele T, Holtappels G, Gevaert P, Bachert C. Differences in initial immunoprofiles between recurrent and nonrecurrent chronic rhinosinusitis with nasal polyps. Am J Rhinol Allergy. 2014;28(3):192–8. https://doi.org/10.2500/ajra.2014.28.4033.
10. Calus L, Van Bruaene N, Bosteels C, Dejonckheere S, Van Zele T, Holtappels G, et al. Twelve-year follow-up study after endoscopic sinus surgery in patients with chronic rhinosinusitis with nasal polyposis. Clin Transl Allergy. 2019;9:30. https://doi.org/10.1186/s13601-019-0269-4.
11. Alsharif S, Jonstam K, van Zele T, Gevaert P, Holtappels G, Bachert C. Endoscopic sinus surgery for type-2 CRS wNP: an endotype-based retrospective study. Laryngoscope. 2019;129(6):1286–92. https://doi.org/10.1002/lary.27815.
12. Jonstam K, Alsharif S, Bogaert S, Suchonos N, Holtappels G, Park J, et al. Extensive type 2 inflammation in chronic rhinosinusitis with nasal polyps is suppressed by complete sinus mucosa removal (reboot surgery). JACI submitted.
13. Bachert C, Zhang N, Holtappels G, De Lobel L, van Cauwenberge P, Liu S, et al. Presence of IL-5 protein and IgE antibodies to staphylococcal enterotoxins in nasal polyps is associated with comorbid asthma. J Allergy Clin Immunol. 2010;126(5):962–8, 8.e1–6. https://doi.org/10.1016/j.jaci.2010.07.007.
14. Sørensen M, Klingenberg C, Wickman M, Sollid JUE, Furberg AS, Bachert C, et al. *Staphylococcus aureus* enterotoxin sensitization is associated with allergic poly-sensitization and allergic multimorbidity in adolescents. Allergy. 2017;72(10):1548–55. https://doi.org/10.1111/all.13175.
15. Khan A, Vandeplas G, Huynh TMT, Joish VN, Mannent L, Tomassen P, et al. The Global Allergy and Asthma European Network (GALEN) rhinosinusitis cohort: a large European cross-sectional study of chronic rhinosinusitis patients with and without nasal polyps. Rhinology. 2019;57(1):32–42. https://doi.org/10.4193/Rhin17.255.
16. Sintobin I, Siroux V, Holtappels G, Pison C, Nadif R, Bousquet J, et al. Sensitisation to staphylococcal enterotoxins and asthma severity: a longitudinal study in the EGEA cohort. Eur Respir J. 2019;54(3). https://doi.org/10.1183/13993003.00198-2019.
17. Heffler E, Blasi F, Latorre M, Menzella F, Paggiaro P, Pelaia G, et al. The severe asthma network in Italy: findings and perspectives. J Allergy Clin Immunol Pract. 2019;7(5):1462–8. https://doi.org/10.1016/j.jaip.2018.10.016.
18. Mahdavinia M, Carter RG, Ocampo CJ, Stevens W, Kato A, Tan BK, et al. Basophils are elevated in nasal polyps of patients with chronic rhinosinusitis without aspirin sensitivity. J Allergy Clin Immunol. 2014;133(6):1759–63. https://doi.org/10.1016/j.jaci.2013.12.1092.
19. Pérez-Novo CA, Watelet JB, Claeys C, Van Cauwenberge P, Bachert C. Prostaglandin, leukotriene, and lipoxin balance in chronic rhinosinusitis with and without nasal polyposis. J Allergy Clin Immunol. 2005;115(6):1189–96. https://doi.org/10.1016/j.jaci.2005.02.029.
20. Dutre T, Al Dousary S, Zhang N, Bachert C. Allergic fungal rhinosinusitis-more than a fungal disease? J Allergy Clin Immunol. 2013;132(2):487–9.e1. https://doi.org/10.1016/j.jaci.2013.02.040.

Regional Difference

21

Kun Du and Xiangdong Wang

Key Points

- The prevalence of type 2 immune reactions among patients with CRSwNP does vary with the geographical region.

Prior to 2005, our existing knowledge of inflammatory patterns in CRS came nearly exclusively from studies with Western patients, and those studies indicated that nasal polyps were "eosinophilic" and characterized by the expression of interleukin (IL)-5 and other type 2 cytokines, whereas CRSsNP resembled a type 1 disease with expression of IFN-gamma [1, 2]. However, less eosinophilic and more neutrophilic inflammation was found in patients with CRSwNP in Asia, when compared with Europe and North America [3]. Chinese patients with CRSwNP demonstrated neutrophil-biased inflammation as compared to their Caucasian counterparts [4]. Approximately 80% of CRSwNP patients in the Western world display a type 2 signature [5, 6], whereas between 20% and 60% display that signature in China, Korea, and Thailand, respectively [3]. By measuring the value of ECP/MPO, Wang et al. [7] found that cases of CRSwNP in regions of Europe, Japan, and Australia showed an eosinophilic dominance (eosinophilic > 50%) rather than a non-eosinophilic dominance (eosinophilic < 50%) such as cases found in Beijing and Chengdu in China. Another study found that <50% of CRSwNP cases in Beijing showed eosinophilic inflammation [8]. The results from different geographic regions indicated that the immunological patterns of CRS were not the same in all ethnic populations [9].

Indeed, the dichotomy of eosinophilic and neutrophilic inflammation does not represent all the immunological responses that occur within the nasal mucosa of patients with CRS (as mentioned in Chap. 20). An extended analysis of transcription factors, cytokines, and cellular infiltrates found in polyps from patients in Belgium compared to polyps from patients in southern China showed that the polyps from Caucasian patients with CRSwNP had significantly higher levels of Th2 transcription factor GATA-3 and Th2 cytokine IL-5 when compared to control subjects, and the polyps from Chinese patients showed a Th1/Th17 cell pattern. Both CRSwNP groups showed a significant downregulation of Foxp3 expression and TGF-β1 protein levels versus their respective control groups [10]. Another study provided an opportunity to learn from regional differences: 83% of the polyp samples from Belgium, but only 20% of the polyp samples from Sichuan province were IL-5 protein positive, and 34% vs. 9% ($P < 0.01$) of the subjects, respectively, suf-

K. Du · X. Wang (✉)
Department of Otolaryngology, Head and Neck Surgery, Beijing Tongren Hospital, Capital Medical University, Beijing, China

Beijing Key Laboratory of Nasal Diseases, Beijing Institute of Otorhinolaryngology, Beijing, China

L. Zhang, C. Bachert (eds.), *Chronic Rhinosinusitis*, https://doi.org/10.1007/978-981-16-0784-4_21

fered from asthma comorbidity [11]. Similarly, Cao et al. found that central southern Chinese patients with CRSsNP had higher levels of IFN-γ expression, and only a subpopulation of eosinophilic CRSwNP patients showed an enhanced expression of GATA-3 and IL-5 [12]. These studies clearly indicated immunological heterogeneity within the same disease phenotype found in different regions.

Endotypes are defined as disease subtypes with unique mechanisms that are functionally and pathologically different from each other due to the involvement of a specific molecule or cell [13, 14]. By using Th1-, Th2-, or Th17-associated inflammatory biomarkers, cases of CRS have been classified into different endotypes as type 1 (T1), type 2 (T2) and type 3 (T3). Tomassen et al. [13] described three endotypes of CRS with and without nasal polyps in European patients based on different expression patterns of Th cytokines, inflammatory biomarkers, and IgE. That investigation showed that CRS can be differentiated into non-type-2 (44%), moderate (38%), and severe type-2 (18%) inflammation endotypes, with a clear increase in the nasal polyp phenotype (from <15% to >90%) and rate of asthma comorbidity from the first endotype (~5%) to the last endotype (60–70%). Liao et al. [15] latterly analysed patients with CRS in the middle region of China and found seven clusters of patients with CRS. These clusters showed much more non-type 2 (83%), but less moderate type 2 (4%) and severe type 2 (13%) endotypes. The above two studies both investigated the endotypes of CRS by collecting samples of nasal polyp tissue and sinus mucosa. In contrast, another recent study reported the CRS endotypes in a North American population based on an analysis of sinonasal mucus samples. That study suggested that a severe, a moderate, and a mild type 2 endotypes with pro-inflammatory signatures were each present in 7%, 8%, and 8% of the patients, respectively; Mild type 2 endotypes without pro-inflammation was present in 62%; however, 15% of the patients showed pro-inflammation but without a distinct Th1-, Th2-, or Th17-associated signature [16]. Furthermore, Wang et al. [7] described Th cytokine in CRS patients and made a comparison among three continents: Asia (China and Japan), Europe (Benelux and Germany), and Australia. Those comparisons revealed a remarkable diversity in Th cytokine signatures among regions, and showed that CRSwNP tissues from Europe and Australia were characterized by a higher expression of type-2 inflammation when compared to CRSwNP tissues in Asia; however, within Asia, the expression patterns varied from low type-2 expression in Chengdu/China to moderate type-2 expression in Beijing and Japan [7]. Those differences were also reflected in CRSsNP tissues, but to a lesser degree. Furthermore, the levels of SE-IgE antibodies within the polyp tissues showed a significant variation, in parallel with the type-2 inflammation signatures. The above studies demonstrated that type 1, type 2, and type 3 associated inflammatory signatures of CRS also appeared to show distinct geographical distributions throughout the world.

As for biomarkers associated with asthma comorbidity, SE-IgE and total IgE in nasal polyp tissues were found to be the most important predictors of asthma in European patients, while IL-5 was an important predictor in Chinese patients [11]. Tomassen et al. [13] investigated CRS samples from 11 European centres and found that the sinus mucosa or nasal polyps from 12.9% of the patients tested positive for SE-IgE. Moreover, patients with higher levels of SE-IgE and total IgE had a higher incidence of asthma (64–71% of the patients). However, the findings were different in China. Bachert et al. [11] found that 37% of Belgian patients tested positive for SE-IgE in their polyps, while only 17% of their Chinese counterparts had nasal polyps that were SE-IgE positive. Furthermore, higher levels of IL-5 and total IgE were predictive of comorbid asthma in the Chinese CRSwNP patients. The study results described above illustrate the central roles played by type-2 immune reactions and IgE in causing asthma comorbidity, and help to explain the difference in asthma comorbidity between the two ethnic groups.

Although the degree of type 2 inflammation was lower in the Asian population as compared to their Western counterparts, a type 2 shift has been detected in several Asian regions (e.g. Thailand, South Korea, and China) over the past 20 years [17–21]. For instance, a longitudinal study from Thailand [17] revealed a significant seven-fold increase in the number of CRS cases with eosinophilic inflammation in 2011 when compared to the values obtained in 1999, the latter of which displayed a neutrophilic character. The type 2 shift was also shown in CRSwNP patients in South Korea, and China [17–21]. These observations may be due to the influence of air pollution. Studies conducted in several large Asian cities have found that a variety of pollutants can adversely affect the nasal mucosa. A longitudinal cohort study of school children indicated that exposure to particulate matter (PM 2.5) might induce neutrophilic nasal inflammation under real-life conditions [22]. Another study reported that short-term haze exposure may lead to nasal inflammation and hypersensitivity in healthy subjects [23]. One recent study found that PM 2.5 could induce a neutrophilic immune response in normal non-inflamed nasal mucosa, but aggravated type-2 responses in vivo and ex vivo in cases of pre-existing type-2 inflammatory disease [23]. These studies suggest that the higher incidence of Th2/Th17/Th1 endotypes in Beijing/China might be related to the population of that city be exposed to higher levels of PM 2.5 when compared to the populations of Chengdu/China and other regions of Europe, Australia, and Japan.

In summary, the endotypes of CRS as based on immunological and inflammatory factors described in the studies cited above confirm that

Table 21.1 Summary of the studies investigating endotypes of CRS

Authors (Publication year)	Population	Associated phenotype (Sample size)	Proportion of endotypes or comparisons between different regions	Ref
Kountakis et al. (2004)	American	CRSwNP (34) CRSsNP (13)	Eosinophilic CRSwNP = 76.5% Eosinophilic CRSsNP = 15.4% Total eosinophilic CRS = 59.6%	[24]
Zhang et al. (2008)	Belgian Chinese	CRSwNP (26 Belgian; 29 Chinese)	ECP/MPO > 2 in Belgian ECP/MPO = 0.25 in Chinese	[10]
Armengot et al. (2010)	Spanish	CRSwNP (40)	Eosinophilic CRSwNP ≥80% Non-eosinophilic CRSwNP ≤20%	[25]
Kim et al. (2007)	Korean	CRSwNP (30)	Eosinophilic CRSwNP = 33.3% Non-eosinophilic CRSwNP = 66.7%	[26]
Cao et al. (2009)	Chinese	CRSwNP (151) CRSsNP (94)	Eosinophilic CRSwNP = 46.4% Eosinophilic CRSsNP = 12% Total eosinophilic CRS = 33.1%	[12]
Kim et al. (2013)	Korean	CRSwNP in 1993 (104) CRSwNP in 2011 (112)	Eosinophilic CRSwNP in 1993 = 24% Eosinophilic CRSsNP in 2011 = 50.9%	[19]
Tomassen et al. (2016)	European	CRS (173)	Non-type-2 = 44% Moderate type-2 = 38% Severe type-2 = 18%	[13]
Turner et al. (2018)	North American	CRS (88)	Non-type-2 = 15% Mild type-2 = 70% Moderate type-2 = 8% Severe type-2 = 7%	[16]
Liao et al. (2018)	Chinese	CRS (246)	Non-type-2 = 83% Moderate type-2 = 4% Severe type-2 = 13%	[15]
Wang et al. (2016)	European; Australian Chinese; Japanese	CRS (139 European; 218 Chinese; 53 Australian; 25 Japanese)	IL-5(+) CRSwNP: 82–84% in Europe; 73% in Australia; 55% in Japan; 20%–61% in China IL-5(+) CRSsNP: 33%–35% in Europe; 40% in Australia; 5%–36% in China	[7]

Abbreviations: *CRS* Chronic rhinosinusitis, *CRSsNP* Chronic rhinosinusitis without nasal polyps, *CRSwNP* Chronic rhinosinusitis with nasal polyps, *ECP* eosinophil cationic protein, *MPO* myeloperoxidase, *Ref* reference

CRS is a heterogeneous inflammatory disease that exists in a variety of patterns in different geographical regions (See Table 21.1 and Fig. 6.1). ENT specialists should be aware of the variations and inflammatory patterns that exist in their region of practice, as this will have impact on the therapeutic approaches used when treating their patents (e.g. treatment with a biologic agent alone or vs. some other form of treatment) [27–31]. With the advent of precision medicine, endotyping will become more important for deciding how to treat severe disease in the near future.

References

1. Van Zele T, Claeys S, Gevaert P, Van Maele G, Holtappels G, Van Cauwenberge P, et al. Differentiation of chronic sinus diseases by measurement of inflammatory mediators. Allergy. 2006;61(11):1280–9. https://doi.org/10.1111/j.1398-9995.2006.01225.x.
2. Mygind N, Dahl R, Bachert C. Nasal polyposis, eosinophil dominated inflammation, and allergy. Thorax. 2000;55(Suppl 2):S79–83. https://doi.org/10.1136/thorax.55.suppl_2.s79.
3. Zhang Y, Gevaert E, Lou H, Wang X, Zhang L, Bachert C, et al. Chronic rhinosinusitis in Asia. J Allergy Clin Immunol. 2017;140(5):1230–9. https://doi.org/10.1016/j.jaci.2017.09.009.
4. Lou H, Wang C, Zhang L. Endotype-driven precision medicine in chronic rhinosinusitis. Expert Rev Clin Immunol. 2019;15(11):1171–83. https://doi.org/10.1080/1744666X.2020.1679626.
5. Rosenfeld RM, Andes D, Bhattacharyya N, Cheung D, Eisenberg S, Ganiats TG, et al. Clinical practice guideline: adult sinusitis. Otolaryngol Head Neck Surg. 2007;137(3 Suppl):S1–31. https://doi.org/10.1016/j.otohns.2007.06.726.
6. Cardell LO, Stjarne P, Jonstam K, Bachert C. Endotypes of chronic rhinosinusitis: impact on management. J Allergy Clin Immunol. 2020;145(3):752–6. https://doi.org/10.1016/j.jaci.2020.01.019.
7. Wang X, Zhang N, Bo M, Holtappels G, Zheng M, Lou H, et al. Diversity of TH cytokine profiles in patients with chronic rhinosinusitis: a multicenter study in Europe, Asia, and Oceania. J Allergy Clin Immunol. 2016;138(5):1344–53. https://doi.org/10.1016/j.jaci.2016.05.041.
8. Lou H, Meng Y, Piao Y, Zhang N, Bachert C, Wang C, et al. Cellular phenotyping of chronic rhinosinusitis with nasal polyps. Rhinology. 2016;54(2):150–9. https://doi.org/10.4193/Rhin15.271.
9. Zhang N, Holtappels G, Claeys C, Huang G, van Cauwenberge P, Bachert C. Pattern of inflammation and impact of *Staphylococcus aureus* enterotoxins in nasal polyps from southern China. Am J Rhinol. 2006;20(4):445–50. https://doi.org/10.2500/ajr.2006.20.2887.
10. Zhang N, Van Zele T, Perez-Novo C, Van Bruaene N, Holtappels G, DeRuyck N, et al. Different types of T-effector cells orchestrate mucosal inflammation in chronic sinus disease. J Allergy Clin Immunol. 2008;122(5):961–8. https://doi.org/10.1016/j.jaci.2008.07.008.
11. Bachert C, Zhang N, Holtappels G, De Lobel L, van Cauwenberge P, Liu S, et al. Presence of IL-5 protein and IgE antibodies to staphylococcal enterotoxinsin nasal polyps is associated with comorbid asthma. J Allergy Clin Immunol. 2010;126(5):962–8, 8.e1–6. https://doi.org/10.1016/j.jaci.2010.07.007.
12. Cao PP, Li HB, Wang BF, Wang SB, You XJ, Cui YH, et al. Distinct immunopathologic characteristics of various types of chronic rhinosinusitis in adult Chinese. J Allergy Clin Immunol. 2009;124(3):478–84, 84.e1–2. https://doi.org/10.1016/j.jaci.2009.05.017.
13. Tomassen P, Vandeplas G, Van Zele T, Cardell LO, Arebro J, Olze H, et al. Inflammatory endotypes of chronic rhinosinusitis based on cluster analysis of biomarkers. J Allergy Clin Immunol. 2016;137(5):1449–56.e4. https://doi.org/10.1016/j.jaci.2015.12.1324.
14. Anderson GP. Endotyping asthma: new insights into key pathogenic mechanisms in a complex, heterogeneous disease. Lancet. 2008;372(9643):1107–19. https://doi.org/10.1016/S0140-6736(08)61452-X.
15. Liao B, Liu JX, Li ZY, Zhen Z, Cao PP, Yao Y, et al. Multidimensional endotypes of chronic rhinosinusitis and their association with treatment outcomes. Allergy. 2018;73(7):1459–69. https://doi.org/10.1111/all.13411.
16. Turner JH, Chandra RK, Li P, Bonnet K, Schlundt DG. Identification of clinically relevant chronic rhinosinusitis endotypes using cluster analysis of mucus cytokines. J Allergy Clin Immunol 2018;141(5):1895–7.e7. https://doi.org/10.1016/j.jaci.2018.02.002.
17. Katotomichelakis M, Tantilipikorn P, Holtappels G, De Ruyck N, Feng L, Van Zele T, et al. Inflammatory patterns in upper airway disease in the same geographical area may change over time. Am J Rhinol Allergy. 2013;27(5):354–60. https://doi.org/10.2500/ajra.2013.27.3922.
18. Shin SH, Ye MK, Kim JK, Cho CH. Histological characteristics of chronic rhinosinusitis with nasal polyps: recent 10-year experience of a single center in Daegu, Korea. Am J Rhinol Allergy. 2014;28(2):95–8. https://doi.org/10.2500/ajra.2014.28.4003.
19. Kim SJ, Lee KH, Kim SW, Cho JS, Park YK, Shin SY. Changes in histological features of nasal polyps in a Korean population over a 17-year period. Otolaryngol Head Neck Surg. 2013;149(3):431–7. https://doi.org/10.1177/0194599813495363.
20. Jiang WX, Cao PP, Li ZY, Zhai GT, Liao B, Lu X, et al. A retrospective study of changes of histopa-

thology of nasal polyps in adult Chinese in central China. Rhinology. 2019;57(4):261–7. https://doi.org/10.4193/Rhin18.070.
21. Wang W, Gao Y, Zhu Z, Zha Y, Wang X, Qi F, et al. Changes in the clinical and histological characteristics of Chinese chronic rhinosinusitis with nasal polyps over 11 years. Int Forum Allergy Rhinol. 2019;9(2):149–57. https://doi.org/10.1002/alr.22234.
22. Chen BY, Chan CC, Lee CT, Cheng TJ, Huang WC, Jhou JC, et al. The association of ambient air pollution with airway inflammation in schoolchildren. Am J Epidemiol. 2012;175(8):764–74. https://doi.org/10.1093/aje/kwr380.
23. Qing H, Wang X, Zhang N, Zheng K, Du K, Zheng M, et al. The effect of fine particulate matter on the inflammatory responses in human upper airway Mucosa. Am J Respir Crit Care Med. 2019;200(10):1315–8. https://doi.org/10.1164/rccm.201903-0635LE.
24. Kountakis SE, Arango P, Bradley D, Wade ZK, Borish L. Molecular and cellular staging for the severity of chronic rhinosinusitis. Laryngoscope. 2004;114(11):1895–905. https://doi.org/10.1097/01.mlg.0000147917.43615.c0.
25. Armengot M, Garin L, de Lamo M, Krause F, Carda C. Cytological and tissue eosinophilia correlations in nasal polyposis. Am J Rhinol Allergy. 2010;24(6):413–5. https://doi.org/10.2500/ajra.2010.24.3549.
26. Kim JW, Hong SL, Kim YK, Lee CH, Min YG, Rhee CS. Histological and immunological features of non-eosinophilic nasal polyps. Otolaryngol Head Neck Surg. 2007;137(6):925–30. https://doi.org/10.1016/j.otohns.2007.07.036.
27. Bachert C, Han JK, Desrosiers M, Hellings PW, Amin N, Lee SF, et al. Dupilumab efficacy and safety in severe chronic rhinosinusitis with nasal polyps in the multicentre, randomised, double-blind, placebo-controlled, parallel group phase 3 trials Liberty NP Sinus-24 and Liberty NP Sinus-52. Lancet. 2019;394(10209):1638–50.
28. Bachert C, Mannent L, Naclerio RM, Mullol J, Ferguson BJ, Gevaert P, et al. Effect of subcutaneous dupilumab on nasal polyp burden in patients with chronic sinusitis and nasal polyposis: a randomized clinical trial. JAMA. 2016;315(5):469–79. https://doi.org/10.1001/jama.2015.19330.
29. Gevaert P, Calus L, Van Zele T, Blomme K, De Ruyck N, Bauters W, et al. Omalizumab is effective in allergic and nonallergic patients with nasal polyps and asthma. J Allergy Clin Immunol, 2013;131:110–6.e1. https://doi.org/10.1016/j.jaci.2012.07.047. Epub 2012 Sep 27. PMID: 23021878.
30. Gevaert P, Lang-Loidolt D, Lackner A, Stammberger H, Staudinger H, Van Zele T, et al. Nasal IL-5 levels determine the response to anti-IL-5 treatment in patients with nasal polyps. J Allergy Clin Immunol. 2006;118:1133–41. https://doi.org/10.1016/j.jaci.2006.05.031.
31. Van Zele T, Gevaert P, Holtappels G, Beule Achim, Wormald PJ, Mayr S, et al. Oral steroids and doxycycline: two different approaches to treat nasal polyps. J Allergy Clin Immunol, 2010;125:1069–1076.e4. https://doi.org/10.1016/j.jaci.2010.02.020.

22 Multimorbidities

David Bedoya, Cristóbal Langdon, Isam Alobid, José Antonio Castillo, and Joaquim Mullol

Key Points

- Allergic rhinitis, asthma, and intolerance to aspirin are well-known and common multimorbidities in the patient with chronic rhinosinusitis.
- Presentation of chronic rhinosinusitis can vary according to multimorbidities. Increase on the impact on severity, quality of life, and control, and therapeutic cost are significant depending on their presence or absence in CRS patients.
- To understand the comorbidities of patients with chronic rhinosinusitis under the concept of Unified Airways is essential to provide them the best and appropriate treatment. Health care providers should take into count those conditions.

22.1 Introduction

Chronic rhinosinusitis (CRS) is defined as a heterogeneous inflammatory disease of the mucosa of the nose and paranasal sinuses. Patients with CRS remain symptomatic for more than 12 weeks, and present alterations in nasal endos-

D. Bedoya
Rhinology Unit and Smell Clinic, Department of Otorhinolaryngology, Hospital Clínic, Universitat de Barcelona, Barcelona, Catalonia, Spain

Clinical & Experimental respiratory Immunoallergy, IDIBAPS, Barcelona, Catalonia, Spain

Sinonasal Inflammatory and Olfactory Research Group (INGENIO), IRCE, IDIBAPS, Barcelona, Catalonia, Spain

I. Alobid
Rhinology Unit & Smell Clinic, Department of Otorhinolaryngology, Hospital Clínic, Universitat de Barcelona, Barcelona, Catalonia, Spain

Clinical & Experimental Respiratory Immunoallergy, Institut d'Investigacions, Biomèdiques August Pi i Sunyer (IDIBAPS), Barcelona, Catalonia, Spain

CIBER of Respiratory Diseases (CIBERES), Barcelona, Catalonia, Spain

C. Langdon · J. Mullol (✉)
Rhinology Unit & Smell Clinic, Department of Otorhinolaryngology, Hospital Clínic, Universitat de Barcelona, Barcelona, Catalonia, Spain

Clinical & Experimental Respiratory Immunoallergy, Institut d'Investigacions, Biomèdiques August Pi i Sunyer (IDIBAPS), Barcelona, Catalonia, Spain

Sinonasal Inflammatory and Olfactory Research Group (INGENIO), IRCE, IDIBAPS, Barcelona, Catalonia, Spain

CIBER of Respiratory Diseases (CIBERES), Barcelona, Catalonia, Spain
e-mail: clangdon@clinic.cat; JMULLOL@clinic.cat

J. A. Castillo
Clinical & Experimental Respiratory Immunoallergy, IDIBAPS, Barcelona, Catalonia, Spain

Respiratory Department, Hospital Universitario Quirón Dexeus, Barcelona, Catalonia, Spain

Rhinitis Group, SEPAR, Barcelona, Catalonia, Spain

L. Zhang, C. Bachert (eds.), *Chronic Rhinosinusitis*, https://doi.org/10.1007/978-981-16-0784-4_22

copy and imaging [1]. It is present in around 11% of the general population [2] and, therefore, it often occurs in the presence of multimorbidities such as allergic rhinitis (AR), asthma, or aspirin sensitivity (N-ERD, NSAID-exacerbated respiratory disease). For them, common or different pathophysiological underlying processes are suggested and named as "endotypes" [3].

Today it is almost impossible to ignore the concept of the Unified Airway. Multiple investigations as well as daily clinical practice prove the tight relationship between interrelated conditions such as asthma and chronic rhinosinusitis with nasal polyps (CRSwNP) [4]. Knowledge about multimorbidities can be determinant to optimize the achievement of better therapeutic outcomes. Patients refractory to medical treatment and who even failed functional endoscopic sinus surgery (FESS) have been found to have more asthma (48.4%), inhalant allergy (38.7%), and NSAID sensitivity (16.0%) [5]. Today's challenge is to find the best treatment for individual CRS patients, under personalized and precision medicine, where the identification of comorbidities is essential.

22.2 Allergic Rhinitis

AR is the most common chronic inflammatory IgE-mediated condition of the nasal mucosa. It is characterized by nasal obstruction, rhinorrhea, nasal itching, sneezing [6], and even loss of smell in the most severe patients [7, 8]. Despite the old concept stating that AR provokes ostiomeatal edema which induces retentions of secretions and facilitates CRS [9], the physiopathological mechanism linking AR and CRS remains unclear [10]. Although it is known that aeroallergens do not penetrate in a significant amount to induce an allergic response in the paranasal sinuses, Baroody et al. [11]demonstrated how a unilateral local stimulus in the nose may trigger a systemic response, able to induce contralateral inflammation in the maxillary sinus, highlighting that systemic response of AR can induce a local inflammatory reaction in the paranasal sinuses [12]. Recently, molecular characterization of the mucosal remodeling effect of AR in CRS had been described and patients with CRS with nasal polyps (CRSwNP) showed enhanced goblet cell hyperplasia, VEGF-A, microvessel density, and MMP-9 expression while patients with CRS without nasal polyps (CRSsNP) showed an increased expression of collagen fibers, TGF-β_1, and MMP-7 [13].

Pathophysiologic mechanisms of CRSwNP and AR as both are related to an immune response through Th2 cells, but an epidemiological relationship still has to be proved. Prevalence of nasal polyps in atopic patients is the same than the general population (more or less 0.5%) [14]. And the prevalence of allergic rhinitis in the general population is the same in CRSwNP patients (25 vs 28%) [15], additionally nasal polyps are not more severe in patients with allergy [16]. Patients with CRS have frequent allergic sensitizations [17] and particularly perennial allergens have been showing a stronger correlation with CRS [14], but the relationship between CRSwNP and allergic sensitization is a controversial issue, still today we do not have sufficient studies to declare the existence of "allergic nasal polyps." In patients with CRSwNP it is possible to find more skin prick test positives than the general population [18]; however, it does not necessarily imply that allergy can modify the presentation or recurrence of nasal polyps [16]. Allergic fungal rhinosinusitis (AFRS) can be considered an endotype of CRSwNP characterized by an allergic response to fungal colonization, particularly *Bipolaris* spp [19]. In a subgroup of patients with localized polyps into middle turbinate, postero-superior septum and superior turbinate have shown almost always sensitization to allergens, it has been denominated Central Compartment Atopic Disease (CCAD) [20].

There are just a few publications about CRSsNP and allergic rhinitis and most of them are not concluding, a recent study found that Lund-Mackay score, duration of symptoms, visual analog score, and the SNOT-22 score were higher in patients with CRSsNP; specifically, facial pain and ostiomeatal complex obstruction showed a 90% and 100% of specificity, respectively, to differentiate CRSsNP and AR [21].

Although allergy does not have a crucial effect on outcomes of patients with CRSwNP [22]; skin prick test and another allergy testing may just be considered in some patients with CRS due to possible benefits with little harm [14]. Immunotherapy is another controversial issue, some studies of low quality have shown that it can reduce symptoms in short term in patient with CRS [23], however, in AFRS show irrelevant effect, despite the known mechanism of hypersensitivity in these patients [24]. Surgical outcomes can be worst in patients with CRS and comorbid allergic rhinitis, in terms of recurrence and surgical failure [25].

22.3 Asthma

Asthma and CRS show similarities, even since definition; both are known as heterogeneous diseases characterized by inflammation with airway related symptoms that vary over time. In case of asthma, the history of respiratory symptoms is related with expiratory airflow limitation, clinically evident as wheeze, shortness of breath, chest tightness, and cough; in CRS, nasal dysfunction manifest as nasal obstruction, decrease in the sense of smell, pain, and changes in normal characteristics of nasal secretions.

CRS is more common in patients with asthma. The prevalence of asthma in CRSsNP (21.16%), CRSwNP (46.91%), and even AFRS patients (73.33%) is higher compared to the general population (9.95%) [26] although comorbid asthma in CRS patients seems to be less frequent in the Asian population [27]. A study founded that 86% of patients with asthma have nasal comorbidities, 50% rhinitis (37% allergic, 13% non-allergic), and 36% CRS (16% without and 20% with nasal polyps) [28]. Comorbid asthma is 12 times more probable if the patient has allergic rhinitis [29]. Loss of smell is frequently disturbed in patients with CRSwNP and asthma [30, 31], and can be considered a predictive symptom of severe asthma [32]. Recently higher serum levels of IL-5 [33] and periostin [34] have been considered as a possible marker of comorbid asthma in patients with CRSwNP. The presence of asthma in patients with CRSwNP also has repercussions in quality of life (QoL) Alobid et al. found worsening of physical functioning, body pain, and vitality [35].

According to the age of onset of symptoms, asthma can be divided into early-onset if symptoms begin before the age of 40 years old and late-onset if the symptoms start later [17]. CRSsNP is more frequent in patients with early-onset asthma and CRSwNP is more frequent in patients with late-onset asthma [27]. Late-onset asthmatics patients have poorer physical function, more frequent nasal polyposis, higher radiological complaints in sinonasal imaging, receive more oral steroid courses frequently and more endoscopic surgeries for CRS management and can be considered as a predictor of severity of disease [36] (Table 22.1).

Physiopathological mechanisms are similar in some patients with asthma and CRS [37] including the role of lymphocytes (Th1 and Th2), profiles of interleukins (IL), and presence of eosinophils (Fig. 22.1). It is known that thymic stromal lymphopoietin (TSLPR), IL- 25, and IL-33 act as triggers of type 2 immunity and IL-5 and IL-13 are important in chemotaxis, differentiation, activation, and survival eosinophils in the upper and lower airway. *Staphylococcus aureus* is a major human pathogen that can produce toxins that act as superantigens, that means simulta-

Table 22.1 Clinical presentation of comorbid asthma in chronic rhinosinusitis patients depending on the onset of asthma

	Onset of disease	CRS phenotype	Disease severity	Multiple surgeries	Impact on QoL	Nasal endoscopic findings	Imaging findings (CT, MRI)	Difficult to treat
Early-onset asthma	<40 years	CRSsNP	++	++	++	+	+	+++
Late-onset asthma	≥40 years	CRSwNP	++++	++++	++++	+++	+++	+/–

Phenotypic manifestation of co-morbid CRS and asthma with clinical implications

CRS chronic rhinosinusitis, *CRS* chronic rhinosinusitis without (CRSsNP) or with (CRSwNP) nasal polyps, *CT* computed tomography, *MRI* magnetic resonance imaging, *QoL* quality of life

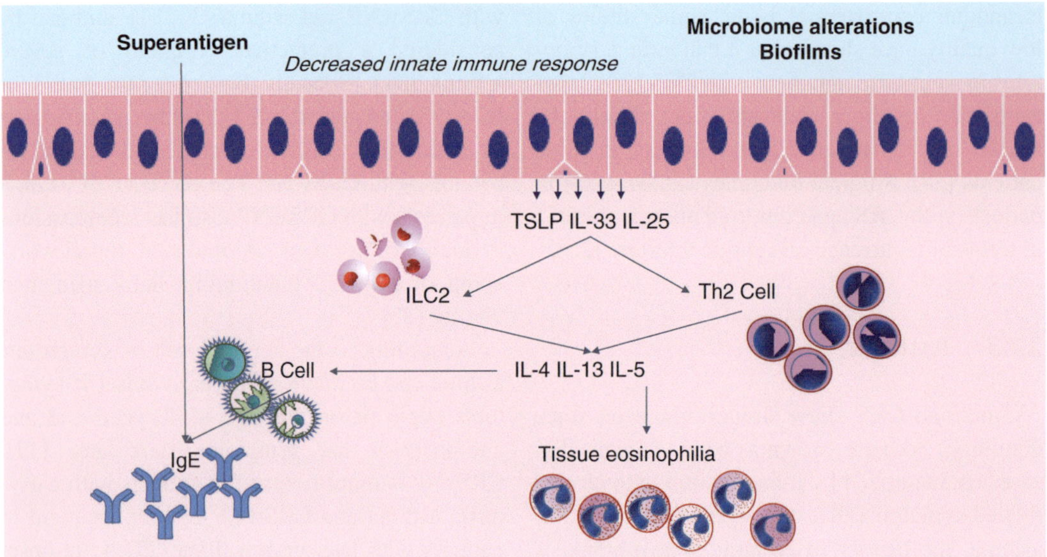

Fig. 22.1 Immunopathology of CRSwNP. Similar mechanisms in immunopathology support the strong relationship between chronic rhinosinusitis and allergic asthma, making promising common therapeutic targets on common mechanisms of both diseases. Abbreviations: *IFN-γ* interferon γ, *IgE* Immunoglobulin E, *IL* interleukin, *ILC2* type 2 innate lymphoid cells, *TSLP* thymic stromal lymphopoietin

neous activations of T-cell receptor and major histocompatibility complex (MHC), inducing a polyclonal response and, finally, a Th2 inflammation imbalance. Had been proving the role of intramucosal *S. aureus* in the physiopathology of nasal polyps and bronchial hyperresponsiveness [38]. Staphylococcal enterotoxin immunoglobulin E (IgE) is associated with persistence and severity of eosinophilic inflammation and is more frequently founded in nasal polyps in patients with asthma [39]. In patients with CRSsNP, a relationship with asthma has been described. T1 T-cell immune response, with neutrophil as the main actor of the inflammation, has been found in these patients by the release of interleukins as IFN-, IL-1, IL-3, IL-6, and IL-8 by dendritic cells. IL-17 can have an important role also [40].

Asthma comorbid in patients with CRS has important implications in treatment and prognosis. The severity, control, and exacerbations of asthma are strongly associated with CRS [29, 41, 42]. Patients with CRS have 3 fold more risk to have asthma, even 45% of patients with CRSwNP will suffer asthma during the course of the disease [43], also the severity and duration of CRS are higher in asthma comorbid patients [44]; sinus opacification is correlated with uncontrolled asthma [45]. Control of both diseases is directly related and dependent [42], asthmatic patients have more severe CRS and polyps are more frequently founded [8]. As for the treatment, nasal steroid and montelukast improve asthma and CRS symptoms in some patients, but without modification in the nose or lung function [46]. Endoscopic sinus surgery in patient with CRS and comorbid asthma had proven to improve not only sinus disease, even an improvement of asthma control, decrease in asthma attack and hospitalizations, as well as a reduction in oral steroid consumption [47]. Comorbid asthma is currently recognized as a predictor of recalcitrant CRS and complete removal of diseased mucosa and Draf type III in primary surgery should be considered [48].

Some special considerations have to take in count due to biologic treatments available on patients with CRSwNP and asthma, especially severe asthma [49]. With omalizumab, some authors have demonstrated similar results to surgery in relation to a reduction in polyp size [50], improvement in CT sinus opacification, QoL [46, 51] and control of asthma and CRS similarly than surgery [52]. Reslizumab decreases the size of polyps in patients with elevated nasal IL-5 [53] and mepolizumab reduces the need for surgery in 30% of the studied cohort [54]. Dupilumab has shown the best results, in June 2019 it was approved by the agency of Food and Drug Administration (FDA) in the USA, for the management of CRSwNP. It has been shown that dupilumab improves the sense of smell and other nasal symptoms, improves endoscopic findings, quality of life, and lung function, and decreases the number of surgeries and its effect is maintained up to 52 weeks [55].

22.4 Non-Steroidal Anti-Inflammatory Drug (NSAID): Exacerbated Respiratory Disease

Today, we know the triad of CRSwNP, severe late-onset asthma, and non-IgE-mediated hypersensitivity to non-steroidal anti-inflammatory drugs (NSAIDS) as a severe subtype of CRS [56, 57]. NSAIDs sensitivity is recognized as a metabolic condition which predispose to eosinophilic inflammation [58] which is present in the general population in 0.3–2.5% [59], in CRSsNP similar to former (3.3%) but in CRSwNP patients is higher (9.6–26%) [60], and in AFRS patients is highest (40%), and a significant relationship has been founded (OR 9.64) [26].

Patients with NSAID-exacerbated respiratory disease (N-ERD) have a proinflammatory imbalance due to an increase of cysteinyl leukotrienes (cysLTs), owing to overexpression of 5-lipoxygenase (5-LO) and LTC_4 synthase besides cyclooxygenase (COX)-2 activity, which is associated with overexpression of cysLT receptors [61] and ultimately leads to increase in mast cell activation and eosinophilic inflammation (Fig. 22.2) [43]. Clinical evolution usually shows a chronological progression of nasal polyps, late-onset asthma and finally intolerance to aspirin.

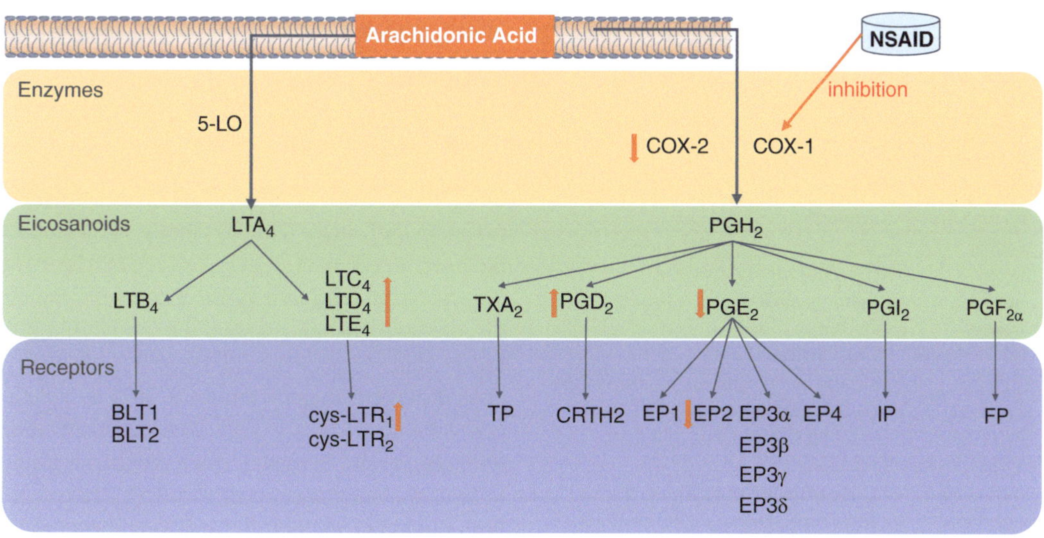

Fig. 22.2 Eicosanoid pathomechanisms of NSAID-exacerbated respiratory disease (N-ERD). Inhibition of cyclooxygenase-1 (COX-1) by NSAID decreases biosynthesis of prostaglandin E_2 (PGE_2) from arachidonic acid (AA). Deficiency of PGE_2, an anti-inflammatory mediator, and its receptor (EP2) is not compensated by the inducible isoenzyme cyclooxygenase-2 (COX-2), which is down-regulated in N-ERD. The production of the chemoattractant prostaglandin D_2 (PGD_2), a proinflammatory mediator, is also up-regulated. Excess of AA substrate is metabolized by 5-lipoxygenase (5-LO) to cysteinyl leukotrienes (*cysLTs*: LTC_4, LTD_4, and LTE_4), also potent proinflammatory mediators [57]. *5-LO 5-lipoxygenase*, *BLT* leukotriene B receptor, CRTH2 Prostaglandin D receptor 2, *cys-LTR* cysteinyl-leukotriene receptor, *EP* E-prostanoid receptor, *IP* prostacyclin receptor, *FP* prostaglandin F receptor, *LTA* leukotriene A, *LTB* leukotriene B, *NSAID* non-steroidal anti-inflammatory drug, *PGH* prostaglandin H, *PGF* prostaglandin F, *PGI* prostaglandin I/prostacyclin, *TP* thromboxane receptor

Although aspirin provocation tests continue as the gold standard for diagnosis of aspirin hypersensitivity, no specific sinus test has been described for N-ERD, a study showed more opacification of ethmoid and frontal sinus in computed tomography (CT) in comparison to CRSwNP patients [62].

Despite dietary recommendations can vary according to geographic locations, culture and availability of foods, a 6-week low-salicylate diet has proven to improve QoL, nasal symptoms, objective nasal endoscopic evaluation scores and asthma control [63] and a 2-week diet high in omega-3 and low in omega-6 fatty acids decrease levels of urinary leukotriene E_4 and urinary prostaglandin D_2 associated with control of asthma and sinus symptoms [64]. Overall low salicylates diet should be included restriction of dried fruits, berries, herbs, and some spices. It is unknown the mechanism, but patients with N-ERD can reproduce their symptoms with alcoholic beverages and also avoiding should be recommended [65] (Table 22.2).

Since medical and surgical treatment is so important, N-ERD patients should include an interdisciplinary approach to achieve the best outcomes. CysLTs are considered the primary markers and the main physiopathological way, pharmacological modification of cysLT cascade can be interesting for patients with N-ERD. Montelukast and zafirlukast act as cysLT-R_1 inhibitors and zileuton inhibits 5-LO activity with consequent decrease of cysLT production [66]. Leukotriene modifiers are usually prescribed in the treatment of asthma and allergic rhinitis with comorbid asthma, however, although zileuton seems to be superior to montelukast in N-ERD patients [67], demonstrated by symptom improvement [68], including smell, decrease of nasal polyp, reduction in the need of systemic steroids, improvement in nasal airflow, and decrease of eosinophils in nasal lavage [69]. Nevertheless, antileukotrienes in N-ERD do not show a differential effect compared with CRSwNP patients [9], and besides, important side effects had been reported, include hepatotoxicity (only with zileuton, 4.4%) and neuropsychiatric alterations such as sleep disturbance, depression, anxiety, psychotic reactions, and even completed suicides in adolescents [70]. Its uses should be limited to patients with N-ERD with persistent symptoms despite intranasal steroid and nasal irrigation treatment [56].

Extended surgery, such as Draf Type III procedure, and subsequently ASA desensitization maintain QoL more than 30 months and decrease the need for revision surgery 9.4% [71]. However, in recalcitrant CRS as in N-ERD, it is important to discuss with patients about the possibilities to repeat sinus surgery during the course of the disease. Revision surgery rates are 37% at 5 years and 89% at 10 years [72]. The desensitization with acetyl salicylic acid (ASA) remains an essential treatment in patients with N-ERD. This procedure includes an oral (most commonly used) challenge with ASA by using incremental doses achieving a maintenance dose. This initial step should be done in a monitored environment due to the risk of severe reactions. To keep the therapeutic effect, maintenance doses should be daily administered, a delay of 24–48 h could not only affect patients missing the therapeutic effect even also can induce severe pseudo allergic reactions

Table 22.2 Dietary recommendations in patients with N-ERD

Dietary modification	Examples
High in omega-3 *Mainly in foods of animal origin*	Vegetable oils: soy, chia seeds, flaxseed, canola, soybean Salmon, albacore, shellfish, trout, sardine Oats, avocado
High in omega-6 *Reduce the consumption*	Diminish: coconut oil, chicken eggs (yolk), corn oil, whole meal bread, meat fat (mainly from poultry), sausage
Foods rich in salicylates *Reduce the consumption*	Olives, blueberries, prunes, dates, strawberry, guava, melon, orange, blackberry, raisins, pineapple, grape, chard, radishes, zucchini, almonds, olive oil, coconut oil, turmeric, ginger, curry
Alcoholic beverages	In general, its restriction is recommended

Dietary modifications to diminish the ingestion of salicylates could be benefic in patients with N-ERD [64, 65]
N-ERD NSAID-exacerbated respiratory disease, *NSAID* non-steroidal anti-inflammatory drug

[73]. Therapeutic effects of desensitization are superior to a strict ASA avoidance [74]; in patients with N-ERD had proved symptomatic improvement, including the sense of smell, nasal polyps decrease, decreased use of intranasal or systemic steroids [75], improvement in health-related QoL, reduction in revision endoscopic sinus surgery [76]. ASA desensitization is indicated in patients with positive aspirin challenge test with persistent symptoms despite endoscopic sinus surgery. It represents a final therapeutic option, especially in patients with an indication of revision surgery or the need of COX-1 inhibitor therapy for cardiovascular protection or anti-inflammatory treatment [76]. Desensitization is contraindicated in pregnancy, unstable asthma, coagulation disorders or anticoagulation therapy, and gastric ulcer.

Monoclonal antibodies treatment has been used N-ERD patients. Although N-ERD it is not an IgE mediated reaction, omalizumab decreases cysLTs and PGD_2 probably by reducing mast cell activation [65]. Mepolizumab studies have reported an improvement in QoL, olfaction, and decrease in polyp size and dupilumab study showed more effective results in several outcomes in N-ERD than in non-N-ERD patients [67, 77].

22.5 Gastroesophageal Reflux

Gastroesophageal reflux disease (GERD) can be defined as a condition that develops when the reflux of stomach contents causes troublesome symptoms and/or complications [78], it has been found to be present in 10–20% of the general population [79], on the other hand, CRS have also known as a high prevalence disease; the above and the fact that a biological mechanism it is not completely determined, still today a strong relation between CRS and GERD is yet to be established. Two systematic reviews of GERD and CRS had been published to try to elucidate this controversial relationship [80, 81].

Possible mechanisms of GERD implicated in CRS can be: (1) direct exposure of gastric acid to the nasal and nasopharyngeal mucosa, with consequent mucosal edema and mucociliary clearance disturbance [82], (2) an autonomic dysregulation originated by esophageal irritation with consequent sinonasal swelling neural mechanism [83]; and (3) through *H. pylori* colonization and proinflammatory induce environment.

In adult patients with CRS the relationship with GERD is controversial. Ph-metry with dual-channel tube (pharynx and esophagus) was positive in 88% and specific activity of pepsin in nasal secretion was detected in 82% of patients with CRS versus 55% and 50% in controls [84]. Patients with recalcitrant CRS can have abnormal pH-metry in the nasopharynx in up to 95%, higher DeMeester score [83] and a more alkaline pH in middle meatus also have been related [85], however pepsin and pepsinogen I were not found different [86]; *H pylori* was found in 28.9% of adult patients with surgery due to CRSwNP in comparison to 3.3% of control patients with nasal surgery for deviated septum [87]. Alteration of mucociliary clearance in patients with GERD had not shown concluding data, studies published had shown normal values [88]. Conventional pH study indicates pathological extraesophageal reflux below 5 in patients with CRS [89] and even greater non-acid episodes also have importance when multichannel impedance-pH monitoring has done [90].

Some studies tried to answer the question regarding GERD as a prognostic factor after functional endoscopic sinus surgery (FESS). Results are not conclusive, some studies found worse outcomes and correlation with refractory CRS [89, 91]and another does not find a correlation [92], or even better [93]. In children with CRS without an adequate response to medical treatment, GERD has shown to be an important element to take in the count before surgery [94].

22.6 Chronic Pulmonary Obstructive Disease

Pulmonary comorbid diseases in patients with CRS are not limited to asthma, also patients with chronic pulmonary obstructive disease (COPD) can be considered as a lower-airway related condition. COPD patients have frequent upper respiratory symptoms and 53–88% of them can be diagnosed with CRS [95]. The association is not only limited to symptoms since COPD can predict the establishment of CRSsNP at 5 years [96]. Patients with multimorbid CRS and COPD have an increased severity of the pulmonary disease [97] and may have overall higher compromise of QoL due to CRS [98] although not related with disease-specific compromise [99]. However, a common physiopathological mechanism is still debated [100] and CRS can be associated with direct exposure of upper-airway to tobacco smoke [101].

22.7 Bronchiectasis

Bronchiectasis is a chronic lower-airway disease characterized by permanent and irreversible destruction and dilatation of small and medium-sized airways as a structural consequence and associated with recurrent lower-airway infections with further progressive alteration of lower-airway anatomy. At least 50% of patients do not have an identifiable etiology and are considered idiopathic [102]. CRS prevalence in bronchiectasis patients, either idiopathic or post-infective, goes from 62% of adults [103] to 77% [7] of adult patients where 26% reported CRSwNP. This lower airway multimorbidity has a significant impact in quality of life of patients with CRS [7, 104]. Although a common mechanism is still unknown, bronchiectasis in patients with CRS should be suspected if chronic cough or unexplained recurrent lower-respiratory infections are present [105].

22.8 Translation into Future Daily Practice

- Allergic rhinitis can be a confounding factor in CRS presentation and differential diagnosis should be performed to provide an appropriate treatment.
- Asthma multimorbidity in patients with CRS, especially with nasal polyps, is determinant for severity and prognosis. All patients with CRS should be actively interrogated lower-airway symptoms.
- N-ERD represents a special subgroup of CRS patients with increased severity and decreased QOL, difficult-to-treat, and poor prognosis.
- GERD remains as a controversial association in CRS. Particularly important in children, this multimorbidity can be related to a recalcitrant presentation of CRS.
- The association of CRS, with/without nasal polyps, with other lower-airway diseases such as bronchiectasis and COPD should be considered as integral management of these patients.
- Given the high prevalence and association of CRS with lower-airway diseases a multidisciplinary approach is also needed to reach patient's optimal management.

References

1. Fokkens WJ, Lund VJ, Mullol J, Bachert C, Alobid I, Baroody F, et al. EPOS 2012: European position paper on rhinosinusitis and nasal polyps 2012. A summary for otorhinolaryngologists. Rhinology. 2012;50(1):1–12. https://doi.org/10.4193/Rhino50E2.
2. Hastan D, Fokkens WJ, Bachert C, Newson RB, Bislimovska J, Bockelbrink A, Bousquet PJ, Brozek G, Bruno A, et al. Chronic rhinosinusitis in Europe – an underestimated disease. A GA^{2}LEN study. Allergy. 2011;66(9):1216–23. https://doi.org/10.1111/j.1398-9995.2011.02646.x.
3. Akdis CA, Bachert C, Cingi C, Dykewicz MS, Hellings PW, Naclerio RM, et al. Endotypes and phenotypes of chronic rhinosinusitis: a PRACTALL document of the European Academy of Allergy and Clinical Immunology and the American Academy of Allergy, Asthma & Immunology. J Allergy Clin Immunol. 2013;131(6):1479–90. https://doi.org/10.1016/j.jaci.2013.02.036.
4. Passalacqua G, Ciprandi G, Canonica GW. The nose-lung interaction in allergic rhinitis and asthma: united airways disease. Curr Opin Allergy Clin Immunol. 2001;1(1):7–13. https://doi.org/10.1097/01.all.0000010978.62527.4e.
5. Batra PS, Tong L, Citardi MJ. Analysis of comorbidities and objective parameters in refractory chronic rhinosinusitis. Laryngoscope. 2013;123 Suppl 7:S1–11. https://doi.org/10.1002/lary.24418.
6. Brożek JL, Bousquet J, Agache I, Agarwal A, Bachert C, Bosnic-Anticevich S, et al. Allergic Rhinitis and its Impact on Asthma (ARIA) guidelines-2016

revision. J Allergy Clin Immunol. 2017;140(4):950–8. https://doi.org/10.1016/j.jaci.2017.03.050.
7. Guilemany JM, Angrill J, Alobid I, Centellas S, Prades E, Roca J, et al. United airways: the impact of chronic rhinosinusitis and nasal polyps in bronchiectasic patient's quality of life. Allergy. 2009;64(10):1524–9. https://doi.org/10.1111/j.1398-9995.2009.02011.x.
8. Langdon C, Mullol J. Nasal polyps in patients with asthma: prevalence, impact, and management challenges. J Asthma Allergy. 2016;9:45–53. https://doi.org/10.2147/jaa.S86251.
9. Lanza DC, Kennedy DW. Adult rhinosinusitis defined. Otolaryngol Head Neck Surg. 1997; 117(3 Pt 2):S1–7. https://doi.org/10.1016/s0194-5998(97)70001-9.
10. Wilson KF, McMains KC, Orlandi RR. The association between allergy and chronic rhinosinusitis with and without nasal polyps: an evidence-based review with recommendations. Int Forum Allergy Rhinol. 2014;4(2):93–103. https://doi.org/10.1002/alr.21258.
11. Baroody FM, Mucha SM, Detineo M. Nasal challenge with allergen leads to maxillary sinus inflammation. J Allergy Clin Immunol. 2008;121(5):1126–32.e7. https://doi.org/10.1016/j.jaci.2008.02.010.
12. Adkins TN, Goodgold HM, Hendershott L, Slavin RG. Does inhaled pollen enter the sinus cavities? Ann Allergy Asthma Immunol. 1998;81(2):181–4. https://doi.org/10.1016/s1081-1206(10)62807-4.
13. Kim SY, Park B, Lim H, Kim M, Kong IG, et al. Gastroesophageal reflux disease increases the risk of chronic rhinosinusitis: a nested case-control study using a national sample cohort. Int Forum Allergy Rhinol. 2019;9(4):357–62. https://doi.org/10.1002/alr.22259.
14. Marcus S, Roland LT, DelGaudio JM, Wise SK. The relationship between allergy and chronic rhinosinusitis. Laryngoscope Investig Otolaryngol. 2019;4(1):13–7. https://doi.org/10.1002/lio2.236.
15. Görgülü O, Ozdemir S, Canbolat EP, Sayar C, Olgun MK, Akbaş Y. Analysis of the roles of smoking and allergy in nasal polyposis. Ann Otol Rhinol Laryngol. 2012;121(9):615–9. https://doi.org/10.1177/000348941212100909.
16. Erbek SS, Erbek S, Topal O, Cakmak O. The role of allergy in the severity of nasal polyposis. Am J Rhinol Allergy. 2007;21(6):686–90. https://doi.org/10.2500/ajr.2007.21.3062.
17. Tan DJ, Walters EH, Perret JL, Lodge CJ, Lowe AJ, Matheson MC, et al. Age-of-asthma onset as a determinant of different asthma phenotypes in adults: a systematic review and meta-analysis of the literature. Expert Rev Respir Med. 2015;9(1):109–23. https://doi.org/10.1586/17476348.2015.1000311.
18. del Castillo FM, Jurado-Ramos A, Fernández-Conde BL, Soler R, Barasona MJ, Cantillo E, et al. Allergenic profile of nasal polyposis. J Investig Allergol Clin Immunol. 2009;19(2):110–6.
19. Collins M, Nair S, Smith W, Kette F, Gillis D, Wormald PJ. Role of local immunoglobulin E production in the pathophysiology of noninvasive fungal sinusitis. Laryngoscope. 2004;114(7):1242–6. https://doi.org/10.1097/00005537-200407000-00019.
20. White LJ, Rotella MR, DelGaudio JM. Polypoid changes of the middle turbinate as an indicator of atopic disease. Int Forum Allergy Rhinol. 2014;4(5):376–80. https://doi.org/10.1002/alr.21290.
21. Koskinen A, Numminen J, Markkola A, Karjalainen J, Karstila T, Seppälä M, et al. Diagnostic accuracy of symptoms, endoscopy, and imaging signs of chronic rhinosinusitis without nasal polyps compared to allergic rhinitis. Am J Rhinol Allergy. 2018;32(3):121–31. https://doi.org/10.1177/1945892418762891.
22. Bonfils P, Avan P, Malinvaud D. Influence of allergy on the symptoms and treatment of nasal polyposis. Acta Otolaryngol. 2006;126(8):839–44. https://doi.org/10.1080/00016480500504226.
23. DeYoung K, Wentzel JL, Schlosser RJ, Nguyen SA, Soler ZM. Systematic review of immunotherapy for chronic rhinosinusitis. Am J Rhinol Allergy. 2014;28(2):145–50. https://doi.org/10.2500/ajra.2014.28.4019.
24. Gan EC, Thamboo A, Rudmik L, Hwang PH, Ferguson BJ, et al. Medical management of allergic fungal rhinosinusitis following endoscopic sinus surgery: an evidence-based review and recommendations. Int Forum Allergy Rhinol. 2014;4(9):702–15. https://doi.org/10.1002/alr.21352.
25. Yacoub M-R, Trimarchi M, Cremona G, Farra SD, Ramirez GA, Canti V, et al. Are atopy and eosinophilic bronchial inflammation associated with relapsing forms of chronic rhinosinusitis with nasal polyps? Clin Mol Allergy. 2015;13(1):23. https://doi.org/10.1186/s12948-015-0026-8.
26. Philpott CM, Erskine S, Hopkins C, Kumar N, Anari S, Kara N, et al. Prevalence of asthma, aspirin sensitivity and allergy in chronic rhinosinusitis: data from the UK National Chronic Rhinosinusitis Epidemiology Study. Respir Res. 2018;19(1):129. https://doi.org/10.1186/s12931-018-0823-y.
27. Won HK, Kim YC, Kang MG, Park HK, Lee SE, Kim MH, et al. Age-related prevalence of chronic rhinosinusitis and nasal polyps and their relationships with asthma onset. Ann Allergy Asthma Immunol. 2018;120(4):389–94. https://doi.org/10.1016/j.anai.2018.02.005.
28. Castillo JA PV, Rodrigo G, Juliá B, Picado C, Mullol J. Asthma with nasal polyps: the "severe" phenotype? Eur Respir J 2014:P4118.
29. Jarvis D, Newson R, Lotvall J, Hastan D, Tomassen P, Keil T, et al. Asthma in adults and its association with chronic rhinosinusitis: the GA2LEN survey in Europe. Allergy. 2012;67(1):91–8. https://doi.org/10.1111/j.1398-9995.2011.02709.x.
30. Alobid I, Cardelus S, Benítez P, Guilemany JM, Roca-Ferrer J, Picado C, et al. Persistent asthma has an accumulative impact on the loss of smell in patients

with nasal polyposis. Rhinology. 2011;49(5):519–24. https://doi.org/10.4193/Rhino10.295.
31. Ehnhage A, Olsson P, Kölbeck K-G, Skedinger M, Dahlén B, Alenius M, et al. Functional endoscopic sinus surgery improved asthma symptoms as well as PEFR and olfaction in patients with nasal polyposis. Allergy. 2009;64(5):762–9. https://doi.org/10.1111/j.1398-9995.2008.01870.x.
32. Lehrer E, Mullol J, Agredo F, Alobid I. Management of chronic rhinosinusitis in asthma patients: is there still a debate? Curr Allergy Asthma Rep. 2014;14(6):440. https://doi.org/10.1007/s11882-014-0440-x.
33. Tomassen P, Vandeplas G, Van Zele T, Cardell L-O, Arebro J, Olze H, et al. Inflammatory endotypes of chronic rhinosinusitis based on cluster analysis of biomarkers. J Allergy Clin Immunol. 2016;137(5):1449–56.e4. https://doi.org/10.1016/j.jaci.2015.12.1324.
34. Asano T, Kanemitsu Y, Takemura M, Yokota M, Fukumitsu K, Takeda N, et al. Serum periostin as a biomarker for comorbid chronic rhinosinusitis in patients with asthma. Ann Am Thorac Soc. 2017;14(5):667–75. https://doi.org/10.1513/AnnalsATS.201609-720OC.
35. Alobid I, Benítez P, Bernal-Sprekelsen M, Roca J, Alonso J, Picado C, et al. Nasal polyposis and its impact on quality of life: comparison between the effects of medical and surgical treatments. Allergy. 2005;60(4):452–8. https://doi.org/10.1111/j.1398--9995.2005.00725.x.
36. John Staniorski C, Price CPE, Weibman AR, Welch KC, Conley DB, Shintani-Smith S, et al. Asthma onset pattern and patient outcomes in a chronic rhinosinusitis population. Int Forum Allergy Rhinol. 2018;8(4):495–503. https://doi.org/10.1002/alr.22064.
37. Fahy JV. Type 2 inflammation in asthma – present in most, absent in many. Nat Rev Immunol. 2015;15(1):57–65. https://doi.org/10.1038/nri3786.
38. Muluk NB, Altın F, Cingi C. Role of superantigens in allergic inflammation: their relationship to allergic rhinitis, chronic rhinosinusitis, asthma, and atopic dermatitis. Am J Rhinol Allergy. 2018;32(6):502–17. https://doi.org/10.1177/1945892418801083.
39. Bachert C, Zhang N, Holtappels G, De Lobel L, van Cauwenberge P, Liu S, et al. Presence of IL-5 protein and IgE antibodies to staphylococcal enterotoxins in nasal polyps is associated with comorbid asthma. J Allergy Clin Immunol 2010;126(5):962–8, 8.e1–6. https://doi.org/10.1016/j.jaci.2010.07.007.
40. Bousquet J, Bachert C, Canonica GW, Casale TB, Cruz AA, Lockey RJ, et al. Unmet needs in severe chronic upper airway disease (SCUAD). J Allergy Clin Immunol. 2009;124(3):428–33. https://doi.org/10.1016/j.jaci.2009.06.027.
41. Pearlman AN, Chandra RK, Chang D, Conley DB, Tripathi-Peters A, Grammer LC, et al. Relationships between severity of chronic rhinosinusitis and nasal polyposis, asthma, and atopy. Am J Rhinol Allergy. 2009;23(2):145–8. https://doi.org/10.2500/ajra.2009.23.3284.
42. Lin DC, Chandra RK, Tan BK, Zirkle W, Conley DB, Grammer LC, et al. Association between severity of asthma and degree of chronic rhinosinusitis. Am J Rhinol Allergy. 2011;25(4):205–8. https://doi.org/10.2500/ajra.2011.25.3613.
43. Dixon AE, Kaminsky DA, Holbrook JT, Wise RA, Shade DM, Irvin CG. Allergic rhinitis and sinusitis in asthma: differential effects on symptoms and pulmonary function. Chest. 2006;130(2):429–35. https://doi.org/10.1378/chest.130.2.429.
44. Hopkins C, Andrews P, Holy CE. Does time to endoscopic sinus surgery impact outcomes in chronic rhinosinusitis? Retrospective analysis using the UK clinical practice research data. Rhinology. 2015;53(1):18–24. https://doi.org/10.4193/Rhin14.077.
45. Kountakis SE, Bradley DT. Effect of asthma on sinus computed tomography grade and symptom scores in patients undergoing revision functional endoscopic sinus surgery. Am J Rhinol. 2003;17(4):215–9.
46. Tiotiu A, Plavec D, Novakova S, Mihaicuta S, Novakova P, Labor M, et al. Current opinions for the management of asthma associated with ear, nose and throat comorbidities. Eur Respir Rev. 2018;27(150):180056. https://doi.org/10.1183/16000617.0056-2018.
47. Vashishta R, Soler ZM, Nguyen SA, Schlosser RJ. A systematic review and meta-analysis of asthma outcomes following endoscopic sinus surgery for chronic rhinosinusitis. Int Forum Allergy Rhinol. 2013;3(10):788–94. https://doi.org/10.1002/alr.21182.
48. Alsharif S, Jonstam K, van Zele T, Gevaert P, Holtappels G, Bachert C. Endoscopic sinus surgery for type-2 CRS wNP: an endotype-based retrospective study. Laryngoscope. 2019;129(6):1286–92. https://doi.org/10.1002/lary.27815.
49. Tsetsos N, Goudakos JK, Daskalakis D, Konstantinidis I, Markou K. Monoclonal antibodies for the treatment of chronic rhinosinusitis with nasal polyposis: a systematic review. Rhinology. 2018;56(1):11–21. https://doi.org/10.4193/Rhin17.156.
50. Gevaert P, Calus L, Van Zele T, Blomme K, De Ruyck N, Bauters W, et al. Omalizumab is effective in allergic and nonallergic patients with nasal polyps and asthma. J Allergy Clin Immunol. 2013;131(1):110–6.e1. https://doi.org/10.1016/j.jaci.2012.07.047.
51. Pinto JM, Mehta N, DiTineo M, Wang J, Baroody FM, Naclerio RM. A randomized, double-blind, placebo-controlled trial of anti-IgE for chronic rhinosinusitis. Rhinology. 2010;48(3):318–24. https://doi.org/10.4193/Rhin09.144.
52. Bidder T, Sahota J, Rennie C, Lund VJ, Robinson DS, Kariyawasam HH. Omalizumab treats chronic rhinosinusitis with nasal polyps and asthma together-a real life study. Rhinology. 2018;56(1):42–5. https://doi.org/10.4193/Rhin17.139.

53. Gevaert P, Lang-Loidolt D, Lackner A, Stammberger H, Staudinger H, Van Zele T, et al. Nasal IL-5 levels determine the response to anti-IL-5 treatment in patients with nasal polyps. J Allergy Clin Immunol. 2006;118(5):1133–41. https://doi.org/10.1016/j.jaci.2006.05.031.
54. Bachert C, Sousa AR, Lund VJ, Scadding GK, Gevaert P, Nasser S, et al. Reduced need for surgery in severe nasal polyposis with mepolizumab: Randomized trial. J Allergy Clin Immunol. 2017;140(4):1024–31.e14. https://doi.org/10.1016/j.jaci.2017.05.044.
55. Bachert C, Mannent L, Naclerio RM, Mullol J, Ferguson BJ, Gevaert P, et al. Effect of subcutaneous dupilumab on nasal polyp burden in patients with chronic sinusitis and nasal polyposis: A Randomized Clinical Trial. JAMA 2016;315:469–79. https://doi.org/10.1001/jama.2015.19330.
56. Levy JM, Rudmik L, Peters AT, Wise SK, Rotenberg BW, Smith TL. Contemporary management of chronic rhinosinusitis with nasal polyposis in aspirin-exacerbated respiratory disease: an evidence-based review with recommendations. Int Forum Allergy Rhinol. 2016;6(12):1273–83. https://doi.org/10.1002/alr.21826.
57. Kowalski ML, Agache I, Bavbek S, Bakirtas A, Blanca M, Bochenek G, et al. Diagnosis and management of NSAID-Exacerbated Respiratory Disease (N-ERD)-a EAACI position paper. Allergy. 2019;74(1):28–39. https://doi.org/10.1111/all.13599.
58. Tint D, Kubala S, Toskala E. Risk factors and comorbidities in chronic rhinosinusitis. Curr Allergy Asthma Rep. 2016;16(2):16. https://doi.org/10.1007/s11882-015-0589-y.
59. Graefe H, Roebke C, Schäfer D, Meyer JE. Aspirin sensitivity and chronic rhinosinusitis with polyps: a fatal combination. J Allergy (Cairo). 2012;2012:817910. https://doi.org/10.1155/2012/817910.
60. Nabavi M, Esmaeilzadeh H, Arshi S, Bemanian MH, Fallahpour M, Bahrami A, et al. Aspirin hypersensitivity in patients with chronic rhinosinusitis and nasal polyposis: frequency and contributing factors. Am J Rhinol Allergy. 2014;28(3):239–43. https://doi.org/10.2500/ajra.2014.28.4034.
61. Sousa AR, Parikh A, Scadding G, Corrigan CJ, Lee TH. Leukotriene-receptor expression on nasal mucosal inflammatory cells in aspirin-sensitive rhinosinusitis. N Engl J Med. 2002;347(19):1493–9. https://doi.org/10.1056/NEJMoa013508.
62. Kim MB, Lim GC, Park JA, Kim YS, Kim JH, Kang JW. Computed tomography findings in patients with samter's triad: an observational study. Open Med (Wars). 2019;14:241–6. https://doi.org/10.1515/med-2019-0018.
63. Sommer DD, Rotenberg BW, Sowerby LJ, Lee JM, Janjua A, Witterick IJ, et al. A novel treatment adjunct for aspirin exacerbated respiratory disease: the low-salicylate diet: a multicenter randomized control crossover trial. Int Forum Allergy Rhinol. 2016;6(4):385–91. https://doi.org/10.1002/alr.21678.
64. Schneider TR, Johns CB, Palumbo ML, Murphy KC, Cahill KN, et al. Dietary fatty acid modification for the treatment of aspirin-exacerbated respiratory disease: a prospective pilot trial. J Allergy Clin Immunol Pract. 2018;6(3):825–31. https://doi.org/10.1016/j.jaip.2017.10.011.
65. Laidlaw TM. Clinical updates in aspirin-exacerbated respiratory disease. Allergy Asthma Proc. 2019;40(1):4–6. https://doi.org/10.2500/aap.2019.40.4188.
66. RG M. Immunomodulatory treatments for aspirin exacerbated respiratory disease 2012;26(2):134–140. https://doi.org/10.2500/ajra.2012.26.3748.
67. Laidlaw TM, Mullol J, Fan C, Zhang D, Amin N, Khan A, Chao J, Mannent LP. Dupilumab improves nasal polyp burden and asthma control in patients with CRSwNP and AERD. 2019;7(7):2462–5.e1. https://doi.org/10.1016/j.jaip.2019.03.044.
68. Parnes SM, Chuma AV. Acute effects of antileukotrienes on sinonasal polyposis and sinusitis. Ear Nose Throat J. 2000;79(1):18–20, 4–5.
69. Schäper C, Noga O, Koch B, Ewert R, Felix SB, Gläser S, et al. Anti-inflammatory properties of montelukast, a leukotriene receptor antagonist in patients with asthma and nasal polyposis. J Investig Allergol Clin Immunol. 2011;21:51–8.
70. Beswick DM, Ramadan H, Baroody FM, Hwang PH. Practice patterns in pediatric chronic rhinosinusitis: a survey of the American Rhinologic Society. Am J Rhinol Allergy. 2016;30(6):418–23. https://doi.org/10.2500/ajra.2016.30.4373.
71. Adappa ND, Ranasinghe VJ, Trope M, Brooks SG, Glicksman JT, Parasher AK, et al. Outcomes after complete endoscopic sinus surgery and aspirin desensitization in aspirin-exacerbated respiratory disease. Int Forum Allergy Rhinol. 2018;8(1):49-53. https://doi.org/10.1002/alr.22036.
72. Mendelsohn D, Jeremic G, Wright ED, Rotenberg BW. Revision rates after endoscopic sinus surgery: a recurrence analysis. Ann Otol Rhinol Laryngol. 2011;120(3):162–6. https://doi.org/10.1177/000348941112000304.
73. Klimek L, Dollner R, Pfaar O, Mullol J. Aspirin desensitization: useful treatment for chronic rhinosinusitis with nasal polyps (CRSwNP) in aspirin exacerbated respiratory disease (AERD)? Curr Allergy Asthma Rep. 2014;14:441. https://doi.org/10.1007/s11882-014-0441-9.
74. Klimek L, Pfaar O. Aspirin intolerance: does desensitization alter the course of the disease? Immunol Allergy Clin North Am. 2009;29:669–75. https://doi.org/10.1016/j.iac.2009.07.008.
75. Xu JJ, Sowerby LJ, Rotenberg BW. Aspirin desensitization for aspirin-exacerbated respiratory disease (Samter's triad): a systematic review of the literature. Int Forum Allergy Rhinol. 2013;3:915–20. https://doi.org/10.1002/alr.21202.

76. Hayashi H, Mitsui C, Nakatani E, Fukutomi Y, Kajiwara K, Watai K, et al. Omalizumab reduces cysteinyl leukotriene and 9α,11β-prostaglandin F2 overproduction in aspirinexacerbated respiratory disease. J Allergy Clin Immunol. 2016;137:1585–7.e4. https://doi.org/10.1016/j.jaci.2015.09.034.
77. Fokkens WJ, Lund V, Bachert C, Mullol J, Bjermer L, Bousquet J, et al. EUFOREA consensus on biologics for CRSwNP with or without asthma. Allergy. 2019 [Epub ahead of print]. https://doi.org/10.1111/all.13875.
78. Vakil N, van Zanten SV, Kahrilas P, Dent J, Jones R, Global Consensus Group. The montreal definition and classification of gastroesophageal reflux disease: a global evidence-based consensus. Am J Gastroenterol. 2006;101(8):1900–20. https://doi.org/10.1111/j.1572-0241.2006.00630.x.
79. El-Serag HB, Sweet S, Winchester CC, Dent J. Update on the epidemiology of gastro-oesophageal reflux disease: a systematic review. Gut. 2014;63(6):871–80. https://doi.org/10.1136/gutjnl-2012-304269.
80. Leason SR, Barham HP, Oakley G, Rimmer J, DelGaudio JM, Christensen JM, et al. Association of gastroesophageal reflux and chronic rhinosinusitis: systematic review and meta-analysis. Rhinology. 2017;55(1):3–16. https://doi.org/10.4193/Rhin16.177.
81. Sella GCP, Tamashiro E, Anselmo-Lima WT, Valera FCP. Relation between chronic rhinosinusitis and gastroesophageal reflux in adults: systematic review. Braz J Otorhinolaryngol. 2017;83(3):356–63. https://doi.org/10.1016/j.bjorl.2016.05.012.
82. Delehaye E, Dore MP, Bozzo C, Mameli L, Delitala G, Meloni F. Correlation between nasal mucociliary clearance time and gastroesophageal reflux disease: our experience on 50 patients. Auris Nasus Larynx. 2009;36(2):157–61. https://doi.org/10.1016/j.anl.2008.06.004.
83. Jecker P, Orloff LA, Wohlfeil M, Mann WJ. Gastroesophageal reflux disease (GERD), extraesophageal reflux (EER) and recurrent chronic rhinosinusitis. Eur Arch Otorhinolaryngol. 2006;263(7):664–7. https://doi.org/10.1007/s00405-006-0022-1.
84. Ozmen S, Yücel OT, Sinici I, Ozmen OA, Süslü AE, Oğretmenoğlu O, et al. Nasal pepsin assay and pH monitoring in chronic rhinosinusitis. Laryngoscope. 2008;118:890–4. https://doi.org/10.1097/MLG.0b013e318165e324.
85. Bhawana GS, Kumar S, Kumar A. Alkaline pH in middle meatus in cases of chronic rhinosinusitis. Am J Otolaryngol. 2014;35(4):496–9. https://doi.org/10.1016/j.amjoto.2014.02.017.
86. Dinis PB, Subtil J. Helicobacter pylori and laryngopharyngeal reflux in chronic rhinosinusitis. Otolaryngol Head Neck Surg. 2006;134(1):67–72. https://doi.org/10.1016/j.otohns.2005.10.013.
87. Siupsinskiene N, Katutiene I, Jonikiene V, Janciauskas D, Vaitkus S. Intranasal Helicobacter pylori infection in patients with chronic rhinosinusitis with polyposis. J Laryngol Otol. 2018;132(9):816–21. https://doi.org/10.1017/s0022215118001299.
88. Durmus R, Naiboglu B, Tek A, Sezikli M, Cetinkaya ZA, Toros SZ, et al. Does reflux have an effect on nasal mucociliary transport? Acta Oto-Laryngol. 2010;130(9):1053–7. https://doi.org/10.3109/00016481003621546.
89. DelGaudio JM. Direct nasopharyngeal reflux of gastric acid is a contributing factor in refractory chronic rhinosinusitis. Laryngoscope. 2005;115(6):946–57. https://doi.org/10.1097/01.Mlg.0000163751.00885.63.
90. Katle EJ, Hatlebakk JG, Grimstad T, Kvaløy JT, Steinsvåg SK. Gastro-oesophageal reflux in patients with chronic rhino-sinusitis investigated with multichannel impedance – pH monitoring. Rhinology. 2017;55(1):27–33. https://doi.org/10.4193/Rhin16.275.
91. Chambers DW, Davis WE, Cook PR, Nishioka GJ, Rudman DT. Long-term outcome analysis of functional endoscopic sinus surgery: correlation of symptoms with endoscopic examination findings and potential prognostic variables. Laryngoscope. 1997;107(4):504-10. https://doi.org/10.1097/00005537-199704000-00014.
92. Deconde AS, Mace JC, Smith TL. The impact of comorbid gastroesophageal reflux disease on endoscopic sinus surgery quality of life outcomes. Int Forum Allergy Rhinol. 2014;4(8):663–9. https://doi.org/10.1002/alr.21333.
93. Jelavic B, Grgic M, Cupic H, Kordic M, Vasilj M, Baudoin T. Prognostic value of Helicobacter pylori sinonasal colonization for efficacy of endoscopic sinus surgery. Eur Arch Otorhinolaryngol. 2012;269(10):2197–202.
94. Phipps CD, Wood WE, Gibson WS, Cochran WJ. Gastroesophageal reflux contributing to chronic sinus disease in children: a prospective analysis. Arch Otolaryngol Head Neck Surg. 2000;126:831–6. https://doi.org/10.1001/archotol.126.7.831.
95. Hurst JR, Wilkinson TM, Donaldson GC, Wedzicha JA. Upper airway symptoms and quality of life in chronic obstructive pulmonary disease (COPD). Respir Med. 2004;98(8):767–70. https://doi.org/10.1016/j.rmed.2004.01.010.
96. Caminha GP, Pizzichini E, Lubianca Neto JF, Hopkins C, Moreira JDS, Pizzichini MMM. Rhinosinusitis symptoms, smoking and COPD: prevalence and associations. Clin Otolaryngol. 2018;43(6):1560–5. https://doi.org/10.1111/coa.13215.
97. Chien CY, Tai SY, Wang LF, Lee CT. Chronic obstructive pulmonary disease predicts chronic rhinosinusitis without nasal polyps: a population-based study. Am J Rhinol Allergy. 2015;29(3):e75–80. https://doi.org/10.2500/ajra.2015.29.4172.
98. Miłkowska-Dymanowska J, Białas AJ, Zalewska-Janowska A, Górski P, Piotrowski WJ. Underrecognized comorbidities of chronic obstructive

pulmonary disease. Int. J. Chron. Obstruct. Pulmon. Dis. 2015;10:1331–41. https://doi.org/10.2147/copd.S82420.
99. Piotrowska VM, Piotrowski WJ, Kurmanowska Z, Marczak J, Górski P, Antczak A. Rhinosinusitis in COPD: symptoms, mucosal changes, nasal lavage cells and eicosanoids. Int. J. Chron. Obstruct. Pulmon. Dis. 2010;5:107–17. https://doi.org/10.2147/copd.s8862.
100. Kelemence A, Abadoglu O, Gumus C, Berk S, Epozturk K, Akkurt I. The frequency of chronic rhinosinusitis/nasal polyp in COPD and its effect on the severity of COPD. COPD. 2011;8(1):8–12. https://doi.org/10.3109/15412555.2010.540272.
101. Hens G, Vanaudenaerde BM, Bullens DM, Piessens M, Decramer M, Dupont LJ, et al. Sinonasal pathology in nonallergic asthma and COPD: 'united airway disease' beyond the scope of allergy. Allergy. 2008;63(3):261–7. https://doi.org/10.1111/j.1398--9995.2007.01545.x.
102. King P, Holdsworth S, Freezer N, Holmes P. Bronchiectasis. Intern Med J. 2006;36(11):729–37. https://doi.org/10.1111/j.1445-5994.2006.01219.x.
103. Handley E, Nicolson CH, Hew M, Lee AL. Prevalence and clinical implications of chronic rhinosinusitis in people with bronchiectasis: a systematic review. J Allergy Clin Immunol Pract. 2019;7(6):2004–12.e1. https://doi.org/10.1016/j.jaip.2019.02.026.
104. Guilemany JM, Alobid I, Angrill J, Ballesteros F, Bernal-Sprekelsen M, Picado C, et al. The impact of bronchiectasis associated to sinonasal disease on quality of life. Respir Med. 2006;100(11):1997–2003. https://doi.org/10.1016/j.rmed.2006.02.016.
105. Guan WJ, Gao YH, Li HM, Yuan JJ, Chen RC, Zhong NS. Impacts of co-existing chronic rhinosinusitis on disease severity and risks of exacerbations in Chinese adults with bronchiectasis. PLoS One. 2015;10(9):e0137348. https://doi.org/10.1371/journal.pone.0137348.

Clinical Diagnosis and Phenotypes 23

Kevin Hur and Robert C. Kern

Key Points
Chronic rhinosinusitis (CRS) is a common disorder characterized by inflammation of the mucosa of the nose and paranasal sinuses affecting up to 12% of the Western population [1–4]. The diagnosis of CRS according to the EPOS 2012 guidelines requires the presence of 2 or more cardinal symptoms for 12 or more consecutive weeks plus objective confirmation by sinus CT or nasal endoscopy. This definition is purposefully broad; therefore, CRS is best viewed as a clinical syndrome or symptom complex rather than a discrete disease. From the standpoint of causation, multiple environmental factors interact with host genetics but the specific elements operative in an individual CRS patient are typically unknown. Nevertheless, this interaction of the host genotype with the environment results in activation of one or more inflammatory pathways or endotypes. This inflammation then manifests as one of the several clinical subgroups or phenotypes based on readily observable characteristics in the patient. Historically, the first attempt at CRS classification utilized nasal endoscopy to delineate two phenotypes: CRS with polyps (CRSwNP) and CRS without nasal polyps (CRSsNP). This chapter will utilize additional observable characteristics, including natural history and response to therapy in order to provide a more current set of CRS phenotypes including aspirin-exacerbated respiratory disease (AERD), allergic fungal rhinosinusitis (AFRS), eosinophilic granulomatosis with polyangiitis (EGPA), cystic fibrosis (CF), odontogenic rhinosinusitis, immunodeficiency, and primary cilia dyskinesia.

K. Hur · R. C. Kern (✉)
Department of Otolaryngology, Head and Neck Surgery, Feinberg School of Medicine, Northwestern University, Chicago, IL, USA
e-mail: kevin.hur@northwestern.edu; Robert.Kern@nm.org

23.1 Aspirin-Exacerbated Respiratory Disease

Aspirin-exacerbated respiratory disease (AERD) is characterized by the clinical triad of nasal polyps, asthma, and sensitivity to cyclooxygenase type 1 inhibitors. The upper and lower airway symptoms are exacerbated by aspirin or other nonsteroidal anti-inflammatory drug (NSAID) ingestion that inhibits cyclooxygenase type 1 [5]. Although the pathophysiology of AERD is not completely clear, dysregulation of arachidonic acid metabolism (higher production of cysteinyl leukotrienes and prostaglandin D2 with lower levels of prostaglandin E2) with increased activation of type 2 effector immune cells such as eosinophils and mast cells is observed. Epithelial cells, ILC2s, basophils, and platelets are also believed to be activated [6, 7].

The prevalence of AERD among adult asthma patients has been reported to range between 7 and

L. Zhang, C. Bachert (eds.), *Chronic Rhinosinusitis*, https://doi.org/10.1007/978-981-16-0784-4_23

21%, whereas 9–16% of patients with CRSwNP have been identified as having AERD [8, 9]. A 2015 systematic review of 1770 publications concluded that the prevalence of AERD in those with asthma was 7%, in those with severe asthma 15%, in those with NP 10%, and in those with CRS 9%. Interestingly, the prevalence of AERD is mostly based on studies of Western and European populations [10]. In Asian populations, the prevalence of AERD has been found to be much lower for unclear reasons [11].

23.1.1 Clinical Presentation and Diagnosis

The clinical diagnosis of AERD relies on the confirmation of the three major components of the disorder: CRSwNP, asthma, and hypersensitivity to aspirin/NSAIDs. These components can be identified with a detailed clinical history and examination that should include endoscopy, radiologic imaging, spirometry, and an aspirin challenge. Patients with AERD tend to present at a younger age and with a more severe clinical presentation compared to the typical patient with nasal polyposis. Typical nasal symptoms of CRS including rhinorrhea and nasal congestion are usually the first symptoms to manifest in the course of the disease and may be difficult to distinguish from other CRS phenotypes. The degree of sinonasal inflammation found on diagnostic CT scans is significantly higher, with a higher rate of polyp recurrence postsurgery compared to other CRSwNP patients [8]. Asthma symptoms most often develop after the presentation of upper airway disease. Studies comparing the pulmonary function of AERD patients versus non-aspirin sensitive asthma have reported that AERD patients have significantly decreased FEV1 compared to other CRS patients with asthma [8, 12]. The unified airway hypothesis suggests that upper and lower airway diseases are linked and an increase in disease severity of the upper airway will likely impact the severity of disease in the lower airway. Therefore, it is reasonable to conclude that since AERD patients are more likely to have more severe and refractory sinonasal disease, they also are more likely to have more severe lower airway disease. Current treatment recommendations include aggressive surgery, ASA desensitization, and the use of newly available biologics that directly target components of type 2 cytokine inflammation.

The key defining feature of AERD that distinguishes it from other CRS phenotypes is aspirin/NSAID hypersensitivity, which may not be easily recognized as the degree of hypersensitivity can be gradual and development and may be missed or difficult to diagnose. A typical presentation of hypersensitivity includes symptoms of rhinorrhea, epiphora, conjunctival edema, nasal congestion, laryngospasm, or bronchospasm typically occurring within hours after ingestion of aspirin/NSAIDs. A history of an asthma attack following ingestion of aspirin or other NSAIDs is suggestive of the diagnosis; however, a clinical history is not necessarily definitive in the diagnosis of an aspirin/NSAID hypersensitivity. In one study, 16% of patients who reported a history of an asthma attack after ingesting aspirin/NSAIDs had a negative oral aspirin provocation challenge. Furthermore, the same study reported that in patients who presented with nasal polyps, CRS, asthma, and a history of avoiding aspirin/NSAIDs, only 43% had a positive oral aspirin challenge [13]. Therefore, an aspirin challenge remains the gold standard for diagnosing AERD as there is no other available form of laboratory testing with similar precision and accuracy currently available. Several methods of provocation challenges have been described, including oral, bronchial inhalation, nasal inhalation, and intravenous [5]. Identification of a more specific biochemical or genetic marker has been elusive.

23.2 Allergic Fungal Rhinosinusitis

Allergic fungal rhinosinusitis (AFRS) is an IgE mediated noninvasive fungal disease of the nasal and paranasal sinuses that accounts for approximately 6–9% of CRSwNP cases [14]. It has a distinctive geographic and demographic profile, occurring more commonly in warm humid climates such as the Southern United States where the mold count is higher. AFRS presents more commonly in younger African Americans and has a male predominance. Patients with AFRS are also more likely to have lower socioeconomic status based on results from retrospective studies [15].

23.2.1 Clinical Presentation and Diagnosis

The presentation of AFRS involves the same symptoms as other phenotypes of CRS including nasal drainage, obstruction, facial pain/pressure, and decreased sense of smell but with a more slow, progressive course that is often unilateral. Age of diagnosis is typically younger than most CRSwNP patients [15]. A unique characteristic of AFRS is the expansile nature of the disease which can remodel the surrounding bones of the paranasal sinuses and skull base, leading to visual changes, proptosis, headaches, and diplopia.

Objective findings on examination that are characteristic of AFRS include the formation of thick brownish allergic mucin classically described as "peanut butter-like" seen on endoscopy along with nasal polyps and proteinaceous debris. The mucin consists of an abundance of eosinophils, eosinophil by-products, and fungal hyphae.

Diagnostic criteria include the following as described by Bent and Kuhn [16] which distinguishes AFRS from other phenotypes of CRS: (1) nasal polyposis; (2) fungi on staining; (3) eosinophilic mucin without fungal invasion into sinus tissue; (4) type 1 hypersensitivity to fungi; (5) characteristic radiological findings with soft tissue differential densities on CT scanning. Other minor criteria include: (1) bone erosion; (2) Charcot–Leyden crystals; (3) unilateral disease; (4) peripheral eosinophilia; (5) positive fungal culture. In AFRS patients, fungal tissue invasion does not occur distinguishing this disorder from acute and chronic invasive fungal rhinosinusitis. In addition, the "fungal mucin" in AFRS is a result of a type 2 reaction to the fungi rather than an accumulation of fungal elements as seen in sinus fungal balls.

Skin testing or RAST testing is necessary to establish a type 1 hypersensitivity to fungal antigens. Other possible laboratory abnormalities include peripheral eosinophilia and elevated total IgE. The most common fungi associated with AFRS include *Aspergillus* species and the dematiaceous fungi [17]. Treatment typically consists of aggressive surgery and postoperative high volume corticosteroid irrigations.

23.3 Eosinophilic Granulomatosis with Polyangiitis

Eosinophilic granulomatosis with polyangiitis (EGPA) is a rare small-vessel vasculitis characterized by asthma and eosinophilia. Formerly called Churg-Strauss syndrome, the incidence of EGPA is 0.5–6.8 cases per 1,000,000 adults per year occurring most often in adults aged 40–60 years of age [18]. The pathophysiology of EGPA is still being elucidated, but some evidence suggests that EGPA is itself a heterogeneous disorder with multiple subtypes that are yet to be clearly defined, thus making diagnosis and treatment challenging [19].

23.3.1 Clinical Presentation and Diagnosis

EGPA has been traditionally characterized as having three phases: allergic, eosinophilic, and vasculitic. The allergic phase presents with symptoms of asthma, allergic rhinitis, and sinusitis. The eosinophilic phase presents with blood and tissue eosinophilia and the vasculitic phase is characterized by peripheral neuropathy, purpura, and pauciimmune necrotizing glomerulonephritis [19]. However, EGPA has several phenotypes and thus not all patients will present in a similar fashion. While asthma commonly presents in 90–95% of EGPA patients, upper airway symptoms also affect a similar percentage. The most common complaints are nasal obstruction, rhinorrhea, loss of smell, and sneezing with nasal polyps found in 70% of patients [20]. Other systems involved include cardiac disease such as pericarditis and cardiomyopathy, skin lesions such as palpable purpura, and renal disease. Patients who present with severe eosinophilic sinonasal inflammation that responds poorly to standard therapy along with the concomitant presence of systemic inflammation should raise the suspicion for EGPA.

There are no universally accepted diagnostic criteria for EGPA but the American College of Rheumatology classifies EGPA as having six distinguishing features: asthma, eosinophilia, neuropathy, pulmonary infiltrate, paranasal sinus abnormality, and extravascular eosinophilic infiltration on biopsy [21]. While a biopsy is not required for diagnosis of EGPA, it can help confirm the presence of vasculitis or an eosinophilic inflammatory process.

For nasal symptoms, nasal saline irrigations and topic intranasal corticosteroids are first line therapy, followed by limited oral corticosteroid bursts as necessary, similar to the management of CRSwNP. Patients who do not respond to medical therapy should be considered for aggressive endoscopic sinus surgery [22]. New biologic medications directed at IL-5 or the IL-5 receptor should also be considered.

23.4 Cystic Fibrosis

Cystic fibrosis (CF) is an autosomal-recessive genetic disease where mutations in the cystic fibrosis transmembrane receptor gene (*CFTR*) lead to defective chloride channels. The defect results in a significant increase in the viscosity of secretions in the upper and lower airways inhibiting mucociliary clearance and increasing the risk for infections. Oftentimes patients are at increased risk of developing *Pseudomonas aeruginosa* and *Staphylococcus aureus* infections which can lead to a decline in lung function. The dysfunction in mucociliary clearance in these patients predisposes them to developing CRS. The disease is most common in populations of European descent, where the incidence is 1 in 3000 births [23].

23.4.1 Clinical Presentation and Diagnosis

Patients with CF differ from other phenotypes of CRS in that patients underreport CRS symptoms. Only 10–15% of the patients with CF will self-report CRS symptoms even though when specifically asked, most patients with CF will fulfill criteria for CRS [1]. Sinonasal clinical features that should place cystic fibrosis higher on the differential diagnosis include nasal polyps found in a child or a sinus infection with culture-proven *Pseudomonas aeruginosa*, *Burkholderia cepacia*, or *Achromobacter xylosoxidans.* These findings in combination with a history of lung infections, pancreatic insufficiency, poor nutrition, and/or chronic diarrhea should raise the suspicion for CF [24].

Nasal polyps are rare in children younger than 6 years but are more prevalent as they age with up to 50% of CF adolescents demonstrating nasal polyps [25]. On radiologic imaging, CF patients have a higher incidence of underdeveloped sinuses compared to other adult patients. In one study, the majority of maxillary and frontal sinuses in CF patients were either aplastic or hypoplastic [26]. The diagnosis of CF involves assessing the results from a sweat chloride test, genetic analysis, and clinical evaluation. A sweat chloride test is performed by placing a solution on the forearm or thigh and through electrical stimulation sweating is induced. The amount of chloride is measured in the sweat with a higher value compared to normal values suggestive of a diagnosis of CF. Genetic testing involves obtaining a blood sample or cells from a cheek swab to identify mutations in the CFTR mutation. The identification of two mutations is considered a positive genetic test for CF. In developed countries, national screening programs for neonates have been implemented in which a heel prick is performed a few days after birth to measure levels of the pancreatic enzyme trypsinogen. Elevated levels are suggestive of CF but not diagnostic. Further evaluation is necessary to establish the diagnosis with a chloride sweat test and genetic testing. Moreover, while CF is very closely tied to the CFTR gene, the genetics of this disorder are more complex with significant clinical relevance. Specifically, the presence of nasal polyps and the severity of CRS symptoms vary in patients with CF. This observation likely stems from the fact that multiple different mutations have been described in CFTR, and the degree of impairment in chloride channel activity is variable [needs reference]. In addition, genetic and epigenetic variation at other sites in the genome may buffer the effect on clinical phenotype.

23.5 Odontogenic Rhinosinusitis

Odonotogenic rhinosinusitis describes the presence of sinonasal disease that is of dental origin. With the rising rates of dental surgery being performed in the general population, the incidence of odontogenic rhinosinusitis from iatrogenic injury will likely only increase. Approximately 10% of maxillary sinusitis cases have been reported to be the result of an odontogenic process. Dental procedures such as extractions, implants, sinus augmentation grafts, and cleft surgery procedures have all been associated with odontogenic sinusitis. Odontogenic rhinosinusitis occurs when the Schneiderian membrane lining the maxillary sinus mucosa is compromised by a dental infection or procedure. This creates a passage for bacterial organisms commonly found in oral flora to spread into and infect the maxillary sinus [27, 28].

23.5.1 Clinical Presentation and Diagnosis

Patients who present with unilateral maxillary sinus disease should be suspected for having odontogenic rhinosinusitis. A detailed clinical history with a thorough dental history is necessary to identify patients who may have odontogenic sinusitis. Ironically, dental pain is not considered specific for odontogenic sinusitis. A careful oral cavity examination of the dentition, periodontal tissue, dental implants, and presence of an oral-antral fistula are important components to the exam. Nasal endoscopy can demonstrate purulence or edema in the middle meatus but this is a nonspecific finding and is not specific for odontogenic rhinosinusitis. Radiologic imaging is almost always necessary in the diagnosis of odontogenic sinusitis. Maxillofacial CT scans are the best imaging modality to provide a high resolution image in multiple planes. One study reported that 70% of unilateral maxillary sinusitis were odontogenic infections [29]. However, odontogenic infections are not necessarily limited to the maxillary sinus. Extension to adjacent paranasal sinuses has been reported in up to 60% of cases and up to 20% of odontogenic rhinosinusitis may be bilateral [27, 30, 31]. As a result, a careful examination for maxillary dental disease is necessary when reviewing radiologic imaging. The most common teeth associated with maxillary sinusitis are the maxillary first and second molars according to a retrospective study of 871 cone-beam CT scans [32]. Evidence of sinonasal disease on imaging in conjunction with a clinical history or radiological evidence of a dental origin are the key components for the diagnosis of odontogenic rhinosinusitis.

Treatment of odontogenic infections initially involves a trial of antibiotics. If there is no improvement, then treating the underlying dental pathology or endoscopic sinus surgery should be considered. A retrospective study of 43 patients with odontogenic sinusitis found that 52% of patients improved with medical and dental treatment, but 48% also needed endoscopic sinus surgery [33]. Sinus surgery can also be considered as the primary surgical intervention because it has demonstrated to result in faster symptom resolution compared to dental treatment for odontogenic sinusitis [34].

23.6 Immunodeficiency

Patients with refractory CRS should raise the clinician's suspicion for a possible immunodeficiency. Although not a solitary phenotype, these patients are linked by the observation that they are less likely to respond to conventional therapies without addressing the underlying immunodeficiency. CRS patients with an immunodeficiency can be further categorized into patients with a primary or secondary immunodeficiency. Secondary immunodeficiencies are a result of other diseases (i.e. HIV) or immunosuppressive medications such as chemotherapy. Primary immunodeficiencies are defects in the immune system affecting the function of B cells, T cells, and/or other components of the immune system. The most common primary immunodeficiency in CRS patients is antibody deficiencies, which are oftentimes the result of genetic mutations that lead to a defect in antibody production or poor antibody function. The prevalence of antibody deficiencies in patients with CRS was 23% in difficult-to-treat CRS and 13% in patients with recurrent CRS in a recent meta-analysis of 13 studies [35].

23.6.1 Clinical Presentation and Diagnosis

The presentation of CRS with an immunodeficiency can be difficult to distinguish from idiopathic CRS. Therefore, the decision to evaluate a patient's immune function is subject to the clinician's judgment based on the history. Clinical features such as rapid recurrence of symptoms after conventional treatment or evidence of other forms of respiratory tract infections such as pneumonia should raise the clinician's suspicion that the patient may have an immunodeficiency. The differential diagnosis for primary immunodeficiencies in CRS is broad and in this section we will review the most commonly described. The initial laboratory test to help distinguish between the various primary immunodeficiencies is the measurement of serum immunoglobulin levels.

Common variable immunodeficiency (CVID) is the most common symptomatic antibody deficiency and is diagnosed by the presence of low IgG levels and low IgA or IgM levels with a lack of functional response to polysaccharide vaccines. CVID is more likely to manifest in adulthood and more than 50% of patients with CVID have CRS [28, 36].

Specific antibody deficiency (SAD) is defined as an impaired response to immunization with polysaccharide antigens such as Pneumovax in the setting of normal quantitative immunoglobulin levels (IgG, IgA, and IgM) and a history of recurrent or prolonged sinopulmonary infections. There is no consensus on what is considered an adequate response to a polysaccharide vaccine; however, 50–70% of pneumococcal serotypes should be above 1.3 mcg/ml after vaccination. In a retrospective review of patients with difficult-to-treat CRS, up to 23% of the patients were noted to have SAD [28, 37].

The most common immunodeficiency in the general population is IgA deficiency with a prevalence of 1–600 [38]. A low IgA level (<7 mg/dl) with normal IgG and IgM levels is diagnostic for the condition. Approximately 7% of CRS patients have IgA deficiency. The clinical significance of IgA deficiency is debatable as most patients with IgA deficiency are asymptomatic.

Other immunodeficiency disorders to consider but not discussed in this chapter include hyperimmunoglobulin E syndrome, IgG subclass deficiency, Wiskott–Aldrich syndrome, ataxia telangiectasia, X-linked immunodeficiency, and X-linked agammaglobulinemia.

The treatment of less severe immunodeficiencies such as SAD and IgA deficiency can be managed symptomatically with prophylactic antibiotics. If refractory, or if the immunodeficiency is more severe such as in CVID, immunoglobulin replacement is recommended. Sinus surgery is generally not considered contraindicated in any immunodeficiency and is an option in patients who meet CRS criteria refractory to medical management [39].

23.7 Primary Ciliary Dyskinesia

In the nose and paranasal sinuses, mucociliary clearance relies on the cilia of the pseudostratified columnar ciliated epithelium to move mucus posteriorly toward the nasopharynx. When there is dysfunction of the cilia, mucus stasis occurs leading to nasal obstruction, rhinorrhea, and a predilection for infections.

Primary ciliary dyskinesias (PCD) is a group of inherited disorders that affect cilia motility. PCD is a rare disorder with the incidence estimated at 1:15,000–30,000 births and consanguinity a risk factor [40].

23.7.1 Clinical Presentation and Diagnosis

Patients with a cilia motility defect present with symptoms secondary to an inability to clear secretions. They typically report having a productive cough, rhinitis, and recurrent upper and lower respiratory infections. Not surprisingly, there is a strong association between PCD and CRS. In a study of PCD patient, all patients had a history of CRS, with one-third having nasal polyps on endoscopy [41]. On exam there may be pooling of mucus on the floor of the nose. These patients will also oftentimes present with multiorgan issues as ciliary movement is involved in several organ systems from neurologic to fertility conditions. Cilia motility can be evaluated with the saccharin test in which a tablet of saccharin is placed on the inferior turbinate and the time to taste the saccharin is noted as the particle is transported along the sinonasal mucosa to the nasopharynx. A prolonged time suggests dysfunction with mucociliary clearance. Nasal nitric oxide in which lower levels of nitric oxide is detected has also been described as a screening test. Diagnosis of a cilia dysfunction oftentimes involves performing a nasal biopsy to examine the cilia with electron microscopy. Defects in the outer and inner dynein arms, radial spokes, or central microtubules of the cilia can be identified. A negative biopsy, however, does not necessarily exclude a cilia motility disorder [38].

High level evidence to help guide the management of PCD is lacking. Sinonasal symptoms are managed similarly to CRS guidelines with nasal saline irrigations and intranasal steroids as first line intervention. Endoscopic sinus surgery can be considered when medical therapy has failed but there are few studies that have studied the outcomes of sinus surgery for PCD [42].

23.8 Conclusion

Chronic rhinosinusitis is a broad clinical syndrome with multiple phenotypes that exhibit relatively distinct clinical profiles that can be used to provide prognostic and therapeutic guidance. AERD and AFRS are the most clear phenotypes, each with type 2 inflammation but with presumably a partially distinct endotype. Other less common phenotypes include CF, EGPA, and PCD but taken together, the totality of these discrete phenotypes comprises a minority of CRS cases. Less well-defined phenotypes have been suggested, proposing that age of onset or the presence of comorbidities are important factors driving clinical course and response to therapy. Typically, CRS is seen as an adult-onset disorder and the relationship, if there is any, between pediatric rhinosinusitis and adult rhinosinusitis is unclear. Nevertheless, some evidence indicates that early onset adult CRS (age < 30) may be linked to atopy and childhood sinonasal problems, suggesting the hypothesis CRS in this setting is a continuation of the atopic march into the sinus cavities [43]. This subgroup of early-onset CRS and atopy may also be milder [44]. CRS with comorbid asthma however, does in general indicate greater severity of both disorders [44, 45]. The effect of childhood-onset asthma, particularly in the CRSsNP subgroup, may be minimal and any independent effect of atopy and age of onset remain unclear. Overall, while there has been some progress in our ability to phenotype CRS patients, the vast majority cases do not fall into discrete phenotypes, resulting in a default to simple polyp status. Continued research into the molecular mechanisms of airway disorders coupled with large scale longitudinal studies will be necessary to permit a more complete and accurate phenotyping of CRS patients in the future.

References

1. Fokkens WJ, Lund VJ, Mullol J, Bachert C, Alobid I, Baroody F, et al. EPOS 2012: European position paper on rhinosinusitis and nasal polyps 2012. A summary for otorhinolaryngologists. Rhinology. 2012;50(1):1–12. https://doi.org/10.4193/Rhino50E2.

2. Orlandi RR, Kingdom TT, Hwang PH, Smith TL, Alt JA, Baroody FM, et al. International consensus statement on allergy and rhinology: rhinosinusitis. Int Forum Allergy Rhinol. 2016;6(Suppl 1):S22–209. https://doi.org/10.1002/alr.21695.
3. Dietz de Loos D, Lourijsen ES, Wildeman MAM, Freling NJM, Wolvers MDJ, Reitsma S, et al. Prevalence of chronic rhinosinusitis in the general population based on sinus radiology and symptomatology. J Allergy Clin Immunol. 2019;143(3):1207–14. https://doi.org/10.1016/j.jaci.2018.12.986.
4. Hirsch AG, Nordberg C, Bandeen-Roche K, Tan BK, Schleimer RP, Kern RC, et al. Radiologic sinus inflammation and symptoms of chronic rhinosinusitis in a population-based sample. Allergy. 2019. https://doi.org/10.1111/all.14106.
5. Lee RU, Stevenson DD. Aspirin-exacerbated respiratory disease: evaluation and management. Allergy Asthma Immunol Res. 2011;3(1):3–10. https://doi.org/10.4168/aair.2011.3.1.3.
6. Stevens WW, Ocampo CJ, Berdnikovs S, Sakashita M, Mahdavinia M, Suh L, et al. Cytokines in chronic rhinosinusitis. Role in Eosinophilia and Aspirin-exacerbated respiratory disease. Am J Respir Crit Care Med. 2015;192(6):682–94. https://doi.org/10.1164/rccm.201412-2278OC.
7. Cahill KN, Bensko JC, Boyce JA, Laidlaw TM. Prostaglandin D(2): a dominant mediator of aspirin-exacerbated respiratory disease. J Allergy Clin Immunol. 2015;135(1):245–52. https://doi.org/10.1016/j.jaci.2014.07.031.
8. Stevens WW, Peters AT, Hirsch AG, Nordberg CM, Schwartz BS, Mercer DG, et al. Clinical characteristics of patients with chronic rhinosinusitis with nasal polyps, asthma, and aspirin-exacerbated respiratory disease. J Allergy Clin Immunol Pract. 2017;5(4):1061–70.e3. https://doi.org/10.1016/j.jaip.2016.12.027.
9. Jenkins C, Costello J, Hodge L. Systematic review of prevalence of aspirin induced asthma and its implications for clinical practice. BMJ. 2004;328(7437):434. https://doi.org/10.1136/bmj.328.7437.434.
10. Rajan JP, Wineinger NE, Stevenson DD, White AA. Prevalence of aspirin-exacerbated respiratory disease among asthmatic patients: a meta-analysis of the literature. J Allergy Clin Immunol. 2015;135(3):676–81.e1. https://doi.org/10.1016/j.jaci.2014.08.020.
11. Ledford DK, Wenzel SE, Lockey RF. Aspirin or other nonsteroidal inflammatory agent exacerbated asthma. J Allergy Clin Immunol Pract. 2014;2(6):653–7. https://doi.org/10.1016/j.jaip.2014.09.009.
12. Mascia K, Haselkorn T, Deniz YM, Miller DP, Bleecker ER, Borish L, et al. Aspirin sensitivity and severity of asthma: evidence for irreversible airway obstruction in patients with severe or difficult-to-treat asthma. J Allergy Clin Immunol. 2005;116(5):970–5. https://doi.org/10.1016/j.jaci.2005.08.035.
13. Dursun AB, Woessner KA, Simon RA, Karasoy D, Stevenson DD. Predicting outcomes of oral aspirin challenges in patients with asthma, nasal polyps, and chronic sinusitis. Ann Allergy Asthma Immunol. 2008;100(5):420–5. https://doi.org/10.1016/S1081-1206(10)60465-6.
14. Bakhshaee M, Fereidouni M, Mohajer MN, Majidi MR, Azad FJ, Moghiman T. The prevalence of allergic fungal rhinosinusitis in sinonasal polyposis. Eur Arch Otorhinolaryngol. 2013;270(12):3095–8. https://doi.org/10.1007/s00405-013-2449-5.
15. Wise SK, Ghegan MD, Gorham E, Schlosser RJ. Socioeconomic factors in the diagnosis of allergic fungal rhinosinusitis. Otolaryngol Head Neck Surg. 2008;138(1):38–42. https://doi.org/10.1016/j.otohns.2007.10.020.
16. Bent JP III, Kuhn FA. Diagnosis of allergic fungal sinusitis. Otolaryngol Head Neck Surg. 1994;111(5):580–8. https://doi.org/10.1177/019459989411100508.
17. Hoyt AE, Borish L, Gurrola J, Payne S. Allergic fungal rhinosinusitis. J Allergy Clin Immunol Pract. 2016;4(4):599–604. https://doi.org/10.1016/j.jaip.2016.03.010.
18. Groh M, Pagnoux C, Baldini C, Bel E, Bottero P, Cottin V, et al. Eosinophilic granulomatosis with polyangiitis (Churg-Strauss) (EGPA) Consensus Task Force recommendations for evaluation and management. Eur J Intern Med. 2015;26(7):545–53. https://doi.org/10.1016/j.ejim.2015.04.022.
19. Wu EY, Hernandez ML, Jennette JC, Falk RJ. Eosinophilic granulomatosis with polyangiitis: clinical pathology conference and review. J Allergy Clin Immunol Pract. 2018;6(5):1496–504. https://doi.org/10.1016/j.jaip.2018.07.001.
20. Goldfarb JM, Rabinowitz MR, Basnyat S, Nyquist GG, Rosen MR. Head and neck manifestations of eosinophilic granulomatosis with polyangiitis: a systematic review. Otolaryngol Head Neck Surg. 2016;155(5):771–8. https://doi.org/10.1177/0194599816657044.
21. Masi AT, Hunder GG, Lie JT, Michel BA, Bloch DA, Arend WP, et al. The American college of rheumatology 1990 criteria for the classification of Churg-Strauss syndrome (allergic granulomatosis and angiitis). Arthritis Rheum. 1990;33(8):1094–100. https://doi.org/10.1002/art.1780330806.
22. Bacciu A, Buzio C, Giordano D, Pasanisi E, Vincenti V, Mercante G, et al. Nasal polyposis in Churg-Strauss syndrome. Laryngoscope. 2008;118(2):325–9. https://doi.org/10.1097/MLG.0b013e318159889d.
23. O'Sullivan BP, Freedman SD. Cystic fibrosis. Lancet. 2009;373(9678):1891–904. https://doi.org/10.1016/S0140-6736(09)60327-5.
24. Hamilos DL. Chronic rhinosinusitis in patients with cystic fibrosis. J Allergy Clin Immunol Pract. 2016;4(4):605–12. https://doi.org/10.1016/j.jaip.2016.04.013.
25. Shwachman H, Kulczycki LL, Mueller HL, Flake CG. Nasal polyposis in patients with cystic fibrosis. Pediatrics. 1962;30:389–401.
26. Orlandi RR, Wiggins RH III. Radiological sinonasal findings in adults with cystic fibrosis. Am J Rhinol

Allergy. 2009;23(3):307–11. https://doi.org/10.2500/ajra.2009.23.3324.
27. Little RE, Long CM, Loehrl TA, Poetker DM. Odontogenic sinusitis: a review of the current literature. Laryngoscope Investig Otolaryngol. 2018;3(2):110–4. https://doi.org/10.1002/lio2.147.
28. Bose S, Grammer LC, Peters AT. Infectious chronic rhinosinusitis. J Allergy Clin Immunol Pract. 2016;4(4):584–9. https://doi.org/10.1016/j.jaip.2016.04.008.
29. Matsumoto Y, Ikeda T, Yokoi H, Kohno N. Association between odontogenic infections and unilateral sinus opacification. Auris Nasus Larynx. 2015;42(4):288–93. https://doi.org/10.1016/j.anl.2014.12.006.
30. Saibene AM, Pipolo GC, Lozza P, Maccari A, Portaleone SM, Scotti A, et al. Redefining boundaries in odontogenic sinusitis: a retrospective evaluation of extramaxillary involvement in 315 patients. Int Forum Allergy Rhinol. 2014;4(12):1020–3. https://doi.org/10.1002/alr.21400.
31. Saibene AM, Vassena C, Pipolo C, Trimboli M, De Vecchi E, Felisati G, et al. Odontogenic and rhinogenic chronic sinusitis: a modern microbiological comparison. Int Forum Allergy Rhinol. 2016;6(1):41–5. https://doi.org/10.1002/alr.21629.
32. Maillet M, Bowles WR, McClanahan SL, John MT, Ahmad M. Cone-beam computed tomography evaluation of maxillary sinusitis. J Endod. 2011;37(6):753–7. https://doi.org/10.1016/j.joen.2011.02.032.
33. Mattos JL, Ferguson BJ, Lee S. Predictive factors in patients undergoing endoscopic sinus surgery for odontogenic sinusitis. Int Forum Allergy Rhinol. 2016;6(7):697–700. https://doi.org/10.1002/alr.21736.
34. Craig JR, McHugh CI, Griggs ZH, Peterson EI. Optimal timing of endoscopic sinus surgery for odontogenic sinusitis. Laryngoscope. 2019;129(9):1976–83. https://doi.org/10.1002/lary.28001.
35. Schwitzguebel AJ, Jandus P, Lacroix JS, Seebach JD, Harr T. Immunoglobulin deficiency in patients with chronic rhinosinusitis: systematic review of the literature and meta-analysis. J Allergy Clin Immunol. 2015;136(6):1523–31. https://doi.org/10.1016/j.jaci.2015.07.016.
36. Quinti I, Soresina A, Spadaro G, Martino S, Donnanno S, Agostini C, et al. Long-term follow-up and outcome of a large cohort of patients with common variable immunodeficiency. J Clin Immunol. 2007;27(3):308–16. https://doi.org/10.1007/s10875-007-9075-1.
37. Kashani S, Carr TF, Grammer LC, Schleimer RP, Hulse KE, Kato A, et al. Clinical characteristics of adults with chronic rhinosinusitis and specific antibody deficiency. J Allergy Clin Immunol Pract. 2015;3(2):236–42. https://doi.org/10.1016/j.jaip.2014.09.022.
38. Naclerio RM, Baroody FM. Other phenotypes and treatment of chronic rhinosinusitis. J Allergy Clin Immunol Pract. 2016;4(4):613–20. https://doi.org/10.1016/j.jaip.2016.03.016.
39. Stevens WW, Peters AT. Immunodeficiency in chronic sinusitis: recognition and treatment. Am J Rhinol Allergy. 2015;29(2):115–8. https://doi.org/10.2500/ajra.2015.29.4144.
40. Bush A, Chodhari R, Collins N, Copeland F, Hall P, Harcourt J, et al. Primary ciliary dyskinesia: current state of the art. Arch Dis Child. 2007;92(12):1136–40. https://doi.org/10.1136/adc.2006.096958.
41. Bequignon E, Dupuy L, Zerah-Lancner F, Bassinet L, Honore I, Legendre M, et al. Critical evaluation of sinonasal disease in 64 adults with primary ciliary dyskinesia. J Clin Med 2019;8(5). https://doi.org/10.3390/jcm8050619.
42. Alanin MC, Aanaes K, Hoiby N, Pressler T, Skov M, Nielsen KG, et al. Sinus surgery can improve quality of life, lung infections, and lung function in patients with primary ciliary dyskinesia. Int Forum Allergy Rhinol. 2017;7(3):240–7. https://doi.org/10.1002/alr.21873.
43. Chang EH, Stern DA, Willis AL, Guerra S, Wright AL, Martinez FD. Early life risk factors for chronic sinusitis: a longitudinal birth cohort study. J Allergy Clin Immunol. 2018;141(4):1291–7.e2. https://doi.org/10.1016/j.jaci.2017.11.052.
44. Wu D, Bleier BS, Li L, Zhan X, Zhang L, Lv Q, et al. Clinical phenotypes of nasal polyps and comorbid asthma based on cluster analysis of disease history. J Allergy Clin Immunol Pract. 2018;6(4):1297–305.e1. https://doi.org/10.1016/j.jaip.2017.09.020.
45. Song WJ, Lee JH, Won HK, Bachert C. Chronic rhinosinusitis with nasal polyps in older adults: clinical presentation, pathophysiology, and comorbidity. Curr Allergy Asthma Rep. 2019;19(10):46. https://doi.org/10.1007/s11882-019-0880-4.

Imaging the Anatomic Landmarks for Safe FESS

24

Simion James Zinreich and Sachin K. Gujar

24.1 Introduction

Functional endoscopic sinus surgery has been practiced worldwide for the past thirty years following the principles established by Messerklinger, Stammberger, Kennedy, and others who have focused this procedure in the stepwise resection of the four ground lamellae [1–3] (Fig. 24.1a–c). This regional anatomy is diverse and varies from person to person. In spite of the technical advances in imaging technology and image guided surgery (IGS) understanding the endoscopically viewed surgical field remains a challenge.

In the early 1980s endoscopic sinus surgery (ESS), now referred to as functional endoscopic sinus surgery (FESS) [2, 3] largely replaced external approaches and today represents the treatment of choice for a long list of sinonasal pathologies, including inflammatory and neoplastic nasal and sinus pathologies, as well as skull base and orbital lesions. The introduction of advanced endoscopes, cutting instruments, and imaging techniques including image guidance facilitated the surgery and aimed to improve the safety of the procedure. Over the past three decades, there has been a steady increase in the number of FESS procedures [4, 5].

The close proximity of the surgical site to the orbit and the cranial compartment, however, continued to associate FESS with a variety of complications. As early as 1929, Mosher noted that intranasal ethmoidectomy was "the easiest way to kill a patient" [6, 7]. One would have hoped that the increasing anatomical knowledge, the introduction of advanced surgical instrumentation, advances in imaging, and the introduction of image guided surgery (IGS) would avoid these complications. However, due to individual anatomic variations and the relative ease of destructing the fine bony structures of the skull base and the orbital wall, FESS results in a broad range of surgical complications [5]. The serious complications have significantly decreased throughout the past decades, but continue to occur [8–20].

The objective of this communication is to address how the imaging information might be better utilized to further aid FESS and to avoid the serious complications. The emphasis therefore will be on identifying, defining, and discussing the most pertinent anatomic variations.

Furthermore, in an attempt to improve the identification of regional landmarks on the imaging information, 3D stereoscopic imaging (3DSI), a new software based technology, will be "sparingly" used to facilitate and enhance the

S. J. Zinreich (✉) · S. K. Gujar
The Russel H. Morgan Department of Radiology, The Johns Hopkins Medical Institutions, Baltimore, MD, USA

Department of Otorhinolaryngology, Head and Neck Surgery, The Johns Hopkins Medical Institutions, Baltimore, MD, USA
e-mail: sjzinreich@jhmi.edu; sgujar1@jhmi.edu

L. Zhang, C. Bachert (eds.), *Chronic Rhinosinusitis*, https://doi.org/10.1007/978-981-16-0784-4_24

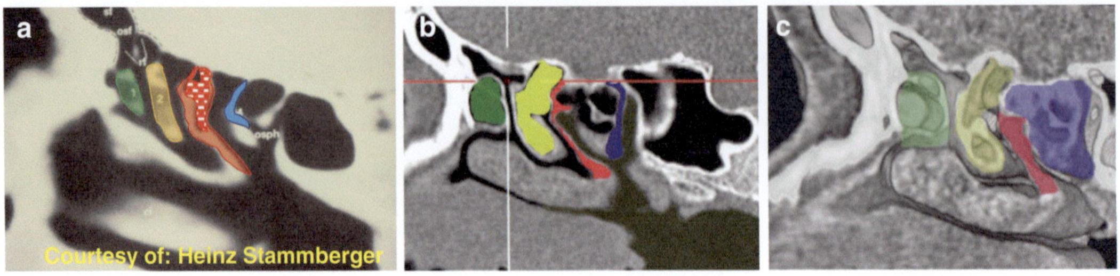

Fig. 24.1 The lamellae within the ethmoid sinus. (**a**) Graphic display by H. Stammberger; (**b**) CT sagittal display; (**c**) 3D stereoscopic display. The color green outlines the uncinate lamella, the color yellow the uncinate lamella, the red color outlines the basal lamella, and the red color the superior lamella

three dimensionality of the regional morphology and aid endoscopic correlation.

24.2 The Use of Imaging to Provide a "Roadmap" for FESS

Since the introduction of endoscopic sinus surgery (ESS) polytomography was used by Messerklinger and Stammberger to replace the imaging information provided by plain films of the sinuses. This planar imaging technology, usually used to evaluate bony structures, providing planar sections of several mms to a centimeter improved the display of the fine bony structures in the nasal cavity and the paranasal sinuses [1, 2, 4]. In turn, in the mid-1980s given the superior resolution of computerized x-ray tomography (CT), it replaced polytomography and rapidly became the choice imaging study to display the regional anatomy and provide a more accurate and detailed guide for FESS [4]. Several publications followed describing the usefulness of CT in guiding FESS, aiding in the diagnosis of pathology, and highlighting risks which could lead to complications [20–24].

More recently, the availability of 3D CT stereoscopic imaging (3DSI) provides a more "intuitive" display of the anatomy, improving the correlation with 3D endoscopy and providing an improved display of the regional "landmarks." The improved imaging display should aid in further decreasing the risk of FESS. This is a new technology, which is not readily available and is still under study. Nevertheless, as stated above, we will use it "sparingly," to aid the description of anatomic detail which needs clarification aiming to address confusion and ambiguity.

24.3 CT Data Acquisition and Technique

The CT equipment currently available is significantly more advanced than at the time it was first introduced to evaluate the nasal cavity and paranasal sinuses and is available worldwide. Also, most of the available CT scanners are equipped with software capable of rendering a multiplanar imaging display (MPR). The following are the important parameters determining a quality CT MPR evaluation of the nasal cavity and paranasal sinuses:

- Slice thickness should be <1.0 mm (preferably 0.75 mm).
- After the performance of a lateral scout view, adjust the field of view to cover the sinuses. The primary images are axial images, parallel to the plane of the hard palate. Subsequently adjust the field of view as follows: **inferiorly**, parallel to the hard palate; **posteriorly**, a coronal plane perpendicular to the hard palate, to include the sella turcica; **anteriorly**, a coronal plane perpendicular to the hard palate, at the tip of the nose; and **superiorly**, a plane parallel to the hard palate, including a few mm of the intracranial compartment above the frontal sinuses. Choosing this field of view will provide proper display (magnification) of the regional anatomy, affording an accurate evaluation.

- Create an MPR data set using the data within the volume of the adjusted field of view. In the rendered dataset confirm that the coronal and sagittal planes are perpendicular to the bony palate.

The "sparingly" used 3D stereoscopic images are rendered volumetrically and as stated earlier still under development. The images you will see are 3D stereo images displayed on a flat surface showing a reduced depth perception and therefore, if we are permitted to say, a 2.5D display.

24.4 The CT Evaluation of Nasal and Paranasal Sinus Anatomy for FESS, According to the Specific Surgical Plan, Which Follows the Four Lamellae Principle

The evaluation of the CT imaging information may be approached in various ways; however, it would be prudent to undertake this task following the "lamellar principle" laid forth by Messerklinger and Stammberger (Fig. 24.1a–c). Stammberger clearly outlines the sequential surgical steps in approaching FESS, starting with: uncinectomy, followed by anterior ethmoidectomy, then the penetration of the basal lamella and removal of posterior ethmoid spaces, so as to then reach and perform a sphenoidotomy. The final step is to perform a frontal sinusotomy. In cases where the posterior ethmoid sinuses and sphenoid sinus remain uninvolved with inflammatory disease, he proposes an uncinectomy followed by partial resection of the ethmoid bulla and then performing a frontal sinusotomy. The imaging evaluation will specifically focus on the structures involved in the performance of the above-mentioned surgical steps, as well as the "tight spots" regulating mucociliary clearance.

24.5 Uncinectomy

Determine the location of the anterior middle turbinate attachment to the lateral nasal wall, the "axilla" on coronal images (Fig. 24.2a–i). Invariably at this location the middle turbinate will be fused to the uncinate process laterally (Fig. 24.3a–c). In Fig. 24.3b, by removal of the middle turbinate the surface relationships between the uncinate process, ethmoid bulla, and basal lamella are clearly visualized. In Fig. 24.3c the nasal tissue anterior to the axilla was removed to reveal the "space" medial to the uncinate process, currently referred to as the "Agger nasi cell" (ANC). In Fig. 24.3b, c in the sagittal plane, the hiatus semilunaris is revealed [the planar "gap" between the uncinate lamella (UP) and the bulla lamella (BL)].

- Scrolling back and forth in the coronal plane and if available using multiplanar CT display, one will be able to determine that: the bony plate of the uncinate process has two components: a turbinal component (TUP) (Fig. 24.4a, b) and an ethmoidal component (EUP) (Fig. 24.5a–f).
- The TUP in 80% of cases arises from the region of the posterior fontanelle, along the medial wall of the maxillary sinus, usually posterior to the ethmoid bulla, and extends from infero-medially to ventro-superiorly to adhere to the lacrimal bone, traversing the surface of the medial nasolacrimal duct to fuse with the fibers of the inferior turbinate. In its course anteriorly it creates a space between the bony plate of the TUP and the medial maxillary wall, increasing in size ventrally as it is in the plane of the lamina papyracea, thus creating the turbinal Infundibulum (Fig. 24.4a, b).
- As the TUP reaches the level of the inferior nasal spine, the sagittal oriented bony plate abruptly turns laterally to begin the creation of a three dimensional space, and the creation of the ethmoidal uncinate process, as the sagittal oriented bony plate fuses: anteriorly, with the medial aspect of the frontal process of the maxilla; posteriorly, with the ventral bulla lamella (creating a common lamella which fuses laterally with the lamina papyracea), and borders the infundibulum; laterally, with the lamina papyracea, which in turn fuses ventrally with the lateral frontal

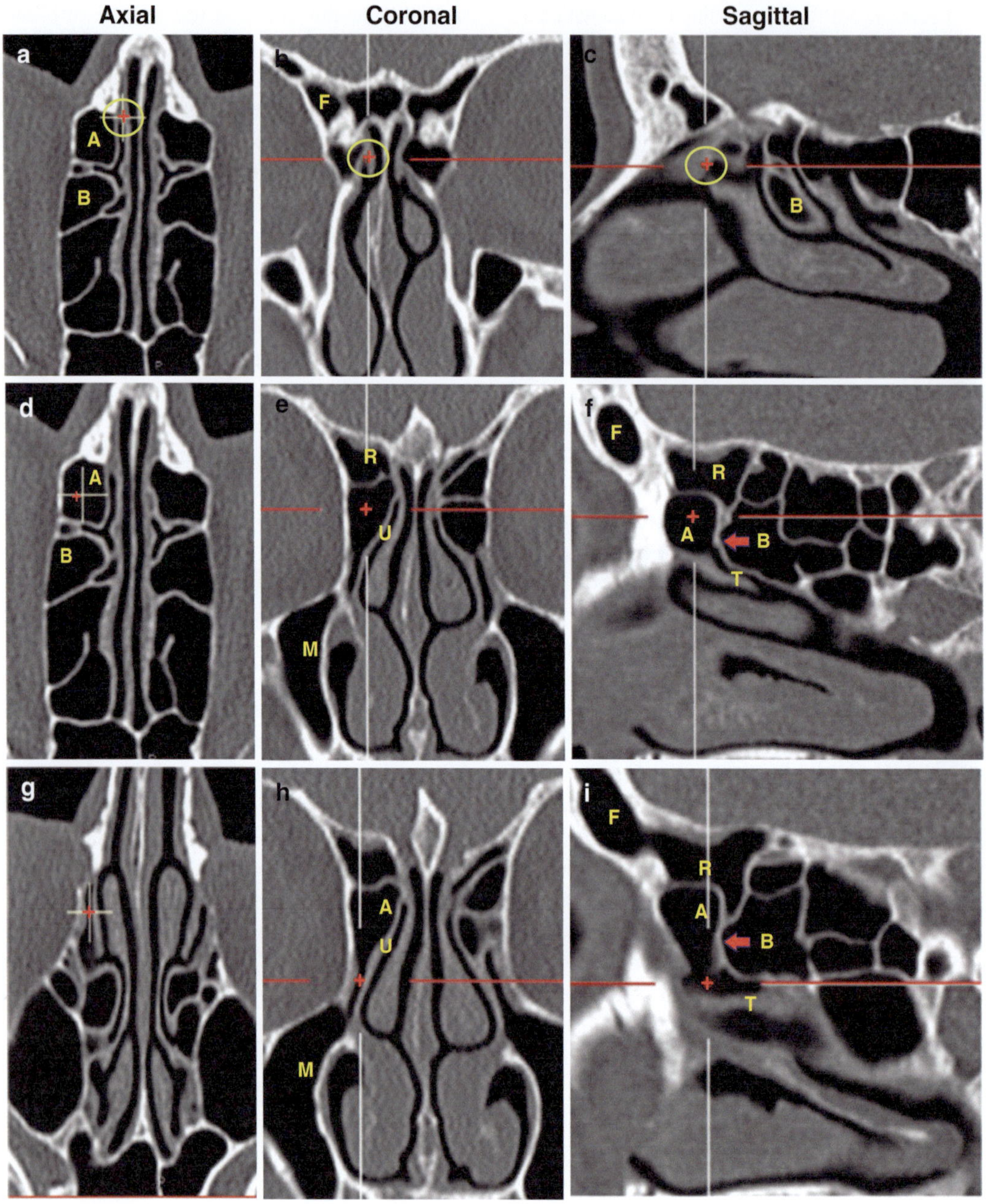

Fig. 24.2 Endoscopic images of the steps in an uncinectomy, performed by H. Stammberger. (**a**) Relationship of the middle turbinate (MT) and the uncinate process (U), (**b**) shows the green perimeter of the planned uncinectomy, (**c**) uncinectomy performed, still showing a green border of remaining uncinate, and the ethmoid bulla is revealed (B)

process of the maxilla; superiorly, usually borders with the floor of the frontal recess, as this union invariably attaches to the superior nasal spine. Inferiorly, the three dimensional space has a horizontally shaped gap affording an opening to the turbinal infundibulum which ultimately communicates with the maxillary sinus. The above described three dimensional space is the ethmoidal uncinate process (EUP), with its

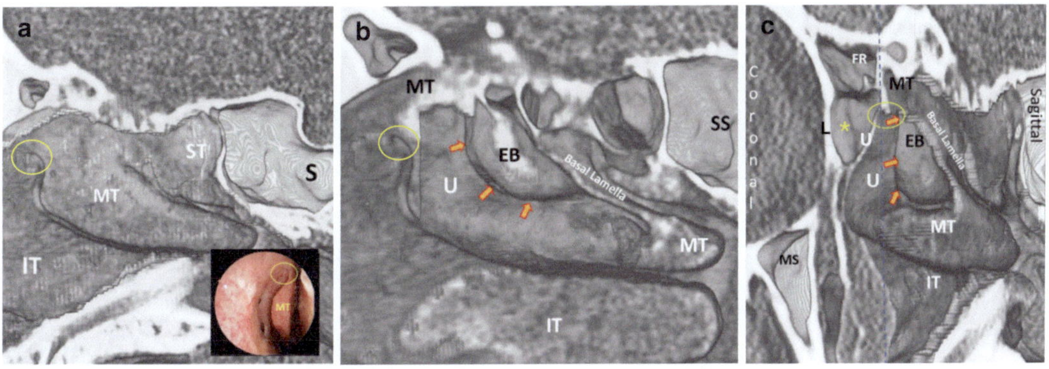

Fig. 24.3 CT MPR images: corresponding axial, coronal, and sagittal images focusing on the "axilla," (attachment of the anterior middle turbinate to lateral nasal wall). (**a**)–(**c**) with red cross hairs, and yellow circle, on the axilla. (**d**)–(**f**) with crosshairs in the infundibular space of the ethmoidal uncinate process (A), currently known as the "Agger Nasi Cell." (**g**)–(**i**) reveals the communication of the EUP with the maxillary sinus (M), and relationship to the front sinus/frontal recess unit (F, frontal sinus, and R, frontal recess). Common lamella between the EUP and the ethmoidal bulla (B) demonstrated in (**f**, **i**), red arrow head: uncinate process (U), turbinal uncinate (T)

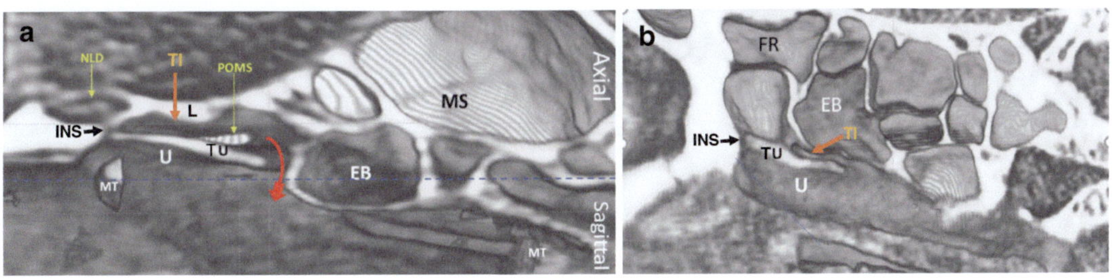

Fig. 24.4 3D stereoscopic images of the lateral nasal wall. (**a**) reveals the lateral nasal wall in the sagittal plane status post a virtual septectomy. Note the region of the "axilla," yellow oval circle, as well as a corresponding endoscopic picture revealing the axilla. (**b**) The lateral nasal wall status post septectomy and partial removal of the middle turbinate revealing the "free edge" of the uncinate process and the hiatus semilunaris (yellow arrows with red outline) note the position of the hiatus semilunaris between the uncinate process (U), and the ethmoid bulla (EB). (**c**), where the sagittally oriented image is angled to the left, and an anterior coronal view is available at the axilla. Note the space denoted by a yellow asterisk, currently known as an Agger Nasi Cell, however, please note that its medial wall is the uncinate process (U), and the lateral wall the lamina papyracea (L). *F* frontal sinus, *FR* frontal recess, *MT* middle turbinate, *EB* ethmoidal bulla, *ST* superior turbinate, *IT* inferior turbinate, *S* sphenoid sinus

infundibular space, currently predominantly being reoffered to as the "Agger Nasi Cell" (Fig. 24.5a–f).

- Note the number of spaces within the EUP, and their communication with the infundibulum, which may be direct, or a confluence of the spaces which communicate with the infundibulum through a single opening.
- Determine how close the uncinate lamella is to the lamina papyracea, the presence of infra bulla ethmoid cells (Haller cells), the presence of bulla within the TUP, the presence of compression from adjacent spaces such as the frontal recess, ethmoid bulla, concha bullosa, and how these changes affect the infundibulum, and in general the drainage pattern of the frontal sinus/frontal recess (Fig. 24.6a–d). Careful attention regarding the superior attachment of the uncinate lamella is needed to ascertain the effect various attachments may have on the infundibulum and the frontal sinus drainage pathway (Fig. 24.7a–c).
- Given that the EUP may be compressed by an expanding ethmoid bulla, frontal recess, concha bullosa, or the presence of an uncinate bulla, specific attention is needed in establish-

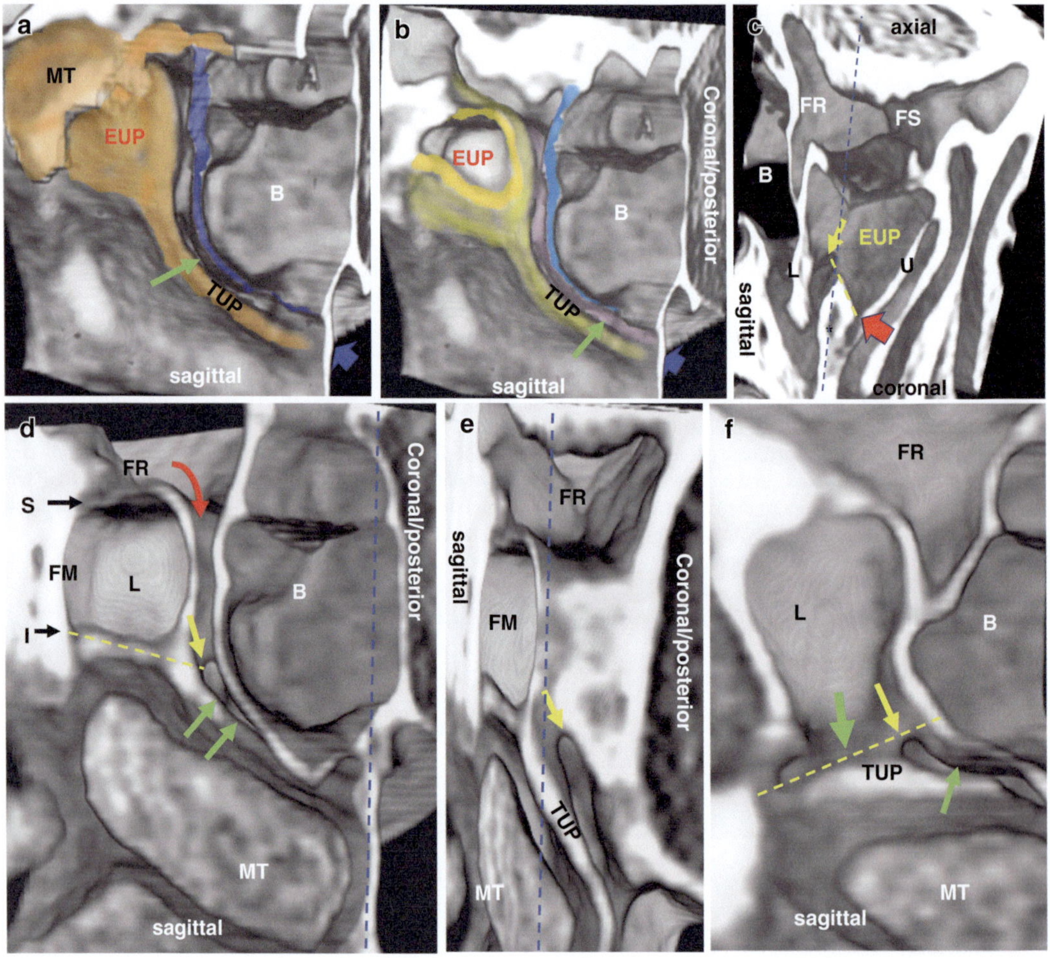

Fig. 24.5 3D stereoscopic images of the turbinal uncinate process. (**a**, **b**) reveals the turbinal uncinate process (TU), arising from the posterior fontanelle area, inferior-laterally, increasing in height as it extends anteriorly to adhere to the lacrimal bone at the inferior nasal spine (INS) and the lamina papyracea (L). As it extends ventrally it creates a steadily increasing space between the bony plate of the turbinal uncinate process (TU), and the lamina papyracea (L), creating the turbinal infundibulum (TI), enclosed ventrally and open dorsally to communicate with the middle meatus (curved red arrow). Nasolacrimal duct (NLD), primary ostium of maxillary sinus (POMS), ethmoid bulla (EB), maxillary sinus (MS), middle turbinate (MT), and frontal recess (FR)

ing the location of the infundibulum and the communication between the frontal sinus/frontal recess "Unit."

24.6 Anterior Ethmoidectomy

This procedure usually follows the uncinectomy. The uncinate process having been partially resected: enlarging the primary ostium of the maxillary sinus; provides a clear view of the anterior "face" of the ethmoid bulla (EB) (Fig. 24.3b, c)

- Establish the width of the EB, easily determined on the coronal and/or the axial images (Fig. 24.8). Determine, whether, the EB extends to the roof of the ethmoid sinus, the presence of supra bulla cells between the EB and the roof of the ethmoid sinus. Understand the vertical distance between the roof of the EB and the skull base (Fig. 24.8a–c).

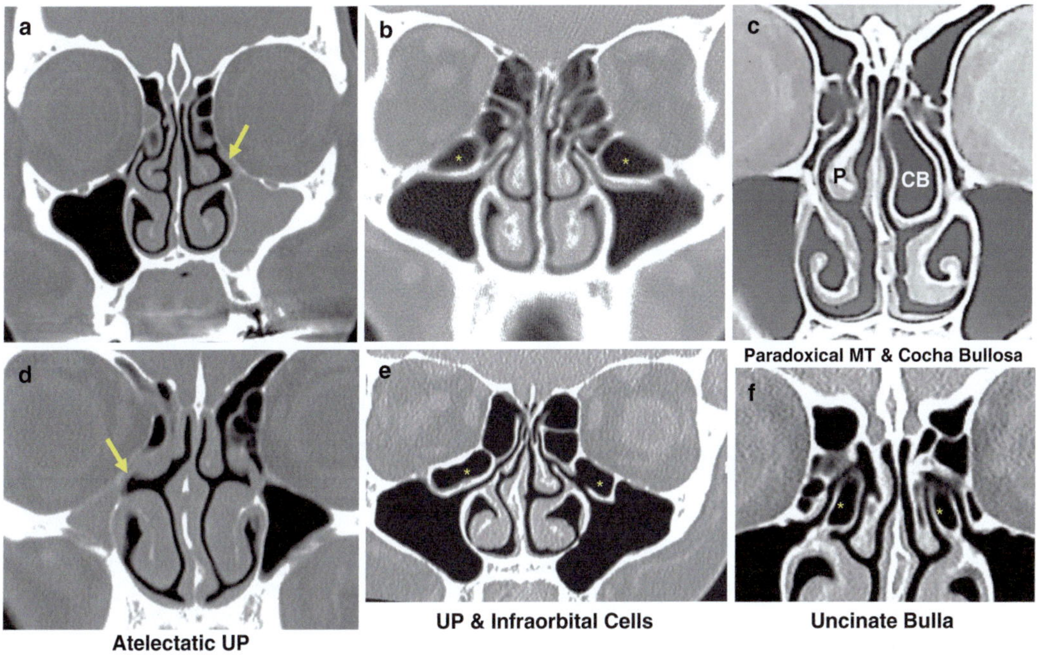

Fig. 24.6 3D stereoscopic images showing the two components of the uncinate process. (**a**, **b**) reveal the 3 dimensionality of the uncinate process, after partially removing the ethmoid bulla (B). The resected plane is colored blue. In (**a**), note in yellow color supero ventrally the fusion between the middle turbinate (MT) and the ethmoidal uncinate process (EUP). An inseparable "tail shaped" extension is visible also in yellow, which courses under the ethmoid bulla and represents the turbinal uncinate process (TUP). The medial border of the EUP as well as the remnant middle turbinate in (**a**) has been removed by "scrolling into the volume from medial to lateral", and (**b**) reveals the space lateral to the agger, the middle turbined, and the uncinate process. This space is surrounded by the bony architecture of the EUP, a superior extension from the turbinal uncinate process (TUP). The plane of separation is shown by the dashed yellow line in (**c**, **d**, **f**). The plane extends from the inferior nasal spine [red arrow, (**c**); I in (**d**)], and posteriorly, the inferior edge of the UP as it fuses with the inferior bulla lamella (yellow arrow, **c**–**f**). Inferior within the space created by the EUP there is an opening affording communication with the turbinal infundibulum (green arrows) which in turn communicates with the maxillary sinus more inferiorly. Anteriorly the space is bordered by the frontal process of the maxilla (FM), laterally with the lamina papyracea (L), dorsally with the infundibulum, and the common lamella as the EUP fuses with the bulla lamella [blue colored edge, (**a**, **b**)]. Superiorly, the uncinate lamella extends in a horizontal plane forward to fuse with the superior nasal spine, (**d**). Given that the space created by the EUP enclosure and communicates with the infundibulum, the space is more accurately called an infundibular space (the term Agger Nasi Cell is likely the result of the surgical penetration into the agger area and thus penetrating into the space within the uncinate bony perimeter). Note is made that fig. © is created by partially removing the lamina papyracea (L) from sagittally and removing the frontal process of the maxilla in the coronal plane, revealing the bony continuity of the EUP dorsally medially and superiorly

- Determine the anterior–posterior distance from the anterior face of the ethmoid bulla to the basal lamella, best measured on the axial and sagittal images. The course of the basal lamella is "tortuous" and its extent and orientation would be best displayed with the use of MPR. Seek the separation point of the superior turbinate from the middle turbinate and view this location on both the sagittal and axial reconstructions. Specifically, on the axial images, scroll to the point of separation between the middle (MT) and superior turbinate (ST). Just below the level of the separation between the MT and the ST, follow the dorsal–lateral extension of the middle turbinate to the lamina papyracea and identify the course of the basal lamella (Fig. 24.8d–f).
- Note the presence of anatomic variations involving the lamina papyracea, whereby the lamina "protrudes" into the volume of the

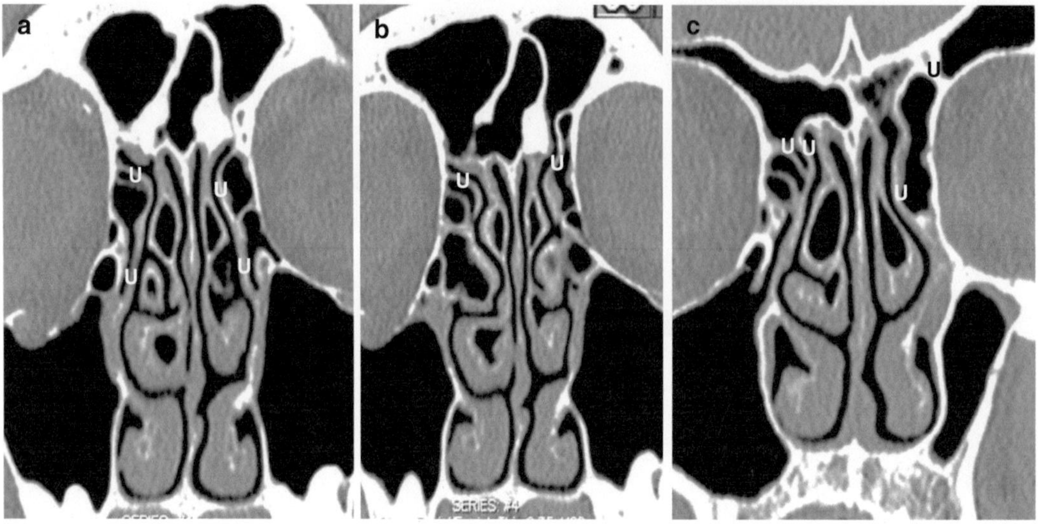

Fig. 24.7 Coronal images displaying atelectatic uncinate process (red arrows) (**a**, **d**), infraorbital cells (yellow asterisks) (**b**, **e**), paradoxical middle turbinate (P), and concha bullosa (B) (**c**) and uncinate bulla (yellow asterisks) (**e**)

anterior ethmoid sinus. These are usually above or below the attachment of the basal lamella (Fig. 24.9a–c). These "invaginations" are anatomic variations and should not be infringed surgically. Establish distance relationships between these "indentations," the middle turbinate, and EB. If present below the attachment of the basal lamella note the relationship to the uncinate process and the infundibulum.

- Use the coronal plane to establish the foramina of the AEA and PEA. MPR images focusing on the foramen and "scrolling" superiorly in the plane of the lamina papyracea will reveal the angulation of the arteries in the axial plane. The AEA foramen and the course of the AEA are commonly associated with the bulla lamella. By medially scrolling in the sagittal plane, establish the medial relationship between the AEA and bulla lamella and/or basal lamella, as these anatomic structures may be used as landmarks and aides in avoiding incursion into the artery during FESS. Not infrequently, medially, the basal lamella will adhere with the medial bulla lamella, and both will adhere with the anterior ethmoidal artery (AEA) (Fig. 24.10a–c).

24.7 Ethmoid Skull Base Height

The most common complication site when performing FESS, is the skull base, and it occurs at its weakest site, where the middle turbinate fuses laterally with the lateral lamella and medially with the cribriform plate [23, 24] (Fig. 24.11a, b). Drawing a horizontal line through the cribriform plate and a horizontal line through the frontal plate provided Keros with a classification based on the distance between these lines (Fig. 24.11a):

1. Keros Type I: 1–3 mm deep.
2. Keros Type II: 4–7 mm deep.
3. Keros Type III: 8–16 mm deep.

The greater the depth (distance) the greater the chance for an intracranial injury. The height of the lateral lamella usually decreases from anterior to posterior [20, 25]. Use coronal planes to determine at which coronal plane is the roof highest and lowest, and where is the asymmetry from side to side most prominent.

The distances in most cases will vary from side to side. In 2/3 of the cases the right lateral lamella is lower than the left. Not surprising, therefore, that most skull base "violations" occur on the right side [24] (Fig. 24.11b).

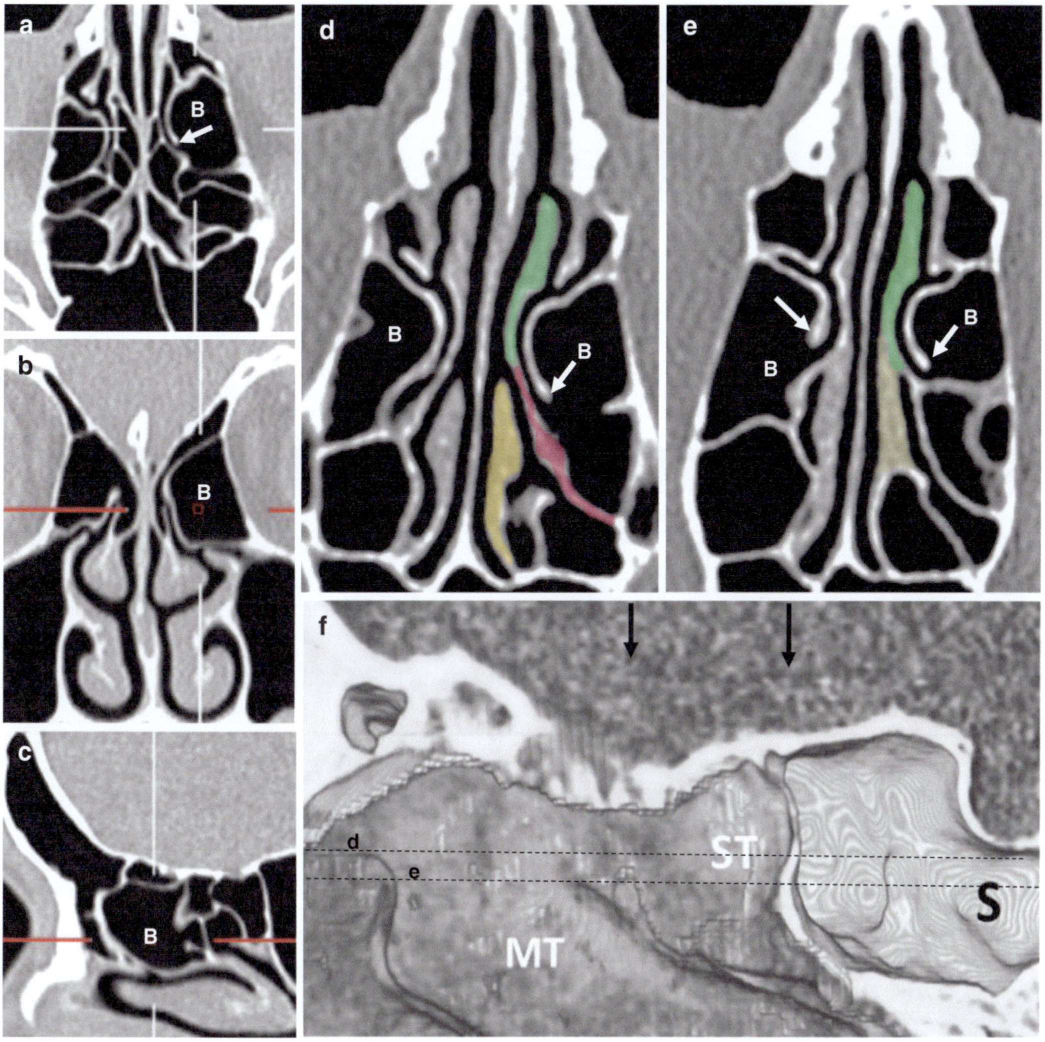

Fig. 24.8 The location and extent of the ethmoid bulla and location of the basal lamella. MPR images (**a–c**), with coronal and sagittal images in the middle of the ethmoidal bulla (B), reveal the location of the ethmoid bulla, and its relation to skull base, lamina papyracea. Note the absence of the posterior wall of the ethmoid bulla (**a**, **d**, **e**), white arrows, at break in the dorsal continuity of the ethmoid bulla wall; B, ethmoid bulla. Also note references to the levels of the axial sections (**d**, **e**) on sagittal image (**f**) at point of separation of the middle turbinate (green), from superior turbinate (yellow), and the dorsal lateral coursing basal lamella (red). On the more superior axial image note the union between the middle turbinate (green) and the superior turbinate (yellow)

24.8 Sphenoidotomy

The identification of the basal lamella as well as its course has been described above. Understanding the dorsal extent of the basal lamella is imperative. It determines the dorsal limit of the anterior ethmoid space, and in sagittal and axial planes it shows the extent of the posterior ethmoid space and its relationship with the "face" of the sphenoid sinus (Fig. 24.8d, f).

One should use the coronal plane to identify the superior turbinate. Not infrequently, a supreme turbinate is readily identified. However, should the supreme turbinate not be readily identified, one should look for a soft tissue "bulge" just above and usually in line with the superior

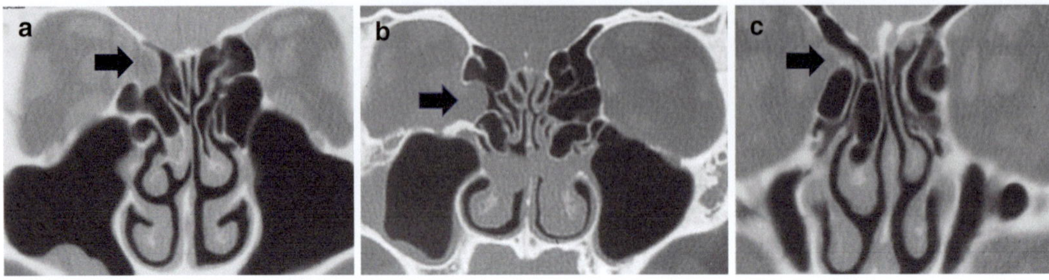

Fig. 24.9 (**a**–**c**) Anatomic variation, with orbital soft tissue "herniating" into the ethmoid space, a "leave me alone lesion." The soft tissue herniation (black arrow) shows the soft tissue "herniation into the ethmoid space", usually adjacent to the basal lamella

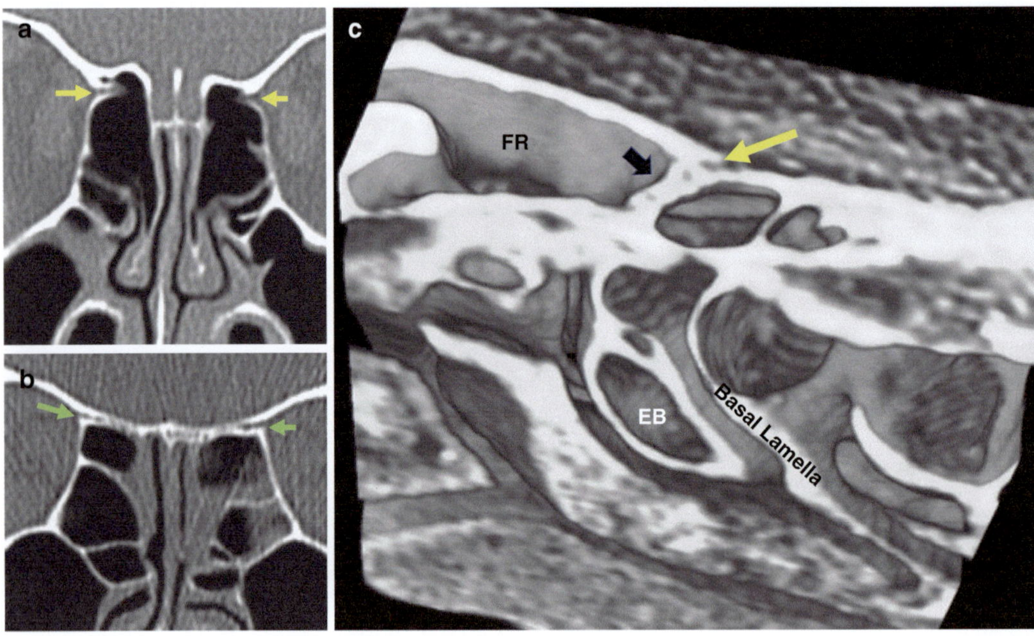

Fig. 24.10 (**a**–**c**) Coronal sections through the anterior ethmoid arteries (yellow arrows) and posterior ethmoid arteries (green arrows). In (**c**) note close relationship between the anterior ethmoid artery and the bulla lamella (black arrow); *FR* frontal recess, *EB* ethmoidal bulla; and the basal lamella

turbinate, to identify "the bulge," which, likely represents an incompletely developed supreme turbinate. In most cases the medial border of this "bulge" or that of the supreme turbinate, in the coronal and at times the sagittal plane is in line or just medial to the sphenoid sinus ostium (Fig. 24.12a–c).

Note the variable aeration of the sinus cavities and the presence and angulation of the intrasinus septum. This may deviate from midline and it should be noted if it adheres to the bony indentations created by the optic canal and the carotid canal. Not infrequently there may be more than one septation within the sphenoid sinus. Septations are vertically oriented, whereas horizontal bony separations represent, sphenoid sinus spaces inferior to this "separation," as the spaces above the horizontal bony structure are posterior ethmoid spaces which have extended above the sphenoid spaces and in several instances may reach the ventral pituitary fossa. In these cases, the optic nerve will be especially vulnerable to

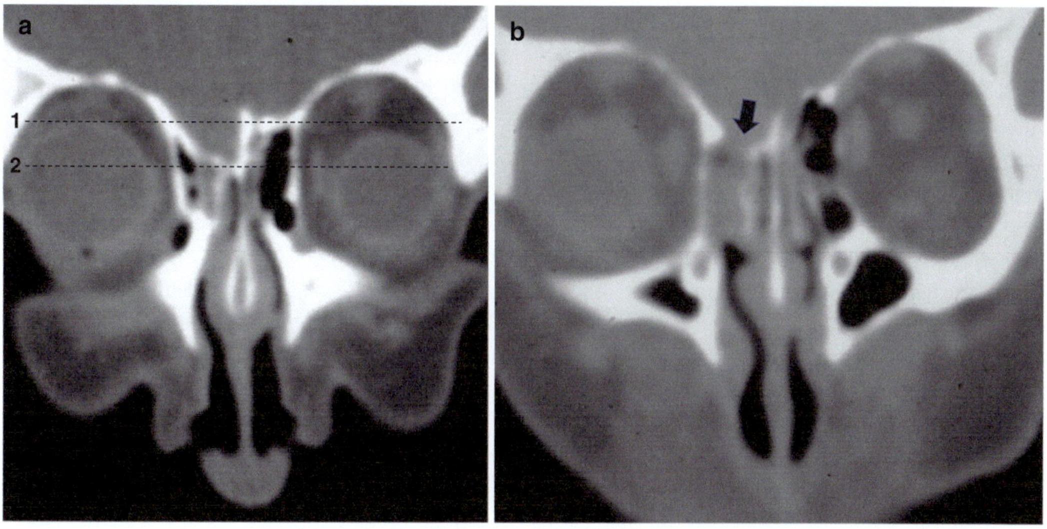

Fig. 24.11 Measurements for Keros classification. (**a**) reveals the planes used to establish the skull base height from the cribriform plate: (plane 1), horizontal to the frontal plate; (plane 2), horizontal to cribriform plate. (**b**) reveals a skull base penetration on the right side, where the plane of the cribriform plate is lower

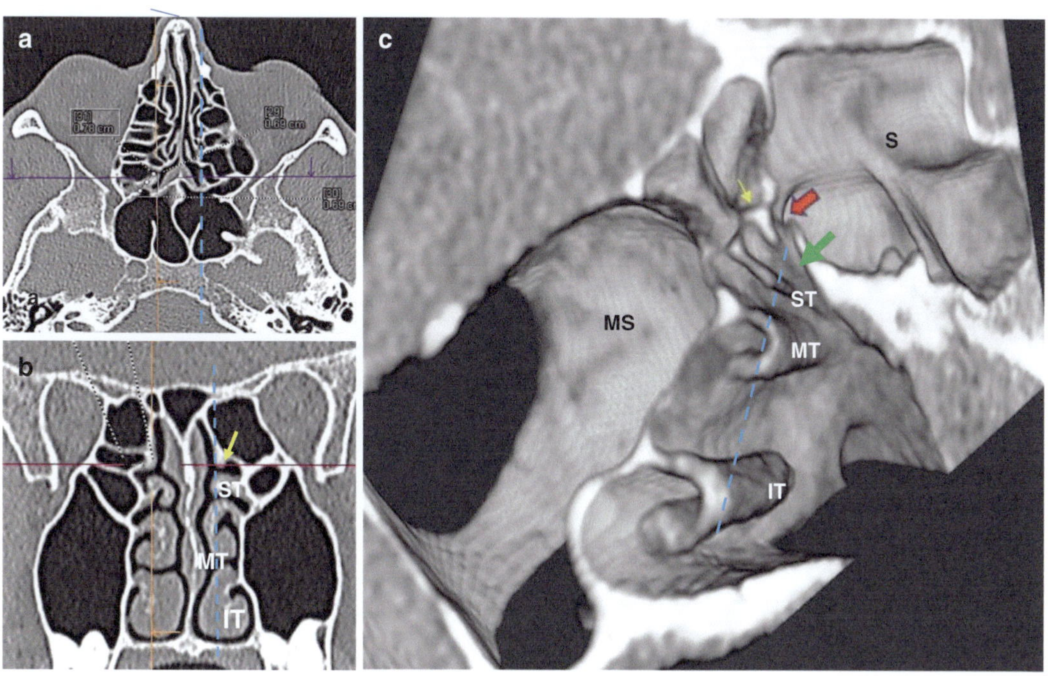

Fig. 24.12 (**a**–**c**) Establishing the path to the sphenoid sinus ostium. In (**a**, **b**) use the coronal plane to identify the superior/supreme turbinate (yellow arrow) and create a vertical plane along the medial borders of the turbinates (blue dashed line) and correlate with sagittal plane crossing through the sphenoid ostium (blue dashed line on axial image). The sagittal plane will be through or just medial to the sphenoid sinus opening. In (**c**), an oblique sagittal 3D stereoscopic view reveals the relationship between the medial turbinates and the sphenoid sinus ostium (blue dashed line); red arrow, ostium of sphenoid sinus; yellow arrow the supreme turbinate; *IT* inferior turbinate, *MT* middle turbinate, *ST* the superior turbinate, *S* the sphenoid sinus, *MS* maxillary sinus

injury (Onodi "sphenoethmoidal cells") (Fig. 24.13a–c).

The bony perimeter of the sphenoid sinus should be carefully evaluated for the presence of dehiscence. These may be present and associated with the indentations created by the carotid artery and the optic nerve canal and should be confirmed. A prominent bulge from the internal carotid artery may be present in up to 80% of patients [15]. The bone overlying the carotid artery may be dehiscent in up to 22% [16]. Additional dehiscence and/or erosion should be considered to be pathologic (Fig. 24.13d, e).

The foramen rotundum and the pterygoid (vidian) canal are in the floor or the lateral wall of the sphenoid sinus. In most cases the pterygoid canal is embedded in the floor of the sphenoid sinus or slightly protruding. In 22%, the canal is suspended from the wall by a bony stalk, almost freely floating in the sinus. In 3%, the canal can be dehiscent and usually anteriorly [17].

The sphenoid sinus may pneumatize posteriorly to variable degrees under and behind the sella turcica into the clivus. The extent of aeration should be noted to avoid intracranial penetration through a thinned sinus wall.

24.9 Frontal Recess/Sinusotomy

Schaeffer states that: "the first evidence of the sinus frontalis must not be sought in the frontal bone, but in the recessus frontalis of the meatus nasi medius." He follows up with the statement that: "The sinus frontalis is in the vast majority a derivative of the recessus frontalis directly" [26, 27].

Considering the above, and the fact that the frontal sinus "funnel" (formerly "infundibulum frontale") and the frontal recess invariably merge completely with potential extension: inferiorly, laterally, and posteriorly, into the space of the anterior ethmoid sinus, without forming an hourglass configuration, as well as the fact that in the adult, there is no identifiable anatomic landmark to define the separation between the frontal sinus and the frontal recess, the airspace, including the frontal sinus and the frontal recess, is and should be considered as a "unit." We therefore refer to

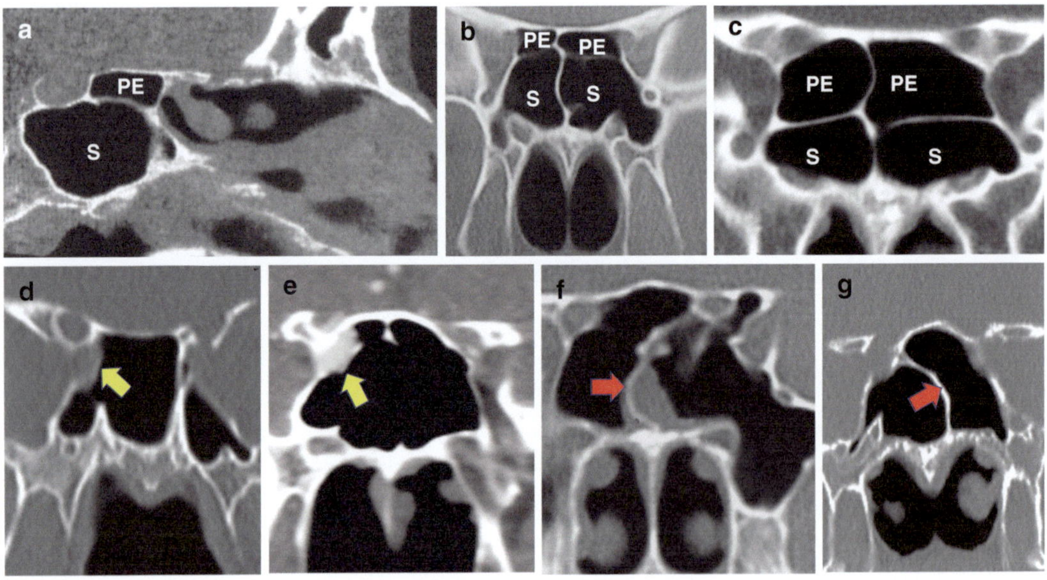

Fig. 24.13 Onodi "sphenoethmoidal cells," dehiscence, and septation adhering to the optic and carotid canals. (**a**)–(**c**) reveal the Onodi sphenoethmoidal cells; (**d**) reveals dehiscence of the carotid canal, yellow arrow; (**e**) contrast in the carotid canal, yellow arrow; (**f**) reveals a septum adhering to the optic canal, red arrow; (**g**) septum adhering to carotid canal, red arrow

the combined space of the frontal sinus and the frontal recess as the frontal sinus/frontal recess unit (FSFRU) (Fig. 24.14a–c).

The FSFRU is bordered superiorly by the skull base; anteriorly by the frontal bone, and at times the frontal process of the maxilla; and medially by the middle turbinate. The posterior border and inferior borders show the more common variability.

- Variability of the posterior border is:
  - Most commonly it is the bulla lamella, extending to skull base (Fig. 24.14b, c, e).
  - The uncinate lamella may extend to skull base anterior to the bulla lamella, creating a suprabullar recess space, with its individual opening to the anterior ethmoid/middle meatus.
- The uncinate lamella and/or a lamella arising from the bony fusion between the uncinate lamella and the bulla lamella may extend into the frontal sinus adhering to the anterior or posterior wall of the frontal sinus, a "frontal bulla space" (Fig. 24.15a–c).
- Variability of the inferior border/floor of the FSFRU:
  - Predominantly, the FSFRU, "space," is horizontally oriented, posteriorly, to the uncinate lamella creating a common border with the roof of the EUP which fuses with the superior nasal spine.
  - The FSFRU "space" may extend posteriorly to the bulla lamella and inferiorly, to a level between the superior and inferior nasal spine. Invariably, in these cases, the posterior extension is primarily lateral, creating a space between the lamina papyracea and the medially displaced lateral wall of the EUP. In virtually all these cases a "gap" is created in the lateral border of the EUP for a direct communication between the FSFRU and the infundibular space within the EUP (Fig. 24.16a–e).

The "opening" of the FSFRU is most commonly to the middle meatus directly and infundibulum indirectly and may also open directly into the infundibulum and middle meatus. The openings are, mostly, medially located whether anterior or posterior in location. Infrequently the FSFRU may open laterally directly into the

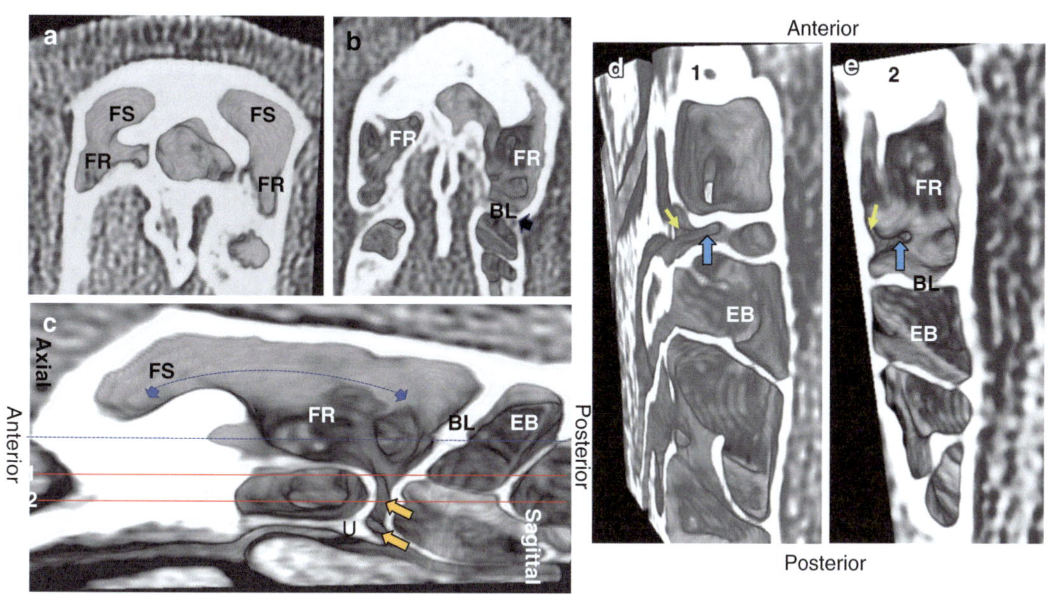

Fig. 24.14 Frontal sinus/frontal recess "unit" w. direct opening to infundibulum and middle meatus. (**a**, **b**) Axial images reveal the continuity of the frontal sinus (FS) and frontal recess (FR) spaces. Image (**c**), a combined axial and sagittal oriented 3D stereoscopic image reveals the path (blue dashed line), to the sphenoid ostium

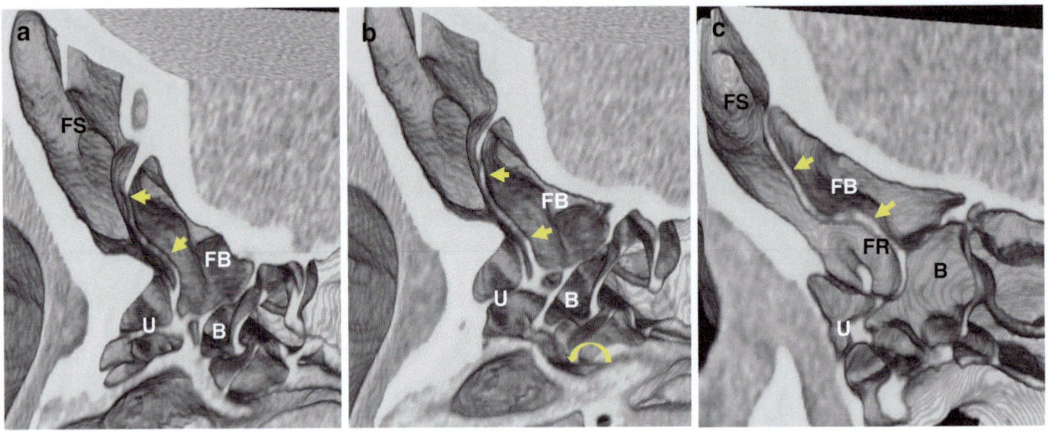

Fig. 24.15 A frontal bulla space. Note lamella arising from the bony fusion between the uncinate lamella and the bulla lamella extending into the frontal sinus adhering to the posterior wall of the frontal sinus (yellow arrows); *FS* frontal sinus, *U* ethmoidal uncinate infundibular space, *B* ethmoidal bulla, *FB* frontal bulla space; curved yellow arrow, primary ostium of maxillary sinus

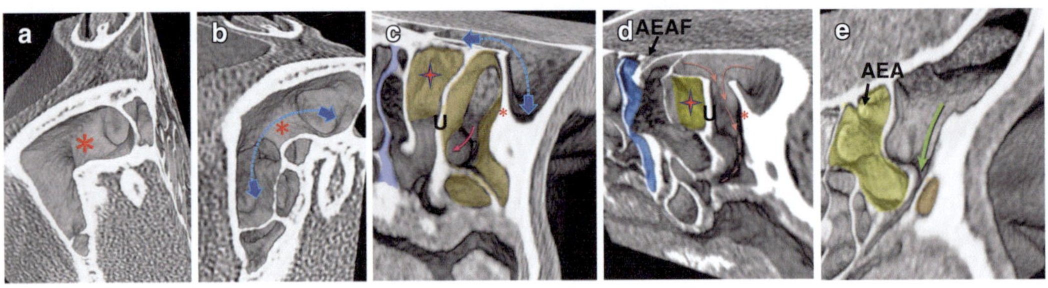

Fig. 24.16 Frontal sinus/frontal recess unit (FS/FRU) extending posterior-laterally, and inferiorly, below level of the superior nasal spine. (**a**)–(**d**) reveal the continuity of the frontal sinus and frontal recess (dashed blue line, and orange arrows). The uncinate lamella (U), superiorly, has a "steeplechase" shape, with its anterior segment attaching to the superior nasal spine (red asterisk). Note the "gap" in the lateral wall of the ethmoidal uncinate process [gap shown in the mustard colored bony architecture of the EUP in (**c**, **d**)]. This "gap" affords direct communication between the FS/FRU and the infundibular space within the EUP [red curved arrow in (**c**) and orange colored arrows in (**d**)]. Note direct/continuous communication between the lateral FS/FRU and the infundibulum, (**e**): yellow area in (**e**), ethmoidal bulla; red star, on a horizontal lamella/bony plate, fusing the uncinate lamella with the bulla lamella; blue colored lamella is the basal lamella; *AEMF* anterior ethmoid artery foramen, *AEA* anterior ethmoid artery

infundibulum and indirectly into the middle meatus (Fig. 24.16e).

24.10 Conclusion

Since X-ray polytomography was replaced by CT for the evaluation of the nasal cavity and paranasal sinuses, given the precarious location of this anatomy, it became clear that performing an endoscopically guided FESS relied on a "road-map," best displayed with CT imaging and more recently CT MPR imaging.

- Given the above, FESS should never be performed without the availability of a previously performed and studied CT evaluation.
- These images and if available image guidance equipment should be available in the OR during the surgical procedure.
- A clear understanding is needed of the lamellae, as landmarks to the "tight spots" which

afford communication of the frontal, maxillary, and sphenoid sinuses, with the ethmoid sinus. The specific tight spots are: the communication of the frontal sinus/frontal recess with the middle meatus; the communication of the maxillary sinus through the infundibulum to the middle meatus; and the drainage from the posterior ethmoid spaces and the sphenoid sinus through the spheno-ethmoid recess to the nasopharynx.

- Being familiar with the anatomy displayed on CT and specifically the ability to correlate the imaging landmarks with the endoscopic information will preclude inadvertent complications.

References

1. Messerklinger W. Role of the lateral nasal wall in the pathogenesis, diagnosis and therapy of recurrent and chronic rhinosinusitis. Laryngol Rhinol Otol. 1987;66(6):293–9.
2. <stammberger1993.pdf>.
3. Kennedy DW. Functional endoscopic sinus surgery. Technique. Arch Otolaryngol (Chicago, Ill: 1960). 1985;111(10):643–9. https://doi.org/10.1001/archotol.1985.00800120037003.
4. Zinreich SJ, Kennedy DW, Rosenbaum AE. Paranasal sinuses: CT imaging requirements for endoscopic sinus surgery. Radiology. 1987;163:769–75.
5. Hosemann W, Draf C. Danger points, complications and medico-legal aspects in endoscopic sinus surgery. GMS Curr Top Otorhinolaryngol Head Neck Surg. 2013;12:Doc06. https://doi.org/10.3205/cto000098.
6. Mosher HP. The applied anatomy and intranasal surgery of the ethmoid labyrinth. Laryngoscope. 1913;23:881–907.
7. Mosher HP. The surgical anatomy of the ethmoidal labyrinth. Ann Otol Rhinol Laryngol. 1929.
8. Stankiewicz JA. Complications of endoscopic intranasal ethmoidectomy. Laryngoscope. 1987;97(11):1270–3. https://doi.org/10.1288/00005537-198711000-00004.
9. Stankiewicz JA. Complications in endoscopic intranasal ethmoidectomy: an update. Laryngoscope. 1989;99(7 Pt 1):686–90. https://doi.org/10.1288/00005537-198907000-00004.
10. Freedman HM, Kern EB. Complications of intranasal ethmoidectomy: a review of 1,000 consecutive operations. Laryngoscope. 1979;89(3):421–34. https://doi.org/10.1288/00005537-197903000-00010.
11. Friedman WH, Katsantonis GP. The role of standard technique in modern sinus surgery. Otolaryngol Clin N Am. 1989;22(4):759–75.
12. Levine HL. Functional endoscopic sinus surgery: evaluation, surgery, and follow-up of 250 patients. Laryngoscope. 1990;100(1):79–84. https://doi.org/10.1288/00005537-199001000-00016.
13. Kennedy DW. Prognostic factors, outcomes and staging in ethmoid sinus surgery. Laryngoscope. 1992;102(12 Pt 2 Suppl 57):1–18.
14. May M, Levine HL, Mester SJ, Schaitkin B. Complications of endoscopic sinus surgery: analysis of 2108 patients – incidence and prevention. Laryngoscope. 1994;104(9):1080–3. https://doi.org/10.1288/00005537-199409000-00006.
15. Gross RD, Sheridan MF, Burgess LP. Endoscopic sinus surgery complications in residency. Laryngoscope. 1997;107(8):1080–5. https://doi.org/10.1097/00005537-199708000-00014.
16. Danielsen A, Olofsson J. Endoscopic endonasal sinus surgery: a review of 18 years of practice and long-term follow-up. Eur Arch Otorhinolaryngol. 2006;263(12):1087–98. https://doi.org/10.1007/s00405-006-0129-4.
17. Eviatar E, Pitaro K, Gavriel H, Krakovsky D. Complications following powered endoscopic sinus surgery: an 11 year study on 1190 patients in a single institute in Israel. Isr Med Assoc J. 2014;16(6):338–40.
18. Krings JG, Kallogjeri D, Wineland A, Nepple KG, Piccirillo JF, Getz AE. Complications of primary and revision functional endoscopic sinus surgery for chronic rhinosinusitis. Laryngoscope. 2014;124(4):838–45. https://doi.org/10.1002/lary.24401.
19. Hudgins PA. Complications of endoscopic sinus surgery. The role of the radiologist in prevention. Radiol Clin N Am. 1993;31(1):21–32.
20. DeLano MC, Fun FY, Zinreich SJ. Relationship of the optic nerve to the posterior paranasal sinuses: a CT anatomic study. AJNR Am J Neuroradiol. 1996;17(4):669–75.
21. Driben JS, Bolger WE, Robles HA, Cable B, Zinreich SJ. The reliability of computerized tomographic detection of the Onodi (Sphenoethmoid) cell. Am J Rhinol. 1998;12(2):105–11. https://doi.org/10.2500/105065898781390325.
22. Keros P. On the practical value of differences in the level of the lamina cribrosa of the ethmoid. Zeitschrift fur Laryngologie, Rhinologie, Otologie und ihre Grenzgebiete. 1962;41:809–13.
23. Kainz J, Stammberger H. The roof of the anterior ethmoid: a locus minoris resistentiae in the skull base. Laryngol Rhinol Otol. 1988;67(4):142–9.
24. Stankiewicz JA, Chow JM. The low skull base: an invitation to disaster. Am J Rhinol. 2004;18(1):35–40.
25. Lund VJ, Wright A, Yiotakis J. Complications and medicolegal aspects of endoscopic sinus surgery. J R Soc Med. 1997;90(8):422–8. https://doi.org/10.1177/014107689709000803.
26. Schaeffer JP. The lateral wall of the cavum nasi in man, with special reference to the various developmental stages. In: J Morphol, vol. 21; 1910. p. 613–707.
27. Schaeffer JP. The genesis, development and adult anatomy of the nasofrontal region in man. Am J Anat. 1916;20:125–46.

Olfactory Function Assessment

25

Meritxell Valls-Mateus, Franklin Mariño-Sánchez, Isam Alobid, Concepció Marin, and Joaquim Mullol

Key Points

- Subjective smell tests allow the qualitative and quantitative assessment of olfactory disorders.
- Smell tests use substances at standardized fixed concentrations identifiable by healthy people, or at different concentrations to determine olfactory threshold.
- There exist rapid, reliable, and low-cost screening tests suitable for differentiating normosmia from smell impairment to be used in daily clinical practice.

M. Valls-Mateus
Servei d'Otorinolaringologia, Hospital Universitari Son Espases, Palma de Mallorca, Illes Balears, Spain

F. Mariño-Sánchez
Unidad de Rinología y Cirugía de Base de Cráneo, Servicio de Otorrinolaringología, Hospital Universitario Ramón y Cajal, Madrid, Spain

I. Alobid
Rhinology Unit & Smell Clinic, Department of Otorhinolaryngology, Hospital Clínic, Universitat de Barcelona, Barcelona, Catalonia, Spain

Clinical & Experimental Respiratory Immunoallergy, Institut d'Investigacions, Biomèdiques August Pi i Sunyer (IDIBAPS), Barcelona, Catalonia, Spain

CIBER of Respiratory Diseases (CIBERES), Barcelona, Catalonia, Spain

C. Marin · J. Mullol (✉)
INGENIO, Immunoal.lèrgia Respiratòria Clínica i Experimental (IRCE), Institut d'Investigacions Biomèdiques August Pi i Sunyer (IDIBAPS), Barcelona, Catalonia, Spain

CIBER de Enfermedades Respiratorias (CIBERES), Barcelona, Catalonia, Spain

Unitat de Rinologia i Clinica de l'Olfacte, Servei d'Otorinolaringologia, Hospital Clínic Barcelona, Universitat de Barcelona, Barcelona, Catalonia, Spain
e-mail: cmarin@clinic.cat; JMULLOL@clinic.cat

25.1 Introduction

The sense of smell is one of the oldest and most important for living organisms. It is responsible for detecting and processing odors, providing critical information about the environment to all species [1]. Assessment of olfactory function is a common problem in otolaryngology and other medical specialties such as neurology. There are diseases of great prevalence in the population that produce smell impairment such as rhinitis, nasal polyposis, Alzheimer's disease, major depression, diabetes mellitus, Parkinson Disease, etc. [2–4].

The olfactory process is initiated when odor particles in the airflow reach the olfactory epithelium and interact with odorant binding proteins (OBP). Perception is completed with cortical processing. Odorants mainly use two different routes to reach the olfactory epithelium: orthonasal and retronasal. Along the orthonasal route, volatile chemical compounds pass through the nostrils via the turbinates and eventually reach the olfactory epithelium. Conversely, the retrona-

L. Zhang, C. Bachert (eds.), *Chronic Rhinosinusitis*, https://doi.org/10.1007/978-981-16-0784-4_25

sal route requires a retrograde direction starting from the oral cavity, continuing through the nasopharynx and choana, ending at the olfactory mucosa [5]. As the orthonasal route serves as the primary source of olfaction, the retronasal route plays an important role in taste perception.

Olfactometry is a test that allows assessing the olfactory status of subjects in a normal or pathological situation, as well as quantifying the results and interpreting them. In clinical practice, smell tests together with an exhaustive physical examination can be useful to determine the presence and intensity of hyposmia, to identify a potentially treatable cause and to monitor its evolution over time. Likewise, it may allow us to establish the severity of the smell loss for legal purposes.

The examination of olfaction consists of electrophysiological and psychophysical tests and measurements. Electrophysiological tests assess cortical neural responses to an odor stimulus. Psychophysical tests, conversely, provide qualitative information about olfaction rather than the objective results obtained from electrophysiological recordings and thus are only employed for clinical symptom assessment [6].

Subjective olfactometry has considerable advantages over conventional methods based on the principles of analytical chemistry, since it allows measuring smell in terms of human perception instead of relying on incomplete assumptions about how odors behave and are perceived.

25.2 Subjective Smell Tests

The active collaboration of the patient is required in subjective smell tests. The subject must remain seated in a noise isolated room in optimal conditions of temperature and humidity. Neither the examiner nor the patient is allowed to use perfumes, lotions, or creams on the day of the test. The patient is given samples of substances to smell that give off different types of odors at different concentrations. The odorant samples are placed approximately at one to three centimeters from the nostrils and the subject is asked to breathe normally and might be asked to recognize certain characteristics of the odor such as: whether the subject identifies the odor and its intensity or perceives it as pleasant or irritating. Several substances are usually used at standardized fixed and identifiable concentrations by healthy people, or at different concentrations to determine the olfactory threshold. These tests have the advantage of using simple and transportable materials, which make them more practical in daily clinical practice. Most olfactometric techniques belong to this group.

25.2.1 Screening Tests

Screening tests for the sense of smell are designed to detect whether a patient has or not an impaired sense of smell. These tests should be fast, reliable, and cheap. A commonly known example is a series of bottles that contain certain odors such as coffee, chocolate, or perfume.

In recent years more sophisticated tests have been developed that are both reliable and easy to use [7]. Some examples are:

- *12-item Cross-Cultural Smell Identification Test* (CC-SIT) [8]: uses 12 selected odorants from the University of Pennsylvania Smell Identification Test (UPSIT). It is a self-administered olfactometry that evaluates the olfactory function in less than 5 min.
- *Japanese Odor Stick Identification Test* [9]: it consists of 13 odorants familiar to the Japanese population, quite different from those used in the other tests marketed. The odors used are described as: condensed milk, curry, hinoki (Japanese cypress wood), Indian ink, Japanese orange, menthol, perfume, rotten smell, toasted garlic, rose, sweaty clothes/natto (fermented soybeans), and wood.
- *Scandinavian Odor Identification Test* (SOIT) [10]: consists of 16 smells with four alternatives for forced-choice identification.
- *The Pocket Smell Test* [11]: very fast test, also derived from the UPSIT, administered in a disposable paper that releases three aromas through the scratch-and-sniff method.

All these tests are validated and well documented in the literature and, therefore, are currently used for the initial approach to an olfactory disorder or to assess the olfactory function before nasal surgery. However, with screening tests you can only distinguish between normal or abnormal olfactory function. For a more detailed evaluation of an olfactory dysfunction, smell identification and threshold tests are required (Table 25.1).

Subjective determination of smell loss can also be quickly obtained by a psychometric scale such as the Likert scale (0–3) or the *Visual Analogue Scale* (VAS, 0–10 cm). VAS has been widely used in studies evaluating the effect of different olfactory disorders such as nasal polyposis

Table 25.1 Subjective smell tests validated for adult populations

Smell test	Author, year (country)	Supraliminar method	Threshold	Test duration (minutes)	Scoring
University of Pennsylvania Smell Identification Test (UPSIT)	Doty et al. [12] (USA)	40 encapsulated odors. Scratch and sniff. 4AFC	–	15	Reference values according to age and gender
Connecticut Olfactory Test (CCCRC)	Cain et al. [13] (USA)	10 odors, in jars. Forced- choice among 20 descriptors Separate nostrils	*n*-butanol. 2AFC. 4-correct-in-a-row	35	0–7 points scale: <2 anosmia 2–5 hyposmia 6–7 normosmia
Smell Diskettes	Briner et al. [14] (Switzerland)	8 diskettes that must be opened to release the odor. 3AFC	–	5	0–8 points scale: 0–6 hyposmia 7–8 normosmia
Sniffin' Sticks	Kobal et al. [15] (Germany)	Identification: 16 odors in felt-tip pens. 4AFC Discrimination: 16 odors in 3AFC. Identify the pen having the different smell	N-butanol in 3AFC. Single staircase method	25	Normosmia if >75% forced-choice identification Updated normative values according to age and gender in Oleszkiewicz A et al. [16]
Barcelona Smell Test (BAST-24)	Cardesin et al. [17] 2006 (Spain)	24 odors (semisolid gel) in glass jars. Evaluates detection, identification, and 4AFC identification	–	20	Reference values according to age, gender and smoking habit
European Test of Olfactory Capabilities (ETOC)	Thomas-Danguin et al. [18] (France, Sweden, The Netherlands)	16 odors in liquid flasks. Evaluates detection and 4AFC identification	–	20	Linear discriminant analysis using both detection and identification for estimating individual probabilities of being anosmic, hyposmic or normosmic [19]
Pocket Smell Test (PST)	Solomon et al. [11] (USA)	Based on UPSIT. Three encapsulated odors, scratch and sniff	–	<5	Normosmia if 2 or 3 correct identifications, hyposmia if 0 or 1 discriminates Alzheimer's dementia from major depression
Odor Stick Identification Test (OSIT-J)	Saito et al. [20] (Japan)	13 odors, solid cream applied in a paraffin paper. Four-plus alternative method and two-step identification method	–	8	0–13 points scale Normative values not available

(continued)

Table 25.1 (continued)

Smell test	Author, year (country)	Supraliminar method	Threshold	Test duration (minutes)	Scoring
Scandinavian Odor Identification Test (SOIT)	Nordin et al. [10] (Sweden)	16 odors in bottles. 4AFC	–	15	0–16 points scale Reference values according to age and gender
Combined olfactory test	Robson et al. [21] (United Kingdom)	Based on CCCRC Nine odors in opaque jars. 4AFC	*n*-butanol in plastic containers. 2AFC	–	0–9 points scale Normative values not available

AFC alternative forced choice paradigm

[22, 23], allergic rhinitis [24], or traumatic brain injury [25].

25.2.2 Smell Identification Tests

Qualitative olfactory tests allow the detection of alterations in perception and are used to evaluate a wide range of olfactory stimuli. The ability to recognize certain odors can be assessed by identification tests, while discrimination tests assess the ability to distinguish between different odors. Subjective smell tests can be performed on one or two nostrils. Some of the most used smell tests are shown in Tables 25.1 and 25.2, and described in detail below:

- *University of Pennsylvania Smell Identification Test* (UPSIT) [12] (Fig. 25.1). The model created by the University of Pennsylvania (USA) is a method that uses strips of paper covered by a layer of resin microspheres that contain the odoriferous substance (scratch-and-sniff method). It explores only the first cranial nerve and does not distinguish between the right or left nostril. It only values the correct knowledge of the smell. It is presented in cases of 40 odors along with response curves, depending on age and sex. The UPSIT has the advantages of not requiring trained personnel to do it, so the patient can perform the test at home, and that it is very easy to handle because of its small size. In addition, there are normative values curves and the containers are sealed, reducing the problem of volatility and the progressive reduction of the concentration of odors.
- *Smell Diskettes* [14] (Fig. 25.2). The Swiss model is simpler. It consists of 8 odorants housed in a disk-shaped case. The concentration of the odor is uniform and unilateral nasal examinations can be carried out. As in the UPSIT model, it only considers the "correct answer" as the sole value of the olfactory function.
- *Sniffin' Sticks* [15] (Fig. 25.3). This test developed in Germany is widely spread for its simplicity and reliability. It uses pen-shaped containers with odorants in different concentrations, which allows to assessing the detection threshold (*n*-butanol) and the discrimination olfactory capacity (forced-choice for 16 pairs of odorants) in addition to the identification and olfactory memory (16 odorants for forced identification from four options). Normative values based on a sample of more than 3000 subjects were defined [35]. Additionally, it has been validated for use in the pediatric population [36].

Recently, an update on the Sniffin' Sticks normative data has been published [16]. Data were obtained from 9139 healthy subjects (aged 5–96 years) and hyposmia was established at a TDI (threshold, discrimination, and identification) score of less than 30.7. Age-related changes were found in each domain, more pronounced for thresholds. Individuals aged 20–30 years performed best, whereas children below the age of 10 years and adults above the age of 71 years

Table 25.2 Subjective smell tests validated for children population

Test name	Author, year (country)	Odorants and methods	Age range (year)	Scoring system	Performance in pre-school children
Pediatric Odorant Identification Task (POIT)	Richman et al. [26] (USA)	Five microencapsulated "scratch and sniff" cards. 5AFC	4–17	Percentage of correct responses is transformed to a logit	The 5 odors were correctly identified by 80% of children as young as 5 years of age
Candy Smell Test (CST)	Renner et al. [27] (Germany)	Retronasal smell. Twenty-three hard candies, containing sorbitol and one unique aroma. 4AFC	4–85	0–23 points scale: Reference values according to age and gender Score < 13 for detecting anosmia in all age groups	Significant lower scores were obtained in children aged 4–6 years These children more often declared items to be unfamiliar
National Institutes of Health (NIH) Toolbox	Dalton et al. [28] (USA)	Six microencapsulated "scratch and sniff" odors. Picture recognition. 4AFC	3–17	0–6 points scale Normative data not available	Time for testing was longer in children <5 years of age Percent of correct identification in 3-4yo children was below 63% for all odorants [29]
Smell Wheel	Cameron et al. [30] (USA)	Cardboard wheel or disk that rotates with 11 scratch and sniff odorants. 4AFC	4–19	0–11 points scale (percentage)	Mean correct identification score was lower than 70% for 4–6 yo children
Sniffin' Kids	Schriever et al. [31] (Germany)	14 odors in felt-tip pens. 4AFC. Descriptors presented in writing and in pictures	6–17	0–14 points scale Normosmia: 6–8 yo >7 9–14 yo >8 15–17 yo >10	Not included
Universal Sniff Test (U-Sniff)	Schriever et al. [32] (multinational)	12 odors in felt-tip pens. 4AFC. Descriptors presented in writing and in pictures	6–17	0–12 points scale Normative data reported for each country	(multicenter study involving 19 countries)
Pediatric Barcelona Olfactory Test (pBOT-6)	Mariño-Sánchez et al. [33] (Spain)	• Identification task: 6 odorants (semisolid gel) in glass jars. • Threshold test: 6 sniff bottles with dilutions of PEA in a geometric series.	6–17	0–6 points scale. Normosmia (IS): 6–11yo >4 12–17yo >5 Normosmia (TS): <2	Not included

AFC alternative forced choice paradigm, *yo* years old, *IS* identification score, *TS* threshold score, *PEA* phenylethyl alcohol

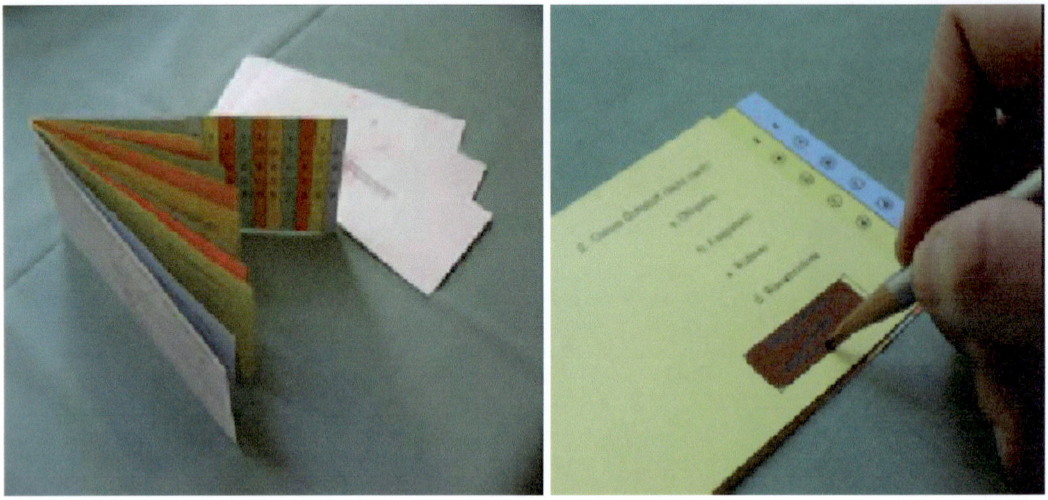

Fig. 25.1 University of Pennsylvania Smell Identification Test (UPSIT) [12]. The picture on the right shows the release of the microencapsulated odorant from the surface of strips by means of a pencil and the four-multiple forced-choice list

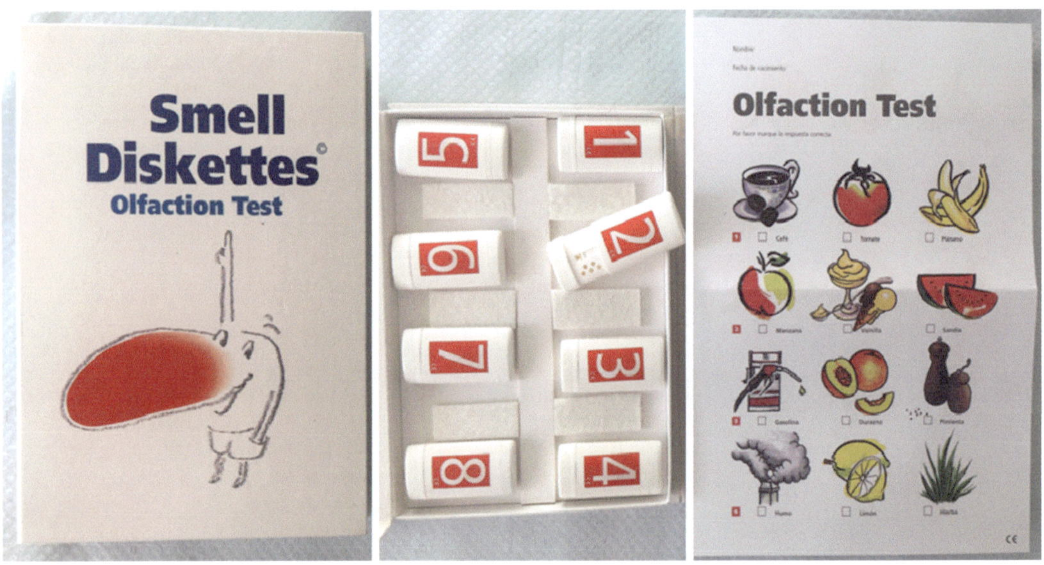

Fig. 25.2 Smell Diskettes test [14]. The eight odorants are presented in a disk-shaped case, when opening it releases the odor. The test includes sheets with pictures and names of the three forced-choice options

scored only half as well. Sex-related differences were also found with women outperforming men.

- *Connecticut Chemosensory Clinical Research Center* (CCCRC) [13]. This American model comprises two parts: the threshold test (with *n*-butanol) and the supraliminar test consisting of eight opaque jars. Subjects then choose from a printed list containing the correct items as well as an equal number of distractor items. It is easy to manufacture and cheap. However, it needs a lot of time to be performed and must be carried out by qualified personnel.
- *Barcelona Smell Test-24* (BAST-24) [17] (Fig. 25.4). It is a model developed in Barcelona (Catalonia, Spain) that consists of 24 semisolid

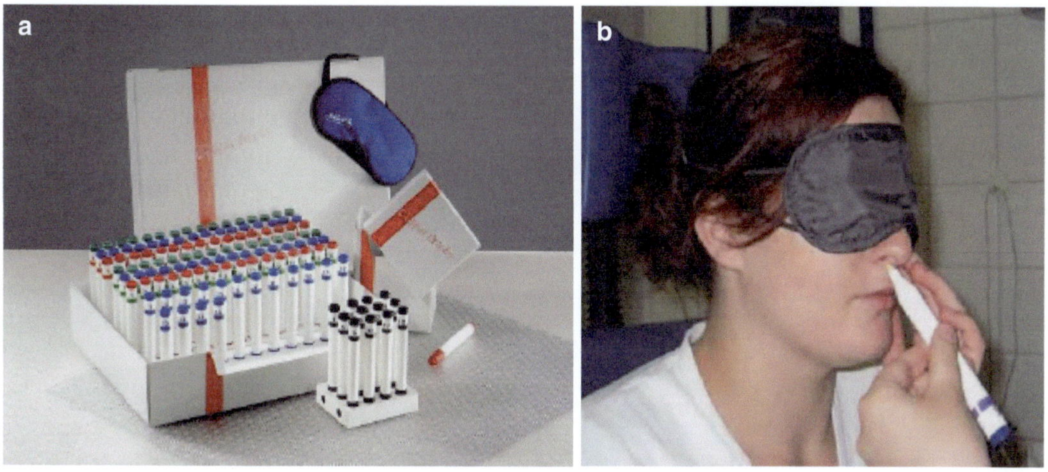

Fig. 25.3 Sniffin' Sticks [15]. Reproduced from Welge-Lüssen et al. [34]. (**a**) Pen-shaped containers with odorants in different concentrations. (**b**) During the threshold test the subject is blind folded to prevent visual identification of the odorants

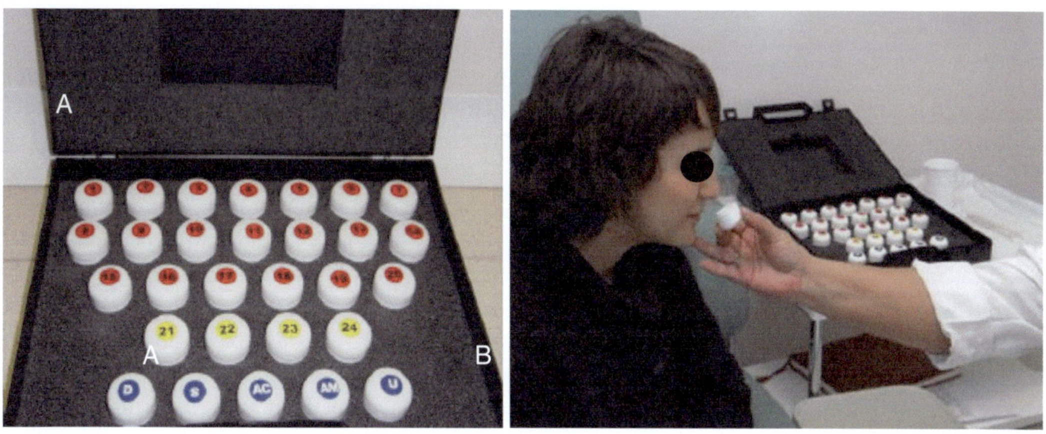

Fig. 25.4 Barcelona Smell Test-24 (BAST-24) [17]. (**a**) BAST-24 briefcase with the 24 odorants (the last 4 predominantly stimulate the trigeminal nerve) and the gustometry (sweet, salty, sour, bitter, and umami). (**b**) Performing the olfactometry, note that the container is a few centimeters apart from the nose of the subject

odorants contained in hermetic glass jars, and 5 additional substances to assess taste. From the 24 odorants, 20 predominantly stimulate the first cranial nerve and the other 4 predominantly stimulate the fifth cranial nerve. The test includes questions for the evaluation of different sensorial aspects of olfaction such as detection, memory, and forced-choice identification among four options (also sensitivity such as odor intensity, irritability, freshness, pleasantness). It differs from American and other European models by its ability to analyze different olfactory characteristics such as quantitative detection, smell memory area, spontaneous recognition, and the correct identification of odors. Any smell assessment should be complemented with a taste examination. BAST-24 includes a chemical gustometry using five substances: sweet, salty, bitter, acid, and umami (glutamate).

25.2.3 Smell Tests in Children

Most of the above-mentioned tests have been used in children despite they are not well suited

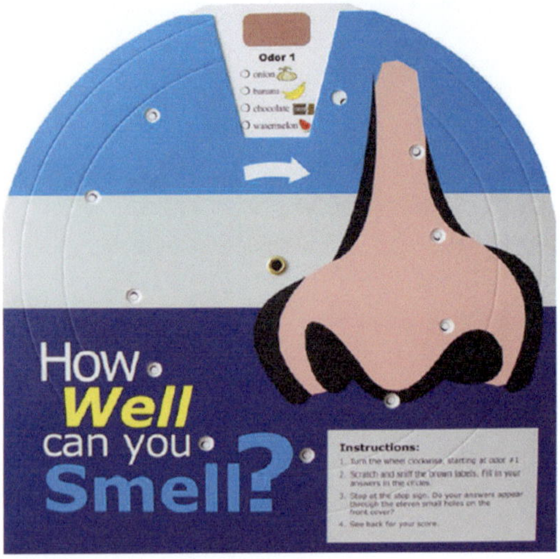

Fig. 25.5 Smell Wheel [30]. This olfactory test specially designed for children has a game-like presentation, the patient has to scratch and sniff the odor and choose between four options

for them due to the lengths of the test and unfamiliarity of some of the odors. To date there are a few odor identification tests, which have been especially developed for children (Table 25.2).

- The "*Sniffin' kids*" [31] and the *Smell Wheel* [30] are two of the most used smell tests in children (Fig. 25.5). The "*Sniffin' kids*" is a 14-item test that includes selected odors from the original Sniffin' Sticks 16-item odor identification test. It has been validated for children aged 6–17 years and normative data for three age groups is available. The *Smell Wheel* is a game-like test presented as a cardboard disk that rotates within an outer jacket, showing one microencapsulated "scratch and sniff" odorant. Both pictures and words are provided in the four-alternative forced choice task to reduce cognitive/linguistic load and potentially to improve performance. Normative values are not available.
- The *U-Sniff* test [32] is a new international odor identification test for children that contains 12 odor items presented as pen-like sniffin' sticks. This test does not include a threshold test. The U-Sniff is administered in a four answer forced choice model using image and name of odors. It has been recently validated across 19 different countries.
- The *pediatric Barcelona Olfactory Test (pBOT-6)* [33] is a smell test recently validated in 6- to 17-year-old Spanish children. It consists of a set of six odorants for a forced-choice identification test and six dilutions phenylethyl alcohol geometric series for the threshold test. It is a fast screening method that distinguishes, with high sensitivity and specificity, between normosmia and smell dysfunction.

25.2.4 Threshold Tests

The quantitative tests measure the threshold levels of smell with certain odorants in order to quantify the olfactory loss. In general, these tests require more time than the smell identification tests, and they are useful to complement the evaluation of the degree of olfactory loss (anosmia, hyposmia, or normosmia).

Nowadays, there are many olfactory threshold tests available; most of them use *n*-butanol as an odorant, although phenylethyl alcohol (rose odor) has also been used. One study [37] compared both substances for threshold tests obtaining similar and reproducible results.

The objective is to find the lowest concentration of an odorant that the patient is able to detect, starting from the weakest dilution. The threshold testing does not require recognition of the smell [38]. Some examples of this type of widely spread tests are the Connecticut Test—CCCRC threshold test [13], which consists of 8 dilutions of *n*-butanol; the Sniffin' Sticks [15], which has 16 dilutions of n-butanol and the Smell Threshold Test that measures the threshold of phenylethyl alcohol in 17 half-log concentration steps [18].

Another instrument to measure olfactory thresholds are the olfactometers. These machines are designed to release odorants at very precise concentrations. Currently olfactory threshold olfactometers are mainly used experimentally [39].

One example of the latter is the T & T Olfactometer [40]. It was developed in Japan and

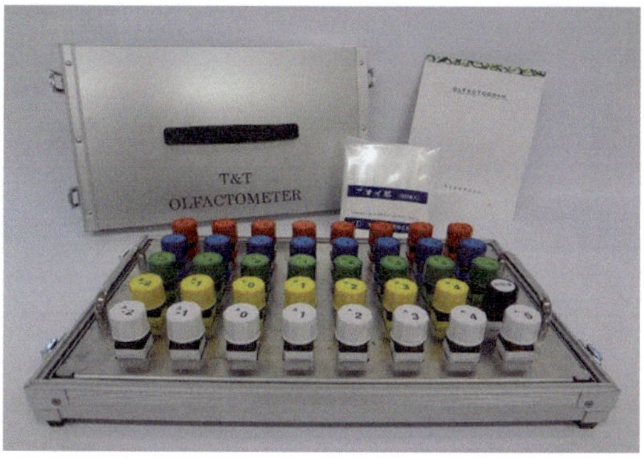

Fig. 25.6 T&T olfactometer [40]. The T&T olfactometer evaluates the detection and recognition thresholds for each of the five odorants. Reproduced from Miwa et al. [41]

consists of five odorants: β-phenylethyl alcohol, methyl cyclopentenolone, isovaleric acid, γ-undecalactone, and scatol and evaluates the detection and recognition thresholds for each stimulus. The detection threshold is defined as the lowest odorant concentration detected by a subject, whereas the recognition threshold is defined as the lowest concentration at which the odor could be identified (Fig. 25.6).

In general terms, these tests measure the olfactory performance and allow us to separate the anosmic and normosmic patients to evaluate in more detail the hyposmic patients. However, the olfactory tests have their limitations, especially when evaluating children, people with cognitive impairment or people from different cultural backgrounds. The complexity of some tests, the cost of the olfactory threshold kits, and the time required to perform the tests have prevented many physicians from adequately evaluating this specific group of patients and, therefore, these tend to be concentrated in specialized centers.

25.2.5 Objective Smell Tests

The objective evaluation of the sense of smell is complex and is based on the detection of changes in the central nervous system caused by olfactory stimulants. In patients who are not able to collaborate or simulators, objective tests are the only way to study for certain sense of smell.

Objective tests do not require the active collaboration of the patient since they register a brain response from an odor stimulus. A single substance is usually used at a very low concentration. They have the advantage of not depending on the active participation of the patient and the inconvenience of needing very complex devices, a lot of time and space, which delays the examination.

- A well-established test is the *Olfactory Event-Related Potentials (OERPs)* [42], which consist of the collection of the electrical activity (olfactory bulb and/or frontal cortex) by means of external electrodes while presenting the patient with odors. Normative data according to age is available [43].
- Another research tool to study smell is the *Olfactory Electrogram* which consists of recording the magnitude of the electrical activity of the nasal olfactory epithelium by applying intranasal electrodes. When an odorant activates the cellular receptor, a negative potential is generated, followed by a recovery potential, and this can be measured using electrodes placed on or near the surface of the olfactory epithelium. There has been little clinical application of olfactory electrogram, due to the low tolerance to intranasal electrodes, and the difficulty of placing them. In addition, reliable responses in the EOG are maintained for very short period of time [24].

New functional imaging techniques include olfactory functional magnetic resonance imaging (fMRI) and functional positron emission tomography that allow direct visualization of central changes caused by olfactory stimuli.

- The olfactory fMRI (Fig. 25.7) allows to study the brain activity in a noninvasive way, while the subject performs a certain task, thanks to the detection of small changes in the signal depending on the level of oxygen in the hemoglobin. The olfactory fMRI identifies the cortical areas that are activated in different areas of the brain in the presence of an olfactory stimuli: entorhinal cortex, tonsil, insula, puta-

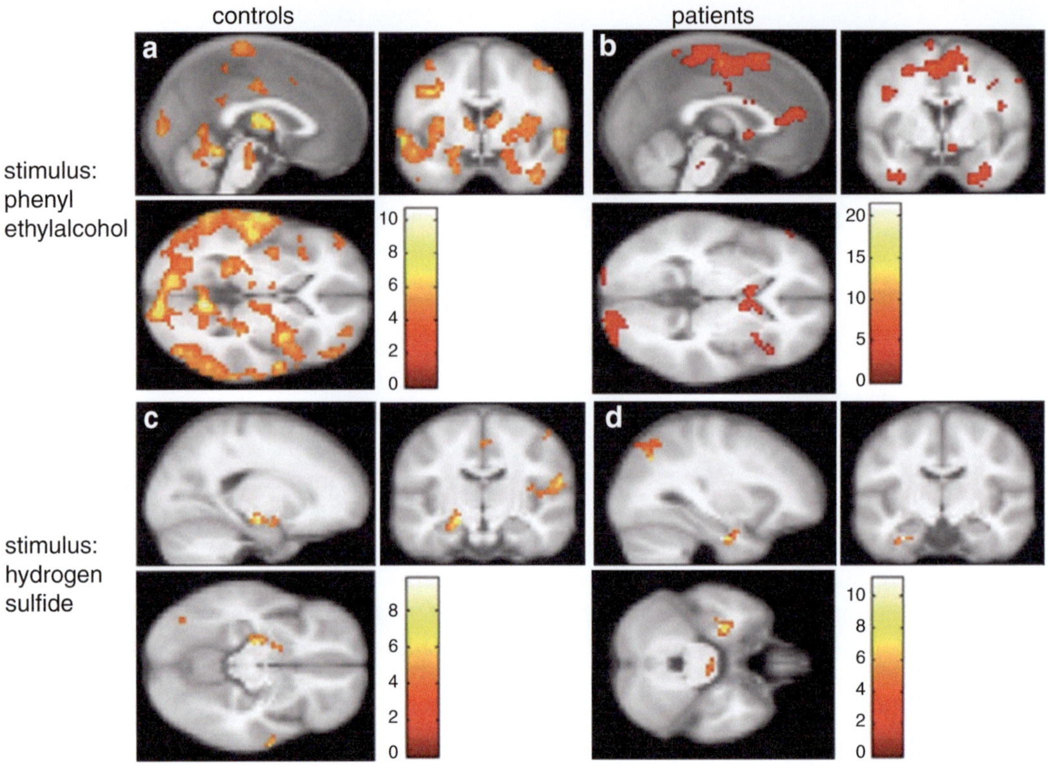

Fig. 25.7 Olfactory fMRI showing brain activation found in controls and in Parkinson Disease after presented of rose odor (phenylethyl alcohol) (**a** and **b**) or the unpleasant odor of rotten (hydrogen sulfide) (**c** and **d**). Reproduced from Hummel et al. [44]

men, and visual cortex [45]. The fMRI has been used very little in the clinical evaluation of olfactory alterations, largely due to the practicality, cost, and the fact that olfactory alterations are easier to detect and quantify through less expensive means [44].

25.3 Translation into Future Daily Practice

- Advances in technology and the proliferation of simple tests to measure olfactory function have improved knowledge of the sense of smell in humans, in both health and disease. To date, multiple smell identification tests have been developed for clinical use, in both adults and children, and validated in different countries.
- All the subjective olfactometries mentioned in this chapter are validated and well documented in the literature and are used today for the first evaluation of olfactory disorders, in clinical trials, or to assess smell function before and after medical or surgical treatment. Globally, olfactometries allow the physician to establish the diagnosis of an olfactory disorder and provide insights into the quantity and diversity of smells that can be detected, recognized, discriminated, or identified by a subject.

References

1. Hadley K, Orlandi RR, Fong KJ. Basic anatomy and physiology of olfaction and taste. Otolaryngol Clin N Am. 2004;37(6):1115–26. https://doi.org/10.1016/j.otc.2004.06.009.
2. Landis BN, Konnerth CG, Hummel T. A study on the frequency of olfactory dysfunction. Laryngoscope. 2004;114(10):1764–9. https://doi.org/10.1097/00005537-200410000-00017.

3. Toledano Muñoz A, González E, Herráiz Puchol C, Plaza Mayor G, Mate Bayón MA, Aparicio Fernández JM, et al. Olfaction disturbances in general ORL practice. Acta otorrinolaringologica espanola. 2002;53(9):653–7. https://doi.org/10.1016/s0001-6519(02)78359-3.
4. Holbrook EH, Leopold DA. Anosmia: diagnosis and management. Curr Opin Otolaryngol Head Neck Surg. 2003;11(1):54–60. https://doi.org/10.1097/00020840-200302000-00012.
5. Özay H, Çakır A, Ecevit MC. Retronasal olfaction test methods: a systematic review. Balkan Med J. 2019;36(1):49–59. https://doi.org/10.4274/balkanmedj.2018.0052.
6. Evren C, Yiğit VB, Çınar F. Subjective assessment of olfactory function. Kulak burun bogaz ihtisas dergisi. 2015;25(1):59–64. https://doi.org/10.5606/kbbihtisas.2015.27136.
7. Fokkens WJ, Lund VJ, Mullol J, Bachert C, Alobid I, Baroody F, et al. European position paper on rhinosinusitis and nasal polyps 2012. Rhinol Suppl. 2012;23:3 p preceding table of contents, 1–298.
8. Doty RL, Marcus A, Lee WW. Development of the 12-item Cross-Cultural Smell Identification Test (CC-SIT). Laryngoscope. 1996;106(3 Pt 1):353–6. https://doi.org/10.1097/00005537-199603000-00021.
9. Hashimoto Y, Fukazawa K, Fujii M, Takayasu S, Muto T, Saito S, et al. Usefulness of the odor stick identification test for Japanese patients with olfactory dysfunction. Chem Senses. 2004;29(7):565–71. https://doi.org/10.1093/chemse/bjh061.
10. Nordin S, Brämerson A, Lidén E, Bende M. The Scandinavian odor-identification test: development, reliability, validity and normative data. Acta Otolaryngol. 1998;118(2):226–34. https://doi.org/10.1080/00016489850154946.
11. Solomon GS, Petrie WM, Hart JR, Brackin HB Jr. Olfactory dysfunction discriminates Alzheimer's dementia from major depression. J Neuropsychiatry Clin Neurosci. 1998;10(1):64–7. https://doi.org/10.1176/jnp.10.1.64.
12. Doty RL, Shaman P, Dann M. Development of the University of Pennsylvania smell identification test: a standardized microencapsulated test of olfactory function. Physiol Behav. 1984;32(3):489–502. https://doi.org/10.1016/0031-9384(84)90269-5.
13. Cain WS, Gent J, Catalanotto FA, Goodspeed RB. Clinical evaluation of olfaction. Am J Otolaryngol. 1983;4(4):252–6. https://doi.org/10.1016/s0196-0709(83)80068-4.
14. Briner HR, Simmen D. Smell diskettes as screening test of olfaction. Rhinology. 1999;37(4):145–8.
15. Kobal G, Hummel T, Sekinger B, Barz S, Roscher S, Wolf S. "Sniffin' sticks": screening of olfactory performance. Rhinology. 1996;34(4):222–6.
16. Oleszkiewicz A, Schriever VA, Croy I, Hähner A, Hummel T. Updated Sniffin' Sticks normative data based on an extended sample of 9139 subjects. Eur Arch Otorhinolaryngol. 2019;276(3):719–28. https://doi.org/10.1007/s00405-018-5248-1.
17. Cardesín A, Alobid I, Benítez P, Sierra E, de Haro J, Bernal-Sprekelsen M, et al. Barcelona Smell Test-24 (BAST-24): validation and smell characteristics in the healthy Spanish population. Rhinology. 2006;44(1):83–9.
18. Thomas-Danguin T, Rouby C, Sicard G, Vigouroux M, Farget V, Johanson A, et al. Development of the ETOC: a European test of olfactory capabilities. Rhinology. 2003;41(3):142–51.
19. Joussain P, Bessy M, Faure F, Bellil D, Landis BN, Hugentobler M, et al. Application of the European Test of Olfactory Capabilities in patients with olfactory impairment. Eur Arch Otorhinolaryngol. 2016;273(2):381–90. https://doi.org/10.1007/s00405-015-3536-6.
20. Saito S, Ayabe-Kanamura S, Takashima Y, Gotow N, Naito N, Nozawa T, et al. Development of a smell identification test using a novel stick-type odor presentation kit. Chem Senses. 2006;31(4):379–91. https://doi.org/10.1093/chemse/bjj042.
21. Robson AK, Woollons AC, Ryan J, Horrocks C, Williams S, Dawes PJ. Validation of the combined olfactory test. Clin Otolaryngol Allied Sci. 1996;21(6):512–8. https://doi.org/10.1111/j.1365-2273.1996.tb01101.x.
22. Alobid I, Benítez P, Bernal-Sprekelsen M, Roca J, Alonso J, Picado C, et al. Nasal polyposis and its impact on quality of life: comparison between the effects of medical and surgical treatments. Allergy. 2005;60(4):452–8. https://doi.org/10.1111/j.1398-9995.2005.00725.x.
23. Benítez P, Alobid I, de Haro J, Berenguer J, Bernal-Sprekelsen M, Pujols L, et al. A short course of oral prednisone followed by intranasal budesonide is an effective treatment of severe nasal polyps. Laryngoscope. 2006;116(5):770–5. https://doi.org/10.1097/01.mlg.0000205218.37514.0f.
24. Mariño-Sanchez F, Valls-Mateus M, Haag O, Alobid I, Bousquet J, Mullol J. Smell loss is associated with severe and uncontrolled disease in children and adolescents with persistent allergic rhinitis. J Allergy Clin Immunol Pract. 2018;6(5):1752–5.e3. https://doi.org/10.1016/j.jaip.2017.12.031.
25. Langdon C, Lehrer E, Berenguer J, Laxe S, Alobid I, Quintó L, et al. Olfactory training in post-traumatic smell impairment: mild improvement in threshold performances: results from a randomized controlled trial. J Neurotrauma. 2018;35(22):2641–52. https://doi.org/10.1089/neu.2017.5230.
26. Richman RA, Wallace K, Sheehe PR. Assessment of an abbreviated odorant identification task for children: a rapid screening device for schools and clinics. Acta Paediatrica (Oslo, Norway: 1992). 1995;84(4):434–7. https://doi.org/10.1111/j.1651-2227.1995.tb13666.x.
27. Renner B, Mueller CA, Dreier J, Faulhaber S, Rascher W, Kobal G. The candy smell test: a new test for retronasal olfactory performance. Laryngoscope. 2009;119(3):487–95. https://doi.org/10.1002/lary.20123.

28. Dalton P, Mennella JA, Maute C, Castor SM, Silva-Garcia A, Slotkin J, et al. Development of a test to evaluate olfactory function in a pediatric population. Laryngoscope. 2011;121(9):1843–50. https://doi.org/10.1002/lary.21928.
29. Dalton P, Doty RL, Murphy C, Frank R, Hoffman HJ, Maute C, et al. Olfactory assessment using the NIH toolbox. Neurology. 2013;80(11 Suppl 3):S32–6. https://doi.org/10.1212/WNL.0b013e3182872eb4.
30. Cameron EL, Doty RL. Odor identification testing in children and young adults using the smell wheel. Int J Pediatr Otorhinolaryngol. 2013;77(3):346–50. https://doi.org/10.1016/j.ijporl.2012.11.022.
31. Schriever VA, Mori E, Petters W, Boerner C, Smitka M, Hummel T. The "Sniffin' Kids" test – a 14-item odor identification test for children. PLoS One. 2014;9(6):e101086. https://doi.org/10.1371/journal.pone.0101086.
32. Schriever VA, Agosin E, Altundag A, Avni H, Cao Van H, Cornejo C, et al. Development of an international odor identification test for children: The Universal Sniff Test. J Pediatr. 2018;198:265–72.e3. https://doi.org/10.1016/j.jpeds.2018.03.011.
33. Mariño-Sánchez F, Valls-Mateus M, Fragola C, de Los Santos G, Aguirre A, Alonso J, et al. Paediatric Barcelona Olfactory Test-6 (pBOT-6): validation of a combined odour identification and threshold screening test in healthy Spanish children and adolescents. J Investig Allergol Clin Immunol. 2020:30(6):439-447. https://doi.org/10.18176/jiaci.0451.
34. Welge-Lüssen A. Re-establishment of olfactory and taste functions. GMS Curr Top Otorhinolaryngol Head Neck Surg. 2005;4:Doc06.
35. Hummel T, Kobal G, Gudziol H, Mackay-Sim A. Normative data for the "Sniffin' Sticks" including tests of odor identification, odor discrimination, and olfactory thresholds: an upgrade based on a group of more than 3,000 subjects. Eur Arch Otorhinolaryngol. 2007;264(3):237–43. https://doi.org/10.1007/s00405-006-0173-0.
36. van Spronsen E, Ebbens FA, Fokkens WJ. Olfactory function in healthy children: normative data for odor identification. Am J Rhinol Allergy. 2013;27(3):197–201. https://doi.org/10.2500/ajra.2013.27.3865.
37. Croy I, Lange K, Krone F, Negoias S, Seo HS, Hummel T. Comparison between odor thresholds for phenyl ethyl alcohol and butanol. Chem Senses. 2009;34(6):523–7. https://doi.org/10.1093/chemse/bjp029.
38. Eibenstein A, Fioretti AB, Lena C, Rosati N, Amabile G, Fusetti M. Modern psychophysical tests to assess olfactory function. Neurol Sci. 2005;26(3):147–55. https://doi.org/10.1007/s10072-005-0452-3.
39. Hellings PW, Scadding G, Alobid I, Bachert C, Fokkens WJ, Gerth van Wijk R, et al. Executive summary of European Task Force document on diagnostic tools in rhinology. Rhinology. 2012;50(4):339–52. https://doi.org/10.4193/Rhino11.252.
40. Takagi SF. A standardized olfactometer in Japan. A review over ten years. Ann N Y Acad Sci. 1987;510:113–8. https://doi.org/10.1111/j.1749-6632.1987.tb43476.x.
41. Miwa T, Ikeda K, Ishibashi T, Kobayashi M, Kondo K, Matsuwaki Y, et al. Clinical practice guidelines for the management of olfactory dysfunction – secondary publication. Auris Nasus Larynx. 2019;46(5):653–62. https://doi.org/10.1016/j.anl.2019.04.002.
42. Auffermann H, Gerull G, Mathe F, Mrowinski D. Olfactory evoked potentials and contingent negative variation simultaneously recorded for diagnosis of smell disorders. Ann Otol Rhinol Laryngol. 1993;102(1 Pt 1):6–10. https://doi.org/10.1177/000348949310200102.
43. Murphy C, Morgan CD, Geisler MW, Wetter S, Covington JW, Madowitz MD, et al. Olfactory event-related potentials and aging: normative data. Int J Psychophysiol. 2000;36(2):133–45. https://doi.org/10.1016/s0167-8760(99)00107-5.
44. Hummel T, Fliessbach K, Abele M, Okulla T, Reden J, Reichmann H, et al. Olfactory FMRI in patients with Parkinson's disease. Front Integr Neurosci. 2010;4:125. https://doi.org/10.3389/fnint.2010.00125.
45. Martínez-Capoccioni GAI. Métodos de exploración objetiva del olfato. Rev Rinol. 2012;12:29–39.

Local and Systemic Biomarkers 26

Nan Zhang

Key Points

- With the opening of a new era of biologics targeting type 2 inflammation, biomarkers with high sensitivity and specificity are the key to identify CRS endotypes.
- Serum/blood rather than tissue/secretion-based biomarkers are needed for predicting the course of disease and monitoring the response to treatment such as biologicals or surgery.
- Serum IgE or blood eosinophils may help to selected patients with severe type 2 CRSwNP endotype who suits for biologics treatment, but cannot be used as marker to monitor the effect of the treatment.

The use of nasal endoscopy and CT scanning, and eventually obtaining a swab or a biopsy for histology, may be insufficient to fully appreciate the pathology of an individual patient. The need for diagnosis, recognizing the disease's natural course, predicting risk for comorbidity and recurrence, and finally the upcoming of biologics drives the quest for biomarkers. The differentiation of chronic rhinosinusitis (CRS) into pathophysiological endotypes—rather than clinical phenotypes—will offer future opportunities to discover genetic, epigenetic, and environmental patterns in the Western hemisphere and Asia [1–3]. Better management of CRS needs a sharpened understanding of disease heterogeneity and mechanisms in relation to clinically significant outcomes. Biomarkers are crucial for the validation of endotypes.

Biomarkers are measurable indicators, such as key molecules or signatures, of a complex biological pathway; ideally, they should be easy to obtain, highly sensitive, specific, and reproducible for identifying disease endotypes in question and should link the disease pathogenic mechanisms (endotypes) to the visible clinical traits (phenotypes) while proving validity (reproducible, easy to measure and cost-efficient) and relatedness to a clinical end-point [4].

26.1 Question-Based Selection of Nasal Biologic Samples and Its Optimal Collecting Techniques (Table 26.1)

Researchers over a decade put their efforts in understanding the pathobiological mechanisms of CRS (Chaps. 5–17). Nose and sinuses offer ease of access for a variety of biological samples to objectively monitor upper and lower airway disease processes and the effect of treatment. It is obvious that the choice of suitable sampling tech-

N. Zhang (✉)
Upper Airways Research Laboratory, Ghent University, Ghent, Belgium
e-mail: nan.zhang@ugent.be

L. Zhang, C. Bachert (eds.), *Chronic Rhinosinusitis*, https://doi.org/10.1007/978-981-16-0784-4_26

Table 26.1 Nasal sampling and applications

Samples	Optimal collecting methods or sample site	Techniques applied for biomarkers in focus
Nasal secretion	Place filter paper or an absorptive matrix into nasal middle meatus for 10 min 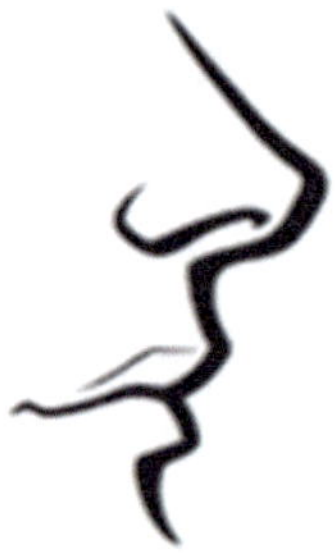 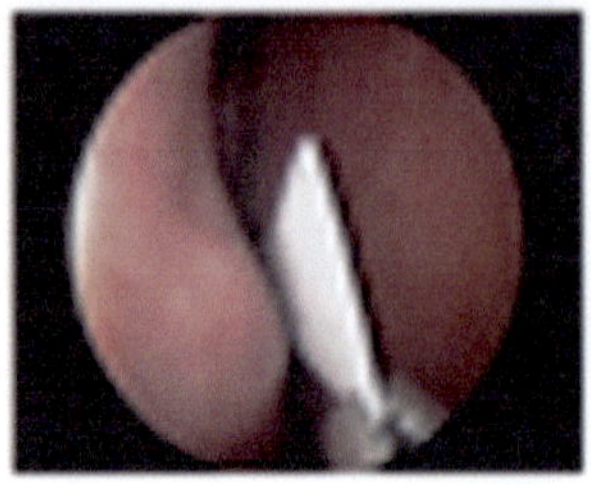	• Secreted biomarkers, extracellular proteins: ECP, leukotrienes, interleukins, chemokines, tryptase, MMPs, elastase, exosomes. • Respiratory microbiology: virus and bacterial detection, DNA sequencing, microbiota characterization. • Transcriptomic and proteomics analysis. • Mucus cytology study: eosinophils, neutrophils leukocytes, basophils, mast cells. • Extrudative response: total protein or alpha-macroglobulin level.
Nasal swab Nasopharyngeal swab	Gently rotate swab in nasal middle meatus or nasopharynx for 5 s	• Microbial identification and quantification. • Virus identification and quantification.
Nasal lavage	Washing nasal cavity with saline	• Luminal cell recruitment, cell activation, and plasma protein extravasation.
Nasal brushing/ scraping	Nylon brush or curettes	• Cytology: mast cells, basophils, eosinophils, neutrophils, leucocytes. • Cell culture: epithelial cells, fibroblasts.
Nasal mucosa biopsy	Procedure requires local or general anesthesia	• Immunohistochemistry: tissue structure, inflammatory cells identification, protein expressions. • Ex vivo mucosa model. • Cell culture. • Microbiology. • Multi-omics studies.

niques and optimal assay is determined by the investigation focus and hypothesis.

A large scale of biomarker candidates have been analyzed in sinonasal mucosal tissue (nasal biopsies), nasal swab, secretions, nasal lavages, peripheral blood, serum, and plasma in order to read the type of mucosal inflammation and correlate to disease endotypes, severity, and treatments (Fig. 26.1).

Non- or less invasive methods are nasal lavage, swab, nasal secretion, brush, or scraping. They can be performed cost-effectively without local anesthesia, and only very mild discomfort is reported from patients. To identify upper airway viruses and microbiota, nasal or nasopharyngeal swab is the easiest and repeatedly sampling method [5]. For nasal cells and mediators, nasal lavage is a suitable way for repeated sampling; it is possible to assess the presence and number of inflammatory cells in the epithelium of the lower nasal turbinate of patients with sinonasal diseases such as allergic and non-allergic rhinitis, or CRSwNP, specifically if severe asthma is associated [6]. For human nasal epithelial cell cultures, nasal brushing or scraping is recommended. For studies which focus on the human innate and

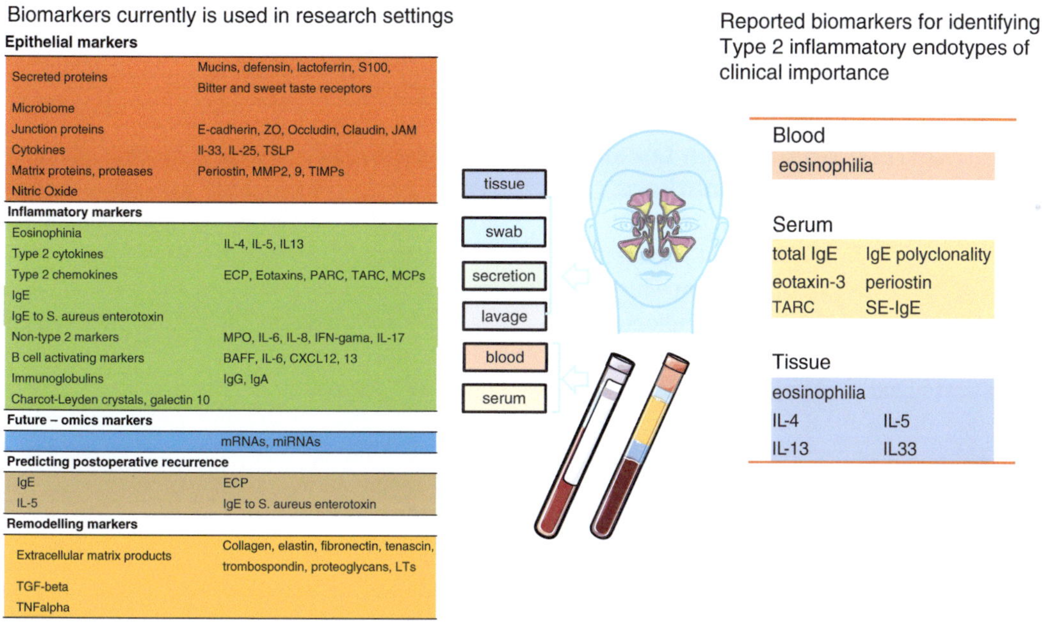

Fig. 26.1 Biomarkers detected from nasal samples. *ZO* zonula occludens, *JAM* junctional adhesion molecules, *IL* interleukin, *TSLP* thymic stromal lymphopoietin, *MMP* matrix metalloproteinases, *TIMP* tissue inhibitors of metalloproteinases, *ECPX* eosinophil cationic protein, *PARC* pulmonary and activation-regulated chemokine, *TARC* thymus and activation-regulated chemokine, *MCPs* monocyte chemotactic proteins, *Ig* immunoglobulin, *SE-IgE* IgE antibody to *Staphylococcus aureus* enterotoxin, *MPO* myeloperoxidase, *BAFF* B cell activating factor, *CXCL* C-X-C motif ligand, *LTs* Leukotrienes, *TGF* transforming growth factor, *TNF* tumor necrosis factor

adaptive defense systems, nasal secretion collected by means of filter paper or a synthetic absorptive matrix (such as Leukosorb, Merocel) would provide detectable concentrations of several secreted extracellular proteins, mucus, immune-related proteins including cytokines, complement factors, immunoglobulins, interleukins, leukotrienes, matrix metalloproteinases. Furthermore nasal secretion can be used for transcriptomic and proteomics analysis to provide molecular characterizes of inflammatory diseases [7, 8].

Nasal cytology as a noninvasive, cheap, and reasonably reproducible technique. Nasal brushings allow a semi-invasive analysis of nasal inflammation, e.g. by measuring increased mRNA levels, e.g. of VEGF, TGF-B2, and periostin in atopic vs. non-atopic asthma patients or healthy subjects [6].

Nasal local tissue is the best biological sample for studying histology, local inflammatory patterns, disease specific immune responses, and biomarkers. Nasal mucosa, sinus mucosa, and nasal polyp tissue sampling is often done under local or general anesthesia, mostly when patients undergo surgical interventions. It has been a concern that anatomic locations play a role, with ethmoid sinuses, maxillary sinuses, and turbinates providing different data in terms of inflammatory cell profile and type 2 cytokine expression compared to inferior turbinates [9]. Other studies have shown that cytokine profiles from the middle meatus mirrors that of nasal olfactory mucosa [10], and increased levels of IL-5 and ECP were observed in ethmoidal and inferior turbinate mucosa in CRSwNP patients, as well as IFN-γ levels were increased in both ethmoidal and inferior turbinate mucosa of CRSsNP patients [11]. Thus, the inflammation of the sinuses can be monitored in the nose, although quantitative differences in mediators are to be expected.

Despite the difference in exact values, there is a variety of techniques of collecting the same biomarkers [12]. Ease of access, cost effectivity, and reproducibility are key factors for biomarkers to be used in daily clinical practice.

26.2 Correlation Between Local and Systemic Biomarkers

When seeking for a biomarker, it is important to consider the clinical specimen from which it will be measured, and techniques for biological sampling should be also taken into consideration. Peripheral blood markers are significantly easier to obtain than a nasal biopsy and require less time, expertise, and expense. However, it may not always reflect local nasal inflammatory processes and is often a poor proxy for the nasal microenvironment. Nasal lavage and nasal secretion are convenient to obtain, and more useful in many situations, serving as a surrogate way to study the local inflammatory response. However, studies [13, 14] which have intended to examine if inflammatory mediators levels measured in nasal lavage fluid or secretion could accurately correlate to the levels in nasal tissue within the same individuals have demonstrated inconsistent correlation between cytokines and proteins in nasal secretions and those in the tissue itself. Different biological sample collection from nasal cavity and sinonasal or nasal polyp mucosa tissue may cause a biased readout [7, 15]. Furthermore, there is regional variability in inflammatory mediator expression within a single sinonasal cavity [16]. Therefore, biomarkers should always be collected from the same location and with the same technique to guarantee comparability, specifically when samples are collected over time. Efforts to link serum and tissue concentrations of markers such as IgE, SE-IgE, IL-5/sIL-5R alpha, periostin, and eosinophil cationic protein failed to show correlations, supporting this notion [17].

For the clinical application, so far, no single validated biomarker has been identified to reliably predict CRS endotypes and the response to treatment, either surgical or biological; however, a combination of markers on a practicable analytical platform and convincing validation cohorts may offer solutions in the future.

26.3 Biomarkers for Endotype Identification

CRS is considered a multidimensional heterogeneous disease with several different inflammatory, clinical, pathological, and physiological involvements. Subsequently, the phenotypic description of CRS patients shifted from a cellular to a molecular level, and the patients were classified according to the type of underlying inflammation and therefore, distinguishing between endotypes.

Four possible endotyping approaches based on different biomarkers have been suggested: a type 2 cytokine-based approach [2, 18], an eosinophil-based approach, an IgE-based approach, and a cysteinyl leukotriene-based approach [19]. These four approaches may of course show substantial overlap, as eosinophils, IgE, and cys-leucotrienes all are a hallmark of type 2 inflammation. Type 2 inflammation is the correct term from an immunology stand point, comprising all these pathways. The currently most accepted endotyping approach [2] is based on an unbiased cluster analysis of inflammatory cytokines and mediators. Another comparable study [18] also based on proteins level in the tissue to identify patients with type 1, 2, or 3 inflammation endotype and confirmed that the majority of CRSwNP patients belong to type 2 immune reactions.

The original analysis divided CRS into three groups, a non-type 2 CRS (mostly CRSsNP, comprising type 1 and type 3 immune reactions), a moderate and a severe type 2 CRS (mostly CRSwNP, predominantly type 2 immune reactions). The severe type 2 CRSwNP demonstrated significantly higher concentrations of inflammatory cytokines compared to the moderate CRSwNP. Interestingly, these groups and endotypes were associated with clinically relevant differences in the expression of polyps, the presence of comorbid asthma, and the recurrence of disease after surgical intervention. Improving the accuracy of diagnosis might guide the decision on specific treatments including drug therapy, surgery, and biologics.

Any of the components of type 2 immune reaction in CRS could potentially serve as source of biomarkers. The term "type 2" includes several key cytokines, IL-4, IL-5, and IL-13 produced by activated T-helper 2 cells and innate lymphocytes 2 (ILC2s); B-cell activation and IgE synthesis [20], eosinophil recruitment, survival and activation [21], epithelial cell activation and mucus production [21–24], as well as macrophage activation and remodeling [25]. Among these events, increased high numbers of blood eosinophils and elevated concentrations of serum total IgE are specifically useful in clinical settings. However, as the nose is a small organ with little impact on the blood compartment, there is a potential risk of underdiagnosing type 2 immune reactions based on these parameters in blood or serum. Other factors such as periostin [17], Cystatins 1 and 2, mucus proteins, Charcot–Leyden crystal forming galectin 10 [26] may be tested for their use as biomarkers in serum. In severe CRSwNP, *Staphylococcus aureus* may colonized on the nasal mucosa, could trigger epithelial cells induced IL-33 release, and initiate the start of type 2 immune response [24], eliciting the formation of IgE to *S. aureus* enterotoxins (SE-IgE), which consequently also can be used as biomarker of severe mucosal inflammation (SE-IgE in serum or tissue). In asthmatics, SE-IgE recently has been shown to be unique in predicting the development of severe asthma and asthma exacerbations within the next 10–20 years [27]. Clinically, the most reliable and easy-to-assess biomarkers to identify type 2 CRSwNP at present are high blood eosinophils counts, high levels of serum total IgE and IgE polyclonality (Fig. 26.1).

26.4 Biomarkers to Monitor Therapeutic Responses

Clinical phenotypes and biomarkers to predict unfavorable mid-to-long term outcome of surgery are comorbid asthma, AERD, AFRS, and high tissue eosinophils, IL-5 and IgE concentrations [28]. The same markers are defining type 2 inflammatory disease and define targets for biologics. The severity of type 2 inflammation has prognostic implications; for example, higher levels of eosinophilic markers predict more rapid polyp recurrence after surgery. This type 2-based endotyping approach clearly is in accordance with the targets of type 2 biologics in clinical trials.

Development of biomarkers for clinical trials in CRSwNP is closely linked to studies assessing the pathophysiology of the disease. For clinical trials of CRSwNP [29], biomarkers can serve several functions:

- As outcome measures they can be used where pre- to post-treatment effects are compared. These markers need to be validated the same way as to clinical and physiologic outcomes and results need to consider the context of all other parameters.
- As predictors of which patients would respond best to therapy. Measuring multi-biomarkers are necessary to reach 70% predictivity. Further extensive work is needed in this field.
- As indicators to provide confirmatory evidence that the treatment in question exerts its expected biologic effect, for example, the level of free IgE should be reduced after anti-IgE antibody treatment, as well as after dupilumab treatment; eosinophils are reduced after anti-IL5/5 receptor treatment.

It may be demanding to obtain tissue samples pre and post the intervention in clinical trials with biologics for CRSwNP. Small tissue biopsies and/or superficial scrapings could be used in combination with single cell analyses, but it is also essential to identify and validate nasal secretion biomarkers that may reflect underlying inflammation. The measured values of type 2 inflammation in nasal mucus collected from the middle meatus, including eosinophils, cytokines, and chemokines, have a certain correlate with nasal tissue parameters. Preliminary data on an analysis using a cluster analysis was demonstrated to identify the type 2 endotype in nasal secretions [17]. However, further work is needed to establish a panel of markers that will most accurately predict underlying tissue endotypes.

Other secretion-based assays demonstrating promise are microparticles and exosomal measures that have been found in small studies to reflect cellular patterns in the tissue [30].

Biomarkers can also be measured in peripheral serum or blood. For example, elevated serum TARC and eotaxin-3 levels before treatment start indicated type 2 disease and were reduced as a consequence of the treatment with dupilumab vs. placebo [17]. This observation also supported the effect of the biologic drug on chemokines as a consequence of anti-IL4 and IL-13 effects, suppressing the migration of eosinophils into the airway tissues. Eosinophil counts and total IgE may be measured routinely and the levels of an array of serum cytokines can be tracked using very sensitive multiplex assays. Blood eosinophils have been considered as a practical way to identify patients with severe eosinophilic non-allergic asthma [31] and have recently included in the clinical management of asthma as a predictor of response to existing biologics. Blood eosinophils have emerged as a reasonable biomarker as they correlate positively with sputum eosinophils, severity of asthma, risk of exacerbation, and negatively with lung function [32]. In patients with adult-onset asthma, those with high eosinophils (classified as blood eosinophils greater than 300/microliter) were more likely to have higher FeNO levels, more sputum eosinophils, have severe fixed airway obstruction, be on frequent oral steroids, have severe fixed airway obstruction, and have a history of CRSwNP [33]. It is clear from clustering analyses, biologic trials, and animal studies that eosinophils are elevated in at least two subtypes of asthma—those with allergic asthma and a strong adaptive immune response and those with a strong ILC2 driven innate response. More advanced work needs to be done in CRSwNP.

Although blood eosinophil counts above 150 or 300 cells/μl in patients with severe uncontrolled asthma identified patients most likely to respond to anti-type 2 monoclonal antibody therapy [including dupilumab (anti-IL-4 receptor alpha), mepolizumab (anti-IL-5), benralizumab (anti-IL-5 receptor), omalizumab (anti-IgE)]. It is not helpful to decide on a specific biologic or monitor responses of individual patients, as blood eosinophil level after drug initiation does not correlate with the clinical response [33].

26.5 Future Multi-omics Biomarkers in Precision Medicine

Novel biological therapies are introduced as a promising treatment option for the management of uncontrolled type 2 CRSwNP patients with or without comorbid asthma, however one therapeutic approach will not be able to offer clinical benefit to all type 2 CRSwNP patients. New biomarkers need to be discovered to predict the response to specific biologics and identify individuals more suitable for a specific drug. With the increasing health care costs, the demand for predictive biomarkers of therapy-success is increasing in order to provide expensive therapies only to those patients who will benefit from the drug.

Recent technological and analytical advances in "omics" science, from DNA microarray to next generation sequencing (NGS) would provide comprehensive monitoring for disease pathophysiology at a molecular level, molecular markers for new sub-endotype identification, and vice versa, new biomarkers can be a novel target for treatments.

"Omics" includes genomics (an entire genome analysis of a cell or organism), transcriptomics (study of the expression of all genes in a cell or organism), epigenomics (epigenetic regulation of the entire genome), proteomics (the analysis of all proteins), metabolomics (the analysis of the metabolites produced by a cell, a tissue, or an organism), and other omics fields [34]. There are increasingly large scale studies performed, and those findings will have huge impact on future inflammatory disease managements. Genomic and transcriptomic studies identified genes associated with inflammation in asthma, e.g. variants at the ORMDL3/GSDMB locus are associated with childhood-onset asthma [35]. In another genome wide large scale study on nasal polyps, CRS and healthy controls found 10 markers associated with NP and 2 with

CRS, and a loss of function variant in ALOX15 to protect against nasal polyp formation, ALOX15 encodes the enzyme 15-lipoxygenase (LO), thus 15-LO would be a potential target for treatment in NP [36].

The majority of "omics" biomarkers currently is used only in research settings, large scale international studies and big data analysis are required to confirm their relevance and effectiveness in precision medicine's daily practice, resulting in an improved selection and satisfaction of patients [37].

References

1. Wang X, Zhang N, Bo M, Holtappels G, Zheng M, Lou H, et al. Diversity of T(H) cytokine profiles in patients with chronic rhinosinusitis: a multicenter study in Europe, Asia, and Oceania. J Allergy Clin Immunol. 2016;138(5):1344–53. https://doi.org/10.1016/j.jaci.2016.05.041.
2. Tomassen P, Vandeplas G, Van Zele T, Cardell LO, Arebro J, Olze H, et al. Inflammatory endotypes of chronic rhinosinusitis based on cluster analysis of biomarkers. J Allergy Clin Immunol. 2016;137(5):1449–56.e4. https://doi.org/10.1016/j.jaci.2015.12.1324
3. Wang W, Gao Z, Wang H, Li T, He W, Lv W, et al. Transcriptome analysis reveals distinct gene expression profiles in eosinophilic and noneosinophilic chronic rhinosinusitis with nasal polyps. Sci Rep. 2016;6:26604. https://doi.org/10.1038/srep26604.
4. Biomarkers and surrogate endpoints: preferred definitions and conceptual framework. Clin Pharmacol Ther. 2001;69(3):89–95. https://doi.org/10.1067/mcp.2001.113989.
5. Kumpitsch C, Koskinen K, Schöpf V, Moissl-Eichinger C. The microbiome of the upper respiratory tract in health and disease. BMC Biol. 2019;17(1):87. https://doi.org/10.1186/s12915-019-0703-z.
6. Gelardi M, Landi M, Ciprandi G. Nasal cytology: a Precision Medicine tool in clinical practice. Clin Exp Allergy. 2018;48(1):96–7. https://doi.org/10.1111/cea.13065.
7. Riechelmann H, Deutschle T, Friemel E, Gross HJ, Bachem M. Biological markers in nasal secretions. Eur Respir J. 2003;21(4):600–5. https://doi.org/10.1183/09031936.03.00072003.
8. Weibman AR, Huang JH, Stevens WW, Suh LA, Price CPE, Lidder AK, et al. A prospective analysis evaluating tissue biopsy location and its clinical relevance in chronic rhinosinusitis with nasal polyps. Int Forum Allergy Rhinol. 2017;7(11):1058–64. https://doi.org/10.1002/alr.22005.
9. Kamil A, Ghaffar O, Lavigne F, Taha R, Renzi PM, Hamid Q. Comparison of inflammatory cell profile and Th2 cytokine expression in the ethmoid sinuses, maxillary sinuses, and turbinates of atopic subjects with chronic sinusitis. Otolaryngol Head Neck Surg. 1998;118(6):804–9. https://doi.org/10.1016/s0194-5998(98)70273-6.
10. Holbrook EH, Rebeiz L, Schwob JE. Office-based olfactory mucosa biopsies. Int Forum Allergy Rhinol. 2016;6(6):646–53. https://doi.org/10.1002/alr.21711.
11. Van Crombruggen K, Van Bruaene N, Holtappels G, Bachert C. Chronic sinusitis and rhinitis: clinical terminology "Chronic Rhinosinusitis" further supported. Rhinology. 2010;48(1):54–8. https://doi.org/10.4193/Rhin09.078.
12. Klimek L, Rasp G. Norm values for eosinophil cationic protein in nasal secretions: influence of specimen collection. Clin Exp Allergy. 1999;29(3):367–74. https://doi.org/10.1046/j.1365-2222.1999.00494.x.
13. Stevens WW, Ocampo CJ, Berdnikovs S, Sakashita M, Mahdavinia M, Suh L, et al. Cytokines in chronic rhinosinusitis. Role in Eosinophilia and Aspirin-exacerbated respiratory disease. Am J Respir Crit Care Med. 2015;192(6):682–94. https://doi.org/10.1164/rccm.201412-2278OC.
14. Oyer SL, Mulligan JK, Psaltis AJ, Henriquez OA, Schlosser RJ. Cytokine correlation between sinus tissue and nasal secretions among chronic rhinosinusitis and controls. Laryngoscope. 2013;123(12):E72–8. https://doi.org/10.1002/lary.24305.
15. Massey CJ, Diaz Del Valle F, Abuzeid WM, Levy JM, Mueller S, Levine CG, et al. Sample collection for laboratory-based study of the nasal airway and sinuses: a research compendium. Int Forum Allergy Rinol. 2020;10(3):303–13. https://doi.org/10.1002/alr.22510.
16. Seshadri S, Rosati M, Lin DC, Carter RG, Norton JE, Choi AW, et al. Regional differences in the expression of innate host defense molecules in sinonasal mucosa. J Allergy Clin Immunol. 2013;132(5):1227–30.e5. https://doi.org/10.1016/j.jaci.2013.05.042.
17. Jonstam K, Westman M, Holtappels G, Holweg CTJ, Bachert C. Serum periostin, IgE, and SE-IgE can be used as biomarkers to identify moderate to severe chronic rhinosinusitis with nasal polyps. J Allergy Clin Immunol. 2017;140(6):1705–8.e3. https://doi.org/10.1016/j.jaci.2017.07.031.
18. Stevens WW, Peters AT, Tan BK, Klingler AI, Poposki JA, Hulse KE, et al. Associations between inflammatory endotypes and clinical presentations in chronic rhinosinusitis. J Allergy Clin Immunol Pract. 2019;7(8):2812–20.e3. https://doi.org/10.1016/j.jaip.2019.05.009.
19. Dennis SK, Lam K, Luong A. A review of classification schemes for chronic rhinosinusitis with nasal polyposis endotypes. Laryngoscope Invest Otolaryngol. 2016;1(5):130–4. https://doi.org/10.1002/lio2.32.
20. Donovan R, Johansson SG, Bennich H, Soothill JF. Immunoglobulins in nasal polyp fluid. Int Arch Allergy Appl Immunol. 1970;37(2):154–66. https://doi.org/10.1159/000230229.

21. Bachert C, Gevaert P, Holtappels G, Johansson SG, van Cauwenberge P. Total and specific IgE in nasal polyps is related to local eosinophilic inflammation. J Allergy Clin Immunol. 2001;107(4):607–14. https://doi.org/10.1067/mai.2001.112374.
22. Kohanski MA, Workman AD, Patel NN, Hung LY, Shtraks JP, Chen B, et al. Solitary chemosensory cells are a primary epithelial source of IL-25 in patients with chronic rhinosinusitis with nasal polyps. J Allergy Clin Immunol. 2018;142(2):460–9.e7. https://doi.org/10.1016/j.jaci.2018.03.019.
23. Nagarkar DR, Poposki JA, Tan BK, Comeau MR, Peters AT, Hulse KE, et al. Thymic stromal lymphopoietin activity is increased in nasal polyps of patients with chronic rhinosinusitis. J Allergy Clin Immunol. 2013;132(3):593–600.e12. https://doi.org/10.1016/j.jaci.2013.04.005.
24. Lan F, Zhang N, Holtappels G, De Ruyck N, Krysko O, Van Crombruggen K, et al. *Staphylococcus aureus* induces a mucosal type 2 immune response via epithelial cell-derived cytokines. Am J Respir Crit Care Med. 2018;198(4):452–63. https://doi.org/10.1164/rccm.201710-2112OC.
25. Svedberg FR, Brown SL, Krauss MZ, Campbell L, Sharpe C, Clausen M, et al. The lung environment controls alveolar macrophage metabolism and responsiveness in type 2 inflammation. Nat Immunol. 2019;20(5):571–80. https://doi.org/10.1038/s41590-019-0352-y.
26. Gevaert E, Delemarre T, De Volder J, Zhang N, Holtappels G, De Ruyck N, et al. Charcot-Leyden crystals promote neutrophilic inflammation in patients with nasal polyposis. J Allergy Clin Immunol. 2020;145(1):427–30.e4. https://doi.org/10.1016/j.jaci.2019.08.027.
27. Bachert C, Humbert M, Hanania NA, Zhang N, Holgate S, Buhl R, et al. Staphylococcus aureus and its IgE-inducing enterotoxins in asthma: current knowledge. Eur Respir J. 2020;55(4):1901592. https://doi.org/10.1183/13993003.01592-2019.
28. Van Zele T, Holtappels G, Gevaert P, Bachert C. Differences in initial immunoprofiles between recurrent and nonrecurrent chronic rhinosinusitis with nasal polyps. Am J Rhinol Allergy. 2014;28(3):192–8. https://doi.org/10.2500/ajra.2014.28.4033.
29. Naclerio R, Baroody F, Bachert C, Bleier B, Borish L, Brittain E, et al. Clinical research needs for the management of chronic rhinosinusitis with nasal polyps in the new era of biologics: a national institute of allergy and infectious diseases workshop. J Allergy Clin Immunol Pract. 2020;8(5):1532–49.e1. https://doi.org/10.1016/j.jaip.2020.02.023.
30. Takahashi T, Kato A, Berdnikovs S, Stevens WW, Suh LA, Norton JE, et al. Microparticles in nasal lavage fluids in chronic rhinosinusitis: potential biomarkers for diagnosis of aspirin-exacerbated respiratory disease. J Allergy Clin Immunol. 2017;140(3):720–9. https://doi.org/10.1016/j.jaci.2017.01.022.
31. Buhl R, Humbert M, Bjermer L, Chanez P, Heaney LG, Pavord I, et al. Severe eosinophilic asthma: a roadmap to consensus. Eur Respir J. 2017;49(5). https://doi.org/10.1183/13993003.00634-2017.
32. Kaur R, Chupp G. Phenotypes and endotypes of adult asthma: moving toward precision medicine. J Allergy Clin Immunol. 2019;144(1):1–12. https://doi.org/10.1016/j.jaci.2019.05.031.
33. Bleecker ER, FitzGerald JM, Chanez P, Papi A, Weinstein SF, Barker P, et al. Efficacy and safety of benralizumab for patients with severe asthma uncontrolled with high-dosage inhaled corticosteroids and long-acting β(2)-agonists (SIROCCO): a randomised, multicentre, placebo-controlled phase 3 trial. Lancet (London, England). 2016;388(10056):2115–27. https://doi.org/10.1016/s0140-6736(16)31324-1.
34. Scelfo C, Galeone C, Bertolini F, Caminati M, Ruggiero P, Facciolongo N, et al. Towards precision medicine: the application of omics technologies in asthma management. F1000Research. 2018;7:423. https://doi.org/10.12688/f1000research.14309.2.
35. Moffatt MF, Gut IG, Demenais F, Strachan DP, Bouzigon E, Heath S, et al. A large-scale, consortium-based genomewide association study of asthma. N Engl J Med. 2010;363(13):1211–21. https://doi.org/10.1056/NEJMoa0906312.
36. Kristjansson RP, Benonisdottir S, Davidsson OB, Oddsson A, Tragante V, Sigurdsson JK, et al. A loss-of-function variant in ALOX15 protects against nasal polyps and chronic rhinosinusitis. Nat Genet. 2019;51(2):267–76. https://doi.org/10.1038/s41588-018-0314-6.
37. Jameson JL, Longo DL. Precision medicine – personalized, problematic, and promising. N Engl J Med. 2015;372(23):2229–34. https://doi.org/10.1056/NEJMsb1503104.

Benign Tumors of the Nose and Sinuses

27

Manuel Bernal-Sprekelsen

Key Points

- Signs and symptoms related to benign tumors in the nose and paranasal sinuses are at initial stages commonly UNILATERAL and UNSPECIFIC.
- Blocked nose and rhinorrhea are most common. The only fact that should raise suspicion is that signs and symptoms are mainly unilateral as compared to CRS.

27.1 Osteoma is the Most Common Benign Sinonasal Tumor

They are usually discovered by chance in routine radiologic examinations of the sinuses in around 1% [1]. The overall incidence of paranasal sinus osteomas in patients with coronal sinonasal CT scans due to sinonasal symptoms has been calculated at 3% [2]. Osteomas can be found starting from the second to the sixth decade, with a predilection of fifth and sixth decades [2, 3]. Male to female ratio is 1.3–2:1. Mostly, the frontal sinus is the most frequently involved site (57%) (of these lesions 37% were close to the fronto-nasal drainage pathway (Fig. 27.1) and 21% above and lateral to the ostium), followed by the maxillary, ethmoid, and the sphenoid sinuses. Maxillary sinuses are affected in about 20% of cases [2, 4].

The most common clinical symptom of osteoma is frontal headache or facial pain. As many as 60% of patients with frontal sinus osteoma complain of headaches [5]. Be aware, that osteomas do NOT produce pain in the sinuses by themselves. Pain may occur secondarily to obstruction of the affected sinus with subsequent sinusitis.

In expanding tumors, this is probably due to an obstruction of the natural drainage of the sinuses, which leads to chronic rhinosinusitis [5]. However, many patients with an osteoma are asymptomatic and the diagnosis is made inciden-

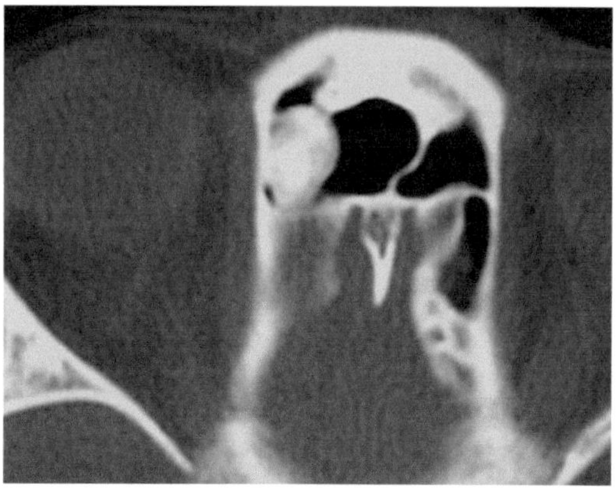

Fig. 27.1 Axial CAT scan. Small osteoma in the outflow tract of the left frontal sinus found incidentally

M. Bernal-Sprekelsen (✉)
Hospital Clinic, University of Barcelona,
Barcelona, Spain
e-mail: mbernal@clinic.cat

L. Zhang, C. Bachert (eds.), *Chronic Rhinosinusitis*, https://doi.org/10.1007/978-981-16-0784-4_27

tally on radiologic imaging obtained for other reasons [6].

Large, expanding osteomas may produce visible external deformities of the face that are strictly unilateral as e.g. compared to broadening of the nasal bones in a Woakes' syndrome. In any case, these deformities appear slowly and without signs of inflammation or infection as compared to an acute complication of a rhinosinusitis.

Growth into the orbit (Fig. 27.2) or intracranially may lead to orbital and/or intracranial complications causing orbital symptoms such as diplopia, epiphora, facial distortion, and even blindness [7, 8].

Intracranial complications may occur when osteomas reach the dura leading to intracranial mucocele, CSF leak, meningitis, brain abscess, or pneumatocele as a first symptom [9–11].

As compared to CRS, osteomas appear as homogenous, very dense, and well-circumscribed lesions in the CAT scans.

Other fibro-osseous lesions, such as fibrous dysplasia or ossifying fibroma tend to rather appear in the mandible and maxilla and in the mandible, respectively. For fibrous dysplasia the age of presentation is the first to second decade, whereas for ossifying fibroma the second to fourth. Radiologically, fibrous dysplasia display as "ground glass" on CT, while ossifying fibroma as an expansile mass with sharp limits [12, 13].

Both fibrous dysplasia and ossifying fibroma are more common in females than in males [5]. Asymptomatic fibrous dysplasia, often found incidentally on X-ray obtained for other reasons, may involve the sphenoid bone and central skull base. Growth speed is variable, and usually slows down after puberty [5].

Aneurysmal bone cysts occur very rarely in craniofacial bones, including ethmoid and orbit [13]. The mandible is mainly involved followed by the maxilla. It is slightly more frequent in females and develops in about 90% of patients during the first two decades of life [14]. Giant cell tumors of the craniofacial bones are rare involving most commonly the sphenoid and ethmoid bones. Osteoblastoma is a benign bone tumor with a clinical presentation similar to other fibro-osseous lesions [13].

Right after osteoma and inverted papilloma, pleomorphic adenoma is the third most common benign tumor of the sinonasal tract [5]. Patients are usually in their fifth decade of life, females are slightly predominant. The nasal septum frequently affected followed by the maxillary sinus [6, 7].

Subsequently, (unspecific) unilateral blockage of the nose may be the leading symptom with isolated mucous discharge.

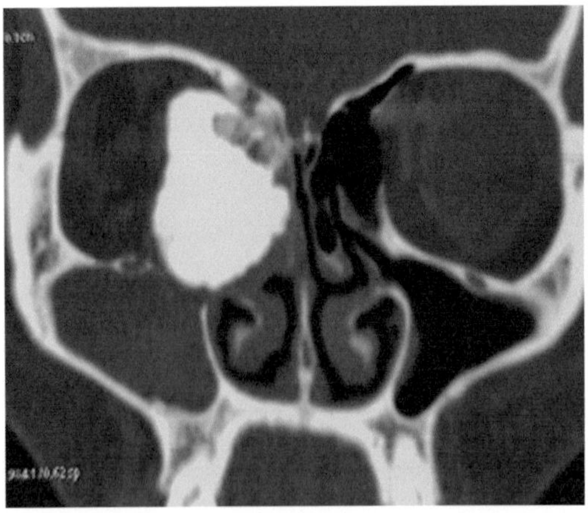

Fig. 27.2 Coronal CAT scan. Large osteoma protruding into the right orbit and producing exophthalmus

27.2 Juvenile Angiofibroma

Juvenile angiofibroma (JA) is a rare benign vascular tumor that accounts for 0.5% of all head and neck tumors with and incidence between 1:5000 and 1:60,000 affecting young males aged 9–19 [15, 16]. The incidence is higher in Middle East countries as well as in India [17].

JAs grow slow and locally from the basisphenoid and sphenopalatine foramen in a dumbbell shape into the pterygopalatine fossa and from there into the infratemporal fossa. The nasal cavity, nasopharynx, paranasal sinuses, and orbit can slowly be occupied eventually reaching the cavernous sinus or an intracranial extension [18]

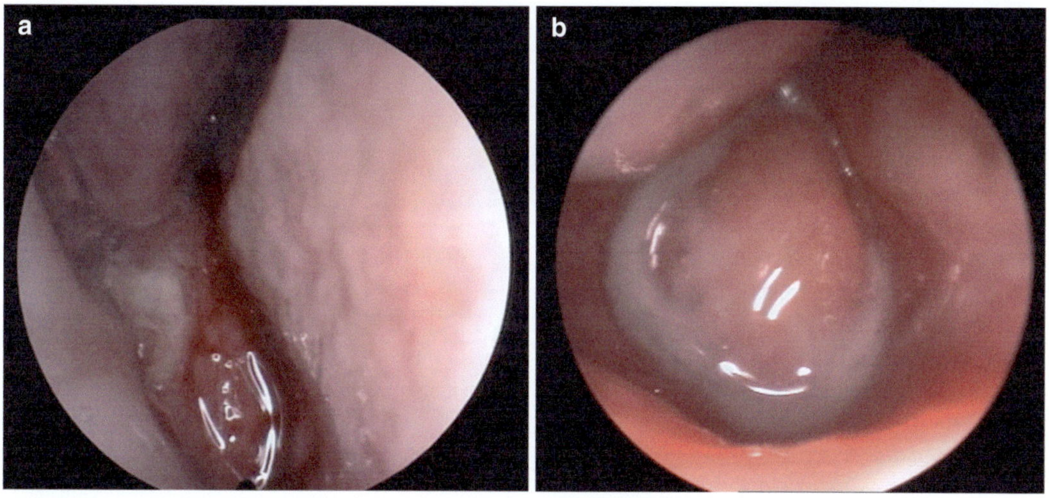

Fig. 27.3 (**a** and **b**) Endoscopic views of two juvenile angiofibromas of the right nasal cavity surrounded by mucous discharge and blocking the choana

(Fig. 27.3a, b). Vascular supply derives from the internal maxillary artery mainly. Among unspecific symptoms there are unilateral nasal obstruction (80–90%) with rhinorrhea and recurrent unilateral epistaxis (45–60%). Headaches (25%) may appear due to the blockage of the paranasal sinuses. Compression of the Eustachian tube produces a secretory otitis media with conductive hearing loss. Growth into the paranasal sinuses and extension beyond may present as chronic rhinosinusitis and swelling of the face/cheek (10–18%). Involvement of the orbit and/or the endocranium display neurologic deficits [17]. Other symptoms are alterations in olfaction, rhinolalia clausa, otalgia, and reduced vision. The submucosal growth and invasion of the cancellous bone of the basisphenoid are typical features that can easily be identified by enhanced CT or MR [19]. "Finger-like projections" with sharp and lobulated margins are the hallmark of JA growth in the soft tissues and along canals and foramina of the skull base (Fig. 27.4). Intradiploic invasion can be better differentiated from normal medullary content on MRI by combining a plain T1 with a post-contrast T1 without or with fat saturation [20]. Signal voids within the lesion on both T1 and T2 sequences indicate major intralesional vessels, corroborating the diagnosis of JA (Figs. 27.3 and 27.4).

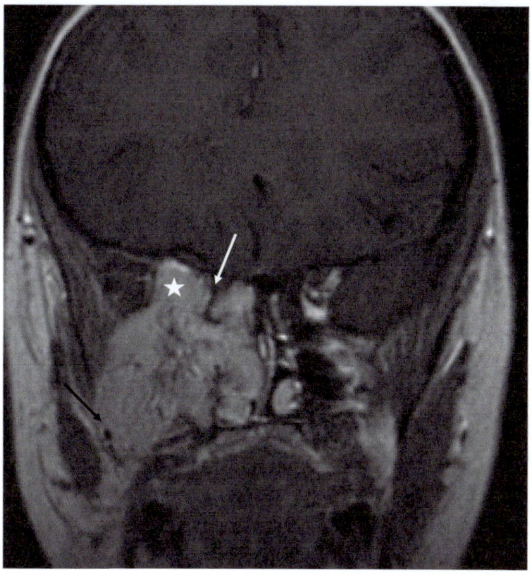

Fig. 27.4 MRI of an extended juvenile angiofibroma. Note the well limited finger-like extensions with isolated voids. *Infratemporal extension; white arrow: cavernous sinus "compressed" between the lateral and medial (sphenoid sinus) tumor extension; black arrow: displaced internal maxillary artery lateral to the tumor extension that fully occupies the right maxillary sinus. The right nasal fossa is blocked by the JA

Clinically, JA produces a unilateral nasal obstruction with recurrent ipsilateral episodes of epistaxis at an early. Full blockage of the china may lead to ipsilateral mucous discharge.

27.3 Schwannomas

Schwannomas are relatively more frequent in the head and neck region (25–45% of all cases). Approximately 4% of these lesions of the head and neck involve the nasal and paranasal cavities. In the paranasal sinuses they are reported mainly as solitary tumors in the naso-ethmoid compartment, less frequently in maxillary sinus, septum, sphenoid, and frontal sinuses. Most cases occur between the second and fifth decade of life; there is no specific association with sex or race. Clinically, they display as a polypoid mass with nasal obstruction.

The risk of malignant transformation is very low; however, in literature there are reports of malignant degeneration in long-standing benign schwannomas, but has been reported to be about 10–15% in von Recklinghausen's disease [17].

27.4 (Acquired) Lobular Capillary Hemangioma (Pyogenic Granuloma)

(Acquired) Lobular capillary hemangioma (pyogenic granuloma) mainly affects the female population in the reproductive period (here known as "granuloma gravidarium") and males younger than 18 years mainly [17]. Sinonasal localization is usually in the anterior portion of the nasal septum (Locus Kiesselbachii/Little's area) and the turbinates [21, 22].

Nasal obstruction and epistaxis are most common clinical features.

There are many other benign tumors such as leiomyoma, paraganglioma, hemangioma, myoepithelioma, oncocytoma, etc. Since they occur sporadically in the sinonasal area, the information in the literature to draw conclusions is scarce. Therefore, they will not be mentioned in detail.

References

1. Mehta BS, Grewal GS. Osteoma of the paranasal sinuses along with a case report of an orbito-ethmoidal osteoma. J Laryngol Otol. 1963;77:601–10. https://doi.org/10.1017/s0022215100061053.
2. Earwaker J. Paranasal sinus osteomas: a review of 46 cases. Skelet Radiol. 1993;22(6):417–23. https://doi.org/10.1007/bf00538443.
3. Strek P, Zagólski O, Składzień J, Kurzyński M, Dyduch G. Osteomas of the paranasal sinuses: surgical treatment options. Med Sci Monit. 2007;13(5):Cr244–50.
4. Gay Escoda C, Bescos Atín MS. Osteomas of the paranasal sinuses. Adv Odontoestomatol. 1990;6(10):587–90. 92-4, 96-8
5. Eller R, Sillers M. Common fibro-osseous lesions of the paranasal sinuses. Otolaryngol Clin N Am. 2006;39(3):585–600. https://doi.org/10.1016/j.otc.2006.01.013.
6. Smith ME, Calcaterra TC. Frontal sinus osteoma. Ann Otol Rhinol Laryngol. 1989;98(11):896–900. https://doi.org/10.1177/000348948909801111.
7. Osma U, Yaldiz M, Tekin M, Topcu I. Giant ethmoid osteoma with orbital extension presenting with epiphora. Rhinology. 2003;41(2):122–4.
8. Mansour AM, Salti H, Uwaydat S, Dakroub R, Bashshour Z. Ethmoid sinus osteoma presenting as epiphora and orbital cellulitis: case report and literature review. Surv Ophthalmol. 1999;43(5):413–26. https://doi.org/10.1016/s0039-6257(99)00004-1.
9. Summers LE, Mascott CR, Tompkins JR, Richardson DE. Frontal sinus osteoma associated with cerebral abscess formation: a case report. Surg Neurol. 2001;55(4):235–9. https://doi.org/10.1016/s0090-3019(01)00344-5.
10. Lunardi P, Missori P, Di Lorenzo N, Fortuna A. Giant intracranial mucocele secondary to osteoma of the frontal sinuses: report of two cases and review of the literature. Surg Neurol. 1993;39(1):46–8. https://doi.org/10.1016/0090-3019(93)90109-e.
11. Umur AS, Gunhan K, Songu M, Temiz C, Yuceturk AV. Frontal sinus osteoma complicated with intracranial inflammatory polyp: a case report and review of the literature. Rev Laryngol Otol Rhinol. 2008;129(4–5):333–6.
12. Lund VJ, Stammberger H, Nicolai P, Castelnuovo P, Beal T, Beham A, et al. European position paper on endoscopic management of tumours of the nose, paranasal sinuses and skull base. Rhinol Suppl. 2010;22:1–143.
13. Mehta D, Clifton N, McClelland L, Jones NS. Paediatric fibro-osseous lesions of the nose and paranasal sinuses. Int J Pediatr Otorhinolaryngol. 2006;70(2):193–9. https://doi.org/10.1016/j.ijporl.2005.09.031.
14. Jaffe HLL. Solitary unicameral bone cyst: with emphasis on the roentgen picture, the pathologic appearance and the patho-genesis. Arch Surg. 1942;44(6):1004–25.
15. Antonelli AR, Cappiello J, Di Lorenzo D, Donajo CA, Nicolai P, Orlandini A. Diagnosis, staging, and treatment of juvenile nasopharyngeal angiofibroma (JNA). Laryngoscope. 1987;97(11):1319–25. https://doi.org/10.1288/00005537-198711000-00014.

16. Batsakis JG. Tumors of the head and neck: clinical and pathological considerations. Baltimore: Williams and Wilkins; 1979.
17. Lund VJ, Howard DJ. Wei WI (eds) Tumors of the nose, sinuses, and nasopharynx. New York, Stuttgart: Thieme; 2014.
18. Chandler JR, Goulding R, Moskowitz L, Quencer RM. Nasopharyngeal angiofibromas: staging and management. Ann Otol Rhinol Laryngol. 1984;93(4 Pt 1):322–9. https://doi.org/10.1177/000348948409300408.
19. Howard DJ, Lloyd G, Lund V. Recurrence and its avoidance in juvenile angiofibroma. Laryngoscope. 2001;111(9):1509–11. https://doi.org/10.1097/00005537-200109000-00003.
20. Maroldi R, Ravanelli M, Borghesi A, Farina D. Paranasal sinus imaging. Eur J Radiol. 2008;66(3):372–86. https://doi.org/10.1016/j.ejrad.2008.01.059.
21. Jafek BW, Wood RP 2nd, Dion M. Granuloma pyogenicum. Ear Nose Throat J. 1977;56(5):228–33.
22. Mills SE, Cooper PH, Fechner RE. Lobular capillary hemangioma: the underlying lesion of pyogenic granuloma. A study of 73 cases from the oral and nasal mucous membranes. Am J Surg Pathol. 1980;4(5):470–9.

28 Sinonasal Inverted Papilloma

Chengshuo Wang, Siyuan Ma, and Luo Zhang

Key Points

- Sinonasal inverted papilloma is one of the most common benign tumors in the nasal cavity and paranasal sinuses, which is characterized by high tendency for recurrence, local aggression, and tendency for malignant transformation.
- MRI is highly efficient for distinguishing sinonasal inverted papilloma lesions preoperatively.
- Complete removal of the tumor, especially resection of the originating site, is the most important procedure for reducing the recurrence rate.

C. Wang · L. Zhang (✉)
Department of Otolaryngology, Head and Neck Surgery, Beijing Tongren Hospital, Capital Medical University, Beijing, China

Beijing Key Laboratory of Nasal Diseases, Beijing Institute of Otolaryngology, Beijing, China

Department of Allergy, Beijing Tongren Hospital, Capital Medical University, Beijing, China

S. Ma
Department of Otolaryngology, Head and Neck Surgery, Beijing Tongren Hospital, Capital Medical University, Beijing, China

Beijing Key Laboratory of Nasal Diseases, Beijing Institute of Otolaryngology, Beijing, China

28.1 Introduction

Sinonasal inverted papilloma (SNIP) , first described in 1854 [1], is one of the most common benign tumors in the nasal cavity and paranasal sinuses. SNIP is characterized by high tendency for recurrence, local aggression, and tendency for malignant transformation [2–5]. These characteristics make it important to differentiate a SNIP from a nasal polyp (NP) in order that appropriate therapy strategies and outcomes can be determined.

28.2 Etiology

The etiology of SNIP has been a matter of much discussion since the first large-scale clinical-pathological study of the SNIP was published in 1971 [6]. Many hypotheses have evolved around this subject over the past nearly half century, but none has been widely accepted.

Although tenuous evidence supports the involvement of human papillomavirus (HPV) as an etiologic factor for SNIP, this has not been shown unequivocally. As HPVs are almost invariably negative when stained for by immunoperoxidase staining techniques, in situ hybridization or the polymerase chain reaction of HPV genomes are widely be used in studies. These have indicated that low-risk subtypes (HPV 6 and 11) are more common in SNIP, although high-

L. Zhang, C. Bachert (eds.), *Chronic Rhinosinusitis*, https://doi.org/10.1007/978-981-16-0784-4_28

risk subtypes (HPV 16 and 18) and HPV 57 have also been detected infrequently. However, the detection rates of HPVs are not consistent and vary from 0% to 100% [7]. While an early meta-analysis has indicated 37.8% of cases of SNIP to be HIV positive [8], a recent study showed this to be the case in only 10.3% of SNIP [9].

Although Epstein–Barr virus (EBV) was also considered as another etiologic factor for SNIP, more negative than positive findings [10–12] have dispelled this hypothesis. A more recent study employing bi-directional Sanger sequencing has suggested that there may be a relationship between epidermal growth factor receptor (EGFR) mutation and SNIP [9].

However, neither the virus infection nor the gene mutation theory can explain some clinical features of SNIP (e.g. unilateral, middle-age adults predilection, no tendency of intimacy contact infection, no effect of anti-virus therapy, etc.). Thus, more studies are required to address this issue.

28.3 Clinical Features

SNIP is more common in the 40- to 70-year old group, with a higher prevalence in men [1, 7]. The progression of SNIP is mild and gentle, which generally results in affected individuals consulting the doctor 1–4 years after the onset of their first symptoms [1].

Although SNIP has mostly been reported to be a unilateral lesion, some previous studies reported bilateral occurrence of SNIP in 0–10% of the cases; which may be caused by a bias of septal erosion or perforation of the unilateral tumor [13].

Usually, unilateral nasal obstruction is the chief complaint, and this can be concomitant with other manifestations including nasal drainage, headaches, epistaxis, anosmia, and some ophthalmic symptoms. Pain is not common, which suggests secondary infection or malignant transformation.

Nasal endoscopic clinical examination shows a granular and lobulated growth, which is pink, tan, or gray in color, and slightly less firm than a NP (Fig. 28.1). The edge of the tumor is very edematous, which make it looks like a nasal polyp; and therefore during endoscopic examination, detailed attention should be paid to the section behind the front of the tumor, especially when there is a unilateral lesion.

Meta-analyses have reported the recurrence rate of SNIP to be between 15% and 20% [14, 15], while the recurrence rates of NPs are much higher, especially for eosinophilic NPs [16]. The

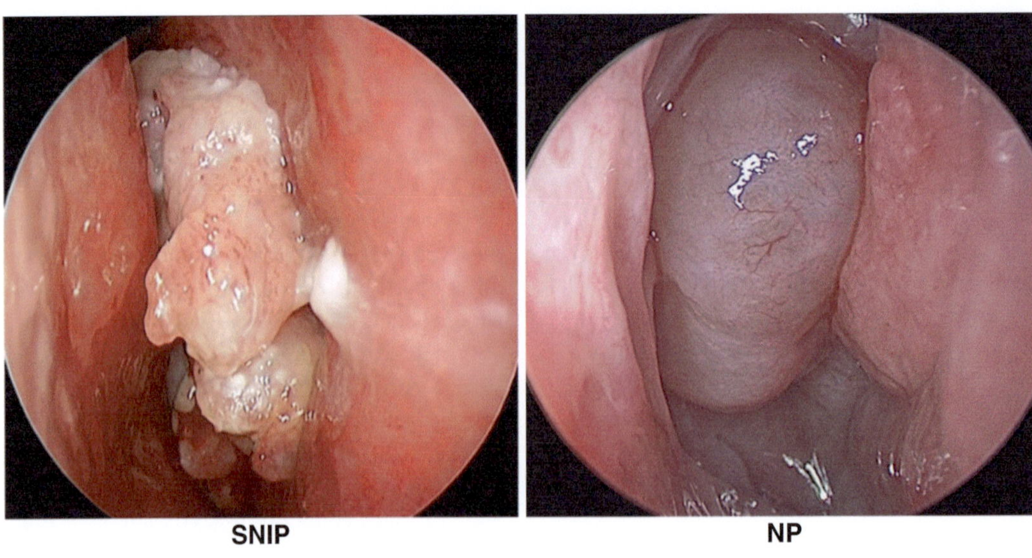

Fig. 28.1 Comparison of SNIP and NP under nasal endoscopic examination

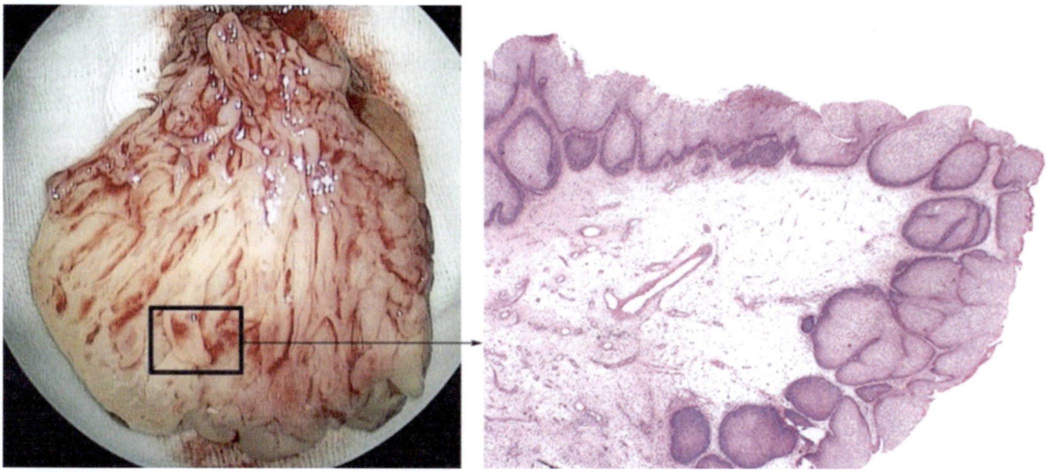

Fig. 28.2 Histological features of SNIP

factors contributing to recurrence of SNIP are still not fully understood. A recent multicenter retrospective study, however, has indicated that the incomplete surgical removal, stage of the disease, site of the lesion, surgical technique, and malignancy rate are the main factors, which affect the recurrence rate [17].

Endoscopic resection surgery or combined endoscopic and external approach is the optimal treatment and gold standard of SNIP. In the case of malignant transformation, chemotherapy or radiation therapy may be suggested after surgery. During the surgery, complete clearance of the tumor, especially resection of the originating site of SNIP, is the most important procedure to reduce the recurrence rate [18, 19]. Identification of the originating site of the tumor, especially ahead of the operation, helps optimize the surgical plan to have a complete resection, so it is important to have a satisfactory surgical outcome and prognosis [20].

28.4 Pathology

The first histological study of inverted papilloma was published in 1975 [4], wherein the author describes the tumor as having a grossly granular and lobulated macroscopic appearance, and a characteristic microscopic feature as the increasing thickness and hyperplastic epithelium inverting into the stroma (Fig. 28.2). Barns and colleagues [13] describe the gross convoluted surface like gyri and sulci of the brain or a wrinkled prune, and upon physical examination as a polypoid growth covered by a convoluted cerebriform mucosa, from which the term "convoluted cerebriform" is derived. Recently, a histological and radiological study has shown that the histological features of SNIP are different between the origin and periphery of the tumor [20]. In particular more edematous stroma and more defective microvessels exist in the periphery of SNIP, whereas more inverted epithelium, more nourishing macrovascular, and more intact-endothelial barrier microvessels exist in the originating site. Furthermore, the periphery of the SNIP is composed of more edematous stroma and less inverted epithelium, making it more like NP, thus necessitating the need to carefully differentiate between the two during pathological examination.

28.5 Imaging

Radiological examination is a very useful non-invasive tool for the diagnosis and identification of the tumor origin [21, 22].

Computed tomography (CT) is used to be overevaluated in the management of SNIP [23]. Focal hyperostosis in the origin of SNIP was first used to diagnose and identify the tumor origin [22]. However, in some cases, ossifying polyps can occur in origin due to trauma, surgery, or bone morphogenetic proteins (BMPs) expression; and thus make it hard to distinguish the polyp from SNIP by CT [24]. Moreover, about 40% SNIP cases present without any osteitis signs [21]. Compared to CT, magnetic resonance imaging (MRI) has been shown to be more useful preoperatively, because it can not only help to distinguish NP from SNIP but can also help to trace the origin of the SNIP more precisely [21].

The diagnosis of inverted papilloma by MRI is mainly based on a typical manifestation of convoluted cerebriform pattern (CCP), which is characterized as striations of high signal intensity in T2 and contrast-enhanced T1 weighted images in the periphery of SNIP. Tracing the CCP back with the striations can determine the origin of the tumor preoperatively. The criteria of the CCP-based reverse tracing method are as follows: (1) CCP always occurs just in the periphery but not in the origin of SNIP, (2) On T2-weighted imaging, the originating site mainly appears as homogeneous equal signal, and on contrast-enhanced T1-weighted imaging shows mild enhancement. However, the periphery site often manifests as low-signal-intensity and relatively high-signal-intensity striations in T2WI, and contrast-enhanced T1WI well enhancement, (3) Typically, the tumor shows a striated septations appearance and spreads in radiating fashion. Tracing the CCP back along the radial texture determines the origin of SNIP.

The key points for the differential diagnosis of sinonasal inverted papilloma and nasal polyps are summarized in Table 28.1.

28.6 Conclusions

In conclusion, SNIP shares many clinical and auxiliary examination features with NP. When a unilateral lesion that looks like NP is encountered, MRI analysis appears to an essential procedure to follow, due to its efficiency to distinguish between the two lesions preoperatively. However, pathological diagnosis is still the golden rule for the differential diagnosis. As therapeutic strategy and prognosis are also different between the two diseases, this further emphasizes the importance of differential diagnosis for SNIP and NP.

Table 28.1 Differential diagnosis of sinonasal inverted papilloma and nasal polyps

	Sinonasal inverted papilloma	Nasal polyps
Age	More common in 40–70 years old group	Increase with age in adults (≥18 age of year)
Gender	Higher prevalence in men	Controversial, no sex predilection, or higher prevalence in men
Symptoms	Unilateral;	Unilateral or bilateral;
	nasal obstruction, nasal drainage, headaches, epistaxis, anosmia, facial pain, ophthalmic symptoms	nasal obstruction, nasal drainage, headaches, anosmia, facial pain or pressure
Endoscopic clinical examination	Granular and lobulated, pink/tan/gray, firmer than nasal polyps	Smooth, yellow/gray/pink, edematous
Recurrence tendency	Yes	Yes
Malignant transformation tendency	Yes	No
Treatment	Resection surgery	Pharmacotherapy or resection surgery
CT	Focal hyperostosis, diffuse hyperostosis, or no osteitis signs	Less likely to have bone erosion
MRI	Convoluted cerebriform pattern in the periphery of SNIP	Homogenization

References

1. Lisan Q, Laccourreye O, Bonfils P. Sinonasal inverted papilloma: From diagnosis to treatment. Eur Ann Otorhinolaryngol Head Neck Dis. 2016;133(5):337–41. https://doi.org/10.1016/j.anorl.2016.03.006.
2. Katori H, Nozawa A, Tsukuda M. Histopathological parameters of recurrence and malignant transformation in sinonasal inverted papilloma. Acta Otolaryngol. 2006;126(2):214–8. https://doi.org/10.1080/00016480500312554.
3. Elliot A, Marklund L, Hakansson N, Song H, Ye W, Stjarne P, et al. Incidence of IP and risk of malignant transformation in the Swedish population 1960-2010. Eur Arch Otorhinolaryngol. 2017;274(3):1445–8. https://doi.org/10.1007/s00405-016-4321-x.
4. Vrabec DP. The inverted Schneiderian papilloma: a clinical and pathological study. Laryngoscope. 1975;85(1):186–220. https://doi.org/10.1288/00005537-197501000-00014.
5. Kasbekar AV, Swords C, Attlmayr B, Kulkarni T, Swift AC. Sinonasal papilloma: what influences the decision to request a magnetic resonance imaging scan? J Laryngol Otol. 2018;132(7):584–90. https://doi.org/10.1017/s0022215118000804.
6. Hyams VJ. Papillomas of the nasal cavity and paranasal sinuses. A clinicopathological study of 315 cases. Ann Otol Rhinol Laryngol. 1971;80(2):192–206. https://doi.org/10.1177/000348947108000205.
7. Barnes L. Schneiderian papillomas and nonsalivary glandular neoplasms of the head and neck. Mod Pathol. 2002;15(3):279–97. https://doi.org/10.1038/modpathol.3880524.
8. Syrjanen K, Syrjanen S. Detection of human papillomavirus in sinonasal papillomas: systematic review and meta-analysis. Laryngoscope. 2013;123(1):181–92. https://doi.org/10.1002/lary.23688.
9. Udager AM, McHugh JB, Goudsmit CM, Weigelin HC, Lim MS, Elenitoba-Johnson KSJ, et al. Human papillomavirus (HPV) and somatic EGFR mutations are essential, mutually exclusive oncogenic mechanisms for inverted sinonasal papillomas and associated sinonasal squamous cell carcinomas. Ann Oncol. 2018;29(2):466–71. https://doi.org/10.1093/annonc/mdx736.
10. Sham CL, To KF, Chan PK, Lee DL, Tong MC, van Hasselt CA. Prevalence of human papillomavirus, Epstein-Barr virus, p21, and p53 expression in sinonasal inverted papilloma, nasal polyp, and hypertrophied turbinate in Hong Kong patients. Head Neck. 2012;34(4):520–33. https://doi.org/10.1002/hed.21772.
11. Dunn ST, Clark GD, Cannon TC, Min KW. Survey of sinonasal inverted papillomata for Epstein-Barr virus. Head Neck. 1997;19(2):98–106.
12. Gaffey MJ, Frierson HF, Weiss LM, Barber CM, Baber GB, Stoler MH. Human papillomavirus and Epstein-Barr virus in sinonasal Schneiderian papillomas. An in situ hybridization and polymerase chain reaction study. Am J Clin Pathol. 1996;106(4):475–82. https://doi.org/10.1093/ajcp/106.4.475.
13. Barnes L, Verbin RS, Gnepp DR. Diseases of the nose, paranasal sinuses, and nasopharynx. In: Barnes L, ed. Surgical pathology of the head and neck, vol. 1. New York: Marcel Dekker,1985:403–51.
14. Peng P, Har-El G. Management of inverted papillomas of the nose and paranasal sinuses. Am J Otolaryngol. 2006;27(4):233–7. https://doi.org/10.1016/j.amjoto.2005.11.005.
15. Busquets JM, Hwang PH. Endoscopic resection of sinonasal inverted papilloma: a meta-analysis. Otolaryngol Head Neck Surg. 2006;134(3):476–82. https://doi.org/10.1016/j.otohns.2005.11.038.
16. Lou H, Zhang N, Bachert C, Zhang L. Highlights of eosinophilic chronic rhinosinusitis with nasal polyps in definition, prognosis, and advancement. Int Forum Allergy Rhinol. 2018;8(11):1218–25. https://doi.org/10.1002/alr.22214.
17. Minni A, Gera R, Bulgheroni C, Ralli M, Cialente F, Candelori F, et al. Endoscopic resection of sinonasal inverted papilloma: a multivariate retrospective analysis of factors affecting recurrence and persistence. Ear Nose Throat J. 2019:145561319890454. https://doi.org/10.1177/0145561319890454.
18. Kim JS, Kwon SH. Recurrence of sinonasal inverted papilloma following surgical approach: a meta-analysis. Laryngoscope. 2017;127(1):52–8. https://doi.org/10.1002/lary.26222.
19. Lisan Q, Laccourreye O, Bonfils P. Sinonasal inverted papilloma: risk factors for local recurrence after surgical resection. Ann Otol Rhinol Laryngol. 2017;126(6):498–504. https://doi.org/10.1177/0003489417705671.
20. Ma S, Xian M, Yang B, Fang G, Lou H, Yu W, et al. Pathological changes from the originating to the peripheral sites of Sinonasal Inverted Papilloma are the underlying mechanisms of preoperative MRI-tumor origin prediction. Rhinol J. 2019;0(0):0. https://doi.org/10.4193/Rhin19.131.
21. Fang G, Lou H, Yu W, Wang X, Yang B, Xian J, et al. Prediction of the originating site of sinonasal inverted papilloma by preoperative magnetic resonance imaging and computed tomography. Int Forum Allergy Rhinol. 2016;6(12):1221–8. https://doi.org/10.1002/alr.21836.
22. Lee DK, Chung SK, Dhong HJ, Kim HY, Kim HJ, Bok KH. Focal hyperostosis on CT of sinonasal inverted papilloma as a predictor of tumor origin. AJNR Am J Neuroradiol. 2007;28(4):618–21.
23. Bhalla RK, Wright ED. Predicting the site of attachment of sinonasal inverted papilloma. Rhinology. 2009;47(4):345–8. https://doi.org/10.4193/Rhin08.229.
24. Yang BT, Wang YZ, Sun FR, Dong JY. Ossifying inverted papilloma and ossifying polyp of the sinonasal tract: comparison of CT and MRI features. Clin Radiol. 2017;72(1):84–90. https://doi.org/10.1016/j.crad.2016.09.018.

Malignant Tumors of the Nose and Sinuses

29

Manuel Bernal-Sprekelsen and Isam Alobid

Key Points

- At initial stages, signs and symptoms related to malignant tumors in the nose and paranasal sinuses, such as blocked nose, nasal discharge, or mild bleedings, are commonly UNILATERAL and UNSPECIFIC. Fleshly or friable tumor masses that may easily bleed are highly suspicious.
- In advanced stages, pain and numbness at terminal branches of the trigéminas nerve, facial deformities, bleeding or orbital symptoms, such as diplopia and exophthalmus, may be present.
- Radiological features differ considerably from those observed in chronic rhinosinusitis with infiltration of tissues, bone destruction, endocranial or orbital invasion.

M. Bernal-Sprekelsen (✉)
Hospital Clinic, University of Barcelona, Barcelona, Spain
e-mail: mbernal@clinic.cat

I. Alobid
Rhinology Unit & Smell Clinic, Department of Otorhinolaryngology, Hospital Clínic, Universitat de Barcelona, Barcelona, Catalonia, Spain

Clinical & Experimental Respiratory Immunoallergy, Institut d'Investigacions, Biomèdiques August Pi i Sunyer (IDIBAPS), Barcelona, Catalonia, Spain

CIBER of Respiratory Diseases (CIBERES), Barcelona, Catalonia, Spain

Sinonasal neoplasms are not very common, as they account only for 1% of all malignancies [1] and for 3% of all upper respiratory tract malignancies and accounting for only 3–5% of all head and neck malignancies [2, 3]. Annual incidence can be relatively high in Asian and African populations, the highest age-adjusted rates, between 2.5 and 2.6 per 100,000 per year occur in Japanese males [4]. Sinonasal malignancies are more common in males [5], whereas in the maxillary sinus it is more common in female.

In 75% of the cases patients are older than 50 years [6]. The sinuses are primarily involved in 75% of the cases, and of all sinus neoplasms 60–80% originate from the maxillary sinus [6].

Tumors affecting the sinonasal region and skull base usually present late as their presenting symptoms are often banal and therefore overlooked by patients and their clinicians, particularly in primary care where these conditions are rarely seen.

The recent onset of unilateral nasal symptoms (blocked nose, rhinorrhea) that do not show improvement with a short course of medical therapy should prompt referral for specialist assessment [7]. Because these tumors are rare they tend be misdiagnosed. Unilateral, fleshy, or friable masses in the nasal fossa or the middle meatus, with a tendency to bleed spontaneously or when manipulated should raise suspicion. Differential diagnosis has to be made with infectious diseases, such as tuberculosis, granulomatosis, fungal rhinosinusitis, among others. Unilateral

L. Zhang, C. Bachert (eds.), *Chronic Rhinosinusitis*, https://doi.org/10.1007/978-981-16-0784-4_29

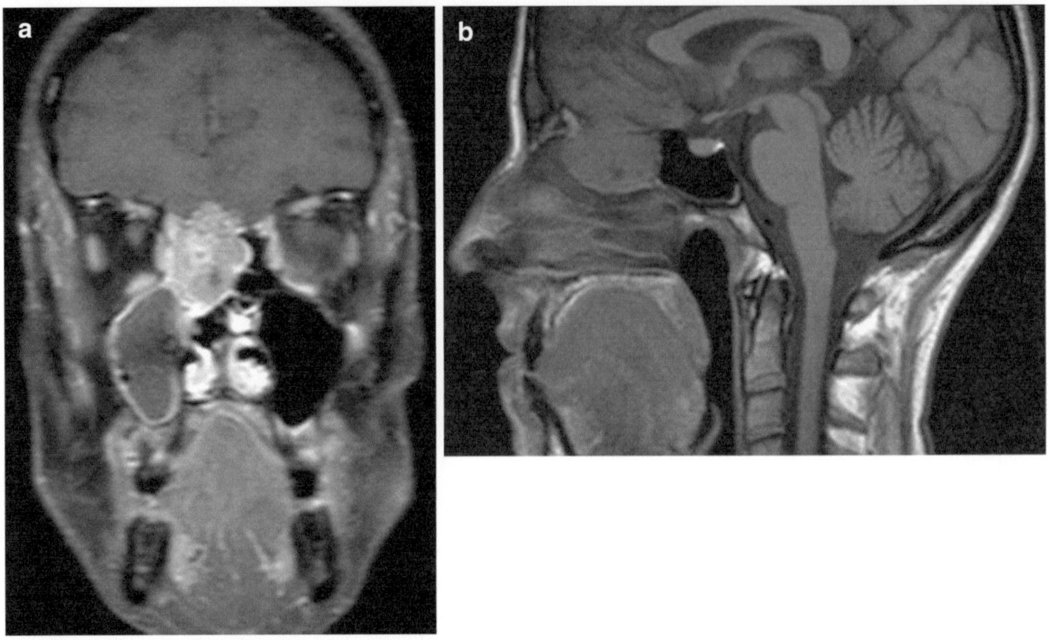

Fig. 29.1 (**a**) Coronal T1-weighted gadolinium enhanced MRI. There is tumor in the right ethmoidal cells with invasion of the anterior cranial fossa, without enhancement of the dura nor infiltration of the brain. Lateral compression of the orbit without infiltration. The middle meatus is obstructed and there are mucous retentions in the right maxillary sinus. (**b**) Sagittal T1-weighted MRI. Tumor mass in the anterior ethmoidal cells with destruction of the skull base

epistaxis, although frequent in elder patients with anticoagulant treatment has to be checked. Once orbital and/or neurological symptoms show up the disease is usually more advanced and should generally be referred immediately. Orbital involvement indicates advanced tumor progression and may present with proptosis, diplopia, or epiphora. Numbness or paresthesia usually indicate infiltration of the infraorbital nerve [8].

Tumors growing downwards in the maxillary sinus may loosen teeth or difficult adaptation of dental prosthesis.

Imaging plays a key role in pretreatment assessment and preoperative planning. Computed tomography (CT) and magnetic resonance imaging (MRI) are indicated in a complementary fashion to accurately assess the loco-regional extent of the tumor including any bone and neurovascular extension or nodal involvement.

The goals of imaging are to differentiate tumor tissue from inflammation and secretions, and map its extent [9]. Soft tissue assessment is best achieved by MR with gadolinium enhancement in T1-weighted and T2-weighted images. As CT is the first investigation commonly obtained in a patient with symptoms suggesting a disease involving the sinonasal tract and/or the adjacent skull base. Fat-saturated T1-weighted techniques help to identify the presence of disease beyond the paranasal sinuses (i.e., perineural spread and/or intracranial extension) [10].

The key issues in imaging are mapping of potential anterior skull base and orbit involvement, and assessment of perineural spread. All these goals are better achieved by MR than with CT (Figs. 29.1, 29.2). When assessing anterior skull base involvement it is crucial to analyze the signal intensity at the interface between the ethmoid and brain: the cribriform plate with its double periosteal layer; the dura mater and the subarachnoid space. Enhanced T1 or fat-saturated T1 (VIBE) display the three layers as a "sandwich" of different signals. A neoplasm abutting against the cribriform plate without interrupting the hypointense signal, the lesion can be considered extracranial. Effacement of the

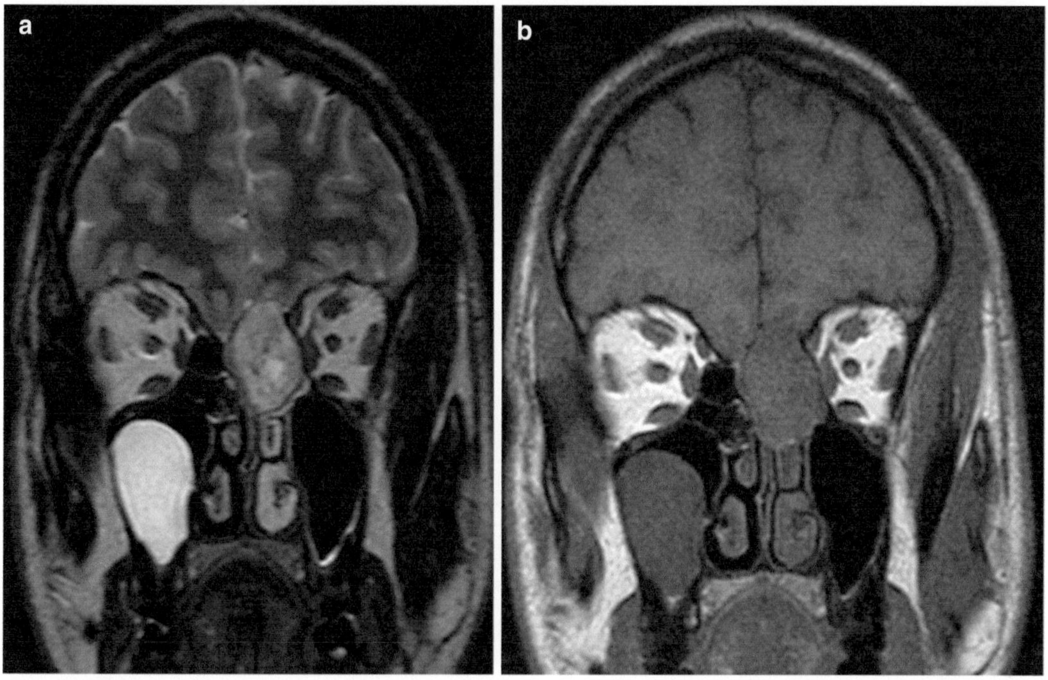

Fig. 29.2 (**a**) Coronal T2-weighted MRI. Tumor mass in the left anterior ethmoidal cells with superior extension. Displacement of the brain without brain invasion. Retention cyst in the right maxillary sinus. (**b**) Coronal T1-weighted MRI of the same case as in figure (**a**). There is a hipointense "halo" that separates the tumor from the brain indication absence of infiltration. Retention cyst in the right maxillary sinus

hypointense signal of the lower layer by tumor implies bone-periosteum penetration. In this case, if an uninterrupted thickened and enhancing dura is visible, the neoplasm may be defined as intracranial-extradural. Focal or more extensive replacement of enhanced thickened dura by tumor signal indicates intracranial-intradural extension. Brain invasion is suggested by the presence of edema [11].

Other sequences may include:

- MR cisternography with thin, T2-weighted (3DFT-CISS, DRIVE) sections (0.6 mm or less) [12] to assess the potential relationships with cisternal cranial nerve segments;
- High resolution sequences with submillimetric isotropic slices (FIESTA; VIBE) to highlight the intraforaminal segment of cranial nerves [11];
- FLAIR (fluid-attenuated inversion recovery), which may help in differentiating CSF from the cystic/fluid content of tumors or secondary mucoceles at the skull base;
- MR angiography, to visualize the entire course (or segments) of the internal carotid artery (ICA) [7].

Orbital walls are frequently involved in both ethmoid and maxillary cancers. A thin and regular hypointensity on T2 images between tumor and orbital fat indicates an intact periorbit [13].

Adenoid cystic carcinoma typically displays a perineural spread, more rarely in squamous cell carcinoma, lymphoma, and melanoma. MR can predict perineural spread with 95% sensitivity [14].

Nerve enhancement and nerve enlargement are indirect signs of perineural spread [11]. Other suggestive features for infiltration are enlargement or destruction of skull base foramina, obliteration of fat planes around a nerve or within a foramen, replacement of the normal CSF signal within the Meckel's cave, and convexity of the lateral cavernous sinus wall. The use of high-spatial resolution post-contrast fat saturation VIBE allows the evaluation of skull base foramina without artifacts with special reference to the discrimination between the nerve and surrounding vascular plexus [11]. Malignant tumors of the sinonasal tract show similar imaging features. Particular radiologic or clinical findings will be listed below for each tumor.

Primary epithelial tumors (squamous cell carcinoma - SCC) originate in 60–73% in the maxillary sinus, 20–30% in the nasal cavity, 10–15% in the ethmoid sinus, and 1% in the sphenoid and frontal sinuses [6, 15, 16]. Early course displays non-specific unilateral symptoms.

At presentation the mean age is around 50 years and the stage is usually advanced. Intranasal inspection may reveal a large intranasal mass, either friable, necrotic, exophytic or papillary that may bleed when biopsied. Facial swelling, symptoms related to infraorbital nerve or orbital infiltration. In about 12% there are lymph nodes present [8].

Primary or secondary sinonasal lymphomas (non-epithelial malignant tumors), mostly non-Hodgkin lymphomas, are the second most common malignant tumor following carcinomas in the sinonasal tract. B-cell lymphomas are predominant and tend to affect paranasal sinuses in the elderly [15]. T or NK cell lymphomas are predominant and the nasal cavity is mainly affecting younger people [16].

Epstein–Barr virus is considered important in the etiopathogenesis of lymphomas, especially for specific lymphomas such as Burkitt lymphoma and nasal NK-T lymphoma. It seems that EBV plays a role in T-cell lymphomas and that the incidence of EBV infection may explain the reported "East-West" difference in the incidence of nasal T-cell lymphomas [15, 16].

Adenoid cystic carcinoma (ACC) accounts for fewer than 1% of all head and neck malignancies and 10% of all salivary gland neoplasms. The maxillary sinus (47%) and the nasal cavity (30%) were the most common primary tumor sites. ACC displays a propensity for perineural spread and bony invasion, which may lead to skull base involvement and intracranial growth. Two other patterns of spread suggest a diagnosis of adenoid cystic carcinoma: subperiosteal bone invasion and extent into fat spaces [15]. Clinical features are unspecific, with unilateral obstruction and serosanguinous discharge. Because of the perineural infiltration patients complain about facial pain and numbness in the branches of the trigeminal nerve. Distant metastasis may develop in the lung on the long-term, even years after treatment [8].

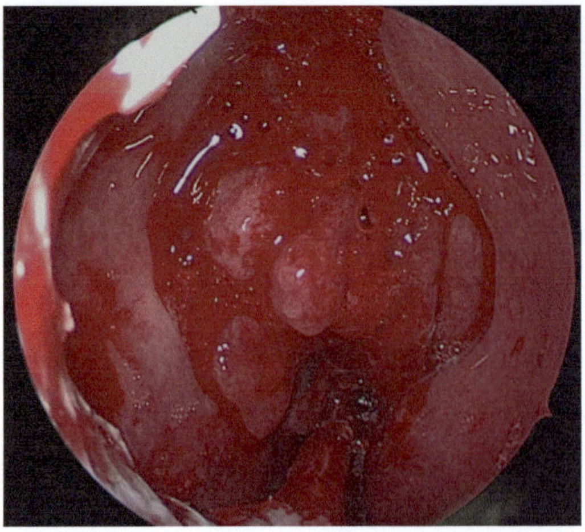

Fig. 29.3 Intraoperative endoscopic view during endoscopic removal of adenocarcinoma. Note that the posterior septum has been removed. Fleshy tumor mass in the midline in between both middle turbinates

Adenocarcinoma is the third most common mucosal epithelial malignancy [17], occurring predominately among men with a mean age of presentation of 60–65 years [18]. Men develop adenocarcinoma four times more frequently than women [19]. The ethmoid sinus is predominately involved (85%) (Fig. 29.3). On sinus CT scans a unilateral expanding opacity of the olfactory cavity should raise the suspicion of nasal adenocarcinoma [20]. Woodworkers have 500 times elevated risk compared to the male population and up to 900 times compared to the population in general [21]. The true risk factor is the direct exposure to wood dust particles, and not the possible exposure to chemical products used in the industry [21]. Hard wood types such as ebony, oak, and beech confer the highest risk of developing sinonasal adenocarcinomas [22]. There is a higher incidence of tumor occurring among workers exposed for longer periods. Because of the occupational exposure to wood dust adenocarcinomas can be multicentric and subsequently bilateral.

In order of decreasing frequency sinonasal mucoepidermoid carcinoma most commonly affects the maxillary sinus followed by nasal cavity, nasopharynx, and ethmoid sinuses [4, 23].

Primary sinonasal tract mucosal malignant melanomas are very rare, but the head and neck represent a common site. The incidence is the same in men and women, although a higher proportion of melanoma was identified in black patients (10.4%) [24]. Malignant melanomas of the sinonasal tract appear later in life (64.3 years) than cutaneous ones. Similarly to cutaneous melanoma, it is a more lethal disease in patients older than 60 years [24]. Melanoma involving the sinus may grow asymptomatically until late in the disease course [25, 26]. A third of patients have neck metastases when diagnosed and distant metastasis is rapidly fatal [27].

Olfactory neuroblastoma (ON) occurs over a wide age range (3–90 years) with peaks in the second and sixth decades of life [28, 29]. Males and females show with similar frequency and can be found in all age groups [30, 31].

ON is commonly found in the upper nasal cavity and/or adjacent ethmoid cells (Fig. 29.4). Radiologically it can display a marginal cyst in the intracranial component or hyperostosis of adjacent bones.

It is rare to find metastasis of malignant tumors and, if so, then at a late stage. Metastasis in the sinonasal tract has an origin in a renal carcinoma in over 50% [32]. Other primary sources, in decreasing order, are lung (12%), urogenital ridge (12%), breast (9%), and gastrointestinal tract (GI tract) (6%) [33]. The maxillary sinus (50%) followed by the ethmoid (18%) and the nasal cavity (15%) is mostly affected [30, 34, 35]. The highest incidence of metastasis is in the sixth decade in men and the seventh decade in women depending on the origin of the primary.

Some recommendations may be helpful when dealing with patients displaying an atypical clinical course of chronic rhinosinusitis that eventually is a malignant tumor.

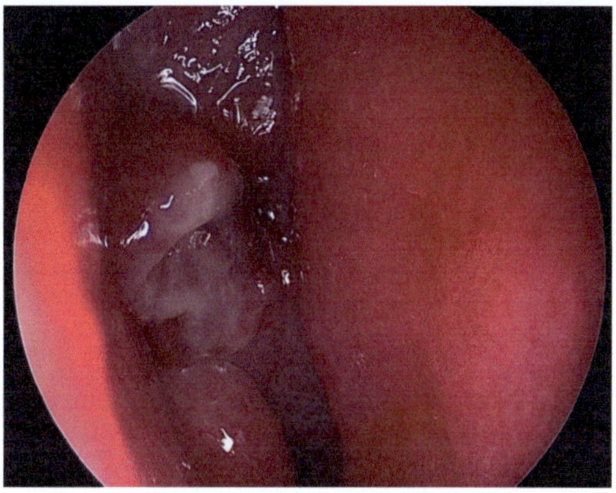

Fig. 29.4 Endoscopic view of the right nasal fossa. Please note the superficial exudation, lack of translucency of the tumor located above the middle turbinate occupying the olfactory cleft. (Histology: olfactory neuroblastoma)

- In an atypical clinical behavior the lesion might be a tumor until the contrary is proven, even when there is no mass or ulceration.
- CT scan or MRI displaying expansive or destructive lesions with infiltration of either skull base, septum or orbit or infiltration of soft tissues are in urgent need of a biopsy.
- When taking a biopsy make sure to avoid necrotic areas and take larger samples. Sometimes, normal polypoid tissue may mask the tumor growing behind.

References

1. Tufano RP, Mokadam NA, Montone KT, Weinstein GS, Chalian AA, Wolf PF, et al. Malignant tumors of the nose and paranasal sinuses: hospital of the University of Pennsylvania experience 1990–1997. Am J Rhinol. 1999;13(2):117–23. https://doi.org/10.2500/105065899782106698.
2. Le QT, Fu KK, Kaplan M, Terris DJ, Fee WE, Goffinet DR. Treatment of maxillary sinus carcinoma: a comparison of the 1997 and 1977 American Joint Committee on cancer staging systems. Cancer. 1999;86(9):1700–11.
3. Tiwari R, Hardillo JA, Mehta D, Slotman B, Tobi H, Croonenburg E, et al. Squamous cell carcinoma of maxillary sinus. Head Neck. 2000;22(2):164–9. https://doi.org/10.1002/(sici)1097-0347(200003)22:2<164::aid-hed8>3.0.co;2-#.
4. Muir CS, Nectoux J. Descriptive epidemiology of malignant neoplasms of nose, nasal cavities, middle

ear and accessory sinuses. Clin Otolaryngol Allied Sci. 1980;5(3):195–211. https://doi.org/10.1111/j.1365-2273.1980.tb01647.x.
5. Zyłka S, Bień S, Kamiński B, Postuła S, Ziołkowska M. Epidemiology and clinical characteristics of the sinonasal malignancies. Otolaryngol Polska—Polish Otolaryngol. 2008;62(4):436–41. https://doi.org/10.1016/s0030-6657(08)70287-7.
6. Olsen KD. Nose and sinus tumours. In: McCaffrey T, editor. Rhinologic diagnosis and treatment. New York: Thieme; 1997. p. 334–59.
7. Lund VJ, Stammberger H, Nicolai P, Castelnuovo P, Beal T, Beham A, et al. European position paper on endoscopic management of tumours of the nose, paranasal sinuses and skull base. Rhinol Suppl. 2010;22:1–143.
8. Valerie JL, David JH, William IW. Tumors of the nose, sinuses, and nasopharynx. New York: Thieme; 2014.
9. Madani G, Beale TJ, Lund VJ. Imaging of sinonasal tumors. Semin Ultrasound, CT, MR. 2009;30(1):25–38. https://doi.org/10.1053/j.sult.2008.10.013.
10. Fatterpekar GM, Delman BN, Som PM. Imaging the paranasal sinuses: where we are and where we are going. Anatomical Rec (Hoboken, NJ: 2007). 2008;291(11):1564–72. https://doi.org/10.1002/ar.20773.
11. Maroldi R, Ravanelli M, Borghesi A, Farina D. Paranasal sinus imaging. Eur J Radiol. 2008;66(3):372–86. https://doi.org/10.1016/j.ejrad.2008.01.059.
12. Yousry I, Moriggl B, Schmid UD, Naidich TP, Yousry TA. Trigeminal ganglion and its divisions: detailed anatomic MR imaging with contrast-enhanced 3D constructive interference in the steady state sequences. AJNR Am J Neuroradiol. 2005;26(5):1128–35.
13. Kim HJ, Lee TH, Lee HS, Cho KS, Roh HJ. Periorbita: computed tomography and magnetic resonance imaging findings. Am J Rhinol. 2006;20(4):371–4. https://doi.org/10.2500/ajr.2006.20.2889.
14. Nemzek WR, Hecht S, Gandour-Edwards R, Donald P, McKennan K. Perineural spread of head and neck tumors: how accurate is MR imaging? AJNR Am J Neuroradiol. 1998;19(4):701–6.
15. Maroldi R, Lombardi D, Farina D, Nicolai P, Moraschi I, Neoplasms M. Imaging in treatment planning for sinonasal diseases. Berlin: Springer; 2005. p. 159–220.
16. Arber DA, Weiss LM, Albújar PF, Chen YY, Jaffe ES. Nasal lymphomas in Peru. High incidence of T-cell immunophenotype and Epstein-Barr virus infection. Am J Surg Pathol. 1993;17(4):392–9.
17. Kleinsasser O, Schroeder HG. Adenocarcinomas of the inner nose after exposure to wood dust. Morphological findings and relationships between histopathology and clinical behavior in 79 cases. Arch Otorhinolaryngol. 1988;245(1):1–15. https://doi.org/10.1007/bf00463541.
18. Llorente JL, Pérez-Escuredo J, Alvarez-Marcos C, Suárez C, Hermsen M. Genetic and clinical aspects of wood dust related intestinal-type sinonasal adenocarcinoma: a review. Eur Arch Otorhinolaryngol. 2009;266(1):1–7. https://doi.org/10.1007/s00405-008-0749-y.
19. Jankowski R, Georgel T, Vignaud JM, Hemmaoui B, Toussaint B, Graff P, et al. Endoscopic surgery reveals that woodworkers' adenocarcinomas originate in the olfactory cleft. Rhinology. 2007;45(4):308–14.
20. Acheson ED, Cowdell RH, Hadfield E, Macbeth RG. Nasal cancer in woodworkers in the furniture industry. Br Med J. 1968;2(5605):587–96. https://doi.org/10.1136/bmj.2.5605.587.
21. Wolf J, Schmezer P, Fengel D, Schroeder HG, Scheithauer H, Woeste P. The role of combination effects on the etiology of malignant nasal tumours in the wood-working industry. Acta Otolaryngol Suppl. 1998;535:1–16.
22. Spiro RH, Huvos AG, Berk R, Strong EW. Mucoepidermoid carcinoma of salivary gland origin. A clinicopathologic study of 367 cases. Am J Surg. 1978;136(4):461–8. https://doi.org/10.1016/0002-9610(78)90262-3.
23. Thompson LD, Wieneke JA, Miettinen M. Sinonasal tract and nasopharyngeal melanomas: a clinicopathologic study of 115 cases with a proposed staging system. Am J Surg Pathol. 2003;27(5):594–611. https://doi.org/10.1097/00000478-200305000-00004.
24. Manolidis S, Donald PJ. Malignant mucosal melanoma of the head and neck: review of the literature and report of 14 patients. Cancer. 1997;80(8):1373–86. https://doi.org/10.1002/(sici)1097-0142(19971015)80:8<1373::aid-cncr3>3.0.co;2-g.
25. Lund VJ. Malignant melanoma of the nasal cavity and paranasal sinuses. Ear Nose Throat J. 1993;72(4):285–90.
26. Dauer EH, Lewis JE, Rohlinger AL, Weaver AL, Olsen KD. Sinonasal melanoma: a clinicopathologic review of 61 cases. Otolaryngol Head Neck Surg. 2008;138(3):347–52. https://doi.org/10.1016/j.otohns.2007.12.013.
27. Walch C, Stammberger H, Anderhuber W, Unger F, Köle W, Feichtinger K. The minimally invasive approach to olfactory neuroblastoma: combined endoscopic and stereotactic treatment. Laryngoscope. 2000;110(4):635–40. https://doi.org/10.1097/00005537-200004000-00018.
28. Morita A, Ebersold MJ, Olsen KD, Foote RL, Lewis JE, Quast LM. Esthesioneuroblastoma: prognosis and management. Neurosurgery. 1993;32(5):706–14.; discussion 14-5. https://doi.org/10.1227/00006123-199305000-00002.
29. Broich G, Pagliari A, Ottaviani F. Esthesioneuroblastoma: a general review of the cases published since the discovery of the tumour in 1924. Anticancer Res. 1997;17(4a):2683–706.
30. Dulguerov P, Calcaterra T. Esthesioneuroblastoma: the UCLA experience 1970-1990.

Laryngoscope. 1992;102(8):843–9. https://doi.org/10.1288/00005537-199208000-00001.
31. Simo R, Sykes AJ, Hargreaves SP, Axon PR, Birzgalis AR, Slevin NJ, et al. Metastatic renal cell carcinoma to the nose and paranasal sinuses. Head Neck. 2000;22(7):722–7. https://doi.org/10.1002/1097-0347(200010)22:7<722::aid-hed13>3.0.co;2-0.
32. Bernstein JM, Montgomery WW, Balogh K Jr. Metastatic tumors to the maxilla, nose, and paranasal sinuses. Laryngoscope. 1966;76(4):621–50. https://doi.org/10.1288/00005537-196604000-00003.
33. Pignataro L, Peri A, Ottaviani F. Breast carcinoma metastatic to the ethmoid sinus: a case report. Tumori. 2001;87(6):455–7.
34. Friedmann I, Osborn DA. Metastatic tumours in the ear, nose and throat region. J Laryngol Otol. 1965;79:576–91. https://doi.org/10.1017/s0022215100064100.
35. Izquierdo J, Armengot M, Cors R, Pérez A, Basterra J. Hepatocarcinoma: metastasis to the nose and paranasal sinuses. Otolaryngol Head Neck Surg. 2000;122(6):932–3. https://doi.org/10.1016/s0194-5998(00)70032-5.

30 Pediatric Chronic Rhinosinusitis: View from Europe

Thibaut van Zele

Key Points

- The prevalence of CRS is lower than in adults (2–4%), but the negative impact on quality of life seems to be similar to that observed in adults.
- Children with CRS refractory to appropriate medical treatment should be evaluated for humoral immune deficiency; if polyps are present, investigations for CF should be performed.
- It is likely that the pathophysiology of pediatric CRS involves both genetic and environmental influences.
- There is no evidence to use either oral or intravenous antibiotics. There is also no evidence to support the utilization of prolonged macrolide therapy in children with uncomplicated CRS.
- Intranasal steroids and nasal lavages are recommended for use in children with CRS despite the absence of good level evidence. There is one study that supports short-term systemic steroid use in children with CRS.
- Adenoidectomy with/without antral irrigation is the simplest and safest first procedure to consider in younger children with symptoms of CRS.
- FESS is a safe and possibly effective surgical modality in children with CRS and can be used after failure of adenoidectomy in older children refractory to medical therapy.

30.1 Prevalence of Pediatric Chronic Rhinosinusitis

Pediatric chronic rhinosinusitis (PCRS) is a commonly encountered condition in otorhinolaryngological practice. The exact incidence and prevalence of PCRS are to date unknown [1]. It is estimated that 5–13% of childhood viral upper respiratory tract infections may progress to acute rhinosinusitis, with a proportion of these progressing to a chronic rhinosinusitis. Estimates from the National Health Interview Survey in the United States in 1996 suggest that young people under the age of 18 years are affected by chronic rhinosinusitis (CRS) at a rate of 63.9 per 1000 individuals showing a lower prevalence than in adults [2].

CT scans in children 3–12 years of age presenting with chronic rhinorrhea, nasal congestion, and cough show [3] maxillary opacification in 63%, ethmoid involvement in 58%, and sphenoidal sinus involvement in 29% of the children of the youngest age groups. In the older age group 13–14 years the incidence of abnor-

T. van Zele (✉)
Upper Airways Research Laboratory and Department of Oto-Rhino-Laryngology, Ghent University, Ghent, Belgium
e-mail: Thibaut.vanzele@ugent.be

L. Zhang, C. Bachert (eds.), *Chronic Rhinosinusitis*, https://doi.org/10.1007/978-981-16-0784-4_30

malities decreased to 10% of the ethmoids, 0% of sphenoids, but still 65% of the maxillaries being involved. The prevalence of rhinosinusitis decreases after age 6–8 years [4] and children with a family history of atopy or asthma attending day-care in the first year of life have 2.2 times higher odds of having doctor-diagnosed sinusitis than children who do not attend day-care [5]. Like adults CRS, PCRS carries a major financial and healthcare resource burden due to its prevalence in the population. The visit burden from chronic rhinosinusitis exceeds that of acute rhinosinusitis [4]. In the USA 3.7–7.5 million visits per year for PCRS are performed. In children 12 years old or younger, $1.8 billion was spent on the treatment of sinusitis in just 1 year [2]. The prevalence of CRS in pediatric patients lies between 2.1 and 4% with children of 10–15 years to be most commonly affected by CRS. CRS was more common than ARS and otitis media in the group between 15 and 20 years (0.9%).

30.2 Quality of Life

CRS in children leads to impaired quality of life, with its related adverse effects potentially exceeding that of children with other common chronic childhood diseases such as asthma, attention deficit hyperactivity disorder, juvenile rheumatoid arthritis, and epilepsy chronic respiratory and arthritic disease. Especially in the physical domains of the quality of life questionnaires such as bodily pain and limitation in physical activity differences were noted. PCRS also has the potential to exacerbate asthma, a condition that negatively affects 2–20% of children [6, 7]. In a group of 85 children aged 2–12 years the SN5 survey has been shown to correlate with CT scan scores in patients with CRS suggesting that it can be used as a substitute for repeated CT scans in clinical follow-up [8].

30.3 Development of the Sinuses

The normal sinus anatomy like in adults is different from the size and shape of the sinuses in children. The sinus cavities continue to grow and pneumatize into teenage years. Ethmoid and maxillary sinuses are already present at birth. They are completely pneumatized around the age of 10 years. The sphenoid and frontal sinus develop at later ages: the sphenoid sinuses pneumatize around 9 months of age while the frontal sinuses start pneumatizing from age 7–8 years. Complete growth for the sphenoid sinus and frontal sinus is achieved by age 12–14 years and 19 years, respectively [7, 9, 10]. Due to this immature development of the sinuses children under the age of 13 are managed differently when presenting with complications of acute rhinosinusitis or chronic rhinosinusitis. On the other hand, children over the age of 13 are having mature sinuses with similar disease processes and can be treated much like an adult [7].

30.4 Clinical Diagnosis and Definition of PCRS

30.4.1 Definition

The clinical diagnosis and definition of PCRS is very similar to adult CRS and consists of both subjective and objective symptoms and features. The EPOS criteria for PCRS define PCRS as an inflammation of the nose and the paranasal sinuses characterized by two or more symptoms, one of which should be either nasal blockage/obstruction/congestion or nasal discharge (anterior/posterior nasal drip): ± facial pain/pressure, ± cough; and either endoscopic signs of disease and/or relevant changes on the CT scan of the sinus [11]. This EPOS definition was adapted in a more recent consensus statement on PCRS in which pediatric chronic rhinosinusitis (PCRS) is defined as at least 90 continuous days of 2 or more symptoms of purulent rhinorrhea, nasal obstruction, facial pressure/pain, or cough and either endoscopic signs of mucosal edema, purulent drainage, or nasal polyposis and/or CT scan changes showing mucosal changes within the ostiomeatal complex and/or sinuses in a pediatric patient aged 18 years or younger [7].

30.4.2 Diagnostic Tools

Although nasal endoscopy is challenging in children, it is a pivotal step in the diagnosis of PCRS as it provides direct visualization of the nasal cavity and middle and superior meatus. Use of topical decongestants and/or anesthetics is at the discretion of the physician [11]. Allergy test can be performed in children by skin prick test or blood test. There is no lower age limit for skin prick testing; however, in young children aeroallergens are best tested in blood for specific IgE for reasons of patient comfort [11].

Nitric oxide is indicated if PCD and to some extent CF is suspected from the age of 5. Taking biopsies is rarely needed in children except in cases of unilateral processes with suspicion for inverted papilloma or malignancy.

CT scan is the imaging modality of choice to evaluate for CRS as it provides detailed information on mucosal inflammation in the sinuses. There are concerns on the potentially high false-positive rates in children as mucosal edema can occur in any child with an upper respiratory tract infection. The presence of mucosal thickening on CT does not necessarily mean that the disease is chronic or that it requires surgical intervention. The impossibility of assessing the chronicity of sinus disease with CT can be circumvented in part by using maximum medical management and assessing the amount of persistent disease [12]. Using the Lund-Mackay scoring system with a cut-off of five gives a sensitivity of 86% and specificity of 85% for PCRS [13]. Although CT scans are recommended to aid in diagnosis of CRS, the risks must be carefully weighed, as one retrospective cohort study found that one head CT before the age of 10 years led to one excess case of brain tumor and one excess case of leukemia per 10,000 patients [14] (Fig. 30.1).

30.5 Predisposing Factors

30.5.1 Anatomical Factors in PCRS

As in adults, the ostiomeatal complex is an important anatomical structure for rhinosinusitis. Impaired drainage through the ostiomeatal complex can occur due to inflammatory changes in the anterior ethmoid and subsequently can impair drainage of the maxillary and frontal sinus. Other anatomical variations that have been found in children are pneumatized middle concha, pneumatization of the superior turbinate and Haller cell; however, these anatomical variations do not correlate to the extent and existence of sinusitis in children and it is not clear whether they have any contribution to CRS in children [15]. Enlarged adenoids can play a role in the development of CRS in children as they can become a reservoir for microbes. These findings have been used to support the role of adenoidectomy for early treatment of children with CRS [16, 17]. Further evidence to support the role of the adenoids in the pathogenesis of PCRS is the fact that there is a high correlation between the bacteria present within the adenoids and within the middle meatus in children with CRS [18]. However, by 12 years of age, the adenoid tissue largely involutes. As a result, adenoid hypertrophy is much less likely to be involved in the pathogenesis of CRS in older patients [19].

30.5.2 Environmental Factors

Environmental factors that play a role in the development and pathophysiology of pediatric CRS are poorly studied and mainly focused on exposure to tobacco. From in vitro studies it is known that exposure to tobacco smoke can inhibit mucociliary clearance and epithelial regeneration. In the adult population active and passive smoking are significant risk factors for the development of CRS [20, 21]. Children exposed to passive smoking have a 68% prevalence of acute rhinosinusitis compared to a prevalence of 1.2% among children without exposure [22]. Passive and/or active smoking lead to worse postoperative outcomes for CRS surgery in children. A second environmental factor is the exposure to viral infection, although poorly studied in children there is up to date no direct evidence to support the importance of viral infections to CRS in children.

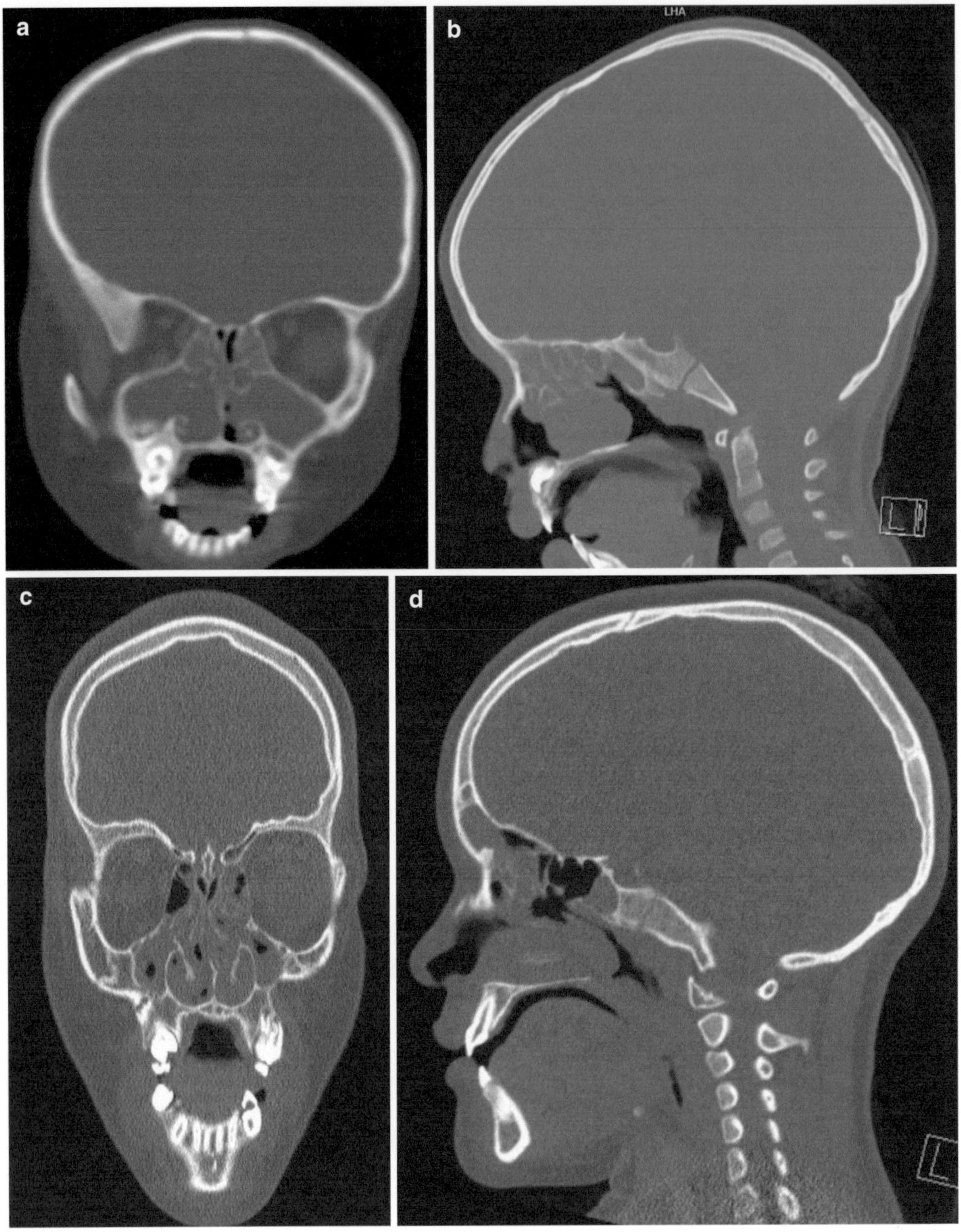

Fig. 30.1 Computed tomography scans (CT scan) from children with chronic rhinosinusitis. (**a**) Coronal image of cystic fibrosis patient (5 year old) with polyposis. (**b**) Sagittal view of same patient, the sphenoidal is underdeveloped as well as the frontal sinus. (**c**) Coronal view of a 12-year-old with chronic rhinosinusitis with no polyposis. (**d**) Sagittal view of same patient of (**c**)

30.5.3 Comorbid Diseases in PCRS

Age is the single most important risk factor associated with chronic rhinosinusitis in children, with 73% of 2–6 year olds, and 74% of 6–10 year olds having sinus CT abnormalities as opposed to the low incidence of sinus abnormalities detected in only 38% of children over 10 years of age. Due to the high prevalence of prevalence of allergic rhinitis in the pediatric population, allergic rhinitis is a common coexisting disease in PCRS; however, the causal relationship between allergic rhinitis and PCRS is highly controversial and probably non-existent [23]. Asthma is also commonly associated with CRS in children. Several studies have shown that pharmacological intervention or surgical intervention for sinusitis has improved asthma control, spirometry, wheezing symptoms [23].

Gastro-esophageal reflux disease (GERD) has been proposed to be a risk factor for pediatric CRS. The rationale behind this idea is the fact that reflux of gastric acid into the nasopharynx and nasal cavity might induce infammation of the sinonasal ostia combined with impaired mucociliary clearance both leading to rhinosinusitis [11]. To date the scientific data are scarce and when available conflicting. Some evidence suggests an association between gastroesophageal reflux disease (GERD) and PCRS; however, the differential diagnosis between GERD and post nasal drip symptoms is difficult [23]. Studies have shown a higher percentage of children with positive 24-h pH probe for reflux in children with PCRS and suggest that treating GERD may improve symptoms of PCRS [24].

It is prudent to screen for immunodeficiencies in children with recurrent or chronic rhinosinusitis. Several immunodeficiencies like IgA, IgG2, IgG3, low immunoglobulin levels with poor response to pneumococcal vaccine have been found in PCRS patients [25]. The rates of deficiency of the immune system appear to be much higher than in adults but vary widely depending on the studied pediatric population. Laboratory investigation in suspected cases should include immunoglobulin quantitation, titers to tetanus, diphtheria, and pneumococcal antibodies after vaccination. If responses are abnormal, these children should be referred to an immunologist [11].

30.5.4 Cystic Fibrosis and PCD

Cystic fibrosis is one of the few causes of nasal polyposis in children. CF is a genetic disease with autosomal recessive inheritance that affects approximately 1 in 3500 new-borns. The prevalence of chronic sinusitis is very high and nasal polyps occur in between 7 and 50% of affected patients [23]. Diagnosis of CF is confirmed by demonstration of elevated sweat chloride, and cases are often identified through newborn screening. However, diagnostic testing may be inconclusive, or not done in patients of higher age. Therefore, CF is not diagnosed until late in adulthood sometimes, when the symptoms are mild to moderate and incomplete.

Primary ciliary dyskinesia is a second autosomal recessive disorder causing PCRS. Half of the children with PCD present with situs inversus, bronchiectasis, and CRS, known as the Kartagener syndrome. PCD is suspected in a child with atypical asthma, bronchiectasis, chronic wet cough and mucus production, rhinosinusitis, chronic and severe otitis media (especially with chronic drainage in children with ear tubes).

30.6 Pathophysiology

30.6.1 Genetics

The pathophysiology of PCRS is still largely unknown but from existing evidence it is clear that it both involves genetic and environmental factors. There is a significant familial risk associated with pediatric CRS as shown by large database studies that show that siblings of patients with CRS have a 57.5-fold increased risk for CRS [19]. Studies on gene mutations show higher rates of heterozygous mutations in the cystic fibrosis transmembrane regulator gene (CFTR) [26]. On the other hand, monozygotic twins are not always both developing polyps, this indicates a combination of environmental and genetic factors plays a role in the occurrence of nasal polyps in children [27].

30.6.2 Inflammatory Mechanisms

In PCRS an upregulation of different inflammatory substances important in adaptive and innate immunity has been found. Eosinophils and CD4 positive lymphocytes play a significant role in tissue inflammation, with eosinophil predominance in the older children and neutrophil predominance in the younger ones [25]. Microarray analysis with subsequent gene mRNA expression analysis by PCR showed that two contributors to the adaptive immune response (cytokine CXCL5, a neutrophil chemoattractant and CXCL13, a B-lymphocyte chemoattractant) were upregulated, as well as serum amyloid A1/A2, serine peptidase inhibitor member 4 (SERPIN B4), and beta-defensin (DEFB1) which are proteins involved in the innate immune system [28]. Serum eosinophil counts and levels of ECP and total IgE tend to be significantly in PCRS that does not respond to antibiotic treatment suggesting that eosinophilic inflammation in the context of allergy is an important factor in children with CRS who do not respond to antibiotics [29]. Although more evidence is emerging to support upregulation of inflammatory markers in paranasal sinus tissues and nasal lavages of children with CRS, the data is relatively limited and heterogeneous and does not yet result in endotyping as has been done in adult CRS [11, 30].

30.6.3 Bacteriology

The presence of bacteria in the sinus cavity has been well established. It is plausible that in CRS, mucociliary clearance and host defenses are impaired to the point that the cavity becomes colonized with greater number of nasal bacterial flora [31]. Antibiotics directed toward the most common causative pathogens should be tried in PCRS. Few studies have ascertained the bacterial causes of PCRS, most have addressed the acute form of the disease. In contrast to the consensus regarding the bacteriology of acute rhinosinusitis, there is no agreement about the bacteriology of CRS due to many issues that confound the reliability of microbiological studies especially in children. These confounding factors may include variability in methods used to sample the sinus cavity; failure to sterilize the area through which the trocar or endoscope is passed; differences in sinuses or areas that are sampled; lack of evaluation of the inflammatory response or quantitation, duration and extent of disease [32]. Using cultures form the ethmoid bullae or maxillary sinus aspirates in children, the principal isolated aerobic organisms were alfa-hemolytic streptococcus, *S. aureus, M. catarrhalis, S. pneumoniae, and H. influenzae* [33, 34]. In children there can be a simultaneous occurrence of chronic otitis media with effusion and maxillary CRS. In the majority (69%) a microbiologic concordance was found between the ear and sinus samples. The most frequent isolates in both locations were *H. influenzae,* S. pneumoniae, *Prevotella spp, and Peptostreptococcus spp.* [31]. In about two thirds of the children affected by CRS anaerobic bacteria have been isolated. In patients with ARS not responding to regular antibiotic therapy repeated cultures revealed antimicrobial resistant anaerobic bacteria including *Prevotella spp, Porphyromonas spp, Fusobacterium nucleatum, and Peptostreptococcus sp.* [31]. If aerobic gram-negative bacilli such as Pseudomonas aeruginosa, Klebsiella pneumoniae, *Enterobacter spp.,* Proteus mirabilis, *and* Escherichia coli are cultured an underlying medical condition like cystic fibrosis (in the case of *Pseudomonas aeruginosa*), diabetes, or immune deficiency (neutropenia, critical illness, diabetes mellitus, or HIV) should be suspected [31].

30.7 Medical Treatment

The initial management of pediatric CRS is medical, with goals that include reducing inflammation, improving drainage, and eradicating pathogens. The most commonly used therapies include antibiotics, intranasal steroids, and saline nasal irrigation [35]. Currently there is no good evidence in the literature to support the use of antibiotics for CRS in children. Some guidelines support the empiric broad-spectrum antibiotic treatment with transition to culture directed antibiotics for 3–12 weeks. Initial empiric treatment should cover *S. pneumoniae*, *M. catarrhalis*, nontypeable *H. influenzae*, S. aureus, and possibly anaerobic bacteria [1, 23]. It is common but unsubstantiated practice to include antibiotics as part of maximal medical therapy in children with CRS. It is likely that, in many of these instances, treatment targets acute exacerbations on top of pre-existing chronic disease [11]. The EPOS guidelines however state that there is currently no evidence to support treatment of children with CRS with either oral or intravenous antibiotics. There is also no evidence to support the utilization of prolonged macrolide usage [11]. There also is no place for topical antibiotics or topical irrigations with antibiotics.

Nasal saline irrigations are a widely used first-line option for treatment of adult and PCRS that are effective and well tolerated with little risk for side effects. Several studies with a broad range of delivery techniques and tonicity of saline have been studied. Overall there is evidence that saline is beneficial in the treatment of symptoms for CRS when used as the sole modality of treatment or as a treatment adjunct [11].

Nasal steroids or topical steroid irrigations can be added to this treatment and are usually included in the initial medical management. Intranasal steroid sprays have been beneficial as they can decrease the amount of mucosal inflammation visualized and also improve symptoms, such as cough and postnasal drainage [35]. Reports on the efficacy of INCS such as fluticasone and mometasone are still conflicting and to date, there is no evidence from randomized controlled trials to support the efficacy of intranasal steroids in pediatric CRS [11]. However, given the low systemic absorption and low risk profile in children with allergic rhinitis and the fact that they are effective in adults with CRS, the use of intranasal steroids can be recommended as first-line therapy in children [1].

Systemic steroids have also been used in children because of their potent anti-inflammatory effects. Systemic corticosteroids in addition to antibiotics can give symptomatic and radiographic improvements in children with CRS [29]. Given the potential for serious side effects with systemic corticosteroid the use and position of systemic steroids is limited because of safety concerns. There is currently no evidence supporting other therapies such as nasal antihistamines, leukotriene modifiers, or decongestants [1, 11]. Treatment of children with CRS for concomitant gastroesophageal reflux disease (GORD) has been suggested with weak evidence showing improvement in rhinosinusitis symptoms and avoidance of surgery; however, routine anti-reflux therapies of children with CRS are not warranted [1, 11].

30.8 Surgery for PCRS

Consideration for surgical intervention is made after failed conservative nasal hygiene and medical management; however, an official definition for appropriate medical therapy and failure of such therapy is lacking. Surgical options are age-dependent and anatomy dependent [1] and can include adenoidectomy with or without antral irrigation and functional endoscopic sinus surgery. A logical surgical algorithm for PCRS begins with adenoidectomy with possible antral irrigation or balloon dilation of the maxillary sinuses, with FESS reserved for treatment failures. Symptomatic children with sinonasal polyposis, cystic fibrosis, allergic fungal rhinosinusitis (AFRS), PCD, or antrochoanal polyps are more likely to require FESS for disease control [23].

30.8.1 Adenoidectomy, Sinus Irrigation, and Balloon Sinuplasty

Adenoidectomy is a simple, well-tolerated procedure that has always been an attractive surgical option to consider for the treatment of PCRS. In children younger than 12 years adenoidectomy is an effective first-line therapy with effects independent from FESS [7, 36]. Multiple studies have shown that this treatment modality is effective in the majority of patients [11]. A meta-analysis that concluded that 69.3% of patients experienced significant improvement following adenoidectomy and that size of the adenoid does not influence success of adenoidectomy [12, 14]. The addition of middle meatal irrigation or balloon dilation may increase the efficacy of adenoid removal in the treatment of PCRS. A non-randomized study in children reported that balloon therapy when combined with adenoidectomy was more effective than adenoidectomy alone. However the balloon sinuplasty included also an antral lavage making it difficult to estimate the effectiveness of the balloon sinuplasty as such [37].

The outcomes of balloon sinuplasty alone versus balloon sinuplasty with concurrent procedures (adenoidectomy, turbinate surgery, ethmoidectomy) showed no difference in symptom control in children who underwent balloon sinuplasty versus children who underwent balloon sinuplasty with other procedures. Although the most recent guidelines acknowledge the safety profile of balloon sinuplasty, given the limited evidence until now, no guideline recommended the use of balloon sinuplasty as a surgical modality in children [11].

30.8.2 Functional Endoscopic Sinus Surgery

In the past physicians opted to use a more conservative approach in children regarding endoscopic sinus surgery. The rationale for this was the small anatomy and development of the sinuses, as well as earlier implications that ESS might interfere with the growth of the midface in children. However later studies have not supported this interference with facial growth. Therefore, controversy has been associated with pediatric ESS since it was introduced [38]. The efficacy of FESS in children has been reported and there is indication that FESS is superior to medical management [38]. A systematic review shows a positive outcome in between 71 and 100% of children after FESS as well as a significant improvement in quality of life after surgery [39]. A limited approach to FESS in children, consisting of the removal of any obvious obstruction (such as polyps and concha bullosa), as well as an anterior bulla ethmoidectomy, and a maxillary antrostomy, has been advocated by many experts [40]. If indicated, FESS is an effective treatment for PCRS with a low complication rate of 0.6% for major complications and 2% for minor complications. In children second-look procedures were common after FESS to clean the cavities; the advent of absorbable packing has made it possible to avoid a second-look procedure. Some studies have found comparable rates of revision sinus surgery in children with and without a second-look procedure, suggesting that it may not be helpful [41]. Besides PCRS there are also absolute indications for pediatric FESS: complete nasal obstruction in cystic fibrosis due to massive polyposis or due to medialization of the lateral nasal wall, orbital abscess, intracranial complications, antrochoanal polyp, mucocoele/mucopyocoele, and fungal rhinosinusitis.

30.9 Translation into Future Daily Practice

Pediatric chronic rhinosinusitis has a lower prevalence than in adults, but with an equal negative impact on quality of life. Appropriate medical therapy is intranasal steroids and nasal lavages; however, strong evidence is lacking. There is currently no strong advice to use either oral or intravenous antibiotics. Children with CRS refractory to appropriate medical treatment should be evaluated for humoral immune deficiency; if polyps are present, investigations for CF should be performed. A first step in the surgical management is adenoidectomy with/without antral irrigation, followed by FESS after failure of adenoidectomy especially in older children who are refractory to medical therapy. In the future further endotyping of PCRS, in analogy to adult CRS, is needed to get more insight in the pathophysiology of PCRS and to look for new or alternative therapeutic options (Fig. 30.2).

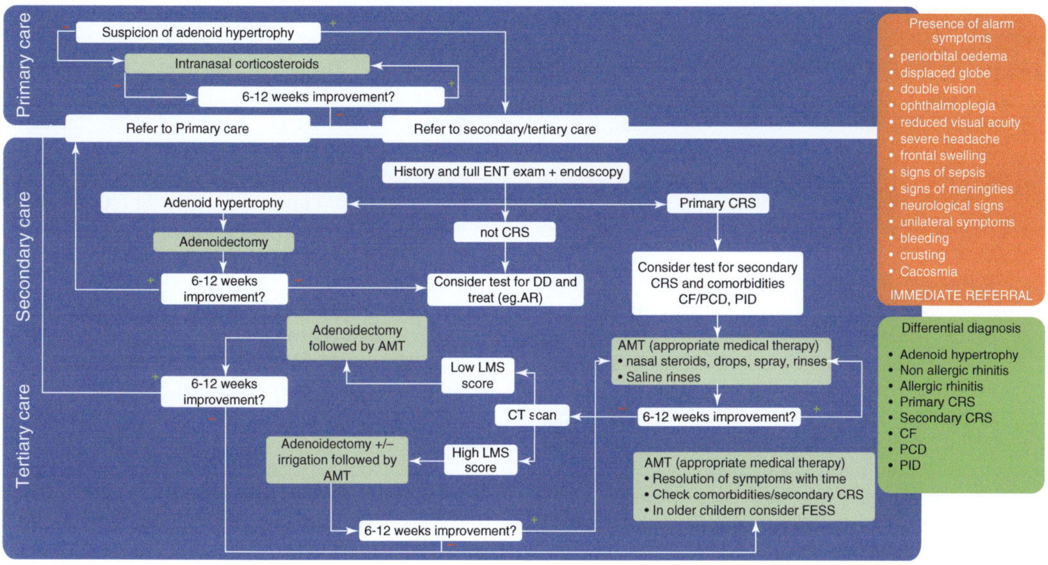

Fig. 30.2 Care pathway for pediatric chronic rhinosinusitis adapted from the EPOS 2020 guidelines

References

1. Orlandi RR, Kingdom TT, Hwang PH, Smith TL, Alt JA, Baroody FM, et al. International Consensus Statement on allergy and rhinology: rhinosinusitis. Int Forum Allergy Rhinol. 2016;6(S1):S22–209.
2. Adams PF, Hendershot GE, Marano MA, Centers for Disease Control and Prevention/National Center for Health Statistics. Current estimates from the National Health Interview Survey, 1996. Vital Health Stat. 1999;10(200):1–203.
3. Van der Veken P, Clement PA, Buisseret T, Desprechins B, Kaufman L, Derde MP. CAT-scan study of the prevalence of sinus disorders and anatomical variations in 196 children. Acta Otorhinolaryngol Belg. 1989;43(1):51–8.
4. Van Buchem FL, Peeters MF, Knottnerus JA. Maxillary sinusitis in children. Clin Otolaryngol Allied Sci. 1992;17(1):49–53.
5. Celedon JC, Litonjua AA, Weiss ST, Gold DR. Day care attendance in the first year of life and illnesses of the upper and lower respiratory tract in children with a familial history of atopy. Pediatrics. 1999;104(3 Pt 1):495–500.
6. Kay DJ, Rosenfeld RM. Quality of life for children with persistent sinonasal symptoms. Otolaryngol Head Neck Surg. 2003;128(1):17–26.
7. Brietzke SE, Shin JJ, Choi S, Lee JT, Parikh SR, Pena M, et al. Clinical Consensus Statement: pediatric chronic rhinosinusitis. Otolaryngol Head Neck Surg. 2014;151(4):542–53.
8. Terrell AM, Ramadan HH. Correlation between SN-5 and computed tomography in children with chronic rhinosinusitis. Laryngoscope. 2009;119(7):1394–8.
9. Magit A. Pediatric rhinosinusitis. Otolaryngol Clin N Am. 2014;47(5):733–46.
10. Badr DT, Gaffin JM, Phipatanakul W. Pediatric rhinosinusitis. Curr Treat Opt Allergy. 2016;3(3):268–81.
11. Fokkens WJ, Lund VJ, Hopkins C, Hellings PW, Kern R, Reitsma S, et al. European position paper on rhinosinusitis and nasal polyps 2020. Rhinology. 2020;58:1–464.
12. Chandy Z, Ference E, Lee JT. Clinical guidelines on chronic rhinosinusitis in children. Curr Allergy Asthma Rep. 2019;19(2):14.
13. Bhattacharyya N, Jones DT, Hill M, Shapiro NL. The diagnostic accuracy of computed tomography in pediatric chronic rhinosinusitis. Arch Otolaryngol Head Neck Surg. 2004;130(9):1029–32.
14. Pearce MS, Salotti JA, Little MP, McHugh K, Lee C, Kim KP, et al. Radiation exposure from CT scans in childhood and subsequent risk of leukaemia and brain tumours: a retrospective cohort study. Lancet. 2012;380(9840):499–505.
15. Sivaslı E, Şirikçi A, Bayazýt Y, Gümüsburun E, Erbagci H, Bayram M, et al. Anatomic variations of the paranasal sinus area in pediatric patients with chronic sinusitis. Surg Radiol Anat. 2002;24(6):399–404.
16. Brietzke SE, Brigger MT. Adenoidectomy outcomes in pediatric rhinosinusitis: a meta-analysis. Int J Pediatr Otorhinolaryngol. 2008;72(10):1541–5.
17. Vandenberg SJ, Heatley DG. Efficacy of adenoidectomy in relieving symptoms of chronic sinusitis in children. Arch Otolaryngol Head Neck Surg. 1997;123(7):675–8.
18. Elwany S, El-Dine AN, El-Medany A, Omran A, Mandour Z, El-Salam AA. Relationship between bacteriology of the adenoid core and middle

meatus in children with sinusitis. J Laryngol Otol. 2011;125(3):279–81.
19. Orb Q, Curtin K, Oakley GM, Wong J, Meier J, Orlandi RR, et al. Familial risk of pediatric chronic rhinosinusitis. Laryngoscope. 2016;126(3): 739–45.
20. Reh DD, Higgins TS, Smith TL. Impact of tobacco smoke on chronic rhinosinusitis: a review of the literature. Int Forum Allergy Rhinol. 2012;2(5): 362–9.
21. Christensen DN, Franks ZG, McCrary HC, Saleh AA, Chang EH. A systematic review of the association between cigarette smoke exposure and chronic rhinosinusitis. Otolaryngol Head Neck Surg. 2018;158(5):801–16.
22. Kakish KS, Mahafza T, Batieha A, Ekteish F, Daoud A. Clinical sinusitis in children attending primary care centers. Pediatr Infect Dis J. 2000;19(11):1071–4.
23. Fokkens WJ, Lund VJ, Mullol J, Bachert C, Alobid I, Baroody F, et al. EPOS 2012: European position paper on rhinosinusitis and nasal polyps 2012. A summary for otorhinolaryngologists. Rhinology. 2012;50(1):1–12.
24. Bothwell MR, Parsons DS, Talbot A, Barbero GJ, Wilder B. Outcome of reflux therapy on pediatric chronic sinusitis. Otolaryngology Head Neck Surg. 1999;121(3):255–62.
25. Berger G, Kogan T, Paker M, Berger-Achituv S, Ebner Y. Pediatric chronic rhinosinusitis histopathology: differences and similarities with the adult form. Otolaryngol Head Neck Surg. 2011;144(1):85–90.
26. Raman V, Clary R, Siegrist KL, Zehnbauer B, Chatila TA. Increased prevalence of mutations in the cystic fibrosis transmembrane conductance regulator in children with chronic rhinosinusitis. Pediatrics. 2002;109(1):E13.
27. Familial Occurrence of Asthma, Nasal Polyps, and Aspirin Intolerance | Annals of Internal Medicine | American College of Physicians [Internet]. https://annals.org/aim/article-abstract/687110/familial-occurrence-asthma-nasal-polyps-aspirin-intolerance. Accessed 26 Feb 2020.
28. Wu X, Ghimbovschi S, Aujla PK, Rose MC, Pena MT. Expression profiling of inflammatory mediators in pediatric sinus mucosa. Arch Otolaryngol Head Neck Surg. 2009;135(1):65–72.
29. Shin YH, Kim HS, Lee EK, Kim YJ, Lee H-S, Jang P-S, et al. Eosinophil related markers and total immunoglobulin E as a predictive marker for antibiotics response in chronic rhinosinusitis: a case-control study. Ann Saudi Med. 2015;35(4):312–7.
30. Bachert C, Zhang N, Hellings PW, Bousquet J. Endotype-driven care pathways in patients with chronic rhinosinusitis. J Allergy Clin Immunol. 2018;141(5):1543–51.
31. Brook I. The role of antibiotics in pediatric chronic rhinosinusitis. Laryngosc Investig Otolaryngol. 2017;2(3):104–8.
32. Brook I. Microbiology of chronic rhinosinusitis. Eur J Clin Microbiol Infect Dis. 2016;35(7):1059–68.
33. Muntz HR, Lusk RP. Nasal antral windows in children: a retrospective study. Laryngoscope. 1990; https://doi.org/10.1288/00005537-199006000-00017. Wiley Online Library [Internet]. Accessed 18 Feb 2020.
34. Hsin C-H, Su M-C, Tsao C-H, Chuang C-Y, Liu C-M. Bacteriology and antimicrobial susceptibility of pediatric chronic rhinosinusitis: a 6-year result of maxillary sinus punctures. Am J Otolaryngol. 2010;31(3):145–9.
35. Heath J, Hartzell L, Putt C, Kennedy JL. Chronic Rhinosinusitis in children: pathophysiology, evaluation, and medical management. Curr Allergy Asthma Rep. 2018;18(7):37.
36. Shay SG, Valika T, Chun R, Rastatter J. Innovations in endonasal sinus surgery in children. Otolaryngol Clin N Am. 2019;52(5):875–90.
37. Ramadan HH, Terrell AM. Balloon catheter sinuplasty and adenoidectomy in children with chronic rhinosinusitis. Ann Otol Rhinol Laryngol. 2010;119(9):578–82.
38. Ramadan HH. Surgical management of chronic sinusitis in children. Laryngoscope. 2004;114(12):2103–9.
39. Vlastarakos PV, Fetta M, Segas JV, Maragoudakis P, Nikolopoulos TP. Functional endoscopic sinus surgery improves sinus-related symptoms and quality of life in children with chronic rhinosinusitis: a systematic analysis and meta-analysis of published interventional studies. Clin Pediatr (Phila). 2013;52(12):1091–7.
40. Chang P-H, Lee L-A, Huang C-C, Lai C-H, Lee T-J. Functional endoscopic sinus surgery in children using a limited approach. Arch Otolaryngol Head Neck Surg. 2004;130(9):1033–6.
41. Walner DL, Falciglia M, Willging JP, Myer CM. The role of second-look nasal endoscopy after pediatric functional endoscopic sinus surgery. Arch Otolaryngol Head Neck Surg. 1998;124(4):425–8.

31 Pediatric Chronic Sinusitis: View from China

Jingying Ma and Bing Zhou

Key Points

- There is a consensus that pediatric chronic rhinosinusitis (CRS) is a medically treatable disease.
- The diagnosis depends mainly on clinical symptoms and routine examination of the nasal cavity. Paranasal sinus computed tomography is indicated only for children with a poor response to appropriate medical treatment and when sinus surgery is a consideration.
- Surgical intervention should be personalized and performed stepwise. The purpose of surgery is to control the symptoms and sinus mucosal inflammation, not to provide a cure. Long-term postoperative follow-up is required.

31.1 Introduction

Pediatric chronic rhinosinusitis (CRS) is a common problem treated by both pediatricians and otorhinolaryngologists. The prevalence of CRS in children is now estimated to be as high as 4% [1]. Pediatric CRS is not as well studied as the same entity in adults. Multiple factors contribute to the disease, including bacteriological and inflammatory factors. Over the last several years, significant advancements have been made in understanding the pathophysiology, diagnosis, and treatment of chronic rhinosinusitis. However, significant controversy still surrounds the medical and surgical management of this disease in children.

31.2 Clinical Characteristics in Children

31.2.1 Definition

The clinical diagnosis of CRS is not easy in childhood because symptoms are similar to symptoms in other common childhood nasal diseases such as lower respiratory tract infections, adenoid hypertrophy/adenoiditis, and allergic rhinitis (cough, wheeze, sputum, nasal blockage, sneeze). Older children may be able to indicate that they have a headache.

CRS in children is defined as chronic inflammation of nasal cavity and sinus mucosa, nasal symptoms lasting more than 12 weeks, cannot be completely relieved or even aggravated [2].

Main symptoms: nasal blockage/obstruction/congestion, nasal discharge (anterior/posterior nasal drip), cough, and headache.

J. Ma · B. Zhou (✉)
Department of Otorhinolaryngology, Head and Neck Surgery, Beijing Tongren Hospital, Capital Medical University, Beijing, China
e-mail: entzhou@263.net

L. Zhang, C. Bachert (eds.), *Chronic Rhinosinusitis*, https://doi.org/10.1007/978-981-16-0784-4_31

Accompanying symptoms: dysosmia, hearing loss, and abnormal behavior (lack of concentration, irritable).

Main signs: inferior nasal concha edema/hyperemia, mucopurulent discharge from the middle meatus, lymphatic hyperplasia of posterior pharyngeal wall, and/or nasal polyps.

Accompanying signs: adenoid and/or tonsil hypertrophy, and/or signs of otitis media with effusion.

31.2.2 Symptoms

Symptoms of pediatric CRS can be variable and age-dependent. In younger patients, the objective witnessed signs are usually described by the parents; an infant might express pain and discomfort only as irritability. There is usually a combination of nasal obstruction, rhinorrhea, and postnasal drip. Studies examining the clinical characteristics of children with CRS suggest that the four most common clinical symptoms are cough, rhinorrhea, nasal congestion, and postnasal drip, with a slightly higher predominance of chronic cough [3, 4]. Older children can provide a more detailed and localized description of their subjective symptoms, such as nasal congestion, otalgia, facial pressure or pain, or hyposmia. Parents often complain about halitosis and epistaxis.

Practically, cough can be the most common manifestation of chronic sinus pathology [5]. A diagnosis is suggested by the cough characteristics as the cough beginning when the child goes to bed and wakes up, which is secondary to drainage of the posterior secretions into the pharynx [6].

In recurrent or chronic sinusitis, isolated nasal obstruction is a rare complaint [7, 8]. This isolated complaint is more frequent in situations such as turbinate hypertrophy (whether from an allergic or infectious etiology), marked septal deviation, or the presence of polyps or a foreign body.

Persistent nasal secretion with different characteristics (aqueous, clear mucoid, purulent, or with blood traces) can be an isolated clinical manifestation of chronic sinusitis [9, 10]. This symptom requires differential diagnosis from multiple sequential colds, allergic rhinitis, foreign body (unilateral secretion), and dysfunction of the respiratory epithelium, as occurs in primary ciliary dyskinesia [11, 12]. Drainage of nasal secretions through the pharynx occurs often in school-age children and can appear as an isolated complaint, but generally, this condition also generates nocturnal cough that can be confirmed by other family members.

Headache and/or facial pain/pressure may be rare manifestations of sinus pathology, and these symptoms can occur when there are points of contact between the lateral nose wall and the septum and in patients with ostiomeatal complex obstruction.

Isolated halitosis is a rare presentation of chronic sinusitis as the odor produced by anaerobic infections also leads to nasal secretions and obstruction. More often, halitosis has another cause such as caseum in the tonsils and, sometimes, foreign bodies.

Allergic manifestations such as nasal/pharyngeal pruritus, sneezing, and respiratory reaction to environmental changes should also be carefully evaluated because these manifestations are an important factor in recurrence and chronicity [13]. Some groups of children are particularly prone to having sinus pathologies and should be identified by their history of cystic fibrosis, immunodeficiency, ciliary motility disorders, and gastroesophageal reflux [14].

31.2.3 Physical Examination

A complete and careful physical exam should follow the obtained medical and family history. The nose is examined using a rhinoscope for signs of mucosal inflammation such as congestion, crusting, and mucopurulent discharge. Flexible endoscopy is required to adequately evaluate the nasal cavity especially when the turbinates are congested. A mixture of topical anesthetic (e.g., lidocaine) and a sympathomimetic drug (e.g., ephedrine) is used topically in the nasal cavity before examination, topical decongestion may improve visualization. A nasal endo-

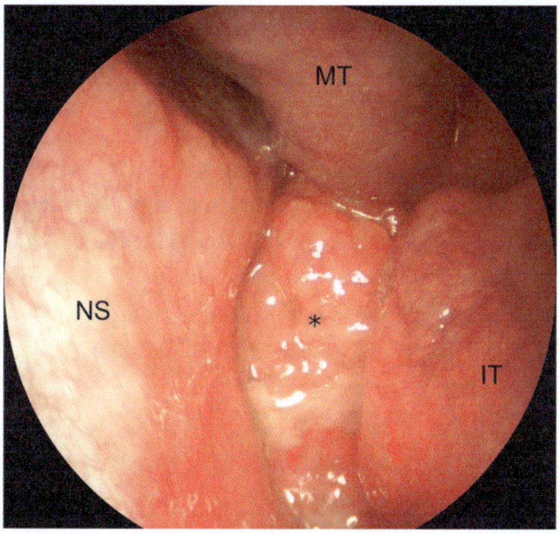

Fig. 31.2 Endoscopic view of adenoid hypertrophy (*), which thoroughly blocks the choana. *NS* nasal septum, *MT* middle turbinate, *IT* inferior turbinate

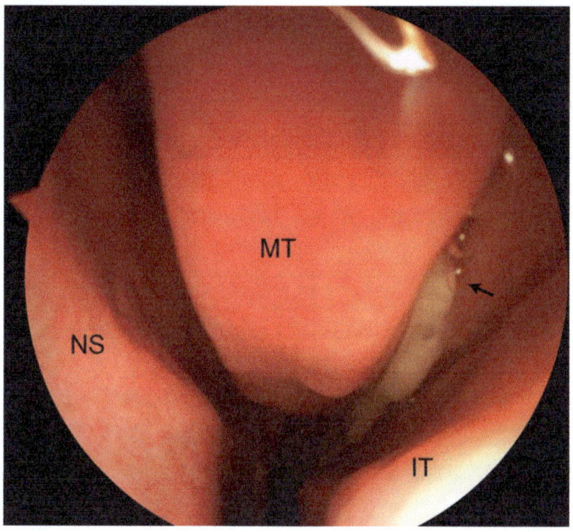

Fig. 31.1 Endoscopic view of purulent secretion in the middle meatus (*arrow*). *NS* nasal septum, *MT* middle turbinate, *IT* inferior turbinate

scope with a diameter of 2.7 mm is recommended to obtain clear visualization of the middle meatus (Fig. 31.1), adenoid bed (Fig. 31.2), and nasopharynx in younger children. Oral examination may reveal retropharyngeal secretions, lymphoid follicular hyperplasia, or tonsillar hypertrophy. Nasal polyps in children are rarely found, and if seen during examination, the suspicion of fibrosis, allergic fungal sinusitis, or choanal polyps should be raised. The middle meatus and sphenoethmoidal recess should be also evaluated for obstruction and discharge, and the nasopharynx can be evaluated for adenoid size and inflammation findings.

The simplest way to examine the nasal cavity of children is to lift the nose tip and using the light of the otoscope [15]. Under these conditions, the nasal cavity can be observed for the presence or absence of secretions, and the size of the inferior turbinate. If the turbinate mucosa is pale, it may be allergic, and if it is hyperemic, infection may be present. Therefore, at least a portion of the differential diagnosis of chronic or recurrent sinusitis can be based on the turbinate examination.

At the end of the clinical suspicion phase, with a history and physical examinations performed, a diagnosis can be established for most patients with chronic or recurrent sinusitis.

31.2.4 Diagnostic Tests

In addition to obtaining a history and performing a physical examination, diagnostic tests such as appropriate laboratory tests should be considered. Allergy serological testing should be considered in children with CRS. Children with recurrent or chronic disease, poor response to medical therapy, a history of other infectious diseases (e.g., recurrent pneumonia or otitis media), or abnormal organisms cultured from sinus secretions should be tested for immunodeficiency.

In patients who do not respond to conventional medical treatment, obtaining a culture may be useful to guide further antimicrobial therapy. For older children who can tolerate rigid endoscopy, nasal secretions can be taken for culture in the outpatient clinic. If general anesthesia is needed, we recommend the gold standard of obtaining a culture from the maxillary sinus itself by antral puncture, a technique that also allows the potential benefit of sinus irrigation. However, antral puncture is not a routine method for all patients with suspected pediatric sinusitis because of its invasiveness and because bacterial infection is not the main pathogenesis for pediatric chronic sinusitis.

31.2.5 Imaging

In uncomplicated CRS, imaging is reserved for evaluating residual disease and anatomical abnormalities after appropriate medical therapy (Fig. 31.3). The imaging study of choice is CT. Abnormalities in the CT images are assessed in the context of their severity and correlation with the clinical picture, and these findings guide the plan for further management, which might include surgical intervention. Plain radiographs tend to be less reliable. The potential risk of exposing a child to radiation should be considered when ordering a CT scan. Current guidelines recommend "imaging gently" because of the reported increased chance of leukemia and brain tumors in children who receive CT scans, with higher risk associated with higher radiation exposure [16].

The key CT features of chronic sinusitis are: (1) The mucoperiosteal thickening of the sinus mucosa and retained secretions contribute to opacification of the involved sinuses. (2) Recurrent or chronic sinusitis leads to osteitis with neo-osteogenesis of the sinus cavity. (3) Most sinonasal polyps are seen as soft tissue masses occupying one or more of the sinonasal cavities. (4) The sinus walls may be eroded by chronic benign inflammation, usually occurring along the medial wall of the maxillary sinus and around the infraorbital canal. (5) If chronic infections occur during childhood, the sinus may remain small and hypoplastic.

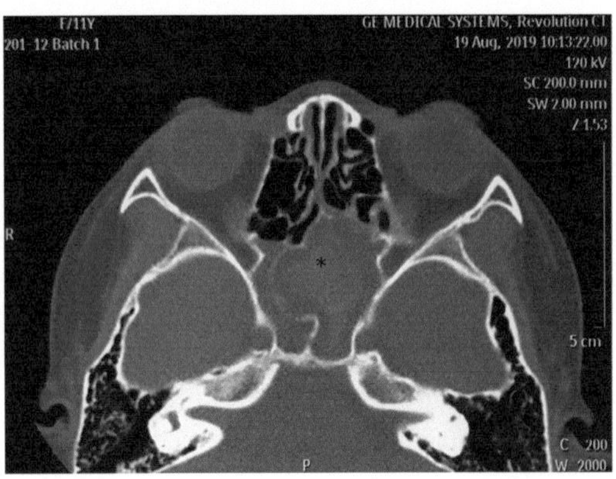

Fig. 31.3 Axial paranasal sinus computed tomography (CT) image in an 11-year-old girl with chronic sphenoid sinusitis. She experienced an intermittent severe headache for 6 months but no nasal symptoms, and she experienced no improvement after medical treatment. CT demonstrated opacification in bilateral sphenoid sinuses

Magnetic resonance imaging (MRI) has not proven useful for evaluating the bony structures of the sinus. However, MRI is performed when differentiation between invasive fungal sinusitis and benign or malignant tumors is in question or when complications of rhinosinusitis are suspected.

The key MRI features of chronic sinusitis are as follows: Thickened mucosa, which is low to intermediate in signal intensity on T1-weighted (T1-W) sequences. On T2-weighted (T2-W) sequences, the thickened mucosa is hyperintense (brighter) in signal intensity. Most polyps are of the same signal intensity as that of water: hypointense on T1W images and hyperintense (bright) on T2W images. Following the administration of gadolinium-diethylenetriamine-penta-acetic acid, there is intense enhancement of the inflamed mucosa [17–19]. Polyps that are bright on T1-W and T2-W images are either secondary to high protein content or to hemorrhage within the polyps.

31.3 Treatment (Essentials of Pediatric Endoscopic Surgery and Medicine) and Prognosis

31.3.1 Introduction

The initial treatment of pediatric CRS should be medical. Exceptions may be considered with adenoid and/or tonsil hypertrophy; nasal polyp, and/or antrochoanal polyp; rhinosinusitis with intracranial and/or orbital complications [2].

31.3.2 Medical Treatment of Chronic Rhinosinusitis in Children

- **Antibiotics**
- There is no good evidence in the literature to support the use of antibiotics in CRS in chil-

dren. Treatment for recurrent acute episodes and exacerbations of CRS (when there are complications in mild acute sinusitis) is approached in the same manner as for severe acute sinusitis [20, 21]. Ideally, the choice of antibiotic is according to culture susceptibility results; however, practically, it is challenging to acquire a reliable culture from a child in the office setting. The first line of therapy is usually amoxicillin (40 mg/kg/day). Another reasonable and safe choice is high-dose amoxicillin (80 mg/kg/day), which can overcome penicillin resistance with *Staphylococcus pneumoniae*. Antibiotic therapy is continued for 2–6 weeks, most often for 2–3 weeks, and should be continued for 1 week after the clinical manifestations of sinusitis have disappeared [22]. When there is no clinical response, fever persists for 3 days, and/or cough persists for 1 week, amoxicillin/clavulanate (30 mg/kg/day) or second-generation cephalosporins (cefuroxime, 30 mg/kg per day) can be used, with the objective of acting against beta-lactamase-producing strains (*Haemophilus sp.*, *Moraxella catarrhalis*, some anaerobes) [23, 24]. Cephalexin is another option in more refractory infections, with the objective of treating *Staphylococcus aureus*. Metronidazole can eventually be added to one of the antibiotics mentioned above to treat mixed infections involving anaerobes [25]. If hypersensitivity to any of these antimicrobials is suspected, alternate choices include trimethoprim/sulfamethoxazole, azithromycin, clarithromycin, or erythromycin, although treatment failure rates may range from 20% to 25% with these antibiotics. Clindamycin is useful if anaerobic organisms are suspected, but this antibiotic provides no coverage against Gram-negative organisms.

- Intravenous antibiotic therapy for resistant CRS has been advocated as an alternative to surgical intervention. Intravenous cefuroxime was most frequently used in previous studies, followed by ampicillin-sulbactam, ticarcillin, clavulanate, and vancomycin. The potential benefits of intravenous therapy must be weighed against the potential for significant complications and morbidity. Furthermore, it is difficult to assign benefits to intravenous antibiotic therapy when other interventions have been used, such as irrigation/aspiration of the sinus and adenoidectomy. Therefore, available data does not justify the use of intravenous antibiotics alone for the treatment of CRS in children.
- **Intranasal corticosteroids**
- There have been no reports of randomized controlled trials assessing the effects of intranasal corticosteroids in children with CRS. However, intranasal corticosteroids have demonstrated efficacy in adults with CRS with and without nasal polyps, and of intranasal corticosteroids have demonstrated efficacy and safety in children with allergic rhinitis. Therefore, intranasal corticosteroids are the first-line treatment for pediatric CRS [26–28]. Nasal corticosteroid sprays are commonly used to decrease inflammation and improve edema and mucociliary clearance. Nasal corticosteroid treatment is a first-line treatment in CRS with and without nasal polyps in children.
- Clinically, corticosteroids are prescribed after antibiotic therapy, when nasal turbinates are hypertrophic and causing nasal obstruction, and when secretions are no longer purulent. Mometasone furoate can be given in a single daily application. In previous studies, children well tolerated the aqueous formulation of some of these steroids [29–32]. Another topical corticosteroid choice is budesonide, which can be used by children between 2 and 4 years of age, as a puff in each nostril twice daily for 1 month, followed by monitoring of signs and symptoms. Other topical corticosteroids are fluticasone propionate, beclomethasone dipropionate, and flunisolide.
- **Ancillary treatments**
- Currently, there is no evidence-based support to indicate a benefit of other adjunct therapies such as oral antihistamines, mucolytic agents, oral steroids, and nasal saline irrigation.
- Systemic steroids have also been used in children with CRS because of their potent anti-inflammatory properties. Ozturk et al.

treated children with CRS with amoxicillin clavulanate for 30 days and with either a prednisone tapering course for 15 days or with placebo [33]. Compared with placebo, treatment with steroids resulted in significant improvements in CT scan scores as well as in the symptoms of cough, nasal obstruction, postnasal discharge, and total symptom score. Even though systemic steroids are effective, for safety reasons, their use for CRS in children is limited.

- Reflux was found to be prevalent in children with CRS resistant to medical treatment, and anti-reflux therapy improved the symptoms in most patients [34].
- Clinicians have certainly tried other treatments for chronic rhinosinusitis, including antihistamines and leukotriene modifiers, especially in light of their effectiveness in treating allergic rhinitis. However, no data exist regarding the potential efficacy of these methods; therefore, their usefulness to treat acute and chronic rhinosinusitis is undetermined. Nonsedating, second-generation antihistamines, which compete with histamine for the H1 receptor, such as loratadine, cetirizine, mizolastine, ebastine, and fexofenadine, can be used orally in rhinosinusitis with a major allergic component [35]. These drugs are effective for sneezing, pruritus, and aqueous rhinorrhea associated with allergic rhinitis, but have little or no action in patients with nasal obstruction. However, prolonged use induces tolerance and adverse effects, such as mood changes and hyperphagia [36]. Thus, the use of these drugs should be limited to short periods in seasons with more clinical manifestations. Topical anti-H1 antihistamines have limited use in children because of local irritation (burning) that can occur immediately after application, leading to low compliance rates.
- Saline nasal irrigation has become the mainstay of CRS treatment in children. Indeed, in a survey of pediatric otolaryngologists and rhinologists in the USA, 93% and 97% of the respondents, respectively, reported using nasal saline irrigations as part of appropriate medical therapy in pediatric CRS [37, 38]. Nasal washing (twice per day) is always recommended to remove secretions and crusts [39]. Additionally, cleaning provides a better area to receive adequate nasal application of other products that are necessary, such as topical corticosteroids [31]. Overall, evidence supports that saline is beneficial in the treatment of CRS symptoms, when used as the sole treatment. A fresh solution should be made every week.
- A minority of children with chronic and recurrent sinusitis, specifically, patients with immunodeficiency, can eventually benefit from immunoglobulin replacement therapy or antibacterial active immunization.

31.3.3 Surgical Treatment

Surgical intervention for rhinosinusitis is usually considered for patients with CRS who have failed appropriate medical therapy (and, less commonly, in complicated acute sinusitis). Surgery is performed stepwise and has been shown to improve symptoms significantly. Parents should be informed that a complete cure is not always possible.

- **Adenoidectomy.**
- Adenoidectomy is often the first-line surgical option in children with CRS, with success rates ranging between 47% and 58% [40]. Adenoidectomy with or without antral irrigation is recommended as a first-line surgery. The adenoids may act as a reservoir for pathogenic bacteria, and the presence of a biofilm may decrease the efficacy of antibiotics to clear the infection [41] (Fig. 31.4). To remove this reservoir, adenoidectomy may be required and has been reported effective in alleviating pediatric CRS, with success rates ranging between 47% and 58% [40].
- **Functional endoscopic sinus surgery, FESS.**
- The current literature supports the use of functional endoscopic sinus surgery (FESS) in children with CRS who fail to respond to appropriate medical treatment and possibly an

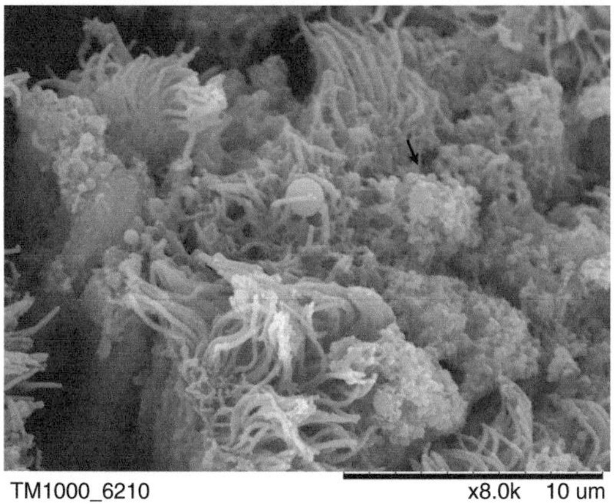

Fig. 31.4 Scanning electron microscopy image showing adherent biofilms (*arrow*) on the surface epithelium of an adenoid

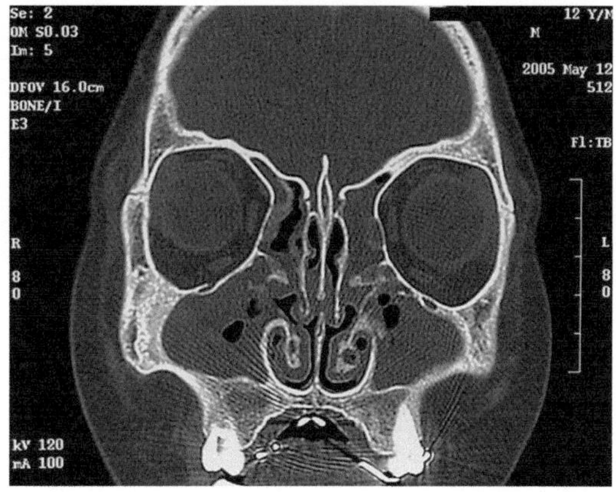

Fig. 31.5 Coronal paranasal sinus computed tomography (CT) in a 12-year-old boy with recurrent chronic rhinosinusitis who underwent limited functional endoscopic sinus surgery. Severe synechiae in the middle meatus and purulent discharge were visible with nasal endoscopy 1 year later. Opacification in the ethmoid and maxillary sinuses, with bone hyperplasia are seen

earlier adenoidectomy, or when anatomical variations are clearly obstructing normal drainage pathways. Other indications include orbital and intracranial complications of acute rhinosinusitis and obstructing nasal polyposis in cases of cystic fibrosis. FESS is considered safe in children regarding midfacial growth [42] and results in symptom improvement in 80–100% of patients [43]. Preoperative CT of the sinuses is essential to provide a surgical "road map" of the nasosinusal complex and to detect structural variants or abnormalities that might increase the risk of injuring adjacent structures. In children, it is important to have a current scan because of ongoing changes in the size and shape of the sinuses during childhood development.

- Many advocate a limited approach to FESS in children, consisting of the removal of any obvious obstruction (such as polyps and concha bullosa), as well as an anterior bulla ethmoidectomy, and a middle meatal antrostomy. This approach typically yields significant improvements in nasal obstruction (91%), rhinorrhea (90%), postnasal drip (90%), headache (97%), hyposmia (89%), and chronic cough (96%) [44]. Nevertheless, the limited approach often causes a series of problems after surgery; e.g. adhesion between the middle turbinates is a very common problem that may lead to surgery failure. In other words, the middle turbinate may often be the main reason for postoperative complications or recurrence (Fig. 31.5). Therefore, the surgical approach should be individualized, and surgery should be considered only when all conservative management measures have not provided good results.
- It is pointed out in the Recommendations for diagnosis and treatment of rhinosinusitis in children [2] that the indications of sinusitis surgery in children are: (1) adenoid hypertrophy and/or almond hypertrophy affecting nasal ventilation and drainage; (2) nasal polyps and/or maxillary sinus choanal polyps cause obstruction to the drainage of the sinonasal complex; (3) intracranial, orbital, or periorbital complications. Other indications were defined in the International Consensus on the Management of Chronic Rhinosinusitis in Children [45], such as: complete nasal obstruction in cystic fibrosis because of massive polyposis or nose closure; mucocele and mucopyocele; traumatic lesions of the optic canal; dacryocystitis refractory to drug treatment and secondary to sinusitis; and fungal sinusitis. The surgical principles of chronic rhinosinusitis in children are small circumference, exquisite and minimally invasive, and

frequent nasal endoscopy and surgical intervention are not appropriate after surgery.
- Postoperative saline irrigation may prevent crusting and facilitate mucosalization, but compliance is expected to be low in young children.
- Special consideration should be taken with CRS patients who have an underlying disease process that interferes with physiological mucociliary clearance (e.g., ciliary dyskinesia, Kartagener syndrome, cystic fibrosis). CRS in this group of patients is difficult to treat and often requires revision surgeries [46]. Additionally, these patients might not benefit from "functional" sinus surgery of the natural ostia, and gravity-based drainage surgery should be considered. Sinonasal polyposis, history of allergic rhinitis, and male sex were seen significantly more often in the group that continued to have problems after ESS.

31.4 Prognosis

A long-term follow-up therapy schedule for patients with recurrent and chronic disease should be established by an otorhinolaryngologist. This schedule is determined by the need to perform nasal fiberscopic examination during diagnosis and follow-up, as well as by sequential evaluation, when there is a surgical indication. To complement the information obtained during follow-up and for consistency, multidisciplinary interaction involving the pediatrician, otorhinolaryngologist, specialized radiologist, and often the immunologist is fundamental from diagnosis to follow-up.

Regarding the treatment of sinusitis in children, the purpose of endoscopic sinus surgery is to control symptoms and sinus mucosal inflammation, not to provide a cure. Long-term postoperative follow-up is necessary in children with CRS.

31.5 Conclusions

Medical treatment for pediatric CRS, including intranasal corticosteroids and saline irrigation, is effective and generally safe in children. Surgery is indicated only for children who fail to respond to appropriate medical treatment. The adenoids may act as a reservoir for pathogenic bacteria, rather than as a source of obstruction. As a stepwise strategy for treating pediatric CRS, adenoidectomy is the first-line surgical procedure. The extent of endoscopic sinus surgery should be personalized once indicated, even for pediatric patients. Our experience showed that postoperative care or second-look surgery after a first surgery is very important.

References

1. Sidell D, Shapiro NL, Bhattacharyya N. Obesity and the risk of chronic rhinosinusitis, allergic rhinitis, and acute otitis media in school-age children. Laryngoscope. 2013;123(10):2360–3. https://doi.org/10.1002/lary.24038.
2. Editorial Board of Chinese Journal of Otorhinolaryngology Head and Neck Surgery, Subspecialty Group of Rhinology and Pediatics, Society of Otorhinolaryngology Head and Neck Surgery, Chinese Medical Association. Recommendations for diagnosis and treatment of rhinosinusitis in children (Kunming, 2012). Chin J Otorhinolaryngol Head Neck Surg. 2013;48(3):177–9.
3. Rachelefsky GS, Goldberg M, Katz RM, Boris G, Gyepes MT, Shapiro MJ, et al. Sinus disease in children with respiratory allergy. J Allergy Clin Immunol. 1978;61(5):310–4. https://doi.org/10.1016/0091-6749(78)90052-0.
4. Rachelefsky GS, Katz RM, Siegel SC. Diseases of paranasal sinuses in children. Curr Probl Pediatr. 1982;12(5):1–57. https://doi.org/10.1016/0045-9380(82)90038-x.
5. Parsons DS. Chronic sinusitis: a medical or surgical disease? Otolaryngol Clin N Am. 1996;29(1):1–9.
6. Havas TE, Motbey JA, Gullane PJ. Prevalence of incidental abnormalities on computed tomographic scans of the paranasal sinuses. Arch Otolaryngol Head Neck Surg. 1988;114(8):856–9. https://doi.org/10.1001/archotol.1988.01860200040012.
7. Wang DY, Clement P, Kaufman L, Derde MP. Fiberoptic examination of the nasal cavity and nasopharynx in children. Acta Otorhinolaryngol Belg. 1991;45(3):323–9.
8. Wang DY, Bernheim N, Kaufman L, Clement P. Assessment of adenoid size in children by fibreoptic examination. Clin Otolaryngol Allied Sci. 1997;22(2):172–7. https://doi.org/10.1046/j.1365-2273.1997.00002.x.
9. Wald ER. Purulent nasal discharge. Pediatr Infect Dis J. 1991;10(4):329–33. https://doi.org/10.1097/00006454-199104000-00013.

10. Wald ER. Sinusitis in children. N Engl J Med. 1992;326(5):319–23. https://doi.org/10.1056/nejm199201303260507.
11. Kronemer KA, McAlister WH. Sinusitis and its imaging in the pediatric population. Pediatr Radiol. 1997;27(11):837–46. https://doi.org/10.1007/s002470050251.
12. Saldiva PH, King M, Delmonte VL, Macchione M, Parada MA, Daliberto ML, et al. Respiratory alterations due to urban air pollution: an experimental study in rats. Environ Res. 1992;57(1):19–33. https://doi.org/10.1016/s0013-9351(05)80016-7.
13. Bergman KE, Bergman RL, Bauer CP, Dorch W, Foster J, Schmidt E, Schulz J, Whan U. Atopy in Deutchland. Deutsches Ärzteblatt. 1993;190:1341–7.
14. Brihaye P, Jorissen M, Clement PA. Chronic rhinosinusitis in cystic fibrosis (mucoviscidosis). Acta Otorhinolaryngol Belg. 1997;51(4):323–37.
15. Handler SD, Myer C. Atlas of ear, nose and throat disorders in children. Hamilton: BC Decker; 1998. p. 44–64.
16. Pearce MS, Salotti JA, Little MP, McHugh K, Lee C, Kim KP, et al. Radiation exposure from CT scans in childhood and subsequent risk of leukaemia and brain tumours: a retrospective cohort study. Lancet (London, England). 2012;380(9840):499–505. https://doi.org/10.1016/s0140-6736(12)60815-0.
17. Jorgensen RA. Endoscopic and computed tomographic findings in ostiomeatal sinus disease. Arch Otolaryngol Head Neck Surg. 1991;117(3):279–87. https://doi.org/10.1001/archotol.1991.01870150047005.
18. Som PM, Curtin HD, editors. Head and neck imaging. 2nd ed. St. Louis: Mosby-Year Book Inc.; 1991.
19. Yousem DM. Imaging of sinonasal inflammatory disease. Radiology. 1993;188(2):303–14. https://doi.org/10.1148/radiology.188.2.8327669.
20. Brook I, Yocum P. Antimicrobial management of chronic sinusitis in children. J Laryngol Otol. 1995;109(12):1159–62. https://doi.org/10.1017/s0022215100132323.
21. Dowelll SFSB, Phillips WR. Appropriate use of antibiotics for URIs in children: Part I. Otitis media and acute sinusitis. The Pediatric URI Consensus Team. Am Pham Phys. 1998;58:1313–8.
22. Giebink GS. Childhood sinusitis: pathophysiology, diagnosis and treatment. Pediatr Infect Dis J. 1994;13(Suppl 1):S55–8. discussion S63–5
23. Pereira MBR. Sinusitis. In: Sih T, editor. Pediatric otorhinolaryngology manual. São Paulo: International Federation of Oto-Rhino-Laryngological Societies; 1998. p. 90–9.
24. Jiang RS, Hsu CY. Bacteriology of chronic sinusitis after ampicillin therapy. Am J Rhinol. 1997;11(6):467–71. https://doi.org/10.2500/105065897780914983.
25. Kluka EA. Medical treatment of rhinosinusitis in children. In: Cotton RT, Myer CM, editors. Practical pediatric otolaryngology. Philadelphia: Lippincott-Raven; 1999. p. 395–404.
26. Seidman MD, Gurgel RK, Lin SY, Schwartz SR, Baroody FM, Bonner JR, et al. Clinical practice guideline: allergic rhinitis executive summary. Otolaryngol Head Neck Surg. 2015;152(2):197–206. https://doi.org/10.1177/0194599814562166.
27. Ratner PH, Meltzer EO, Teper A. Mometasone furoate nasal spray is safe and effective for 1-year treatment of children with perennial allergic rhinitis. Int J Pediatr Otorhinolaryngol. 2009;73(5):651–7. https://doi.org/10.1016/j.ijporl.2008.12.025.
28. Schenkel EJ, Skoner DP, Bronsky EA, Miller SD, Pearlman DS, Rooklin A, et al. Absence of growth retardation in children with perennial allergic rhinitis after one year of treatment with mometasone furoate aqueous nasal spray. Pediatrics. 2000;105(2):E22. https://doi.org/10.1542/peds.105.2.e22.
29. Waldner DL, Falciglia M, Willging JP, Myer CM 3rd. The role of second-look nasal endoscopic after pediatric functional endoscopic surgery. Arch Otolaryngol Head Neck Surg. 1998;124:425–8.
30. Wang DSJ, DeWaele M, Clement P. Effect of topical applications of budesonide and azelastine on nasal allergen challenge during the pollen season. Int Arch Allergy Immunol. 1997;114:185–92.
31. Barlan IB, Erkan E, Bakir M, Berrak S, Başaran MM. Intranasal budesonide spray as an adjunct to oral antibiotic therapy for acute sinusitis in children. Ann Allergy Asthma Immunol. 1997;78(6):598–601. https://doi.org/10.1016/s1081-1206(10)63223-1.
32. Meltzer EO, Berger WE, Berkowitz RB, Bronsky EA, Dvorin DJ, Finn AF, et al. A dose-ranging study of mometasone furoate aqueous nasal spray in children with seasonal allergic rhinitis. J Allergy Clin Immunol. 1999;104(1):107–14. https://doi.org/10.1016/s0091-6749(99)70121-1.
33. Ozturk F, Bakirtas A, Ileri F, Turktas I. Efficacy and tolerability of systemic methylprednisolone in children and adolescents with chronic rhinosinusitis: a double-blind, placebo-controlled randomized trial. J Allergy Clin Immunol. 2011;128(2):348–52. https://doi.org/10.1016/j.jaci.2011.04.045.
34. Phipps CD, Wood WE, Gibson WS, Cochran WJ. Gastroesophageal reflux contributing to chronic sinus disease in children: a prospective analysis. Arch Otolaryngol Head Neck Surg. 2000;126(7):831–6. https://doi.org/10.1001/archotol.126.7.831.
35. McCormick DP, John SD, Swischuk LE, Uchida T. A double-blind, placebo-controlled trial of decongestant-antihistamine for the treatment of sinusitis in children. Clin Pediatr. 1996;35(9):457–60. https://doi.org/10.1177/000992289603500905.
36. Sibbald B. Epidemiology of allergic rhinitis. In: Burr ML, editor. eEiCABK; 1993. p. 61–79.
37. Beswick DM, Messner AH, Hwang PH. Pediatric chronic rhinosinusitis management in rhinologists and pediatric otolaryngologists. Ann Otol Rhinol Laryngol. 2017;126(9):634–9. https://doi.org/10.1177/0003489417719717.
38. Beswick DM, Ramadan H, Baroody FM, Hwang PH. Practice patterns in pediatric chronic rhinosinusitis: a survey of the American Rhinologic Society.

Am J Rhinol Allergy. 2016;30(6):418–23. https://doi.org/10.2500/ajra.2016.30.4373.
39. Shoseyov D, Bibi H, Shai P, Shoseyov N, Shazberg G, Hurvitz H. Treatment with hypertonic saline versus normal saline nasal wash of pediatric chronic sinusitis. J Allergy Clin Immunol. 1998;101(5):602–5. https://doi.org/10.1016/s0091-6749(98)70166-6.
40. Vandenberg SJ, Heatley DG. Efficacy of adenoidectomy in relieving symptoms of chronic sinusitis in children. Arch Otolaryngol Head Neck Surg. 1997;123(7):675–8.
41. Shin KS, Cho SH, Kim KR, Tae K, Lee SH, Park CW, et al. The role of adenoids in pediatric rhinosinusitis. Int J Pediatr Otorhinolaryngol. 2008;72(11):1643–50. https://doi.org/10.1016/j.ijporl.2008.07.016.
42. Bothwell MR, Piccirillo JF, Lusk RP, Ridenour BD. Long-term outcome of facial growth after functional endoscopic sinus surgery. Otolaryngol Head Neck Surg. 2002;126(6):628–34. https://doi.org/10.1067/mhn.2002.125607.
43. Ramadan HH. Surgical management of chronic sinusitis in children. Laryngoscope. 2004;114(12):2103–9.
44. Chang P-H, Lee L-A, Huang C-C, Lai C-H, Lee T-J. Functional endoscopic sinus surgery in children using a limited approach. Arch Otolaryngol Head Neck Surg. 2004;130(9):1033–6.
45. Clement PA, Bluestone CD, Gordts F, Lusk RP, Otten FW, Goossens H, et al. Management of rhinosinusitis in children: consensus meeting, Brussels, Belgium, September 13, 1996. Arch Otolaryngol Head Neck Surg. 1998;124(1):31–4. https://doi.org/10.1001/archotol.124.1.31.
46. Ramadan HH. Revision endoscopic sinus surgery in children: surgical causes of failure. Laryngoscope. 2009;119(6):1214–7. https://doi.org/10.1002/lary.20230.

Wegener's Granulomatosis

32

Jichao Sha and Dongdong Zhu

Key Points

Wegener's granulomatosis (WG) or granulomatosis with polyangiitis (GPA) is the local malignant manifestation of systemic disorder. Otorhinolarygologists have the responsibility for recognizing the early onset and make the definite diagnosis by biopsy of lesion in nasal cavity.

32.1 Introduction

Wegener's granulomatosis (WG) or granulomatosis with polyangiitis (GPA), firstly described by Friedrich Wegener as rhinogenic granulomatosis in 1936 [1], is a rare long-term systemic disorder which involves the formation of granulomas and inflammation of blood vessels. The disorder is an anti-neutrophil cytoplasmic antibody (ANCA) associated granuloma forming vasculitis affecting small- and medium-size vessels in many organs but most commonly affecting the upper respiratory tract, lungs, and kidneys. Up to 85% of the patients have evidence of nasal or sinus disease [2, 3], causing the complaints of stuff, purulent, bloody discharge, and pain in nasal cavity [4].

J. Sha · D. Zhu (✉)
Department of Otolaryngology, Head and Neck Surgery, China-Japan Union Hospital of Jilin University, Changchun, China
e-mail: shajichao@jlu.edu.cn; zhudd@jlu.edu.cn

32.2 Pathogenesis

The pathogenesis of WG remains unknown. As an ANCA-associated vasculitis disease, WG patients have a predisposing genetic background who have been exposed to causative environmental factors [5]. Neutrophils are the sources of the autoantigen targeted in ANCA vasculitides that release inflammatory cytokines, reactive oxygen species, and lytic enzymes. The excessive activation of neutrophils by ANCAs also induces formation of neutrophil extracellular traps (NETs) [6]. In addition, some evidences suggest that Bruton's tyrosine kinase (BTK) in B cells may play a role in the pathogenesis [7]. The histopathological features of WG include necrosis, granulomatous inflammation, and vasculitis [8].

32.3 Clinical Manifestations

WG is an autoimmune disease with multiple organs lesions. The typical presentations involve upper airways, lungs, and kidneys. Less common affected sites include skin, central nervous system, heart, salivary gland, orbit and eye, breast, spleen, thyroid gland, alimentary tract, and pituitary gland and urogenital tract [9, 10] . The symptoms include fever, malaise, bloody secretion, cough, pain, hoarseness, salivary gland enlargement, arthritis, and ulcers.

L. Zhang, C. Bachert (eds.), *Chronic Rhinosinusitis*, https://doi.org/10.1007/978-981-16-0784-4_32

It is noteworthy that otorhinolaryngologic symptoms may be the first clinical manifestation, because the nasal cavity and the paranasal sinuses are the most common involved sites in the head and neck area (85–100%) [11] . Some warning symptoms for WG include persistent nasal discharges, blood discharge, epistaxis, crusting, mucosal ulceration, nasal bridge collapse, nasal granulomatous lesions, sinusitis, and regional tenderness.

32.4 Diagnosis

The diagnosis of WG is based on clinical history, serological tests for ANCA, and pathohistological analysis. Imaging also plays an important role in diagnosis as well as the management of patients with small and medium vessel vasculitis [12]. Early diagnosis can be difficult as the nonspecific manifestations [13]. The ANCA testing *is* a sensitive *and* specific marker for WG.

32.5 Treatment

Corticosteroids and immunosuppressive agents are the mainstay of therapy for WG. In recent study, the immunologically specific therapeutic agents such as rituximab, a monoclonal antibody directed against B cells, has been shown to be effective for WG patients [14]. The mean survival time is 5 months and 1-year mortality rate is up to 82% if untreated and the limited treatment options exist [15]. Therefore, further study is necessary to better clarify the pathophysiology and to develop innovative target therapies for WG.

32.6 Summary

WG is an autoimmune disease with multiple organs lesions, and methods of the diagnosis and treatment for WG are rapidly developing. However, it still remains a huge clinical challenge. Otorhinolarygologists have the responsibility for recognizing the early onset and for starting an appropriate therapy for this disease.

References

1. Wegener F. 50 years of Wegener's granulomatosis. Immun Infekt. 1990;18(1):11–9.
2. Trimarchi M, Sinico RA, Teggi R, Bussi M, Specks U, Meroni PL. Otorhinolaryngological manifestations in granulomatosis with polyangiitis (Wegener's). Autoimmunity Rev. 2013;12(4):501–5. https://doi.org/10.1016/j.autrev.2012.08.010.
3. D'Anza B, Langford CA, Sindwani R. Sinonasal imaging findings in granulomatosis with polyangiitis (Wegener granulomatosis): a systematic review. Am J Rhinol Allergy. 2017;31(1):16–21. https://doi.org/10.2500/ajra.2017.31.4408.
4. Coordes A, Loose SM, Hofmann VM, Hamilton GS III, Riedel F, Menger DJ, et al. Saddle nose deformity and septal perforation in granulomatosis with polyangiitis. Clin Otolaryngol. 2018;43(1):291–9. https://doi.org/10.1111/coa.12977.
5. Nakazawa D, Masuda S, Tomaru U, Ishizu A. Pathogenesis and therapeutic interventions for ANCA-associated vasculitis. Nat Rev Rheumatol. 2019;15(2):91–101. https://doi.org/10.1038/s41584-018-0145-y.
6. Pruchniak MP, Ostafin M, Wachowska M, Jakubaszek M, Kwiatkowska B, Olesinska M, et al. Neutrophil extracellular traps generation and degradation in patients with granulomatosis with polyangiitis and systemic lupus erythematosus. Autoimmunity. 2019;52(3):126–35. https://doi.org/10.1080/08916934.2019.1631812.
7. von Borstel A, Abdulahad WH, Sanders JS, Rip J, Neys SFH, Hendriks RW, et al. Evidence for enhanced Bruton's tyrosine kinase activity in transitional and naïve B cells of patients with granulomatosis with polyangiitis. Rheumatology (Oxford). 2019;58(12):2230–9. https://doi.org/10.1093/rheumatology/kez205.
8. Hong Y, Shi P, Liu X, Yang L, Li K, Xu F, et al. Distinction between MPO-ANCA and PR3-ANCA-associated glomerulonephritis in Chinese patients: a retrospective single-center study. Clin Rheumatol. 2019;38(6):1665–73. https://doi.org/10.1007/s10067-019-04458-9.
9. Kühn D, Hospowsky C, Both M, Hey M, Laudien M. Manifestation of granulomatosis with polyangiitis in head and neck. Clin Exp Rheumatol. 2018;36(Suppl 111(2)):78–84.
10. Sfiniadaki E, Tsiara I, Theodossiadis P, Chatziralli I. Ocular manifestations of granulomatosis with polyangiitis: a review of the literature. Ophthal Ther. 2019;8(2):227–34. https://doi.org/10.1007/s40123-019-0176-8.

11. Greco A, Marinelli C, Fusconi M, Macri GF, Gallo A, De Virgilio A, et al. Clinic manifestations in granulomatosis with polyangiitis. Int J Immunopathol Pharmacol. 2016;29(2):151–9. https://doi.org/10.1177/0394632015617063.
12. Singhal M, Gupta P, Sharma A. Imaging in small and medium vessel vasculitis. Int J Rheumatic Dis. 2019;22(Suppl 1):78–85. https://doi.org/10.1111/1756-185x.13390.
13. Nasser M, Cottin V. The respiratory system in autoimmune vascular diseases. Respiration: Int Rev Thorac Dis. 2018;96(1):12–28. https://doi.org/10.1159/000486899.
14. Lynch JP III, Derhovanessian A, Tazelaar H, Belperio JA. Granulomatosis with polyangiitis (Wegener's Granulomatosis): evolving concepts in treatment. Semin Respir Crit Care Med. 2018;39(4):434–58. https://doi.org/10.1055/s-0038-1660874.
15. Flossmann O. Risks of treatments and long-term outcomes of systemic ANCA-associated vasculitis. Presse Med (Paris, France: 1983). 2015;44(6 Pt 2):e251–7. https://doi.org/10.1016/j.lpm.2015.02.019.

33 IgG4-Related Disorders

Yingshi Piao

Key Points

- IgG4-related CRS has been recognized as systemic disease.
- It may be related to genetics, autoimmunity, environment, and allergy.
- It can be mistaken for malignancies by damaging the bone and skull base of the sinus wall.
- To date, there is no consensually agreed criteria for diagnosis.

33.1 Introduction

Immunoglobulin (Ig)G4-related disease (IgG4-RD) is an independent clinical pathological entity. IgG4-RD first described as autoimmune pancreatitis (AIP) [1] is an immune-mediated disease. Histopathology is characterized by a large number of lymphocytes and plasma cells infiltration, storiform fibrosis, and occlusive phlebitis. The characteristics of IgG4-related chronic rhinosinusitis (IgG4-related CRS) have not been widely investigated [2–20]. To date, there is no consensually agreed criteria for diagnosis and still a lack of large sample clinical research data.

Y. Piao (✉)
Department of Pathology, Beijing Tongren Hospital, Capital Medical University, Beijing, China

33.2 Pathogenesis

The etiology and pathogenesis are unclear. It is related to genetics, autoimmunity, environment, and allergy.

33.2.1 Genetic Phenotypes

HLA DRB1*0405, DQB1*0401, BRB1*0701, and DQB1*0202 haplotype are associated with autoimmune pancreatitis in the Japanese and South Korea's population [21, 22]. Cytotoxic T lymphocyte antigen 4 (CTLA-4) polymorphism may be one of the risk factors of AIP [23].

33.2.2 Autoimmunity

Several autoantibodies including those to pancreatic trypsin inhibitor (PSTI), lactoferrin (LF), and carbonic anhydrase (CA) have been reported in patients with IgG4-related AIP [24]. However, they are not the specific molecular markers. The idea that autoantibodies may play a major role in IgG4-related disease has been questioned. Nevertheless, several studies involving autoantibodies in IgG4-RD against different antigens have been reported one after another in Europe, USA, China, and Japan. Recently, self-antigens including Laminin 511 E8, Galectin-3, Annexin A11, and Prohibitin have been reported as auto-

L. Zhang, C. Bachert (eds.), *Chronic Rhinosinusitis*, https://doi.org/10.1007/978-981-16-0784-4_33

antigens which may be involved in the pathogenesis of IgG4-RD [25–28].

33.2.3 Environment

IgG4-RD trigger factors may be associated with microorganisms. Guarneri et al. [29] reported that human carbonic anhydrase II and helicobacter pylori alpha-carbonic anhydrase have homologous structures. Frulloni et al. [30] found that the amino acid sequence of helicobacter pylori's plasminogen binding protein has structural homology with the ubiquitin protein ligase on human pancreatic acini suggesting that helicobacter pylori infection may be involved in the occurrence of AIP through molecular simulation mechanism. As the nasal cavity is exposed to the external environment, microorganisms might also be involved in its pathogenesis.

33.2.4 Allergy

IgG4-RD patients often accompanied by allergic characteristics, such as asthma, eczema, and peripheral blood eosinophilia granulocyte increased. Zen et al. [31] found that Th2 and regulatory immune reactions are increased in IgG4-related sclerosing pancreatitis and cholangitis. Takeuchi et al. [32] confirmed that Th2 and Treg cells factor from mast cells plays a key role in the course of illness. Above results support the IgG4- RD is probably an allergic disease.

33.3 Clinical Features

33.3.1 Symptoms

Most IgG4-RD patients are adults, mainly middle-aged and elderly people, while adolescents are rarely affected. Clinical symptoms include nasal congestion, epistaxis, hyposmia, facial pain, etc. Endoscopic examination reveals a mass of medium or firm texture. In a few cases, nasal symptoms are absent, with only facial pain and exophthalmus. Rare cases may be associated with optic neuritis and blindness [10]. The disease may be accompanied by symptoms in other areas, such as swelling/mass in the eyelid, parotid or submandibular gland, and palpable enlargement in the neck, armpit, or other lymph nodes.

33.3.2 Imaging Features

Imaging findings show unilateral or bilateral sinus involvement, most commonly involving the maxillary sinus, followed by ethmoid sinus, sphenoid sinus, and nasal septum. CT examination may reveal uniform soft tissue density shadow with or without bone destruction. MRI may indicate T2-hypointense soft tissue in the nasal cavity and paranasal sinuses, which showed homogeneous enhancement on post-contrast scans. Lesions can be mistaken for malignancies by damaging the bone and skull base of the sfinus wall and invading nerve and bone marrow tissue [5, 6]. In addition to nasal and paranasal sinus lesions, lacrimal gland mass shadow is often seen, mostly bilateral. Some of them involve a wide range, including extraocular muscle, pterygopalatine fossa and cavernous sinus, etc. [33].

33.3.3 Laboratory Examinations

IgG and IgG4 concentrations may be higher in IgG4-RD than in other diseases. However, some diseases such as allergic dermatitis, parasitic infection, pemphigus vulgaris, deciduous pemphigus, pancreatic cancer, and others can also be increased [1]. Elevated serum IgG4 may also be seen in nasal polyps, fungal sinusitis, and granulomatosis with polyangiitis [33]. Therefore, serum IgG4 can be used as a reference biomarker rather than a specific biomarker in IgG4-RD.

Some studies found that the count of plasmablasts (PB) in peripheral blood of some patients was significantly higher and decreased after the treatment of glucocorticoid and rituximab, so it was suggested that PB level might be more appropriate than serum IgG4 level as a diagnostic marker for IgG4-RD. PB may be a potential biomarker for diagnosis, and evaluation of treatment efficacy and disease activity [34]. In some cases, IgE, erythrocyte sedimentation rate, C-reactive protein were increased, and C3 and C4 complement levels were decreased [33].

33.3.4 Histopathological Features

Histopathology is the most important diagnostic criterion. As suggested by the 2011 Boston criteria, histological diagnosis of IgG4-RD should be based on the presence of the characteristic morphological features [35]. Moteki and colleagues [36] first proposed the concept that IgG4-related CRS was a new clinical entity of nasal disease.

A large number of lymphocyte and plasma cell infiltration can be seen in the nasal mucosa of IgG4-related CRS, which are distributed in the lamina propria below the surface respiratory epithelium and around the intrinsic glands and ducts. Infiltration can also be diffused, and some cases form lymphoid follicles. The interstitium shows patchy storiform or collagen fibrosis. Local sclerosis is common around the intrinsic glands or ducts in the early stage, presenting a "collagen sheath" like change (Fig. 33.1). Extensive fibrosis can be seen with the progression of the disease. Different degrees of fibrosis were observed around the diffuse proliferated nest of lymphocytes and plasma cells, with the glands atrophy (Fig. 33.2). In some cases a small amount of eosinophilic infiltration can be seen and occlusive phlebitis is rare in IgG4-related CRS [37].

The significance of IgG+ and IgG4+ plasma cell count in the diagnosis of IgG4-related CRS is controversial. Moteki et al. [36] believed that there was no significant difference in the number of IgG4+ plasma cells between IgG4-related

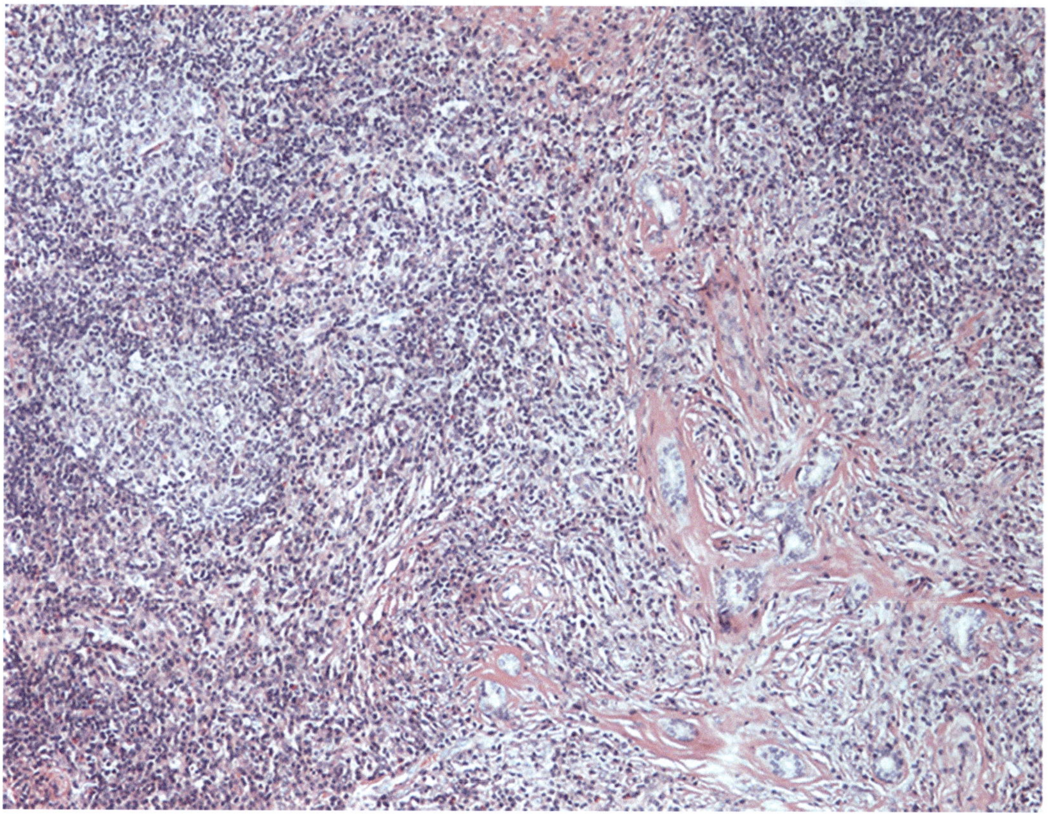

Fig. 33.1 A large number of the lymphocytes and plasma cells infiltrated the lamina propria of nasal mucosa and exhibited sporadic lymphoid follicles locally. Local sclerosis is common around the intrinsic glands or ducts, presenting a "collagen sheath" like change (hematoxylin and eosin staining, original magnification 10×)

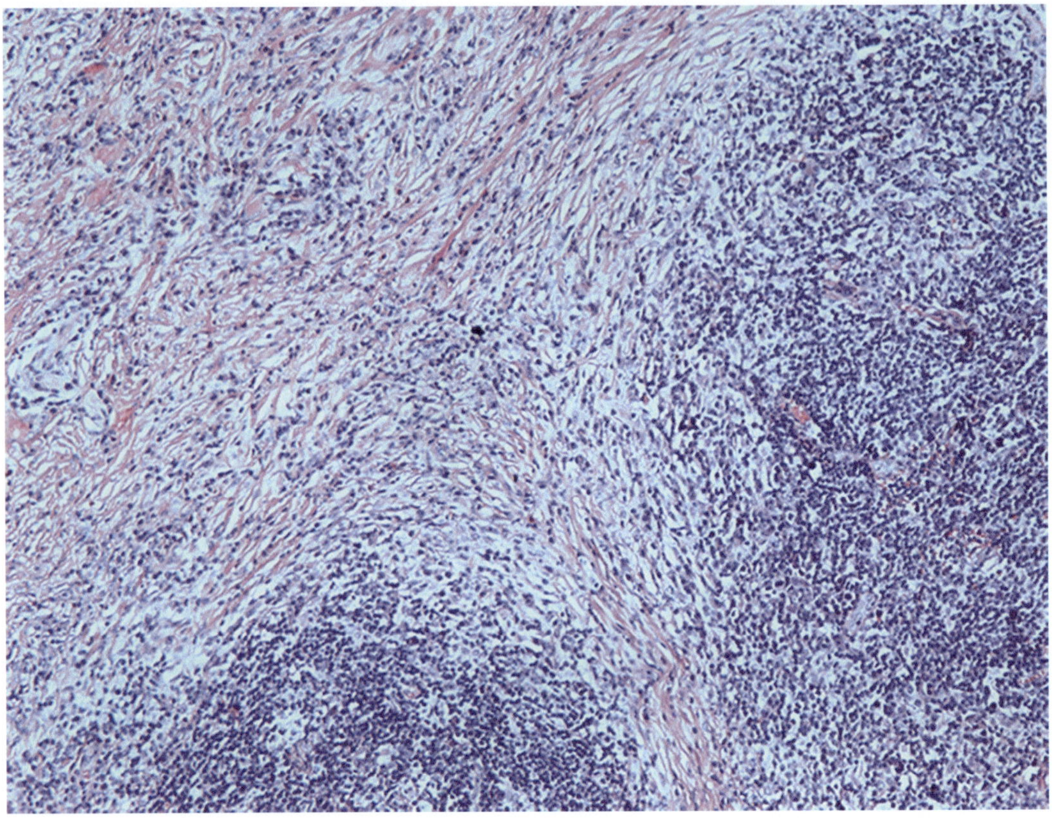

Fig. 33.2 Wide storiform fibrosis existed in the nasal mucosa. Different degrees of fibrosis were observed around the diffuse proliferated nest of lymphocytes and plasma cells, with the glands atrophy (hematoxylin and eosin staining, original magnification 10×)

CRS and common CRS, and the diagnosis mainly depended on serum IgG4 concentration. However, Piao et al. [37] found that a relatively large number of IgG4+ plasma cells infiltrated the nasal mucosa in IgG4-related CRS (Fig. 33.3), and it was significantly increased compared with the common CRS, so it was considered that the number of plasma cells of IgG+ and IgG4+ was one of the important indicators for the diagnosis of the disease, but their specificity still needed to be further studied. Lv et al. [38] selected 103 patients with inflammatory diseases of nasal sinuses, observed the number of IgG+ and IgG4+ plasma cells, and found that 22 patients met the diagnostic criteria of IgG4-RD, including chronic sinusitis, nasal polyps, inflammatory pseudotumor, fungal sinusitis, granulomatous with polyangiitis, Rosai-Dorfman disease, etc. It is suggested that the increase of IgG+ and IgG4+ plasma cells alone cannot diagnose IgG4-related CRS, and specific infection should be excluded first.

33.3.5 Diagnostic Criteria

There are no specific diagnostic criteria for IgG4-related CRS . At present, the comprehensive diagnostic standard of IgG4-RD revised by Umehara et al. [39] in 2012 is mostly adopted. The following three indicators should be integrated: (1) Diffuse/local swelling or masses in single or multiple organs; (2) Elevated serum IgG4 concentration (≥1350 mg/L); (3) Histopathology showed significant lymphocyte/plasma cell infiltration and fibrosis, and IgG4+

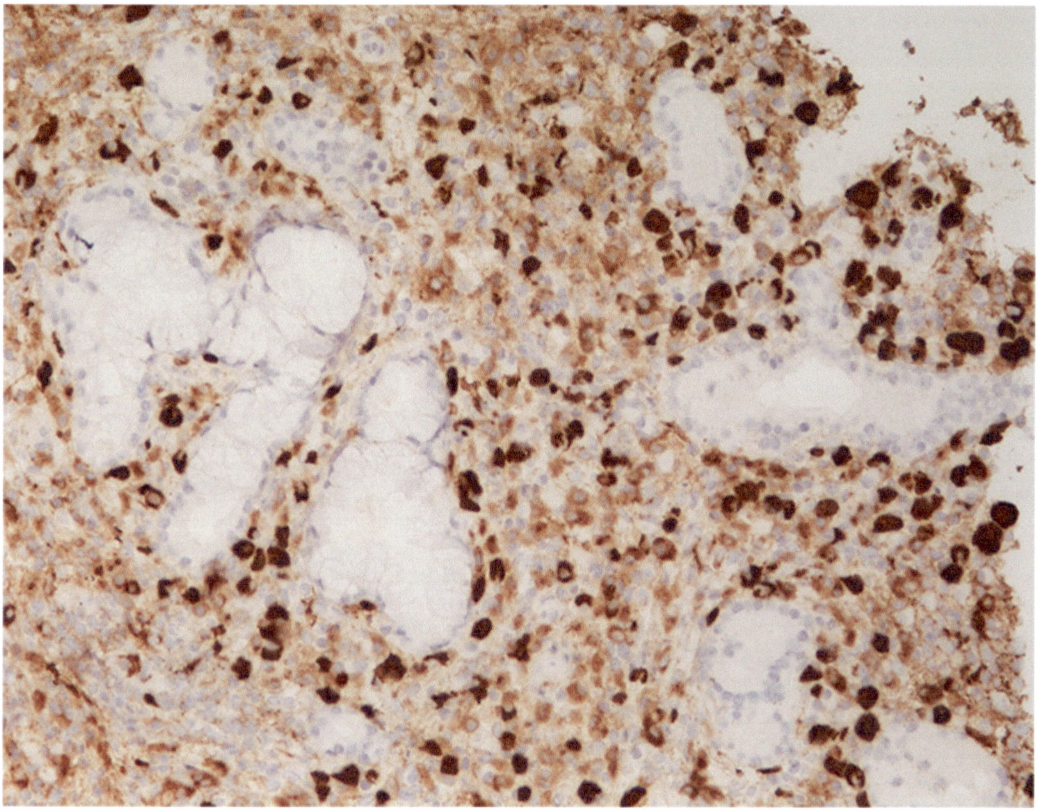

Fig. 33.3 A relatively large number of IgG4-positive plasma cells infiltrated the nasal mucosa (immunohistochemical staining, original magnification 10×)

plasma cell number >10/HPF, IgG4+/IgG+ plasma cells >40%.

Diagnosis was classified as "Definite" when criteria (1) + (2) + (3) were demonstrable; "probable" when criteria (1) + (3) were demonstrable, and "possible" when criteria (1) + (2) were demonstrable.

A comprehensive consideration combining the clinical signs and symptoms with a histopathological assessment may provide accurate diagnoses of IgG4-related CRS.

It should be noted that IgG4+ plasma cell count >10/HPF is the minimum standard in this standard, inconsistent with the critical value (50/HPF) required by the international consensus of histopathology of IgG4-RD [35]. The diagnostic critical value of different organs and different specimen types (needle puncture or resection) is different; therefore, the diagnostic critical value of IgG4-related CRS needs to be further studied in large samples to develop the diagnostic criteria of organ specificity.

33.4 Treatment

At present, no standardized treatment procedure for IgG4-related CRS has been established, and the current protocol is based on the treatment method of IgG4-RD of other organs. The treatment principle is to inhibit abnormal immune response, fibrosis, and organ function damage. Glucocorticoid is the first-line therapy to induce remission and prednisone 30–40 mg/day is recommended for early treatment and moderate adjustment is required when the disease progresses rapidly [40]. It has been reported that patients' symptoms can be completely relieved after 1 year of low-dose glucocorticoid maintenance therapy, while some studies suggest that patients should be given low-dose glucocorticoid maintenance therapy for 3 years [41]. The efficacy of low-dose glucocorticoids varies from study to study, and there is a risk of relapse during discontinuities [40].

Treatment of IgG4-related CRS is still being explored. In addition to glucocorticoid therapy, for some patients who fail to respond to glucocorticoid therapy, combination immunosuppressant or rituximab is given. Some patients who cannot apply glucocorticoids due to diabetes and other diseases can use local nasal spray or nasal irrigation, and most patients get better after treatment. For patients with extensive fibrosis, external volume reduction surgery and postoperative combined treatment with glucocorticoids and immunosuppressants can be performed.

33.5 Translation into Future Daily Practice

- Serum IgG4 can be used as a reference biomarker rather than a specific biomarker in IgG4-RD.
- A comprehensive consideration combining the clinical signs and symptoms with a histopathological assessment may provide accurate diagnoses of IgG4-related CRS.
- The treatment principle is to inhibit abnormal immune response, fibrosis, and organ function damage.

References

1. Hamano H, Kawa S, Horiuchi A, Unno H, Furuya N, Akamatsu T, et al. High serum IgG4 concentrations in patients with sclerosing pancreatitis. N Engl J Med. 2001;344(10):732–8. https://doi.org/10.1056/nejm200103083441005.
2. Ishida M, Hotta M, Kushima R, Shibayama M, Shimizu T, Okabe H. Multiple IgG4-related sclerosing lesions in the maxillary sinus, parotid gland and nasal septum. Pathol Int. 2009;59(9):670–5. https://doi.org/10.1111/j.1440-1827.2009.02425.x.
3. Ikeda R, Awataguchi T, Shoji F, Oshima T. A case of paranasal sinus lesions in IgG4-related sclerosing disease. Otolaryngol Head Neck Surg. 2010;142(3):458–9. https://doi.org/10.1016/j.otohns.2009.09.019.
4. Pace C, Ward S. A rare case of IgG4-related sclerosing disease of the maxillary sinus associated with bone destruction. J Oral Maxillofac Surg. 2010;68(10):2591–3. https://doi.org/10.1016/j.joms.2009.07.073.
5. Alt JA, Whitaker GT, Allan RW, Vaysberg M. Locally destructive skull base lesion: IgG4-related sclerosing disease. Allergy Rhinol (Providence, RI). 2012;3(1):e41–5. https://doi.org/10.2500/ar.2012.3.0026.
6. Sasaki T, Takahashi K, Mineta M, Fujita T, Aburano T. Immunoglobulin G4-related sclerosing disease mimicking invasive tumor in the nasal cavity and paranasal sinuses. AJNR Am J Neuroradiol. 2012;33(2):E19–20. https://doi.org/10.3174/ajnr.A2495.
7. Lindau RH, Su YB, Kobayashi R, Smith RB. Immunoglobulin G4-related sclerosing disease of the paranasal sinus. Head Neck. 2013;35(10):E321–4. https://doi.org/10.1002/hed.23175.
8. Hu EK, Parrish C, Wrobel B, Deshpande V, Stone JH. Immunoglobulin G4-related disease presenting as an ethmoid and maxillary mass. Ann Allergy Asthma Immunol. 2013;111(1):75–7. https://doi.org/10.1016/j.anai.2013.05.007.
9. Suzuki M, Nakamaru Y, Akazawa S, Mizumachi T, Maeda M, Takagi D, et al. Nasal manifestations of immunoglobulin G4-related disease. Laryngoscope. 2013;123(4):829–34. https://doi.org/10.1002/lary.23792.
10. Chandrasekharan R, Mathew V, Ashish G, Tyagi AK, Job AK. Isolated IgG4-related disease of sphenoid sinus manifesting as blindness. Int J Otorhinolaryngol Clin. 2013;5(3):178–81.
11. Cain RB, Colby TV, Balan V, Patel NP. Lal D. Perplexing lesions of the sinonasal cavity and skull base: IgG4-related and similar inflammatory diseases. Otolaryngol Head Neck Surg. 2014;151(3):496–502. https://doi.org/10.1177/0194599814533648.
12. Lee YS, Cho HJ, Yoo HS, Shin YS, Park HS. A case of IgG4-related disease with bronchial asthma and chronic rhinosinusitis in Korea. J Korean Med Sci. 2014;29(4):599–603. https://doi.org/10.3346/jkms.2014.29.4.599.
13. Prabhu SM, Yadav V, Irodi A, Mani S, Varghese AM. IgG4-related disease with sinonasal involvement: a case series. Indian J Radiol Imaging. 2014;24(2):117–20. https://doi.org/10.4103/0971-3026.134384.
14. Song BH, Baiyee D, Liang J. A rare and emerging entity: sinonasal IgG4-related sclerosing disease. Allergy Rhinol (Providence, RI). 2015;6(3):151–7. https://doi.org/10.2500/ar.2015.6.0136.
15. Suliman OA, Aidarous T, Marglani O, Banjar A. Diagnostic and therapeutic challenges in IgG4-related disease in the sphenoid sinus. J Clin Exp Oncol. 2015;4(1):1–2.
16. Morris C, Ng T, Kevin P, Singh N. Immunoglobulin G4 related disease isolated to the nasal cavity: a rare cause of nasal obstruction. J Laryngol Otol.

2015;129(Suppl 1):S57–9. https://doi.org/10.1017/s0022215114001911.
17. Inoue A, Wada K, Matsuura K, Osafune H, Ida Y, Kosakai A, et al. IgG4-related disease in the sinonasal cavity accompanied by intranasal structure loss. Auris Nasus Larynx. 2016;43(1):100–4. https://doi.org/10.1016/j.anl.2015.05.005.
18. Chen BN. IgG4-related disease presenting with destructive sinonasal lesion mimicking malignancy. Eur Arch Otorhinolaryngol. 2016;273(11):4027–9. https://doi.org/10.1007/s00405-016-4033-2.
19. Vandjelovic ND, Humphreys IM. Immunoglobulin G4-related sclerosing disease of the paranasal sinuses: a case report and literature review. Allergy Rhinol (Providence, RI). 2016;7(2):85–9. https://doi.org/10.2500/ar.2016.7.0154.
20. Bashyam A, Nagala S, Tahir F, Mirza S. Immunoglobulin G4-related disease of the paranasal sinuses. BMJ Case Rep. 2018:2018. https://doi.org/10.1136/bcr-2018-224472.
21. Kawa S, Ota M, Yoshizawa K, Horiuchi A, Hamano H, Ochi Y, et al. HLA DRB10405-DQB10401 haplotype is associated with autoimmune pancreatitis in the Japanese population. Gastroenterology. 2002;122(5):1264–9. https://doi.org/10.1053/gast.2002.33022.
22. Park DH, Kim MH, Oh HB, Kwon OJ, Choi YJ, Lee SS, et al. Substitution of aspartic acid at position 57 of the DQbeta1 affects relapse of autoimmune pancreatitis. Gastroenterology. 2008;134(2):440–6. https://doi.org/10.1053/j.gastro.2007.11.023.
23. Chang MC, Chang YT, Tien YW, Liang PC, Jan IS, Wei SC, et al. T-cell regulatory gene CTLA-4 polymorphism/haplotype association with autoimmune pancreatitis. Clin Chem. 2007;53(9):1700–5. https://doi.org/10.1373/clinchem.2007.085951.
24. Okazaki K, Uchida K, Miyoshi H, Ikeura T, Takaoka M, Nishio A. Recent concepts of autoimmune pancreatitis and IgG4-related disease. Clin Rev Allergy Immunol. 2011;41(2):126–38. https://doi.org/10.1007/s12016-010-8214-2.
25. Shiokawa M, Kodama Y, Sekiguchi K, Kuwada T, Tomono T, Kuriyama K, et al. Laminin 511 is a target antigen in autoimmune pancreatitis. Sci Transl Med 2018;10(453). https://doi.org/10.1126/scitranslmed.aaq0997.
26. Perugino CA, SB AS, Mattoo H, Della-Torre E, Mahajan V, Ganesh G, et al. Identification of galectin-3 as an autoantigen in patients with IgG(4)-related disease. J Allergy Clin Immunol. 2019;143(2):736–45.e6. https://doi.org/10.1016/j.jaci.2018.05.011.
27. Du H, Shi L, Chen P, Yang W, Xun Y, Yang C, et al. Prohibitin Is Involved in patients with IgG4 related disease. PLoS One. 2015;10(5):e0125331. https://doi.org/10.1371/journal.pone.0125331.
28. Hubers LM, Vos H, Schuurman AR, Erken R, Oude Elferink RP, Burgering B, et al. Annexin A11 is targeted by IgG4 and IgG1 autoantibodies in IgG4-related disease. Gut. 2018;67(4):728–35. https://doi.org/10.1136/gutjnl-2017-314548.
29. Guarneri F, Guarneri C, Benvenga S. Helicobacter pylori and autoimmune pancreatitis: role of carbonic anhydrase via molecular mimicry? J Cell Mol Med. 2005;9(3):741–4. https://doi.org/10.1111/j.1582-4934.2005.tb00506.x.
30. Frulloni L, Lunardi C, Simone R, Dolcino M, Scattolini C, Falconi M, et al. Identification of a novel antibody associated with autoimmune pancreatitis. N Engl J Med. 2009;361(22):2135–42. https://doi.org/10.1056/NEJMoa0903068.
31. Zen Y, Fujii T, Harada K, Kawano M, Yamada K, Takahira M, et al. Th2 and regulatory immune reactions are increased in immunoglobin G4-related sclerosing pancreatitis and cholangitis. Hepatology (Baltimore, MD). 2007;45(6):1538–46. https://doi.org/10.1002/hep.21697.
32. Takeuchi M, Sato Y, Ohno K, Tanaka S, Takata K, Gion Y, et al. T helper 2 and regulatory T-cell cytokine production by mast cells: a key factor in the pathogenesis of IgG4-related disease. Mod Pathol. 2014;27(8):1126–36. https://doi.org/10.1038/modpathol.2013.236.
33. Piao Y, Zhang Y, Yue C, Wang C, Zhang L. Immunoglobulin G4-related chronic rhinosinusitis: a pitfall in the differential diagnosis of granulomatosis with polyangiitis, Rosai-Dorfman disease, and fungal rhinosinusitis. Hum Pathol. 2018;73:82–8. https://doi.org/10.1016/j.humpath.2017.12.011.
34. Lin W, Zhang P, Chen H, Chen Y, Yang H, Zheng W, et al. Circulating plasmablasts/plasma cells: a potential biomarker for IgG4-related disease. Arthritis Res Ther. 2017;19(1):25. https://doi.org/10.1186/s13075-017-1231-2.
35. Deshpande V, Zen Y, Chan JK, Yi EE, Sato Y, Yoshino T, et al. Consensus statement on the pathology of IgG4-related disease. Mod Pathol. 2012;25(9):1181–92. https://doi.org/10.1038/modpathol.2012.72.
36. Moteki H, Yasuo M, Hamano H, Uehara T, Usami S. IgG4-related chronic rhinosinusitis: a new clinical entity of nasal disease. Acta Otolaryngol. 2011;131(5):518–26. https://doi.org/10.3109/00016489.2010.533699.
37. Piao Y, Wang C, Yu W, Mao M, Yue C, Liu H, et al. Concomitant occurrence of Mikulicz's disease and immunoglobulin G4-related chronic rhinosinusitis: a clinicopathological study of 12 cases. Histopathology. 2016;68(4):502–12. https://doi.org/10.1111/his.12775.
38. Lü J, Liu HG. Expression and significance of IgG4 in inflammatory disease of nasal cavity and paranasal sinuses. Zhonghua bing li xue za zhi = Chin J Pathol. 2013;42(6):386–91. https://doi.org/10.3760/cma.j.issn.0529-5807.2013.06.007.
39. Umehara H, Okazaki K, Masaki Y, Kawano M, Yamamoto M, Saeki T, et al. Comprehensive diagnostic criteria for IgG4-related disease (IgG4-RD), 2011. Mod Rheumatol. 2012;22(1):21–30. https://doi.org/10.1007/s10165-011-0571-z.
40. Khosroshahi A, Wallace ZS, Crowe JL, Akamizu T, Azumi A, Carruthers MN, et al. International

Consensus Guidance statement on the management and treatment of IgG4-related disease. Arthritis Rheumatol (Hoboken, NJ). 2015;67(7):1688–99. https://doi.org/10.1002/art.39132.
41. Masaki Y, Matsui S, Saeki T, Tsuboi H, Hirata S, Izumi Y, et al. A multicenter phase II prospective clinical trial of glucocorticoid for patients with untreated IgG4-related disease. Mod Rheumatol. 2017;27(5):849–54. https://doi.org/10.1080/14397595.2016.1259602.

34 Eosinophilic Granulomatosis with Polyangiitis

Yujie Cao and Huabin Li

Key Points

- Eosinophilic granulomatosis with polyangiitis (EGPA), formerly called Churg-Strauss syndrome (CSS), is a systemic small-vessel vasculitis commonly presenting with upper airway tract and lung involvement, peripheral neuropathy, cardiac lesions, etc.
- Some drugs (e.g., montelukast) are considered potential triggers of CSS that may unmask a pre-existing pathologic condition (*forme fruste* CSS) or cause progresses of disease because of the withdrawal or decrease of systemic corticosteroids.
- EGPA develops through a prodromic allergic phase characterized by asthma and rhinosinusitis, an eosinophilic phase marked by peripheral eosinophilia and organ involvement, and a vasculitic phase with clinical manifestations due to small vessel vasculitis.
- Glucocorticoids are recommended for all patients, and for those with severe/refractory disease and Five-Factor Score (FFS)-defined poor prognoses, immunosuppressants should be used (cyclophosphamide for induction and azathioprine for maintenance therapy).

Y. Cao · H. Li (✉)
Department of Otolaryngology, Head and Neck Surgery, Affiliated Eye and ENT Hospital, Fudan University, Shanghai, China
e-mail: caoyj7@mail2.sysu.edu.cn

Eosinophilic granulomatosis with polyangiitis (EGPA), formerly called Churg-Strauss syndrome(CSS) is a rare vasculitis characterized by a history of asthma and frequently allergic rhinitis and sinusitis, blood eosinophilia, and extrapulmonary manifestations [1, 2]. The estimated incidence is approximately 0.11–2.66 new cases per 1 million people per year, with an overall prevalence of 10.7–14 per 1 million adults [3]. EGPA may occur at all ages, without significant gender predominance [4].

34.1 Pathogenesis

The pathogenesis of EGPA is still largely unknown and different environmental factors have been reported as potential triggers of CSS, such as allergens, infections, vaccinations, and medications [3]. Some drugs, mainly leukotriene-receptor antagonists (e.g., montelukast) or anti-IgE antibodies (e.g., omalizumab), are considered potential triggers [5–8]. *Forme fruste* indicates that the signs and symptoms of CSS are (inadvertently) suppressed by corticosteroids [9]. And the antiasthma agents may unmask a pre-existing pathologic condition (*forme fruste* CSS) or cause progresses of disease because of the withdrawal or decrease of systemic corticosteroids. However, the mechanism is not entirely resolved.

In addition, genetic predisposition and immune dysregulation are also involved in

L. Zhang, C. Bachert (eds.), *Chronic Rhinosinusitis*, https://doi.org/10.1007/978-981-16-0784-4_34

pathogenesis of EGPA [2]. The HLADRB1*04 and *07 alleles and the related HLADRB4 gene are associated with an increased risk of EGPA [3]. As to immune dysregulation, Th2 responses are prominent with eosinophils activated and granule proteins being released. Moreover, IgG4 and IgE responses are dysregulated [10]. IgG4 levels are markedly increased in active CSS patients. As well, serum IgG4 correlated with the number of disease manifestations and the Birmingham vasculitis activity score [1]. Furthermore, anti-neutrophil cytoplasmic antibodies (ANCA) have been found in around 40–70% of EGPA patients with a main perinuclear immunofluorescence pattern [3, 9]. Eosinophil infiltration and ANCA-induced endothelial damage are probably the most crucial mechanisms of disease pathogenesis [3].

34.2 Pathology

EGPA has traditionally been described to develop through a prodromic allergic phase characterized by asthma and rhinosinusitis, an eosinophilic phase marked by peripheral eosinophilia and organ involvement, and a vasculitic phase with clinical manifestations due to small vessel vasculitis [11]. Once the disease progresses to the vasculitic phase, lesions will be observed in small- to medium-sized vessel walls including fibrinoid necrosis and eosinophilic vessel wall infiltration [3].

34.3 Main Clinical Manifestations

Asthma is the major EGPA manifestation, affecting 91–100% of the patients, most often before diagnosis (mean interval: 9.3–10.8 years) [10, 12]. Patients with EGPA frequently have ear, nose, and throat (ENT) manifestations often occurring at the onset of disease and may indicate relevant clues for the diagnosis. Allergic rhinitis and nasal polyposis are the most common ENT manifestations [13, 14]. Other otolaryngological manifestations include secretive otitis media, chronic ear drainage, sensorineural hearing loss, and facial nerve palsy [10]. The eosinophilic phase is characterized by lung, cardiac, and gastrointestinal involvement. The vasculitic phase is characterized by constitutional symptoms such as fever, weight loss, fatigue, and often by an apparently paradoxical improvement of asthma. In vasculitic phase, peripheral neuropathy is a main feature affecting ~70% of the patients. And renal manifestations are found in ~25% of the patients ranging from isolated urinary abnormalities (i.e., microscopic hematuria, proteinuria) to rapidly progressive glomerulonephritis [10]. EGPA patients differ according to their ANCA status, ANCA+ patients had significantly more frequent ENT manifestations, peripheral neuropathy, and/or renal involvement, but less frequent cardiac manifestations than ANCA-patients [12].

34.4 Laboratory Findings

Active EGPA is characterized by peripheral eosinophilia (usually >1500 cells/μl or >10%) [3]. Eosinophilia correlates with disease activity, and its increase often indicates relapses [10]. C-reactive protein and erythrocyte sedimentation rate are also high in the active phase [10, 11]. Perinuclear immunofluorescence is the main pattern in ANCA+ EGPA patients [3, 9]. A recent study demonstrated that serum eotaxin-3 is a sensitive and specific marker for the diagnosis of active CSS with a sensitivity and specificity of 87.5% and 98.6%, respectively, at a cut-off level of 80 pg/ml [15]. Eosinophil cationic protein (ECP) is also reported to be a potential disease activity marker in CSS [16].

34.5 Diagnosis

In 1990, the American College of Rheumatology (ACR) defined the classification criteria to distinguish the different vasculitides and there were six criteria for EGPA, namely asthma, eosinophilia >10%, neuropathy (mononeuropathy, or polyneuropathy), non-fixed lung infiltrates, paranasal sinus abnormalities, and extravascular eosinophils on biopsy. Diagnosis can be made when four of the six criteria are met with a sensitivity of 85% and a specificity of 99.7% [17]. More recently, the Chapel Hill Consensus Conference Nomenclature defined EGPA as an "eosinophil-rich and necrotizing granulomatous inflammation, frequently involving the respiratory tract, and necrotizing vasculitis predominantly affecting small- to medium-size vessels, and associated with asthma and eosinophilia" [18]. Of note, all those criteria above are used for classification once vasculitis has been diagnosed.

34.6 Treatment

Treatment decisions should be made according to each EGPA patient's characteristics, such as disease severity, organ involvement, prognosis, age, and comorbidities [2]. The Five-Factor Score (FFS) is the most widely used prognostic score in EGPA [10]. The revised FFS, based on a new analysis of 1108 vasculitis patients, including 230 with EGPA demonstrated that the following factors were significantly associated with higher 5-year mortality: age >65 years, cardiac symptoms, gastrointestinal involvement, and renal insufficiency (stabilized peak creatinine ≥150 μmol/l); the presence of each was accorded +1 point. ENT symptoms, affecting patients with Wegener granulomatosis (WG) and CSS, were associated with a lower relative risk of death and the presence of each was accorded −1 point. An FFS of 0, 1, or 2 was associated with respective 5-year mortality rate of 9%, 21%, or 40%, respectively [19]. The FFS was initially devised to assess disease prognosis and using it to make treatment decisions remains debated internationally. For patients without poor prognosis factors (FFS = 0), glucocorticoids alone were recommended at start, which were effective and safe to induce and maintain remissions. For EGPA patients with poor prognosis factors (FFS ≥ 1) and/or when other life-threatening manifestations are present, even those not included in the FFS (e.g., possible blindness due to eye involvement, severe alveolar hemorrhage, and/or fulminant mononeuritis multiplex), immunosuppressants were recommended to join with glucocorticoids [2].

Other treatments including immunoglobulins, therapeutic plasma exchanges, interferon-α, and newer biologic therapies such as rituximab, omalizumab, mepolizumab are being evaluated.

References

1. Vaglio A, Strehl JD, Manger B, Maritati F, Alberici F, Beyer C, et al. IgG4 immune response in Churg-Strauss syndrome. Ann Rheum Dis. 2012;71(3):390–3. https://doi.org/10.1136/ard.2011.155382.
2. Nguyen Y, Guillevin L. Eosinophilic granulomatosis with polyangiitis (Churg-Strauss). Semin Respir Crit Care Med. 2018;39(4):471–81. https://doi.org/10.1055/s-0038-1669454.
3. Greco A, Rizzo MI, De Virgilio A, Gallo A, Fusconi M, Ruoppolo G, et al. Churg-Strauss syndrome. Autoimmun Rev. 2015;14(4):341–8. https://doi.org/10.1016/j.autrev.2014.12.004.
4. Mouthon L, Dunogue B, Guillevin L. Diagnosis and classification of eosinophilic granulomatosis with polyangiitis (formerly named Churg-Strauss syndrome). J Autoimmun. 2014;48-49:99–103. https://doi.org/10.1016/j.jaut.2014.01.018.
5. Bibby S, Healy B, Steele R, Kumareswaran K, Nelson H, Beasley R. Association between leukotriene receptor antagonist therapy and Churg-Strauss syndrome: an analysis of the FDA AERS database. Thorax. 2010;65(2):132–8. https://doi.org/10.1136/thx.2009.120972.
6. Nathani N, Little MA, Kunst H, Wilson D, Thickett DR. Churg-Strauss syndrome and leukotriene antagonist use: a respiratory perspective. Thorax. 2008;63(10):883–8. https://doi.org/10.1136/thx.2007.093955.
7. Ruppert AM, Averous G, Stanciu D, Deroide N, Riehm S, Poindron V, et al. Development of Churg-Strauss syndrome with controlled asthma during omalizumab treatment. J Allergy Clin Immunol. 2008;121(1):253–4. https://doi.org/10.1016/j.jaci.2007.10.040.
8. Solans R, Bosch JA, Selva A, Orriols R, Vilardell M. Montelukast and Churg-Strauss syndrome. Thorax. 2002;57(2):183–5. https://doi.org/10.1136/thorax.57.2.183.
9. Lilly CM, Churg A, Lazarovich M, Pauwels R, Hendeles L, Rosenwasser LJ, et al. Asthma therapies and Churg-Strauss syndrome. J Allergy Clin Immunol. 2002;109(1):S1–S19. https://doi.org/10.1067/mai.2002.120854.
10. Vaglio A, Buzio C, Zwerina J. Eosinophilic granulomatosis with polyangiitis (Churg-Strauss): state of the art. Allergy. 2013;68(3):261–73. https://doi.org/10.1111/all.12088.

11. Noth I, Strek ME, Leff AR. Churg-Strauss syndrome. Lancet. 2003;361(9357):587–94. https://doi.org/10.1016/s0140-6736(03)12518-4.
12. Comarmond C, Pagnoux C, Khellaf M, Cordier JF, Hamidou M, Viallard JF, et al. Eosinophilic granulomatosis with polyangiitis (Churg-Strauss): clinical characteristics and long-term followup of the 383 patients enrolled in the French Vasculitis Study Group cohort. Arthritis Rheum. 2013;65(1):270–81. https://doi.org/10.1002/art.37721.
13. Bacciu A, Bacciu S, Mercante G, Ingegnoli F, Grasselli C, Vaglio A, et al. Ear, nose and throat manifestations of Churg-Strauss syndrome. Acta Otolaryngol. 2006;126(5):503–9. https://doi.org/10.1080/00016480500437435.
14. Bacciu A, Buzio C, Giordano D, Pasanisi E, Vincenti V, Mercante G, et al. Nasal polyposis in Churg-Strauss syndrome. Laryngoscope. 2008;118(2):325–9. https://doi.org/10.1097/MLG.0b013e318159889d.
15. Zwerina J, Bach C, Martorana D, Jatzwauk M, Hegasy G, Moosig F, et al. Eotaxin-3 in Churg-Strauss syndrome: a clinical and immunogenetic study. Rheumatology (Oxford). 2011;50(10):1823–7. https://doi.org/10.1093/rheumatology/keq445.
16. Guilpain P, Auclair JF, Tamby MC, Servettaz A, Mahr A, Weill B, et al. Serum eosinophil cationic protein: a marker of disease activity in Churg-Strauss syndrome. Ann N Y Acad Sci. 2007;1107:392–9. https://doi.org/10.1196/annals.1381.041.
17. Masi AT, Hunder GG, Lie JT, Michel BA, Bloch DA, Arend WP, et al. The American College of Rheumatology 1990 criteria for the classification of Churg-Strauss syndrome (allergic granulomatosis and angiitis). Arthritis Rheum. 1990;33(8):1094–100. https://doi.org/10.1002/art.1780330806.
18. Jennette JC, Falk RJ, Andrassy K, Bacon PA, Churg J, Gross WL, et al. Nomenclature of systemic vasculitides. Proposal of an international consensus conference. Arthritis Rheum. 1994;37(2):187–92. https://doi.org/10.1002/art.1780370206.
19. Guillevin L, Pagnoux C, Seror R, Mahr A, Mouthon L, Le Toumelin P, et al. The Five-Factor Score revisited: assessment of prognoses of systemic necrotizing vasculitides based on the French Vasculitis Study Group (FVSG) cohort. Medicine. 2011;90(1):19–27. https://doi.org/10.1097/MD.0b013e318205a4c6.

35 Oral Corticosteroids

Chengshuo Wang, Yifan Meng, and Luo Zhang

Key Points

- Many rhinologists consider oral corticosteroids as "maximal" medical therapy in CRS.
- Oral corticosteroids are highly effective in the treatment of CRSwNP.
- The use of oral corticosteroids as sole drugs in the treatment of CRSsNP lacks indisputable evidence to support this.
- The risks of oral corticosteroid need to be taken under consideration.

C. Wang (✉)
Department of Otolaryngology, Head and Neck Surgery, Beijing Tongren Hospital, Capital Medical University, Beijing, China

Beijing Key Laboratory of Nasal Diseases, Beijing Institute of Otolaryngology, Beijing, China

Y. Meng
Department of Otolaryngology, Head and Neck Surgery, Beijing Tongren Hospital, Capital Medical University, Beijing, China

L. Zhang
Department of Otolaryngology, Head and Neck Surgery, Beijing Tongren Hospital, Capital Medical University, Beijing, China

Beijing Key Laboratory of Nasal Diseases, Beijing Institute of Otolaryngology, Beijing, China

Department of Allergy, Beijing Tongren Hospital, Capital Medical University, Beijing, China

Oral corticosteroids (OCS) are a mainstay of treatment in the management of chronic rhinosinusitis (CRS) and are considered by many doctors to constitute a key component of "maximal" medical therapy [1]. Corticosteroids are used in CRS for their anti-inflammatory effects, which are complex but vitally involve in the regulation of prostaglandin secretion [2]. Their anti-fibroblast effects are commonly utilized to reduce postoperative scar formation [1]. Mechanistically, corticosteroids bind to the glucocorticoid receptor and lead to gene transcriptional changes, which result in several effects, including changes in carbohydrate and fat metabolism, reduced protein synthesis, increased fat redistribution and protein breakdown [2]. Calcium absorption is reduced and excretion might increase the risk of osteoporosis. Moreover, corticosteroids can have a negative feedback effect on the anterior pituitary gland and hypothalamus, thereby resulting in depressed secretion of adrenocorticotropic hormone and corticotropin-releasing hormone, which can take several weeks to start once the corticosteroids are stopped [3].

35.1 Chronic Rhinosinusitis with Nasal Polyps (CRSwNP)

The therapy efficacy of OCS in the CRSwNP has been verified in the recent decade. Van Zele et al. [4] conducted a randomized control trial (RCT),

L. Zhang, C. Bachert (eds.), *Chronic Rhinosinusitis*, https://doi.org/10.1007/978-981-16-0784-4_35

which enrolled 47 CRSwNP patients to receive oral methylprednisolone taper, doxycycline, or placebo for 3 months. The study concluded a significant reduction in the polyps size, nasal congestion improvement, loss of sense of smell, and postnasal drip in the steroid group as well as the doxycycline group compared to placebo. Meanwhile, the steroid group demonstrated significant decreases in blood eosinophil counts, eosinophilic cationic protein, immunoglobulin E (IgE), and interleukin 5 (IL-5). Vaidyanathan et al. [5] conducted a RCT in which 60 CRSwNP patients were randomized to receive 25 mg of prednisolone or identical placebo daily for 2 weeks. During the follow-up period, the polyps showed significant reductions in size at 2 weeks and 10 weeks follow-up. Nineteen patients in the steroid group and 18 in the placebo group reported adverse events, none of which were considered serious as defined by the protocol. Kirtsreesakul et al. [6] investigated 109 patients with nasal polyposis, randomized to treat it with 50 mg of prednisolone or placebo daily for 2 weeks. The authors suggested although subjective symptoms were improved in the two groups that the steroid group had significantly greater improvements in all subjective variants than the placebo group. Furthermore, the steroid group also showed significant improvements in the peak expiratory flow index. Similarly, a study by Hissaria et al. [7] has also found clinically significant improvements in symptoms and pathology of nasal polyposis with a short course of oral corticosteroids. A recent meta-analysis by Zhang et al. [8] has suggested that OCS provides significant improvements in nasal symptoms and reduction in nasal polyp size in patients with CRSwNP. Prednisone dose of less than 50 mg/day was recommended when efficacy of oral corticosteroids in CRSwNP was balanced against potential adverse effects.

With the development of endoscopic sinus surgery (ESS), the efficacy of a combination of ESS and OCS has been increasingly investigated. González-Castro et al. [9] performed a national survey of active members of the American Rhinologic Society (ARS) and showed that nearly 90% of the respondents in the cohort saw an advantage in the use of preoperative OCS in ESS. Furthermore, the most common diagnosis among the respondents for using preoperative OCS was CRSwNP. A meta-analysis conducted by Pundir et al. [10] has recently reported that preoperative use of corticosteroids in ESS resulted in significantly reduced blood loss, shorter operative time, and improved surgical field quality. Similarly, postoperative corticosteroids improved postoperative endoscopic scores in CRS and recurrence rates in cases of CRSwNP. Studies from our department have also demonstrated that 2 weeks' treatment with OCS dramatically decreases polyp recurrence following ESS (Fig. 35.1). However, not all studies have shown the efficacy of postoperative OCS in the treatment of CRWwNP. A more recent study by Shen et al. [11] has shown that postoperative OCS did not provide additional improvements in VAS and SNOT-22 scores, despite an improvement trend in Lund-Kennedy endoscopic scores at 6 months postoperatively.

35.2 Chronic Rhinosinusitis Without Nasal Polyps (CRSsNP)

Compared to CRSwNP, quality evidence has been lacking to support the use of oral corticosteroids in the management of CRSsNP in the recent decade. Indeed, despite common use of oral corticosteroids for CRSsNP, no study has evaluated its efficacy as a single agent for CRSsNP and also oral steroid use in CRSsNP is considered optional due to insufficient solid evidence to support this [12, 13]. Lal and Hwang et al. [14] have recently conducted a systematic review of the literature on the use of oral corticosteroids for CRSsNP and demonstrated most of the studies described the use of OCS in combination with oral antibiotics and nasal steroids, with no randomized controlled trial elucidating the effect of only oral steroid use in CRSsNP. Hessler et al. [15] performed a prospective study in which CRS patients were followed up monthly to evaluate the effect of medication using the Sino-Nasal Outcomes Test-20 plus olfaction (SNOT-20 + 1) health questionnaire. Patients were managed by combination use of medical therapy besides prednisone. The

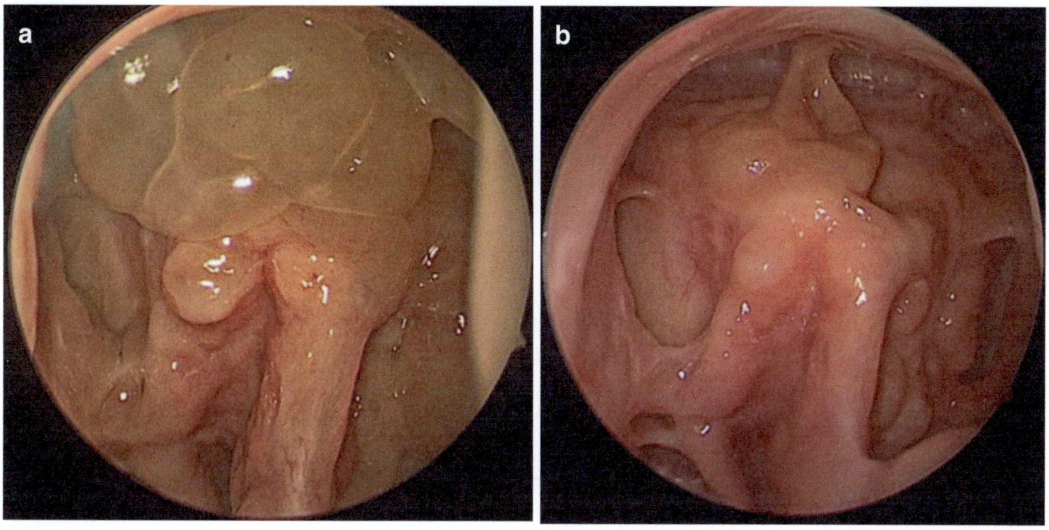

Fig. 35.1 Efficacy of oral corticosteroids in combination with Draf 3 surgery in CRSwNP with asthma. (**a**) Recurrent nasal polyps at 5 years after Draf 3 surgery in patient with CRSwNP and comorbid asthma. (**b**) Nasal polyps disappeared after 2 weeks of oral corticosteroids treatment post-surgery

authors demonstrated a significant overall improvement in the SNOT-20 + 1 scores in patients using prednisone for more than 11 days. A study by Lal et al. [16] that enrolled CRSsNP and CRSwNP patients showed that after a 12-day OCS taper besides other therapies 55% of CRSsNP patients were "symptoms control."

35.3 The Dose of Oral Corticosteroid in Chronic Rhinosinusitis

The dosage of OCS varies greatly in treatment of CRS patients. A recent study evaluating appropriateness criteria for ESS during management of uncomplicated adult chronic rhinosinusitis has indicated that in patients with uncomplicated CRSwNP, requirement for a short course (1–3 week) of OCS would make the patient a candidate for endoscopic sinus [17]. However, an online survey by Scott et al. [18] of all American Rhinologic Society members to evaluate their prescribing habits for CRS patients has demonstrated that the starting dose (median, mg/day) of OCS in the therapy of CRS ranges from 25 to 60 over a duration ranging from 3 to 45 days. Although some studies have verified the efficacy and safety of OCS in the CRS therapy [1, 4, 6, 7], RCTs are still needed to establish the effective dosage of OCS and its safety in CRSwNP and CRSsNP patients. To date, significant heterogeneity exists in OCS prescribing habits for CRS. Furthermore, discrepancies have been observed between survey results and evidence-based recommendations [18]. Thus, developing standardized OCS treatment methods for CRS might not only improve the quality of care, but also reduce the risk of complications.

35.4 Risks of Oral Corticosteroid

Despite most studies reporting benefits of prescribing OCS in the treatment of CRS, many studies are not familiar with the risks of oral corticosteroid [1]; thus, necessitating the need for special attention to these risks during CRS treatment to avoid complications.

35.5 Bone Metabolism

The adverse effect of steroids in bone metabolism has been well documented. It may occur through several mechanisms. Steroids reduce intestinal calcium absorption and increase urinary calcium excretion. Meanwhile, steroids may also inhibit osteoblast activity [19, 20] and suppress the production of adrenal androgens, which decreases the effect on bone formation [19]. Additionally, steroids have been reported to cause apoptosis of osteoblasts and osteocytes [21], an effect that slows after 6 months. Winblad et al. [22] have recently carried out a systematic review of studies including adult patients with CRSwNP treated with oral steroids to evaluate the effect of steroids on bone mineral density (BMD) and prevalence of fractures in relation to dose and duration of oral steroids. The authors demonstrated that when the dose and duration of oral steroids was 1 mg/kg body weight/day for 6–10 days for ≥4 courses/year, the prevalence of low bone mass was high up to 61%. Furthermore, no studies evaluated prevalence of fracture. Despite the conflict about whether the dose has a more significant clinical effect on bone density, several studies have demonstrated that supplemental calcium and vitamin D and bisphosphonates can help reduce the corticosteroid-induced loss of bone mineral density [23].

35.6 Adrenal Suppression

Exogenous steroids can increase the circulating corticosteroid levels, and thereby lead to a negative feedback on the hypothalamic-pituitary-adrenal (HPA) axis [24]. A study has shown atrophy of adrenal glands after as few as 5 days of corticosteroid therapy [22]. However, two earlier studies showed no definitive cases of adrenal suppression if the prednisone dose taken was <5 mg/day, even after several months. In contrast, when the doses were high up to 10 mg daily for 4 days, there was a significant decrease in plasma cortisol [25, 26].

35.7 Gastrointestinal

Although some CRS patients are thought to suffer from stomach ulcers after taking OCS, a large meta-analysis has not shown an association between steroid and peptic ulcer [27, 28]. However, these studies demonstrated that patients used prednisone had peptic ulcer symptoms more frequently than did the controls. Thus, the side effects of the gastrointestinal tract need to be clarified in RCT or multicenter studies in the future.

35.8 Others

Other risks of OCS such as morphologic change [22, 29], hyperglycemia [30], increased intraocular pressure, posterior-subcapsular cataract formation or glaucoma [31], and psychiatric [1] have also been reported.

35.9 Translation into the Future Daily Practice

OCS is one of the most important therapies for the CRSwNP or CRSsNP patients besides ESS, especially for refractory CRS (aspirin tolerant triad, CRS with asthma recurrence, nasal polyps, etc.) or eosinophilic CRS, which are highly associated with eosinophil infiltration. For CRS patients falling in these categories, OCS should be applied throughout the perioperative period. After surgery, the OCS therapy should be replaced with intranasal corticosteroid (INS) or nebulization corticosteroid. However, during the OCS treatment, supplemental calcium, vitamin D, gastric mucosal protective agent, and other appropriate medications should be used to reduce the possible side effects of OCS therapy. Tapered use of OCS is also important because it can avoid the rebound phenomenon. Serum cortisol level should also be checked intermittently during the OCS treatment.

References

1. Poetker DM. Oral corticosteroids in the management of chronic rhinosinusitis with and without nasal polyps: risks and benefits. Am J Rhinol Allergy. 2015;29(5):339–42. https://doi.org/10.2500/ajra.2015.29.4223.
2. Campbell RG. Risks and management of long-term corticosteroid use in chronic rhinosinusitis. Curr

Opin Otolaryngol Head Neck Surg. 2018;26(1):1–7. https://doi.org/10.1097/moo.0000000000000421.
3. Rang HP, Dale MM, Ritter JM, RJ F. Rang and Dale's pharmacology. Philadelphia: Elsevier Ltd.; 2007.
4. Van Zele T, Gevaert P, Holtappels G, Beule A, Wormald PJ, Mayr S, et al. Oral steroids and doxycycline: two different approaches to treat nasal polyps. J Allergy Clin Immunol. 2010;125(5):1069–76.e4. https://doi.org/10.1016/j.jaci.2010.02.020.
5. Vaidyanathan S, Barnes M, Williamson P, Hopkinson P, Donnan PT, Lipworth B. Treatment of chronic rhinosinusitis with nasal polyposis with oral steroids followed by topical steroids: a randomized trial. Ann Intern Med. 2011;154(5):293–302. https://doi.org/10.7326/0003-4819-154-5-201103010-00003.
6. Kirtsreesakul V, Wongsritrang K, Ruttanaphol S. Clinical efficacy of a short course of systemic steroids in nasal polyposis. Rhinology. 2011;49(5):525–32. https://doi.org/10.4193/Rhino11.140.
7. Hissaria P, Smith W, Wormald PJ, Taylor J, Vadas M, Gillis D, et al. Short course of systemic corticosteroids in sinonasal polyposis: a double-blind, randomized, placebo-controlled trial with evaluation of outcome measures. J Allergy Clin Immunol. 2006;118(1):128–33. https://doi.org/10.1016/j.jaci.2006.03.012.
8. Zhang Y, Wang C, Huang Y, Lou H, Zhang L. Efficacy of short-term systemic corticosteroid therapy in chronic rhinosinusitis with nasal polyps: a meta-analysis of randomized controlled trials and systematic review. Am J Rhinol Allergy. 2019;33(5):567–76. https://doi.org/10.1177/1945892419851312.
9. González-Castro J, Pascual J, Busquets J. National survey on the use of preoperative systemic steroids in endoscopic sinus surgery. Int Forum Allergy Rhinol. 2013;3(6):497–503. https://doi.org/10.1002/alr.21122.
10. Pundir V, Pundir J, Lancaster G, Baer S, Kirkland P, Cornet M, et al. Role of corticosteroids in functional endoscopic sinus surgery—a systematic review and meta-analysis. Rhinology. 2016;54(1):3–19. https://doi.org/10.4193/Rhin15.079.
11. Shen KH, Wang YH, Hsu TW, Hsieh LC, Sun FJ, Wang YP. Differential effects of postoperative oral corticosteroid on eosinophilic vs. non-eosinophilic CRSwNP subtypes. Am J Otolaryngol. 2019;40(1):22–9. https://doi.org/10.1016/j.amjoto.2018.09.005.
12. Poetker DM, Jakubowski LA, Lal D, Hwang PH, Wright ED, Smith TL. Oral corticosteroids in the management of adult chronic rhinosinusitis with and without nasal polyps: an evidence-based review with recommendations. Int Forum Allergy Rhinol. 2013;3(2):104–20. https://doi.org/10.1002/alr.21072.
13. Howard BE, Lal D. Oral steroid therapy in chronic rhinosinusitis with and without nasal polyposis. Curr Allergy Asthma Rep. 2013;13(2):236–43. https://doi.org/10.1007/s11882-012-0329-5.
14. Lal D, Hwang PH. Oral corticosteroid therapy in chronic rhinosinusitis without polyposis: a systematic review. Int Forum Allergy Rhinol. 2011;1(2):136–43. https://doi.org/10.1002/alr.20024.
15. Hessler JL, Piccirillo JF, Fang D, Vlahiotis A, Banerji A, Levitt RG, et al. Clinical outcomes of chronic rhinosinusitis in response to medical therapy: results of a prospective study. Am J Rhinol. 2007;21(1):10–8. https://doi.org/10.2500/ajr.2007.21.2960.
16. Lal D, Scianna JM, Stankiewicz JA. Efficacy of targeted medical therapy in chronic rhinosinusitis, and predictors of failure. Am J Rhinol Allergy. 2009;23(4):396–400. https://doi.org/10.2500/ajra.2009.23.3334.
17. Rudmik L, Soler ZM, Hopkins C, Schlosser RJ, Peters A, White AA, et al. Defining appropriateness criteria for endoscopic sinus surgery during management of uncomplicated adult chronic rhinosinusitis: a RAND/UCLA appropriateness study. Rhinology. 2016;54(2):117–28. https://doi.org/10.4193/Rhin16.023.
18. Scott JR, Ernst HM, Rotenberg BW, Rudmik L, Sowerby LJ. Oral corticosteroid prescribing habits for rhinosinusitis: The American Rhinologic Society membership. Am J Rhinol Allergy. 2017;31(1):22–6. https://doi.org/10.2500/ajra.2017.31.4396.
19. Allen DB, Bielory L, Derendorf H, Dluhy R, Colice GL, Szefler SJ. Inhaled corticosteroids: past lessons and future issues. J Allergy Clin Immunol. 2003;112(3 Suppl):S1–40. https://doi.org/10.1016/s0091-6749(03)01859-1.
20. Keenan GF. Management of complications of glucocorticoid therapy. Clin Chest Med. 1997;18(3):507–20. https://doi.org/10.1016/s0272-5231(05)70398-1.
21. Ton FN, Gunawardene SC, Lee H, Neer RM. Effects of low-dose prednisone on bone metabolism. J Bone Miner Res. 2005;20(3):464–70. https://doi.org/10.1359/jbmr.041125.
22. Winblad L, Larsen CG, Håkansson K, Abrahamsen B, von Buchwald C. The risk of osteoporosis in oral steroid treatment for nasal polyposis: a systematic review. Rhinology. 2017;55(3):195–201. https://doi.org/10.4193/Rhin15.367.
23. Fardet L, Kassar A, Cabane J, Flahault A. Corticosteroid-induced adverse events in adults: frequency, screening and prevention. Drug Saf. 2007;30(10):861–81. https://doi.org/10.2165/00002018-200730100-00005.
24. Weifeng Guo. The adrenal medulla and adrenal cortex. New York: McGraw-Hill; 2007. p. 356–81.
25. Wilson AM, McFarlane LC, Lipworth BJ. Systemic bioactivity profiles of oral prednisolone and nebulized budesonide in adult asthmatics. Chest. 1998;114(4):1022–7. https://doi.org/10.1378/chest.114.4.1022.
26. LaRochelle GE Jr, LaRochelle AG, Ratner RE, Borenstein DG. Recovery of the hypothalamic-pituitary-adrenal (HPA) axis in patients with rheumatic diseases receiving low-dose prednisone. Am J Med. 1993;95(3):258–64. https://doi.org/10.1016/0002-9343(93)90277-v.
27. Conn HO, Poynard T. Corticosteroids and peptic ulcer: meta-analysis of adverse events during steroid

therapy. J Intern Med. 1994;236(6):619–32. https://doi.org/10.1111/j.1365-2796.1994.tb00855.x.
28. Piper JM, Ray WA, Daugherty JR, Griffin MR. Corticosteroid use and peptic ulcer disease: role of nonsteroidal anti-inflammatory drugs. Ann Intern Med. 1991;114(9):735–40. https://doi.org/10.7326/0003-4819-114-9-735.
29. Fardet L, Cabane J, Lebbé C, Morel P, Flahault A. Incidence and risk factors for corticosteroid-induced lipodystrophy: a prospective study. J Am Acad Dermatol. 2007;57(4):604–9. https://doi.org/10.1016/j.jaad.2007.04.018.
30. Hirsch IB, Paauw DS. Diabetes management in special situations. Endocrinol Metab Clin North Am. 1997;26(3):631–45. https://doi.org/10.1016/s0889-8529(05)70271-1.
31. Carnahan MC, Goldstein DA. Ocular complications of topical, peri-ocular, and systemic corticosteroids. Curr Opin Ophthalmol. 2000;11(6):478–83. https://doi.org/10.1097/00055735-200012000-00016.

36 Nasal Spray Corticosteroids

Yujie Cao, Huabin Li, and Dehui Wang

Key Points

- Topical and systemic corticosteroids constitute the first step in therapy in CRSwNP and CRSsNP. Endoscopic sinus surgery is recommended only when medical treatment fails.
- There is evidence from five meta-analyses that standard topical steroid therapy contributes to both patient based and objective clinical improvements in CRSwNP and CRSsNP.
- Compared with nasal delivery (simple sprays/low volume) methods, sinus delivery (direct sinus cannulation or postoperative sinonasal irrigation) methods can achieve greater symptom improvements.

Anti-inflammatory therapy plays a critical role in the treatment of chronic rhinosinusitis. This includes corticosteroids and low-dose macrolides [1]. Topical corticosteroids are more widely used compared with systemic corticosteroids because of not only the longer periods it can be given without associated systemic side effects but also the potentially achievement of better drug concentration in sinonasal mucosa [2]. Classes of topical corticosteroids include first-generation intranasal steroids (beclomethasone dipropionate, triamcinolone acetonide, flunisolide, and budesonide) and newer preparations (fluticasone propionate, mometasone furoate, ciclesonide, and fluticasone furoate) [1].

Effective distribution of topical corticosteroids into sinonasal mucosa depends not only on the anatomically remodeled sinus cavity by surgery but also on the effective delivery of corticosteroids that together brings about the optimal context for disease control.

Y. Cao · H. Li · D. Wang (✉)
Department of Otolaryngology, Head and Neck Surgery, Affiliated Eye and ENT Hospital, Fudan University, Shanghai, China
e-mail: caoyj7@mail2.sysu.edu.cn

36.1 Mechanism

The corticosteroids play various roles to achieve anti-inflammatory effects, including reducing proinflammatory or increasing anti-inflammatory gene transcription, to reduce the infiltration of inflammatory cell, such as eosinophils, T cells, mast cells, and dendritic cells, as well as to suppress the production of proinflammatory mediators, cell chemotactic factors, and adhesion molecules. Different steroids, delivered in different ways (such as sprays versus drops) may differ in their effectiveness [1].

36.2 Efficacy

In CRSwNP and CRSsNP, medical treatment, including topical and systemic corticosteroids, constitutes the first step in therapy. Endoscopic

L. Zhang, C. Bachert (eds.), *Chronic Rhinosinusitis*, https://doi.org/10.1007/978-981-16-0784-4_36

sinus surgery is recommended only when medical treatment fails.

Luke Rudmik et al. based on the available evidence draw the conclusion that standard topical nasal steroid therapy is recommended in the topical treatment of CRS. Standard topical nasal steroid therapies are U.S. Food and Drug Administration (FDA)-approved metered-dose nasal spray delivery of steroid agents including the following: mometasone furoate, fluticasone propionate, fluticasone furoate, budesonide, beclomethasone dipropionate monohydrate, ciclesonide, flunisolide, and triamcinolone acetonide [3]. This review identified five meta-analyses evaluating the role of standard topical nasal steroid therapy on clinical outcomes for both CRSwNP and CRSsNP. All studies were level 1a quality.

The studies by Joe et al. [4], Rudmik et al. [5], and Snidvongs et al. [6] evaluated the effect of topical steroid therapy in CRSwNP patients. Joe et al. [4] combined the data from six RCTs that evaluated the treatment effect on the change in polyp size and found significant improvement in polyp size in the treatment group as compared to controls. In Rudmik et al.'s [5] study, a total of 12 studies were combined for quantitative analysis and demonstrated a significant improvement in nasal symptoms in patients with CRSwNP. The study by Snidvongs et al. [6] demonstrated that topical steroid therapy for CRSwNP resulted in improved overall symptom scores and a higher proportion of responders. Reduction in polyp scores and polyp recurrence after surgery were also recorded. Of note, subgroup analyses according to sinus surgery status revealed that patients with sinus surgery responded to topical steroid more than patients without sinus surgery in polyp score reduction.

The studies by Kalish et al. [7] and Snidvongs et al. [8] evaluated the effect of topical steroid therapy in patients with CRSsNP. Kalish et al. [7] combined the results from five RCTs and concluded that there was insufficient evidence to demonstrate a clear overall benefit for topical steroids in CRSsNP. However, total symptom score was reported in three trials with a standardized mean difference favoring topical steroids. The study conducted by Snidvongs et al. [8] combined the results from ten RCTs and demonstrated that topical steroid therapy results in improved symptom scores and a higher proportion of symptom responders. With a limited number of studies, the subgroup analyses based on sinus surgery status was not significant. A subgroup analysis demonstrated a greater symptom improvement with direct sinus delivery of topical steroid compared to simple nasal delivery.

A prospective, randomized controlled clinical trial comparing the efficacy of a drug-eluting stent (DES) and topical intranasal corticosteroid spray therapy in CRS patients demonstrates that both treatments significantly improved the quality of life with no significant difference between the two groups, except the greater increase in the total nasal cavity volumes favoring the nasal spray group [9].

36.3 Safety

Although nasal topical corticosteroids are very safe in general, they are not completely free of systemic and local side effects. Potential side effects of topical steroid therapy occur in <5% of patients and most commonly including headache, epistaxis, and cough [3].

36.4 Limits

The topical delivery method significantly affects the amount of corticosteroids that comes into then contact with the sinonasal mucosa [1]. The edematous inflammatory mucosa and ostiomeatal occlusion allows <1% of solution volume to enter the sinus cavities before surgery. An adequate ostial opening is necessary for appropriate topical drug distribution [2]. Simple nasal delivery methods such as drops, sprays, and nebulizers provide good nasal cavity contact but poor sinus delivery. Nasal irrigation as well as direct sinus cannulation is likely to provide better delivery to the sinuses, especially after sinus surgery. Compared with nasal delivery (simple sprays/low volume) methods, sinus delivery (direct sinus cannulation or postoperative sinonasal irrigation) methods can achieve greater symptom improvements. No significant difference was found according to reducing polyp size between nasal spray and nasal drops [2]. The poorer performance of the corticosteroid nasal spray, despite the higher dose used, may be due to the fact that corticosteroids are not reaching the sinonasal mucosa effectively [10].

References

1. Chong LY, Head K, Hopkins C, Philpott C, Burton MJ, Schilder AG. Different types of intranasal steroids for chronic rhinosinusitis. Cochrane Database Syst Rev. 2016;(4):CD011993. https://doi.org/10.1002/14651858.CD011993.pub2.
2. Snidvongs K, Kalish L, Sacks R, Sivasubramaniam R, Cope D, Harvey RJ. Sinus surgery and delivery method influence the effectiveness of topical corticosteroids for chronic rhinosinusitis: systematic review and meta-analysis. Am J Rhinol Allergy. 2013;27(3):221–33. https://doi.org/10.2500/ajra.2013.27.3880.
3. Rudmik L, Hoy M, Schlosser RJ, Harvey RJ, Welch KC, Lund V, et al. Topical therapies in the management of chronic rhinosinusitis: an evidence-based review with recommendations. Int Forum Allergy Rhinol. 2013;3(4):281–98. https://doi.org/10.1002/alr.21096.
4. Joe SA, Thambi R, Huang J. A systematic review of the use of intranasal steroids in the treatment of chronic rhinosinusitis. Otolaryngol Head Neck Surg. 2008;139(3):340–7. https://doi.org/10.1016/j.otohns.2008.05.628.
5. Rudmik L, Schlosser RJ, Smith TL, Soler ZM. Impact of topical nasal steroid therapy on symptoms of nasal polyposis: a meta-analysis. Laryngoscope. 2012;122(7):1431–7. https://doi.org/10.1002/lary.23259.
6. Kalish L, Snidvongs K, Sivasubramaniam R, Cope D, Harvey RJ. Topical steroids for nasal polyps. Cochrane Database Syst Rev. 2012;(12):CD006549. https://doi.org/10.1002/14651858.CD006549.pub2.
7. Kalish LH, Arendts G, Sacks R, Craig JC. Topical steroids in chronic rhinosinusitis without polyps: a systematic review and meta-analysis. Otolaryngol Head Neck Surg. 2009;141(6):674–83. https://doi.org/10.1016/j.otohns.2009.08.006.
8. Snidvongs K, Kalish L, Sacks R, Craig JC, Harvey RJ. Topical steroid for chronic rhinosinusitis without polyps. Cochrane Database Syst Rev. 2011;(8):CD009274. https://doi.org/10.1002/14651858.CD009274.
9. Taulu R, Bizaki AJ, Numminen J, Rautiainen M. A prospective, randomized clinical study comparing drug eluting stent therapy and intranasal corticoid steroid therapy in the treatment of patients with chronic rhinosinusitis. Rhinology. 2017;55(3):218–26. https://doi.org/10.4193/Rhino16.070.
10. Harvey RJ, Snidvongs K, Kalish LH, Oakley GM, Sacks R. Corticosteroid nasal irrigations are more effective than simple sprays in a randomized double-blinded placebo-controlled trial for chronic rhinosinusitis after sinus surgery. Int Forum Allergy Rhinol. 2018;8(4):461–70. https://doi.org/10.1002/alr.22093.

Nebulization Corticosteroids

37

Chengshuo Wang, Yifan Meng, and Luo Zhang

Key Points

- Nebulization of corticosteroids is a relatively new treatment in the management of CRS.
- The efficacy and safety of nebulized corticosteroids have been evaluated in several studies.
- Few studies have studied the nebulization of biologics in CRS.

Inhalation drug delivery is a commonly recommended route of administration for the treatment of airway disease [1]. In this regard, nebulization has been a widely used means of drug delivery to both the upper and lower airways [2], particularly in the treatment of asthma [1, 3, 4].

37.1 History, Categories, and Principle of Nebulization

Nebulization therapy is a relatively new method in the treatment of CRS. The first pressurized inhaler was invented 160 years ago by Sales-Girons in France [5]; with the first nebulization device invented to atomize liquid medicine in the early 1860s. In 1950, pneumonia was treated with inhaled corticosteroid as anti-inflammatory agent and 20 years later, beclomethasone was marketed as the first inhaled steroid. Subsequently, numerous steroids were developed for inhalation therapy, including budesonide, which was launched in 1987 by Astra Zeneca. Presently, the modern inhalation devices can generally be classified into three categories: nebulizers, pressurized metered-dose inhalers (pMDI), and dry powder inhalers [5]. Nebulizers are the most historical devices for aerosol therapy and comprise two main types: the jet and ultrasonic nebulizers, respectively, (Fig. 37.1) [6, 7]. However, the nebulizers have a major drawback in that they are noisy, less portable, time-consuming, and inefficient, with up to 50% drug wastage occurring during continuous operation [5]. The pMDI is a portable outpatient aerosol delivery device that is widely used currently. However, a major drawback in pMDI use is that it requires proper hand–mouth coordination, which if not done properly results in less medication getting into the lungs than intended. The breath-actuated dry powder inhaler is another portable outpatient aerosol delivery device that requires no hand–mouth coordination, but has the drawback that it is not suitable for elderly patients and young children, especially as the respirable dose delivered

C. Wang · Y. Meng
Department of Otolaryngology, Head and Neck Surgery, Beijing Tongren Hospital, Capital Medical University, Beijing, China

L. Zhang (✉)
Department of Otolaryngology, Head and Neck Surgery, Beijing Tongren Hospital, Capital Medical University, Beijing, China

Beijing Key Laboratory of Nasal Diseases, Beijing Institute of Otolaryngology, Beijing, China

L. Zhang, C. Bachert (eds.), *Chronic Rhinosinusitis*, https://doi.org/10.1007/978-981-16-0784-4_37

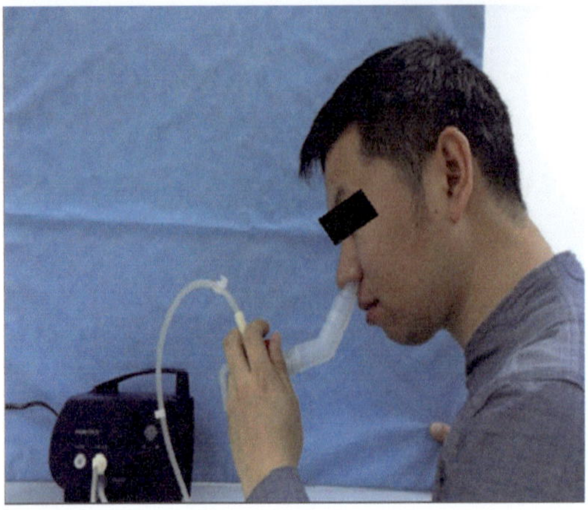

Fig. 37.1 A representative image of ultrasonic transnasal nebulization with corticosteroids

depends on the inspiratory flow rate attained by the user [8].

The efficacy of nebulization evaluated in a study can generally be affected by the dose delivered to the study participant and the site of deposition in the airway [5]. As a first step of topical therapy, although the amount of drug deposited in the nasal mucosa is greater with nasal sprays, nebulization increases the volume of delivery with relatively higher quantities of steroids compared with nasal spray [5–7]. It has been estimated that a 1-min pulsating aerosol delivery can deposit comparable amounts to two puffs of a nasal pump spray in the nasal cavity and 10–15 ml of the nebulized solution into the sinus [5]. Furthermore, evidence suggests that the amount of drug lost through systemic absorption in the nose, due to the vascular nature of the nasal mucosa, is markedly low when delivered by nebulization than when delivered by nasal spray [5]. Thus, transnasal nebulization is likely to be an ideal treatment option for CRS.

37.2 Mechanisms Underlying Efficacy of Steroid Nebulization in the Treatment of CRS

The anti-inflammatory mechanisms underlying corticosteroid therapy generally include reduction in inflammatory cells, suppression of inflammatory cell-associated cytokines and chemotactic factors, and regulation of tissue remodelling [5]. A study by Wang et al. [9] investigating the effect of treatment for 2 weeks with budesonide transnasal nebulization (1 mg twice daily) in patients with eosinophilic CRS has demonstrated that this significantly inhibited eosinophil infiltration, accompanied by lower eotaxin production. Concomitantly, Th2-biased inflammation was also significantly attenuated, as evidenced by reduction of Th2 cell numbers and decrease of IL-5 levels in nasal polyps. Similarly, Van Zele et al. [10] have shown that oral steroids significantly reduced the levels of ECP and IL-5 in nasal secretions of patients with CRSwNP [10]. However, Th1/Th17-mixed inflammation, which is highly associated with neutrophils, has been shown to exhibit reduced sensitivity to corticosteroids [9]. Indeed, treatment with budesonide transnasal nebulization was not found to significantly alter the levels of cytokines IFN-g and IL-17 compared with placebo nebulization, but was found to significantly increase the frequencies of natural regulatory T (Treg) cells and Tr1 cells [9]. Similarly, the cytokine transforming growth factor beta (TGF-b) has also been shown to be increased after treatment with topical corticosteroids and to be associated with elevation of regulatory T cells and suppression of ongoing inflammatory responses [9]. Additionally, excessive collagen deposition in nasal polyp after budesonide transnasal nebulization has been shown to coincide with a significant increase in TGF-b, as well as a significant decrease in matrix metalloproteinases (MMPs) and significant increase in tissue inhibitors of metalloproteinases (TIMPs) [9, 11].

37.3 The Efficacy and Safety of Steroid Nebulization in CRS

Topical corticosteroids have been recommended as an integral part of the strategy for the management of CRS [12]. Clinically, transnasal nebulization of corticosteroids has been shown to be a new option for topical corticosteroids treatment in the CRS (Fig. 37.1). A RCT by Wang et al. [9] has recently indicated that twice-daily administration of budesonide inhalation suspension via a pulsating atomization device (i.e., budesonide transnasal nebulization) was an effective treatment in patients with eosinophilic CRS with nasal polyps, as evidenced by significant improvements in symptom scores, reduction of nasal polyp size, and improvements in several inflammatory markers. A similar earlier study [13] also showed that topical nebulized budesonide effectively reduced the need for systemic prednisone and improved global assessment scores in refractory postoperative CRS patients. Another recent study has shown that nebulized budesonide was significantly more effective than budesonide administered by nasal spray, and equally effective as oral prednisolone, in improving olfactory function in CRS patients [14]. Moreover, nebulization has been shown to provide a wider area of action in the sinonasal mucosa than nasal spray. Indeed, Reychler et al. [14] have demonstrated a significantly greater improvement in olfactory function with budesonide transnasal nebulization, compared with intranasal budesonide delivered with nasal spray. Similarly, Wang et al. [9] have demonstrated that reduction in polyp sizes after 2 weeks' budesonide transnasal nebulization was comparable with that obtained after 4 weeks' treatment with budesonide nasal spray [9], suggesting that steroid treatment by transnasal nebulization may possibly confer a faster onset of action in CRS patients.

Safety of nebulized steroids is a major clinical concern because steroids at high doses have been shown to be associated with systemic side effects, such as suppression of hypothalamic-pituitary-adrenal (HPA) axis and reduction of endogenous cortisol levels. Thamboo et al. [15] have suggested that use of nebulized budesonide (1 mg twice daily for 60 days) is a safe and potentially an ideal treatment option for CRS patients because this did not result in adrenal suppression. In accordance with these findings, Wang et al. [9] have demonstrated that transnasal nebulized budesonide (1 mg twice daily for 2 weeks) is a clinically well-tolerated treatment option in patients with eosinophilic CRS, as neither HPA axis suppress nor any clinically relevant adverse effects were found. However, long-term dose-dependent RCT studies with nebulized steroids are needed to verify the safety of this treatment option for management of CRS.

37.4 Nebulization of Other Drugs in CRS

Antibiotic nebulization has also been used in the CRS treatment; however, few studies have reported the efficacy and safety of this form of treatment. One prospective double-blind, placebo-controlled study has assessed the effect of nebulization of either physiological saline or 80 mg tobramycin three times daily for 4 weeks in CRS patients after failure of medical and surgical treatment [16]. CRS symptoms, quality of life, and endoscopic parameters were assessed at the end of treatment and at 4 weeks' follow-up. The authors found that symptoms and quality of life showed significant improvements in both groups; with tobramycin nebulization associated with faster resolution of pain at 2 weeks but no significant difference by 4 weeks [16]. Similarly, Scheinberg et al. [17] have reported a prospective study of antibiotic nebulization for 3–6 weeks in 41 exacerbated CRS patients resistant to surgical and medical therapy. Antibiotics comprised cefuroxime (285 mg twice daily), ciprofloxacin (70 mg twice daily), or tobramycin (90 mg twice daily), and improved symptoms in 83% of cases [17]. Videler et al. [18] have reported a double-blind prospective, randomized cross-over study investigating the efficacy of bacitracin/colimycin nebulization versus placebo in 14 exacerbated CRS patients resistant to surgical and medical treatment. All patients received 500 mg levofloxacin twice daily for 2 weeks prior to nebulization of either bacitracin/colimycin (6.64 mg/5.12 mg/8 ml) or physiological saline twice daily for 8 days. The authors showed that facial pain was reduced in both treatment groups at the end of the study [18].

37.5 Translation into the Future Daily Practice

Nebulization of corticosteroids is a relatively new treatment option in the management of CRS. Based on available evidence for efficacy and safety of nebulized corticosteroids in the literature, 2 mg budesonide nebulization twice daily should be performed. For CRS patients who need surgical intervention, 2 mg budesonide nebulization twice daily should be performed during the entire peri-operation period, and for the refractory CRS patients (recurrence patients, ASA patients), the dose of nebulized budesonide should be increased accordingly. Some refractory CRS patients may need to be treated by both nebulization and oral corticosteroid to control the inflammation and the serum cortisol levels should be checked intermittently during the OCS treatment.

References

1. Basu K, Nair A, Williamson PA, Mukhopadhyay S, Lipworth BJ. Airway and systemic effects of soluble and suspension formulations of nebulized budesonide in asthmatic children. Ann Allergy Asthma Immunol. 2009;103(5):436–41. https://doi.org/10.1016/s1081-1206(10)60365-1.
2. Prulière-Escabasse V, Michel J, Percodani J, Serrano E, Gilain L, Crampette L, et al. Consensus document for prescription of nebulization in rhinology. Eur Ann Otorhinolaryngol Head Neck Dis. 2014;131(6):371–4. https://doi.org/10.1016/j.anorl.2014.07.004.
3. Chow AH, Tong HH, Chattopadhyay P, Shekunov BY. Particle engineering for pulmonary drug delivery. Pharm Res. 2007;24(3):411–37. https://doi.org/10.1007/s11095-006-9174-3.
4. Ely L, Roa W, Finlay WH, Löbenberg R. Effervescent dry powder for respiratory drug delivery. Eur J Pharm Biopharm. 2007;65(3):346–53. https://doi.org/10.1016/j.ejpb.2006.10.021.
5. Lou H, Wang C, Zhang L. Steroid transnasal nebulization in the treatment of chronic rhinosinusitis. Curr Opin Allergy Clin Immunol. 2016;16(1):39–44. https://doi.org/10.1097/aci.0000000000000230.
6. Sanders M. Inhalation therapy: an historical review. Prim Care Respir J. 2007;16(2):71–81. https://doi.org/10.3132/pcrj.2007.00017.
7. Labiris NR, Dolovich MB. Pulmonary drug delivery. Part II: The role of inhalant delivery devices and drug formulations in therapeutic effectiveness of aerosolized medications. Br J Clin Pharmacol. 2003;56(6):600–12. https://doi.org/10.1046/j.1365-2125.2003.01893.x.
8. Dolovich MB, Ahrens RC, Hess DR, Anderson P, Dhand R, Rau JL, et al. Device selection and outcomes of aerosol therapy: evidence-based guidelines: American College of Chest Physicians/American College of Asthma, Allergy, and Immunology. Chest. 2005;127(1):335–71. https://doi.org/10.1378/chest.127.1.335.
9. Wang C, Lou H, Wang X, Wang Y, Fan E, Li Y, et al. Effect of budesonide transnasal nebulization in patients with eosinophilic chronic rhinosinusitis with nasal polyps. J Allergy Clin Immunol. 2015;135(4):922–29.e6. https://doi.org/10.1016/j.jaci.2014.10.018.
10. Van Zele T, Gevaert P, Holtappels G, Beule A, Wormald PJ, Mayr S, et al. Oral steroids and doxycycline: two different approaches to treat nasal polyps. J Allergy Clin Immunol. 2010;125(5):1069–76.e4. https://doi.org/10.1016/j.jaci.2010.02.020.
11. Li X, Meng J, Qiao X, Liu Y, Liu F, Zhang N, et al. Expression of TGF, matrix metalloproteinases, and tissue inhibitors in Chinese chronic rhinosinusitis. J Allergy Clin Immunol. 2010;125(5):1061–8. https://doi.org/10.1016/j.jaci.2010.02.023.
12. Fokkens WJ, Lund VJ, Mullol J, Bachert C, Alobid I, Baroody F, et al. EPOS 2012: European position paper on rhinosinusitis and nasal polyps 2012. A summary for otorhinolaryngologists. Rhinology. 2012;50(1):1–12. https://doi.org/10.4193/Rhino50E2.
13. Kanowitz SJ, Batra PS, Citardi MJ. Topical budesonide via mucosal atomization device in refractory postoperative chronic rhinosinusitis. Otolaryngol Head Neck Surg. 2008;139(1):131–6. https://doi.org/10.1016/j.otohns.2008.03.009.
14. Reychler G, Colbrant C, Huart C, Le Guellec S, Vecellio L, Liistro G, et al. Effect of three-drug delivery modalities on olfactory function in chronic sinusitis. Laryngoscope. 2015;125(3):549–55. https://doi.org/10.1002/lary.24937.
15. Thamboo A, Manji J, Szeitz A, Santos RD, Hathorn I, Gan EC, et al. The safety and efficacy of short-term budesonide delivered via mucosal atomization device for chronic rhinosinusitis without nasal polyposis. Int Forum Allergy Rhinol. 2014;4(5):397–402. https://doi.org/10.1002/alr.21280.
16. Desrosiers MY, Salas-Prato M. Treatment of chronic rhinosinusitis refractory to other treatments with topical antibiotic therapy delivered by means of a large-particle nebulizer: results of a controlled trial. Otolaryngol Head Neck Surg. 2001;125(3):265–9. https://doi.org/10.1067/mhn.2001.117410.
17. Scheinberg PA, Otsuji A. Nebulized antibiotics for the treatment of acute exacerbations of chronic rhinosinusitis. Ear Nose Throat J. 2002;81(9):648–52.
18. Videler WJ, van Drunen CM, Reitsma JB, Fokkens WJ. Nebulized bacitracin/colimycin: a treatment option in recalcitrant chronic rhinosinusitis with *Staphylococcus aureus*? A double-blind, randomized, placebo-controlled, cross-over pilot study. Rhinology. 2008;46(2):92–8.

Steroid-Eluting Stent Placement 38

Chengshuo Wang, Longgang Yu, and Luo Zhang

Key Points

- Topical treatment is an integral part of the CRS management plan; with steroid-eluting stent placement recommended as a useful adjuvant therapy.
- Steroid-eluting stents can not only achieve locally controlled release of steroids at known doses, but also separate the raw edges of mucosal wounds and prevent adhesion formation and stenosis.
- The effectiveness and safety of steroid-eluting stents have been demonstrated in several prospective, randomized, controlled trials.
- Steroid-eluting stents significantly reduce postoperative polyposis, adhesions, middle turbinate lateralization, the need for postoperative interventions, systemic steroids, and revision surgery.

C. Wang
Department of Otolaryngology, Head and Neck Surgery, Beijing Tongren Hospital, Capital Medical University, Beijing, China

Beijing Key Laboratory of Nasal Diseases, Beijing Institute of Otolaryngology, Beijing, China

L. Yu
Department of Otolaryngology, Head and Neck Surgery, The Affiliated Hospital of Qingdao University, Qingdao, China

L. Zhang (✉)
Department of Otolaryngology, Head and Neck Surgery, Beijing Tongren Hospital, Capital Medical University, Beijing, China

Beijing Key Laboratory of Nasal Diseases, Beijing Institute of Otolaryngology, Beijing, China

Department of Allergy, Beijing Tongren Hospital, Capital Medical University, Beijing, China

38.1 Introduction

Chronic rhinosinusitis is a common and challenging entity in clinical practice. Medical treatment is the primary treatment modality for chronic rhinosinusitis, and if medical treatment fails, functional endoscopic sinus surgery (FESS) is the next step [1]. Endoscopic sinus surgery has been shown to be an effective way to maintain patency of flow pathways in the ciliated respiratory epithelium, as well as to create a dosing channel for postoperative saline irrigation and local administration of steroids. Although FESS has proven to be an effective treatment for chronic rhinosinusitis, surgery cannot treat the underlying predisposing causes that affect the disease. Moreover, surgical treatment may fail for a variety of reasons, including adhesion formation, recurrent nasal polyps, mucosal inflammation, middle turbinate lateralization, and surgical ostial stenosis [2].

Thus, postoperative medical therapy is as important for long-term control of the disease as the surgery itself. Topical or systemic corticosteroids are currently indispensable for the treat-

L. Zhang, C. Bachert (eds.), *Chronic Rhinosinusitis*, https://doi.org/10.1007/978-981-16-0784-4_38

ment of chronic rhinosinusitis and postoperative management of FESS [3]. Systemic steroids are highly effective in reducing postoperative edema and promoting postoperative healing, however, there may be significant side effects, including aseptic necrosis of the femoral head, uncontrolled hyperglycemia in diabetic patients, and orbital and psychiatric complications. Although topical steroid spray administration has no systemic side effects, the rate of middle meatus penetration appears to be low, and its benefits can be further reduced by poor adhesion and postoperative edema, secretions, or crusting. In addition, most steroid drug delivery systems cannot successfully reach the frontal sinus due to its anatomical location. In addition, other problems arise with the use of corticosteroid nasal sprays, such as incorrect dosing technique and lack of motivation to use the recommended medications regularly and for extended periods. The original topical approach to intranasal steroid delivery is therefore suboptimal, and new methods of delivering corticosteroids and other drugs directly to the nasal mucosa in a controlled manner have emerged.

38.2 Review of Steroid-Eluting Stents

A stent is defined as a device that is temporarily placed in the body cavity to keep the cavity open, promote wound healing, and relieve obstruction. A drug-eluting stent is a surgically implanted stent that helps heal the affected tissue by releasing the loaded drug locally and continuously in a controlled manner over an intended period of time [4]. Drug-eluting stents can be constructed from rigid and pliable absorbable or nonabsorbable (metal) materials. The biodegradable absorbable drug-eluting devices are superior to metal stents because their bioabsorbability does not result in late stent thrombosis. Biodegradable implants consist of biodegradable polymeric materials, which degrade in vivo over long periods of time. The main advantage of these implants is that they do not require additional surgery for their removal.

Drugs loaded onto nasal stents include: corticosteroids such as dexamethasone, fluticasone, and mometasone, as well as antibiotics for bacterial infections. Steroid-eluting stents have now been introduced in the clinic as a novel approach to optimize surgical outcomes by delivering locally sustained release of corticosteroids directly to inflamed sinus tissue for the treatment of recurrent nasal polyposis after surgery. The advantage of this targeted application is the precise delivery of high concentrations of the drugs to the diseased mucosa in a controlled manner, while reducing the risk of systemic absorption and the accompanying complications.

The most studied steroid-eluting stent is the absorbable implant with mometasone furoate, which consists of three components: a polymer stent, a polyethylene glycol coating, and mometasone furoate embedded in the coating. Because of its long history of safety and efficacy in humans, biodegradable polymers such as polylactic acid (PLA) or polylactic-co-glycolic acid (PLGA) are used in the framework system of nasal implants. Polylactic-co-glycolide is an inert monofilament that is woven into a mesh. The lamellar structure on the monofilament is a drug-eluting formulation of polyethylene glycol and the active ingredient mometasone furoate. Mometasone furoate, a highly lipophilic compound with good anti-inflammatory effects and biosafety, is one of the most commonly used topical corticosteroids for the treatment of chronic sinusitis. Polyethylene glycol helps regulate the release of mometasone furoate and also has mild anti-inflammatory properties. A dose of mometasone furoate embedded in polyethylene glycol is released in a controlled manner as the implant dissolves.

The method of stent implantation involves the following steps: Prior to implantation, the steroid-eluting stent is compressed in the delivery sheath, which has a suitable length and angle. The front end of the delivery sheath is introduced into the ethmoid sinus or frontal recess, under the vision of an endoscope. The implant is then advanced through a syringe-like mechanism, and after delivery the device expands like a spring to fit the contour of the implanted site. The stent can be placed at the desired site intraoperatively or during the early postoperative period [5].

38.3 Efficacy of Steroid-Eluting Stents

Since FDA approval of steroid stents for the treatment of nasal polyps in 2011 [6], three major clinical trials have demonstrated the effectiveness of mometasone nasal stents.

Murr and colleagues [7] conducted a prospective, multicenter, randomized, double-blind clinical trial involving a total of 43 CRS patients, who had undergone functional endoscopic sinus surgery (FESS). Following surgery, 38 patients acted as intrapatient controls, with drug-eluting stents placed on one side and non-drug-eluting stents on the opposite side, and 5 patients had drug-eluting stents placed in bilateral cavities to evaluate the systematic safety. Endoscopic follow-up was performed at 7, 14, 21, 30, 45, and 60 days after operation for assessment of inflammation, polyp formation, adhesions, and middle turbinate position. Within 30 days after operation, the drug-eluting stents significantly reduced the frequency of inflammation, polyp formation, and obvious adhesion, compared to control stents. Additionally, the frequency of middle turbinate lateralization also decreased; however, the difference was not statistically significant between the active and control stents.

Similarly, Forwith and colleagues [8] conducted the ADVANCE study, a prospective, multicenter clinical trial investigating the efficacy and safety of steroid-eluting nasal stents in 10 patients with unilateral stents and 40 patients with bilateral stents post-FESS. Follow-up assessments were scheduled 7, 14, 21, 30, 60 days and 6 months after surgery for grading of inflammation, polyp formation, adhesions, and middle turbinate position. Consistent with Murr's findings [7], steroid stents lowered the inflammation scores, fewer polypoid edema, adhesion formation and middle turbinate lateralization. Furthermore, questionnaires such as SNOT-22 (the SinoNasal Outcome Test-22) and RSDI (The Rhinosinusitis Disability Index) showed significant improvements in patient-reported outcomes.

To determine whether steroid-eluting nasal stents could reduce the need for post-surgical oral steroids and post-surgical adhesions in CRS patients, Marple and colleagues [9] conducted another prospective, multicenter, randomized, controlled, double-blind trial, using an intrapatient control design (ADVANCE II). 105 patients who had undergone bilateral ESS surgery were implanted with drug-releasing and non-drug-releasing stents in opposite sides and followed up at days 14, 30, 60, and 90 for evaluation of postoperative interventions, polyposis, and adhesions. This study showed that, compared with non-drug-releasing implants, drug-releasing implants provided a relative decrease of 29.0% ($P = 0.028$) in postoperative interventions and 52% ($P = 0.005$) in lysis of adhesions. The relative reduction rate of frank polyposis was 44.9% ($P = 0.002$).

With the increase in the variety of steroid-eluting stents, more drug-loaded and longer-lasting stents have been used to treat recurrent nasal polyps after ESS. Several major clinical trials have demonstrated the effectiveness of this new generation of stents.

A prospective multicore pilot study conducted by Lavigne and colleagues [10] showed that bioabsorbable steroid-eluting implants improved patients' polyp endoscopic grading, patient-reported outcomes, and reduced the need for revision surgery. At 1 month after surgery, the mean bilateral polyp grade decreased from 4.5 at baseline to 2.3 ($P = 0.008$) and sustained through 6 months (2.33; $P = 0.008$). The mean SNOT-22 score was significantly improved from 2.19 at baseline to 0.90 ($P = 0.001$) within 1 month and persisted to 6 months (1.03; $P = 0.012$) and 64% of patients no longer needed revision ESS at 6 months.

RESOLVE, a randomized, controlled, double-blind trial conducted by Han and colleagues [11, 12], involved a total of 100 patients, including 53 patients with steroid-eluting stents and 47 patients with sham stents. At 3 and 6 months after operation, both polyp grading and ethmoid sinus obstruction in the treatment group were significantly reduced and nasal congestion/congestion scores were significantly improved compared to the control group. At 6 months, the risk of remaining "indicated for ESS" in the control group was 3.6 times higher than that in the treatment group.

RESOLVE 2, another randomized, double-blind, sham-controlled trial was undertaken in 300 patients with refractory chronic rhinosinusitis with NPs (CRSwNP), who were likely to require repeat surgery [13]. The patients were randomized to in-office placement of two corticosteroid-eluting sinus implants or a sham procedure, and assessed for the change from baseline to day 30 in nasal obstruction/congestion score, and change from baseline to day 90 in bilateral polyp grade. Compared with the control group, patients treated with implants had significantly lower nasal obstruction/obstruction scores ($P = 0.0074$) and bilateral polyp grading ($P = 0.0073$). At day 90, the implants also significantly reduced the proportion of patients still indicated for repeat sinus surgery ($P = 0.0004$), percent ethmoid sinus obstruction ($P = 0.0007$), nasal obstruction/congestion ($P = 0.0248$), and decreased olfaction ($P = 0.0470$). Significant improvements in subjective and objective indicators suggest that mometasone sinus implants may play an important role in the treatment of recurrent nasal polyps.

38.4 Safety of Steroid-Eluting Stents

Almost all of the above-mentioned clinical trials monitored the possible adverse reactions of steroid stent implantation and indicated that the incidence of adverse reactions was satisfactorily low. Moreover, the study by Murr and colleagues [7] showed that the concentration of mometasone in plasma was lower than the quantitative limit of detection of the liquid chromatography technique, and the average cortisol concentration was at normal level in all five patients with bilateral stents at baseline and other follow-up time points. This suggests that steroid stents did not cause adrenal suppression.

The systemic absorption and ocular safety of steroid-eluting stents, however, are of particular concern to researchers. Consequently, a number of clinical trials have focused on the effects of implants on the eyes, as assessed by changes in intraocular pressure and slit lamp examination of lens opacity, but have not found significant increases in neither intraocular pressure nor nuclear sclerosis or cataract grading. However, other reported adverse reactions include epistaxis, nasal discomfort, nasal pain, decreased sense of smell, and other minor complaints. The Kern study [13], for example, reported that one patient developed severe epistaxis.

38.5 Use of Stents in the Frontal Sinus Ostia

Treatment of frontal sinuses in patients with chronic sinusitis is a challenge for otolaryngologists. Greater anatomical complexity, proximity to important structures such as the skull base and orbit, narrow and angular vision make the surgical management of the frontal sinus much more difficult than that of other sinuses. Moreover, due to the action of gravity, it is difficult for local drugs to reach the frontal sinus. Therefore, inflammation and restenosis of frontal sinus ostia are prone to occur after surgery. This provides broad prospects for the use of steroid-eluting stents in frontal sinus (Fig. 38.1).

Currently, two double-blind randomized controlled trials have investigated the effectiveness and safety of bioabsorbable steroid-releasing sinus implants for the frontal sinus opening. The two RCTs shared the same study protocol, using an intrapatient control design in 80 patients who underwent the same endoscopic frontal sinus surgery for CRS, to compare frontal sinus implants with contralateral frontal sinus without the implants. Smith and colleagues [14] found that compared with the control group, oral steroids and surgical intervention requirements in the steroid implant study group were reduced by 55.6% and 75%, and inflammation scores and restenosis rates were decreased by 16.7% and 54.3%, respectively, 30 days after surgery. Furthermore,

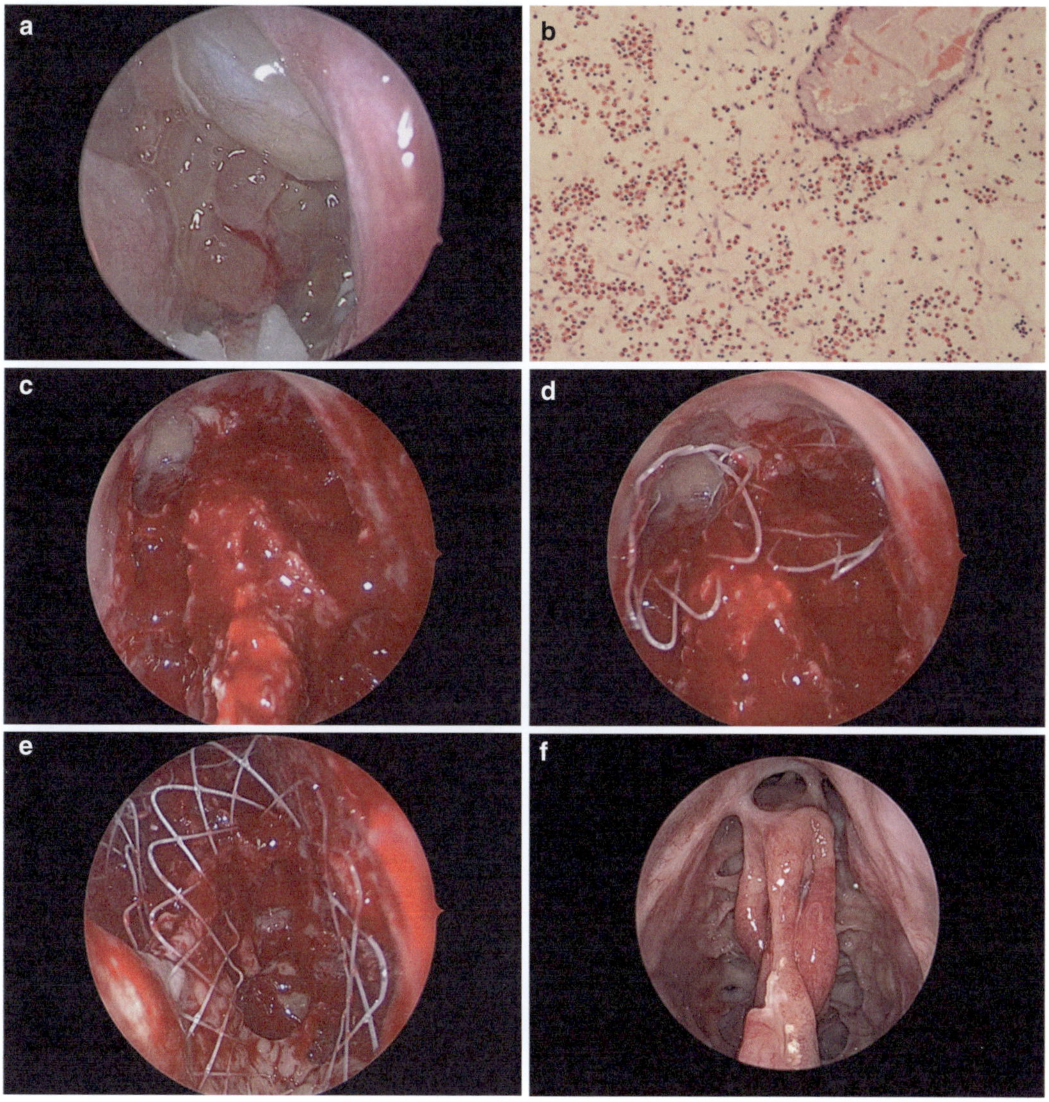

Fig. 38.1 (**a**) Nasal polyps in a patient with recurrent rhinosinusitis with comorbid asthma prior to surgery. (**b**) Histological assessment of polyps of the patient, demonstrating infiltration by a large number of eosinophils. (**c**) Intraoperative endoscopic view of frontal sinus after the Draf 3 procedure. (**d**) Steroid-eluting sinus stents in the frontal sinuses. (**e**) Steroid-eluting sinus stents in the ethmoid sinuses. (**f**) Endoscopic view of the frontal sinus, 6 months post-surgery

in the steroid implant group the frontal sinus diameter was increased by 32.2% and there was a significant reduction in the need for intervention 90 days post-ESS, compared to the control group.

In another study Luong and colleagues [15] evaluated the safety and efficacy of another hourglass steroid-releasing sinus implant. These authors demonstrated that on the 30th day following surgery, there were significantly fewer patients requiring intervention, lower inflammatory scores, and fewer restenosis occlusion rates in the active treatment group than in the control group. Moreover, at 90 days postoperatively, the reduction in the need for postoperative intervention and frontal sinus occlusion were still maintained.

More recently, Singh and colleagues [16] have pooled and analyzed the data from the studies by Smith and colleagues [14] and Luong and colleagues [15]. Analysis of the pooled data showed that at 30 days after surgery, the demand for postoperative intervention in the steroid stent study group was significantly decreased by 46.8%, surgical intervention was decreased by 51.2%, and oral steroid intervention decreased by 37.2%. The effect of steroid sinus implants was also maintained until day 90 after surgery; with the combined data showing postoperative intervention requirements and restenosis/occlusion rate of the sinus opening to be significantly reduced, and the diameter of the frontal sinus opening significantly larger than in the control group. No implant-related adverse reactions occurred.

38.6 Conclusions and Future Perspectives

At present, it is more recognized that the treatment of CRS is aimed at reducing symptoms, improving quality of life, and preventing disease progression or recurrence. Topical treatment is an integral part of the CRS management plan, which has good safety and can be repeated or sustained over a long period of time; thus avoiding the risk of long-term oral corticosteroids, antibiotics, and repeat surgery. Most commonly used topical treatment includes topical saline irrigations and topical corticosteroids. In the past 10 years, increasing attention has been paid to the use of steroid-eluting stents as a new topical therapy strategy. These stents are efficacious, well tolerated and demonstrate no obvious adverse reactions. Steroid-eluting sinus implants are unique in that they achieve locally controlled release of known doses of steroids and are also used to separate the healing sinus tissues and reduce adhesion and restenosis.

Previous studies have shown that steroid-eluting stents can be used after ESS to reduce postoperative adhesion and polyp formation, lateralization of the middle turbinate, and the need for oral steroids and intervention. Steroid-eluting stents can also be used to treat recurrent nasal polyps, relieve sinus inflammation, nasal congestion, and surgical needs. Over time, different types of stents suitable for ethmoid sinus, frontal sinus, and other sinuses have been developed, and stents containing different dosages of drugs have been gradually introduced in clinical practice. Steroid-eluting stents are a useful complement to medical devices for CRS management, especially in patients with refractory nasal polyps, and have the potential to combine with more minimally invasive surgery such as sinus balloon dilation to control inflammatory processes. Thus, use of steroid-eluting sinus implants is recommended as a useful adjuvant therapy for CRS.

At present, steroid-eluting stents are only used in a few countries and the cost of stent placement is still relatively high. Rudmik et al. [17] used the decision tree model to confirm the cost-effectiveness of mometasone steroid-eluting sinus implants after ESS in refractory chronic rhinosinusitis, which can prevent clinical intervention within 60 days after ESS. Rizzo et al. [18] found that the upfront cost of implants in patients with refractory chronic rhinosinusitis was largely offset by savings associated with polyp recurrence, adhesion release, and subsequent treatment.

Current evidence suggests that steroid-eluting stents reduce the need for postoperative surgical intervention and polyp formation and significantly improve early postoperative outcomes. Unfortunately, these randomized controlled trial [7–9, 11–15] studies were followed up for no more than 6 months. Taulu et al. [19] conducted a prospective randomized clinical trial following up for more than 6 months and found that ethmoid drug-eluting stents were not superior to nasal corticosteroid sprays in the prevention of nasal endoscopic surgery. In the future, it is necessary to conduct further randomized controlled trials to evaluate the safety and long-term efficacy of steroid-eluting stents.

Overall, drug-eluting stent implantation is a promising new technique in the treatment of CRS. In the future, new stents loaded with other drug components such as anti-infective agents, anti-interleukin drugs, anti-IgE medications or different drug combinations, larger doses of corticosteroids or longer drug elution time need to be further developed.

References

1. Fokkens WJ, Lund VJ, Mullol J, Bachert C, Alobid I, Baroody F, et al. European position paper on rhinosinusitis and nasal polyps 2012. Rhinol Suppl. 2012;23:3 p preceding table of contents, 1–298.
2. Bernstein JM, Lebowitz RA, Jacobs JB. Initial report on postoperative healing after endoscopic sinus surgery with the microdebrider. Otolaryngol Head Neck Surg. 1998;118(6):800–3.
3. Shen J, Welch K, Kern R. Mometasone furoate sinus implant – a new targeted approach to treating recurrent nasal polyp disease. Expert Rev Clin Pharmacol. 2018;11(12):1163–70.
4. Parikh A, Anand U, Ugwu MC, Feridooni T, Massoud E, Agu RU. Drug-eluting nasal implants: formulation, characterization, clinical applications and challenges. Pharmaceutics. 2014;6(2):249–67.
5. Bury S, Singh A. Evaluation of a steroid releasing sinus implant for the treatment of patients undergoing frontal sinus surgery for chronic rhinosinusitis. Expert Rev Med Devices. 2017;14(2):93–101.
6. Santarelli GD, Han JK. Evaluation of the PROPEL((R)) mini sinus implant for the treatment of frontal sinus disease. Expert Opin Drug Deliv. 2016;13(12):1789–93.
7. Murr AH, Smith TL, Hwang PH, Bhattacharyya N, Lanier BJ, Stambaugh JW, et al. Safety and efficacy of a novel bioabsorbable, steroid-eluting sinus stent. Int Forum Allergy Rhinol. 2011;1(1):23–32.
8. Forwith KD, Chandra RK, Yun PT, Miller SK, Jampel HD. ADVANCE: a multisite trial of bioabsorbable steroid-eluting sinus implants. Laryngoscope. 2011;121(11):2473–80.
9. Marple BF, Smith TL, Han JK, Gould AR, Jampel HD, Stambaugh JW, et al. Advance II: a prospective, randomized study assessing safety and efficacy of bioabsorbable steroid-releasing sinus implants. Otolaryngol Head Neck Surg. 2012;146(6):1004–11.
10. Lavigne F, Miller SK, Gould AR, Lanier BJ, Romett JL. Steroid-eluting sinus implant for in-office treatment of recurrent nasal polyposis: a prospective, multicenter study. Int Forum Allergy Rhinol. 2014;4(5):381–9.
11. Han JK, Forwith KD, Smith TL, Kern RC, Brown WJ, Miller SK, et al. RESOLVE: a randomized, controlled, blinded study of bioabsorbable steroid-eluting sinus implants for in-office treatment of recurrent sinonasal polyposis. Int Forum Allergy Rhinol. 2014;4(11):861–70.
12. Forwith KD, Han JK, Stolovitzky JP, Yen DM, Chandra RK, Karanfilov B, et al. RESOLVE: bioabsorbable steroid-eluting sinus implants for in-office treatment of recurrent sinonasal polyposis after sinus surgery: 6-month outcomes from a randomized, controlled, blinded study. Int Forum Allergy Rhinol. 2016;6(6):573–81.
13. Kern RC, Stolovitzky JP, Silvers SL, Singh A, Lee JT, Yen DM, et al. A phase 3 trial of mometasone furoate sinus implants for chronic sinusitis with recurrent nasal polyps. Int Forum Allergy Rhinol. 2018;8(4):471–81.
14. Smith TL, Singh A, Luong A, Ow RA, Shotts SD, Sautter NB, et al. Randomized controlled trial of a bioabsorbable steroid-releasing implant in the frontal sinus opening. Laryngoscope. 2016;126(12):2659–64.
15. Luong A, Ow RA, Singh A, Weiss RL, Han JK, Gerencer R, et al. Safety and effectiveness of a bioabsorbable steroid-releasing implant for the paranasal sinus ostia: a randomized clinical trial. JAMA Otolaryngol Head Neck Surg. 2017;144(1):28–35.
16. Singh A, Luong AU, Fong KJ, Ow RA, Han JK, Gerencer R, et al. Bioabsorbable steroid-releasing implants in the frontal sinus ostia: a pooled analysis. Int Forum Allergy Rhinol. 2019;9(2):131–9.
17. Rudmik L, Smith TL. Economic evaluation of a steroid-eluting sinus implant following endoscopic sinus surgery for chronic rhinosinusitis. Otolaryngol Head Neck Surg. 2014;151(2):359–66.
18. Rizzo JA, Rudmik L, Mallow PJ, Palli SR. Budget impact analysis of bioabsorbable drug-eluting sinus implants following endoscopic sinus surgery. J Med Econ. 2016;19(9):829–35.
19. Taulu R, Sillanpaa N, Numminen J, Rautiainen M. Ethmoidal drug-eluting stent therapy is not superior to nasal corticosteroid spray in the prevention of endoscopic sinus surgery: results from a randomised, clinical trial. Clin Otolaryngol. 2020;45(3):402–8.

Steroid Infiltrated Packing Materials

39

Yueqi Sun and Jianbo Shi

Key Points

- Steroid infiltrated packing materials could improve clinical symptoms and wound healings post-ESS, but evidence of their long-term benefits is lacking.
- Steroid-impregnated packing materials may suppress serum cortisol levels during the early postoperative period.

Since the use of oral steroids in the post-ESS period has shown promising results in reducing inflammation and recurrence [1], there has been an interest in the use of steroid infiltrated packing materials for their potentially better anti-inflammatory effect in the sinus cavity than oral steroids while avoiding the side effects of systemic steroids. A variety of commercially available nasal packing materials, both nonabsorbable and absorbable, have been used as steroid delivery systems (Table 39.1). No studies have directly compared efficacy of nonabsorbable to absorbable materials for steroid delivery, although many practitioners consider absorbable materials more efficacious and convenient because there is no need to remove the pack postoperatively.

Merocel (Medtronic Inc., Minneapolis, MN, USA) is one of the most common nonabsorbable nasal packing materials. It is a compressed, dehydrated sponge made of hydroxylated polyvinyl acetate. When rehydrated with normal saline, it becomes enlarged and swollen and compresses a bleeding vessel within the nasal cavity. In a double-blinded, randomized, controlled trial of 64 patients with CRS who were randomized to a medication-soaked Merocel (either one of budesonide, gentamicin, or Manuka honey) in one nostril or a nonmedicated Merocel in the contralateral side for 7 days following ESS [2] (Table 39.2), however, all three medication-soaked interventions did not reach significant difference in tissue inflammation as determined by histology, endoscopic score of mucosal wound healing, and pain on pack removal compared with the nonmedicated intervention, although budesonide-soaked Merocel showed a trend toward reduced inflammation and decreased pain on removal.

NasoPore (Stryker, Kalamazoo, Michigan, USA) is one of the most commonly used biodegradable nasal packing materials that consists of fully synthetic biodegradable, fragmenting foam. It can provide pressure against bleeding

Y. Sun
Department of Otolaryngology, The Seventh Affiliated Hospital, Sun Yat-sen University, Shenzhen, China

Otorhinolaryngology Hospital, The First Affiliated Hospital, Sun Yat-sen University, Guangzhou, China

J. Shi (✉)
Otorhinolaryngology Hospital, The First Affiliated Hospital, Sun Yat-sen University, Guangzhou, China

L. Zhang, C. Bachert (eds.), *Chronic Rhinosinusitis*, https://doi.org/10.1007/978-981-16-0784-4_39

Table 39.1 Commercially available nasal packing materials

	Brand	Compounds	Corporation
Nonabsorbable	Merocel	Expandable polyvinyl acetate foam tampons	Medtronic (USA)
Absorbable	NasoPore	Synthetic polyurethane foam	Stryker (USA)
	Surgicel	Oxidized cellulose	ETHICOM (USA)
	Sinu-Foam	Carboxymethyl cellulose	ArthroCare ENT (USA)
	Gelfoam	Gelatin	Pfizer (USA)
	Algi-Pack	Calcium alginate	MD Pharm (South Korea)

vessels within the nasal cavity after absorbing water or blood. Within several days after placing, NasoPore starts to dissolve and can be suctioned from the nasal cavity. Three randomized, double-blinded, placebo-controlled studies have evaluated effect of steroid-impregnated NasoPore on clinical symptoms and wound healings post-ESS with consistent results (Table 39.2). Zhao et al. [3] studied 64 patients with CRSwNP who were randomized to a mometasone-impregnated NasoPore in one nostril or a nonmedicated NasoPore in the contralateral side. They found patients who received the 8-mL mometasone-impregnated packing for 2 weeks had significantly improved Perioperative Sinus Endoscopy score and Lund-Kennedy score at 1, 2, and 3 postoperative months. Côté et al. [4] found significantly improved Perioperative Sinus Endoscopy score and Lund-Kennedy score up to 6 months postoperatively among 19 patients with CRSwNP who were randomized to receive triamcinolone-impregnated NasoPore in one nostril and saline-impregnated NasoPore contralaterally. Xu et al. [5] evaluated 80 patients with CRSwNP who were randomized to receive triamcinolone-impregnated or unmedicated NasoPore and found that patients who received the triamcinolone-impregnated packing had significantly decreased Sino-Nasal Outcome Test 20 (SNOT-20), Perioperative Sinus Endoscopy score and Lund-Kennedy score and improved olfactory dysfunction determined by Korean Version of the Sniffin' Stick (KVSS) II test at postoperative 1 and 3 months. In addition, More et al. [6] found no statistical difference in Sinonasal Assessment Questionnaire (SNAQ-11) and Perioperative Sinus Endoscopy score at postoperative 4 and 8 weeks among 41 patients with CRSwNP in a retrospective case–control study where the cavities in one arm were treated triamcinolone-impregnated NasoPore, while the others received a short course of oral steroids (starting at 24 mg/day and tapered over 6 days).

There are few studies that have evaluated side effects of steroid-impregnated nasal packing materials. In an another randomized, double-blinded, placebo-controlled study (Table 39.2), Hong et al. [7] evaluated the systemic effects and safety of steroid-impregnated NasoPore post-ESS. Twenty patients with CRS were randomized to receive nasal packing with triamcinolone-soaked or unmedicated-impregnated NasoPore after ESS. Nasal packing materials were removed at postoperative 10 days. They found that triamcinolone-impregnated nasal packing suppressed serum cortisol levels during the early postoperative period and this systemic effect resolved by postoperative day 10. This study suggests that although significant HPA axis suppression is unlikely, systemic steroid absorption might occur when using steroid-impregnated nasal packing materials post-ESS. Furthermore, the clinical effects of steroid-impregnating absorbable nasal packing reported by other studies [4–6] might be because of systemic absorption as well as direct topical effects of the steroids.

There were also other commercially available nasal packing materials, such as Stammberger Sinu-Foam, Gelfoam and Algi-Pack, that have been reported to be used as steroid delivery systems [9–11]. Largely consistent results were found across those studies (Table 39.2).

Table 39.2 Efficacy of steroid infiltrated packing materials in postoperative CRS

References	Packing materials	Sample size, n	Comparison method	Study outcomes	Efficacy comparisons
Change et al. [2]	Merocel® with budesonide	48	Intrapatient	Comfort: VAS on pack removal Wound healing: endoscopic score Anti-inflammation: mucosal biopsy	=Unmedicated Merocel for comfort, wound healing, and anti-inflammation
Zhao et al. [3]	NasoPore® with mometasone	64	Intrapatient	Wound healing: Perioperative sinus endoscopy and Lund-Kennedy score	>Unmedicated NasoPore for wound healing
Côté et al. [4]	NasoPore® with triamcinolone	19	Intrapatient	Wound healing: Perioperative sinus endoscopy and Lund-Kennedy score	>Unmedicated NasoPore for wound healing
Xu et al. [5]	NasoPore® with triamcinolone	80	Interpatient	Comfort: SNOT-20 and olfactory dysfunction Wound healing: Perioperative sinus endoscopy and Lund-Kennedy score	>Unmedicated NasoPore for comfort and wound healing
More et al. [6]	NasoPore® with triamcinolone	41	Interpatient	Comfort: Sinonasal Assessment Questionnaire Wound healing: Perioperative sinus endoscopy score	=Oral steroids for comfort and wound healing
Hong et al. [7]	NasoPore® with triamcinolone	20	Interpatient	Safety: Serum cortisol, 12-h urine cortisol, serum adrenal-corticotropic hormone (ACTH), and serum osteocalcin	>Unmedicated NasoPore for safety on serum cortisol levels during the early postoperative period
Wataru et al. [8]	Surgicel® with triamcinolone	43	Interpatient	Comfort: olfactory dysfunction Wound healing: CT score Anti-inflammation: polyp score Need for oral steroid intake	>Topical steroid for comfort, wound healing and need for oral steroid intake, but not anti-inflammation
Rudmik et al. [9]	Sinu-Foam® with dexamethasone	36	Interpatient	Wound healing: Lund-Kennedy score	=Unmedicated Sinu-Foam for wound healing
Mohammad et al. [10]	Gelfoam with triamcinolone	60	Interpatient	Comfort: olfactory dysfunction	>Unmedicated Gelfoam for comfort
Hwang et al. [11]	Algi-Pack with triamcinolone	22	Intrapatient	Wound healing: Perioperative Sinus Endoscopy score	>Unmedicated calcium alginate packing for wound healing

39.1 Translation into Future Daily Practice

Steroid infiltrated packing materials have an acceptable safety profile and show promising results with improved clinical symptoms and wound healings after ESS. The long-term benefits that these steroid-soaked materials may have on the CRS course still need further studies.

References

1. Wright ED, Agrawal S. Impact of perioperative systemic steroids on surgical outcomes in patients with chronic rhinosinusitis with polyposis: evaluation with the novel Perioperative Sinus Endoscopy (POSE) scoring system. Laryngoscope. 2007;117(11 Pt 2 Suppl 115):1–28. https://doi.org/10.1097/MLG.0b013e31814842f8.
2. Chang EH, Alandejani T, Akbari E, Ostry A, Javer A. Double-blinded, randomized, controlled trial of medicated versus nonmedicated merocel sponges for functional endoscopic sinus surgery. J Otolaryngol Head Neck Surg. 2011;40(Suppl 1):S14–9.
3. Zhao KQ, Yu YQ, Yu HM. Effects of mometasone furoate-impregnated biodegradable nasal dressing on endoscopic appearance in healing process following endoscopic sinus surgery: a randomized, double-blind, placebo-controlled study. Int Forum Allergy Rhinol. 2018;8(11):1233–41. https://doi.org/10.1002/alr.22213.
4. Cote DW, Wright ED. Triamcinolone-impregnated nasal dressing following endoscopic sinus surgery: a randomized, double-blind, placebo-controlled study. Laryngoscope. 2010;120(6):1269–73. https://doi.org/10.1002/lary.20905.
5. Xu J, Park SJ, Park HS, Han R, Rha KS, Kim YM. Effects of triamcinolone-impregnated nasal dressing on subjective and objective outcomes following endoscopic sinus surgery. Eur Arch Otorhinolaryngol. 2016;273(12):4351–7. https://doi.org/10.1007/s00405-016-4185-0.
6. More Y, Willen S, Catalano P. Management of early nasal polyposis using a steroid-impregnated nasal dressing. Int Forum Allergy Rhinol. 2011;1(5):401–4. https://doi.org/10.1002/alr.20067.
7. Hong SD, Kim JH, Dhong HJ, Kim HY, Chung SK, Chang YS, et al. Systemic effects and safety of triamcinolone-impregnated nasal packing after endoscopic sinus surgery: a randomized, double-blinded, placebo-controlled study. Am J Rhinol Allergy. 2013;27(5):407–10. https://doi.org/10.2500/ajra.2013.27.3924.
8. Konno W, Kashiwagi T, Tsunemi Y, Goto K, Haruna S. Long-term postoperative control of eosinophilic chronic rhinosinusitis recurrence by inserting a steroid-eluting, sinus-bioabsorbable device reduces the dosage of oral steroid. Auris Nasus Larynx. 2019;46(3):365–73. https://doi.org/10.1016/j.anl.2018.09.001.
9. Rudmik L, Mace J, Mechor B. Effect of a dexamethasone Sinu-Foam middle meatal spacer on endoscopic sinus surgery outcomes: a randomized, double-blind, placebo-controlled trial. Int Forum Allergy Rhinol. 2012;2(3):248–51. https://doi.org/10.1002/alr.21011.
10. Bardaranfar MH, Ranjbar Z, Dadgarnia MH, Atighechi S, Mirvakili A, Behniafard N, et al. The effect of an absorbable gelatin dressing impregnated with triamcinolone within the olfactory cleft on polypoid rhinosinusitis smell disorders. Am J Rhinol Allergy. 2014;28(2):172–5. https://doi.org/10.2500/ajra.2014.28.4016.
11. Hwang CS, Al Sharhan SS, Kim BR, Kim SI, Kim JW, Cho HJ, et al. Randomized controlled trial of steroid-soaked absorbable calcium alginate nasal packing following endoscopic sinus surgery. Laryngoscope. 2018;128(2):311–6. https://doi.org/10.1002/lary.26871.

Corticosteroids Resistance

40

Yujie Cao, Dehui Wang, and Huabin Li

Key Points

- Usually, corticosteroids are particularly effective in patients with a Th2-dominated and eosinophilic inflammation.
- The mechanism of corticosteroids resistance includes the abnormality of glucocorticoid receptor (GR), the abnormality of transcription factor, increased neutrophil infiltration, *Staphylococcus aureus* superantigen, and dysfunction of histone deacetylase.
- Anti-IgE monoclonal antibodies (e.g., omalizumab) and anti-IL5 monoclonal antibodies (e.g., mepolizumab) could be used in CRSwNP patients with corticosteroids resistance. In addition, vitamin D can also improve the sensitivity of corticosteroid-resistant patients to corticosteroid.

40.1 Introduction

CRSwNP is characterized by a predominantly Th2 and eosinophilia-mediated inflammatory process. Topical corticosteroids are more widely used compared with systemic corticosteroids because of not only the longer periods it can be given with nearly negligible systemic effects but also potentially achievement of better drug concentration in sinonasal mucosa [1]. Although systemic corticosteroids have shown benefit in managing CRSwNP, the need for long period of treatment and associated side effects precludes their use beyond intermittent therapy for most patients [2]. Both topical and systemic corticosteroids are effective in the treatment of CRS and act as the first step in therapy. However, a subset of patients do not respond to the maximal treatment with disease progressing despite the treatment of corticosteroids [3]. The rate of response to corticosteroids in CRS reportedly varies from 50% to 80% [4]. The insensitivity to corticosteroids therapy is called corticosteroids resistance. There is no consistent definition of corticosteroid resistance in treatment of CRSwNP at present. In Milara et al.'s [5] study, CRSwNP subjects with no clinical and endoscopic response to intranasal corticosteroids for 3 months were recruited and then started oral corticosteroid at 1 mg/kg/day for 8 days followed by 0.5 mg/kg/day for other 7 days according to routine clinical practice. Corticosteroid resistance was evaluated at day 15 after corticosteroid therapy. Patients who reduced less than 1 NP endoscopic score after oral corticosteroid course were considered resistant to corticosteroid. In general, corticosteroids are particularly effective in patients with a Th2-

Y. Cao · D. Wang · H. Li (✉)
Department of Otolaryngology, Head and Neck Surgery, Affiliated Eye and ENT Hospital, Fudan University, Shanghai, China
e-mail: caoyj7@mail2.sysu.edu.cn

L. Zhang, C. Bachert (eds.), *Chronic Rhinosinusitis*, https://doi.org/10.1007/978-981-16-0784-4_40

dominated and eosinophilic inflammation [6]. The more the eosinophilic component, the better the response to corticosteroids [2].

40.2 Mechanism

The mechanism of corticosteroids resistance has not been fully investigated yet. It is generally believed the mechanism involved are as follows.

- **The abnormality of glucocorticoid receptor (GR)**

Corticosteroids bind to the GR and cause downstream gene transcriptional changes which result in several effects [6]. GRα has widespread distribution and acts as a transcription factor with the participation of numerous cofactors. It is responsible for induction and repression of target genes. GRβ acts as a dominant negative inhibitor of GRα-mediated transactivation and transrepression in certain cell types [7]. Studies on glucocorticoid resistance have reported that the abnormal expression level of GR, especially the overexpression of the GRβ subtype contributes to corticosteroids resistance [3]. Other hypotheses that could account for corticosteroids resistance include alterations in GR binding to ligand, nuclear translocation, and binding to glucocorticoid response element (GRE) [7].

- **The abnormality of transcription factor**

A large number of transcription factors are involved in the pathogenesis of CRSwNP, including nuclear factor κB (NF-κB) and signal transduction activated transcription factor (STAT). These transcription factors mediate the expression of T cells and other relevant inflammatory genes. Corticosteroids can inhibit inflammatory gene transcription mediated by transcription factors such as NF-κB, thus inhibiting inflammatory response. Previous study has demonstrated that abnormal activation of transcription factors can lead to corticosteroids resistance [8].

- **Increased neutrophil infiltration**

Patients with neutrophilic phenotype have less response to corticosteroids treatment according to symptom scores [9]. Corticosteroids are known to effectively inhibit the action of eosinophils; however, they can hardly inhibit the inflammatory processes mediated by neutrophils.

- **Other factors**

Staphylococcus aureus superantigen and dysfunction of histone deacetylase may also contribute to corticosteroid resistance in CRSwNP [3, 8].

40.3 Treatment

It is important to categorize whether a patient is sensitive or resistant to corticosteroids, which is helpful to make the most effective treatment decision. Treatment strategies for corticosteroid-resistant patients mainly consist of alternative anti-inflammatory drugs and reversing the molecular pathway of corticosteroids resistance. In addition, selective glucocorticoid receptor agonists can also be chosen to enhance the anti-inflammatory effect of corticosteroid [8].

At present, anti-IgE monoclonal antibodies (e.g., omazumab) and anti-IL5 monoclonal antibody (e.g., mepolizumab) can be used in corticosteroid-resistant CRSwNP. In addition, vitamin D can also improve the sensitivity of corticosteroid-resistant patients to corticosteroid [8].

Further research on the molecular mechanism of corticosteroids resistance will help to develop new therapeutic targets to better control the occurrence and development of diseases.

References

1. Snidvongs K, Kalish L, Sacks R, Sivasubramaniam R, Cope D, Harvey RJ. Sinus surgery and delivery method influence the effectiveness of topical corticosteroids for chronic rhinosinusitis: systematic review and meta-analysis. Am J Rhinol Allergy. 2013;27(3):221–33. https://doi.org/10.2500/ajra.2013.27.3880.

2. Oakley GM, Harvey RJ. Topical steroids. Adv Otorhinolaryngol. 2016;79:121–30. https://doi.org/10.1159/000445148.
3. Wang M, Shi P, Chen B, Shi G, Li H, Wang H. Superantigen-induced glucocorticoid insensitivity in the recurrence of chronic rhinosinusitis with nasal polyps. Otolaryngol Head Neck Surg. 2011;145(5):717–22. https://doi.org/10.1177/0194599811413859.
4. Gurrola J II, Borish L. Chronic rhinosinusitis: endotypes, biomarkers, and treatment response. J Allergy Clin Immunol. 2017;140(6):1499–508. https://doi.org/10.1016/j.jaci.2017.10.006.
5. Milara J, Morell A, Ballester B, Armengot M, Morcillo E, Cortijo J. MUC4 impairs the anti-inflammatory effects of corticosteroids in patients with chronic rhinosinusitis with nasal polyps. J Allergy Clin Immunol. 2017;139(3):855–62.e13. https://doi.org/10.1016/j.jaci.2016.06.064.
6. Campbell RG. Risks and management of long-term corticosteroid use in chronic rhinosinusitis. Curr Opin Otolaryngol Head Neck Surg. 2018;26(1):1–7. https://doi.org/10.1097/moo.0000000000000421.
7. Pujols L, Mullol J, Picado C. Importance of glucocorticoid receptors in upper and lower airways. Front Biosci (Landmark Ed). 2010;15:789–800.
8. Zhang YY, Lou HF, Wang CS, Zhang L. Mechanisms underlying glucocorticoid resistance in chronic rhinosinusitis with nasal polyps. Zhonghua er bi yan hou tou jing wai ke za zhi = Chinese J Otorhinolaryngol Head Neck Surg. 2018;53(2):154–60. https://doi.org/10.3760/cma.j.issn.1673-0860.2018.02.017
9. Wen W, Liu W, Zhang L, Bai J, Fan Y, Xia W, et al. Increased neutrophilia in nasal polyps reduces the response to oral corticosteroid therapy. J Allergy Clin Immunol. 2012;129(6):1522–8.e5. https://doi.org/10.1016/j.jaci.2012.01.079.

Leukotriene Receptor Antagonists

41

Rui Zheng, Tian Yuan, and Qintai Yang

Key Points

- More and more evidences have indicated the role of cysteinyl leukotrienes (Cys-LTs) in the pathogenesis of chronic rhinosinusitis (CRS).
- Leukotriene receptor antagonists (LTRAs) play a role mainly through blocking the interaction between leukotrienes and leukotriene receptors.
- CRS patients with asthma, aspirin intolerance and eosinophilia may benefit more from LTRAs.

Cysteinyl leukotrienes (Cys-LTs) are a class of lipid mediators with the same cysteinyl structure, which are generated from arachidonic acid (AA) via the 5-lipoxygenase (5-LO) pathway, including leukotriene C_4 (LTC_4), D_4 (LTD_4), E_4 (LTE_4), etc. [1]. Cys-LTs play an important role in chronic airway inflammatory diseases such as asthma, allergic rhinitis (AR), and chronic rhinosinusitis (CRS). The main pathophysiological role of Cys-LTs is vascular permeability and vasodilation, resulting in mucosal swelling, which causes rhinorrhea and nasal congestion. In addition, Cys-LTs can promote chemotaxis and adhesion of inflammatory cells (particularly eosinophils), as well as prolonged cell survival and activation, which aggravate airway inflammation. LTRAs, such as montelukast, by competitively binding to the cysteinyl LT1 (Cys-LT1) receptor and blocking the activity of Cys-LTs, can improve the symptoms of some allergic diseases [2].

Allergy plays a certain role in the pathogenesis of CRS [3, 4] and is an important factor of refractory CRS [5]. Cys-LTs play a critical role in both the rapid and delayed phases of allergic reactions. Currently, LTRAs have been used as a first-line treatment for AR [6].

In recent years, more and more evidences have indicated the role of Cys-LTs in the pathogenesis of CRSwNP. Levels of Cys-LTs and their receptors in nasal sinus mucosa of CRSwNP patients, especially eosinophilic CRSwNP, have been found to be significantly increased in several studies [7, 8]. Cys-LTs promote airway inflammation by encouraging eosinophil infiltration, collagen deposition, mucus secretion, and cytokines release, which can be blocked by LTRAs [9]. A recent meta-analysis finds that LTRAs are superior to placebo in improving symptoms of CRSwNP patients, including headache, facial pain, sneezing, nasal itching, postnasal drip, and olfaction disorders, decreasing the degree of polyposis and reducing eosinophils counting in peripheral blood or nasal mucosa [10]. LTRAs, as an integral part of systemic anti-inflammatory treatment, can be effective to control the inflammation in nasal and paranasal

R. Zheng · T. Yuan · Q. Yang (✉)
Department of Otorhinolaryngology, Head and Neck Surgery, The Third Affiliated Hospital, Sun Yat-sen University, Guangzhou, China

L. Zhang, C. Bachert (eds.), *Chronic Rhinosinusitis*, https://doi.org/10.1007/978-981-16-0784-4_41

sinuses mucosa. Pre- and post-operative use of LTRAs may have benefit in controlling symptoms, reducing surgical intervention and recurrence [7, 8, 11, 12].

Aspirin-exacerbated respiratory disease (AERD) is characterized by the presence of eosinophilic rhinosinusitis, nasal polyposis, bronchial asthma, and nonsteroidal anti-inflammatory drugs hypersensitivity, and Cys-LTs play an integral role in driving the disease process. LTRAs have shown a decrease in asthma symptoms, a reduced frequency in the use of bronchodilators, improvement of pulmonary function evaluated through FEV_1, and an increase in quality of life [13]. Key features of aspirin intolerant CRS patients include the presence of eosinophilic infiltrates in the respiratory tract and the overproduction of Cys-LTs. Compared with aspirin tolerant patients, levels of Cys-LTs and their receptors in mucosal tissue of aspirin intolerant CRS patients are further elevated, and these patients may benefit even more from anti-leukotrienes [13–16].

The overall safety and tolerability of montelukast are high, even in children and the elderly, and no dosage adjustment is required in elderly patients, patients with renal insufficiency, and patients with mild-to-moderate hepatic insufficiency [15, 17]. Montelukast is Category B in the US Food and Drug Administration (FDA) pregnancy category ratings and no teratogenic effects were seen [18].

41.1 Translation into Practice

For CRS patients who have concomitant asthma, aspirin intolerance, or eosinophilia, LTRAs can play an active role in comprehensive treatment (Fig. 41.1). Recommendation: orally once daily in the evening; the treatment is not less than 4 weeks.

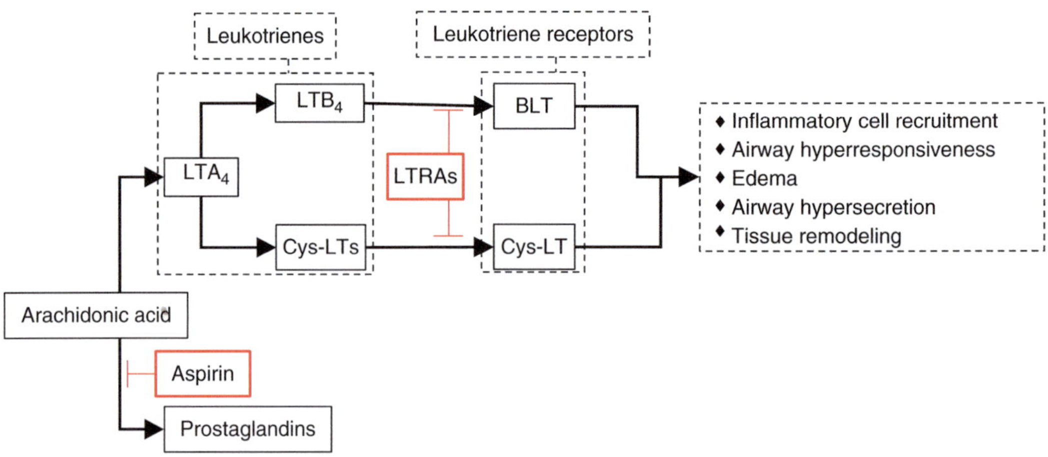

Fig. 41.1 Leukotrienes synthesis, function and inhibitor. Firstly, arachidonic acid is converted into leukotriene A_4 (LTA_4) and prostaglandins. Then LTA_4 can be further converted into leukotriene B_4 (LTB_4) and cysteinyl leukotrienes (Cys-LTs), which include leukotriene C_4 (LTC_4), D_4 (LTD_4) and E_4 (LTE_4). LTA_4, LTB_4, and Cys-LTs are members of leukotrienes. At last, leukotrienes function through leukotriene receptors, which include BLT (BLT1, BLT2) and Cys-LT (Cys-LT1, Cys-LT2). BLT and Cys-LT are receptors of LTB4 and Cys-LTs, respectively. Through these receptors, leukotrienes contribute to pathological processes such as tissue remodeling and edema. In this progress, aspirin inhibits the conversion of arachidonic acid into prostaglandins, and leukotriene receptor antagonists (LTRAs) block interaction between leukotrienes and leukotriene receptors. Montelukast is one of LTRAs and is an inhibitor of Cys-LT1 receptor

References

1. Liu M, Yokomizo T. The role of leukotrienes in allergic diseases. Allergol Int. 2015;64(1):17–26. https://doi.org/10.1016/j.alit.2014.09.001.
2. Cingi C, Muluk NB, Ipci K, Şahin E. Antileukotrienes in upper airway inflammatory diseases. Curr Allergy Asthma Rep. 2015;15(11):64. https://doi.org/10.1007/s11882-015-0564-7.
3. Kennedy JL, Borish L. Chronic sinusitis pathophysiology: the role of allergy. Am J Rhinol Allergy. 2013;27(5):367–71. https://doi.org/10.2500/ajra.2013.27.3906.
4. Fokkens WJ, Lund VJ, Hopkins C, Hellings PW, Kern R, Reitsma S, et al. European position paper on rhinosinusitis and nasal polyps 2020. Rhinology. 2020;58(Suppl S29):1–464. https://doi.org/10.4193/Rhin20.600.
5. S MA, Zuo KJ, Shi JB, Xu G. Investigation of relevant factors on refractory chronic rhinosinusitis. Zhonghua er bi yan hou tou jing wai ke za zhi = Chin J Otorhinolaryngol Head Neck Surg. 2010;45(12):1003–7.
6. Cheng L, Chen J, Fu Q, He S, Li H, Liu Z, et al. Chinese society of allergy guidelines for diagnosis and treatment of allergic rhinitis. Allergy, Asthma Immunol Res. 2018;10(4):300–53. https://doi.org/10.4168/aair.2018.10.4.300.
7. Du J, Ba L, Zhou J, Yu L, Liu R, Zhang J, et al. The role of cysteinyl leukotrienes and their receptors in refractory nasal polyps. Prostaglandins Leukot Essent Fatty Acids. 2017;126:39–48. https://doi.org/10.1016/j.plefa.2017.09.009.
8. Wu X, Hong H, Zuo K, Han M, Li J, Wen W, et al. Expression of leukotriene and its receptors in eosinophilic chronic rhinosinusitis with nasal polyps. Int Forum Allergy Rhinol. 2016;6(1):75–81. https://doi.org/10.1002/alr.21625.
9. Holgate ST, Peters-Golden M, Panettieri RA, Henderson WR Jr. Roles of cysteinyl leukotrienes in airway inflammation, smooth muscle function, and remodeling. J Allergy Clin Immunol. 2003;111(1 Suppl):S18–34; discussion S-6. https://doi.org/10.1067/mai.2003.25.
10. Wentzel JL, Soler ZM, DeYoung K, Nguyen SA, Lohia S, Schlosser RJ. Leukotriene antagonists in nasal polyposis: a meta-analysis and systematic review. Am J Rhinol Allergy. 2013;27(6):482–9. https://doi.org/10.2500/ajra.2013.27.3976.
11. Yelverton JC, Holmes TW, Johnson CM, Gelves CR, Kountakis SE. Effectiveness of leukotriene receptor antagonism in the postoperative management of chronic rhinosinusitis. Int Forum Allergy Rhinol. 2016;6(3):243–7. https://doi.org/10.1002/alr.21649.
12. Van Gerven L, Langdon C, Cordero A, Cardelús S, Mullol J, Alobid I. Lack of long-term add-on effect by montelukast in postoperative chronic rhinosinusitis patients with nasal polyps. Laryngoscope. 2018;128(8):1743–51. https://doi.org/10.1002/lary.26989.
13. Rodríguez-Jiménez JC, Moreno-Paz FJ, Terán LM, Guaní-Guerra E. Aspirin exacerbated respiratory disease: current topics and trends. Respir Med. 2018;135:62–75. https://doi.org/10.1016/j.rmed.2018.01.002.
14. Halderman AA, Lane AP. Immunomodulators in the treatment of nasal polyposis. Adv Otorhinolaryngol. 2016;79:103–13. https://doi.org/10.1159/000445141.
15. Mion OG, Mello JF Jr, Dutra DL, Andrade NA, Almeida WL, Anselmo-Lima WT, et al. Position statement of the Brazilian Academy of Rhinology on the use of antihistamines, antileukotrienes, and oral corticosteroids in the treatment of inflammatory sinonasal diseases. Braz J Otorhinolaryngol. 2017;83(2):215–27. https://doi.org/10.1016/j.bjorl.2017.01.002.
16. Kennedy JL, Stoner AN, Borish L. Aspirin-exacerbated respiratory disease: prevalence, diagnosis, treatment, and considerations for the future. Am J Rhinol Allergy. 2016;30(6):407–13. https://doi.org/10.2500/ajra.2016.30.4370.
17. Beswick DM, Gray ST, Smith TL. Pharmacological management of chronic rhinosinusitis: current and evolving treatments. Drugs. 2017;77(16):1713–21. https://doi.org/10.1007/s40265-017-0803-4.
18. Lal D, Jategaonkar AA, Borish L, Chambliss LR, Gnagi SH, Hwang PH, et al. Management of rhinosinusitis during pregnancy: systematic review and expert panel recommendations. Rhinology. 2016;54(2):99–104. https://doi.org/10.4193/Rhin15.228.

42 Antihistamine

Hongfei Lou, Yanran Huang, and Luo Zhang

Key Points

- Evidence for antihistamines in treating rhinosinusitis is limited and controversial.
- The second-generation H1 antihistamines are well tolerated, compared to first-generation antihistamines, and have fewer potential adverse effects on cognition.
- For CRS patients with comorbid AR, use of an antihistamine is a viable option for treatment strategy.

To date the evidence for use of antihistamines in the treatment of rhinosinusitis has been limited and controversial. A meta-analysis of randomized control trials (RCTs) investigating the effect of antihistamines in 184 patients with rhinosinusitis has recently demonstrated that the antihistamine loratadine significantly reduced nasal obstruction in allergic rhinitis (AR) patients with acute rhinosinusitis, but did not improve total nasal symptom score or rhinorrhea symptom [1]. Similarly, another meta-analysis involving 18 RCTs with 4342 patients suffering from acute viral rhinosinusitis has shown that antihistamines have a limited beneficial effect on severity of overall symptoms in adults in the short-term (days 1 and 2 of treatment), but not in mid to long term [2]. Braun and colleagues [3] have evaluated the adjunct effect of loratadine in acute exacerbation of sinusitis in patients with AR and found that loratadine provided additional improvement in control of sinusitis symptoms [3]. A study by McCormick and colleagues [4], however, has demonstrated that the effect of antihistamines was not significantly different compared to placebo in patients with acute rhinosinusitis. Desloratadine, a second-generation H1-antihistamine, has been found to inhibit cell activation in nasal polyps, indicating that this antihistamine might be useful in modulating the development of nasal polyps [5]. Indeed, another study has shown that desloratadine could also inhibit eosinophil inflammation in vitro, and that this effect was amplified in combination with mometasone furoate [6]. One clinical trial has demonstrated that while cetirizine also significantly reduces nasal sneezing and rhinorrhea compared to placebo, it does not have any effect on the number or size of polyps [7].

H. Lou (✉) · Y. Huang
Department of Otolaryngology, Head and Neck Surgery, Beijing Tongren Hospital, Capital Medical University, Beijing, China

Beijing Key Laboratory of Nasal Diseases, Beijing Institute of Otolaryngology, Beijing, China

L. Zhang
Department of Otolaryngology, Head and Neck Surgery, Beijing Tongren Hospital, Capital Medical University, Beijing, China

Beijing Key Laboratory of Nasal Diseases, Beijing Institute of Otolaryngology, Beijing, China

Department of Allergy, Beijing Tongren Hospital, Capital Medical University, Beijing, China

L. Zhang, C. Bachert (eds.), *Chronic Rhinosinusitis*, https://doi.org/10.1007/978-981-16-0784-4_42

It is well documented that histamine is released by mast cells and can provoke nasal symptoms in the early phase of the allergic reactions. Consequently, both oral and topical antihistamines are approved as the first-line treatment for allergic rhinitis, targeting symptoms such as rhinorrhea, nasal itching, and sneezing [8]. Topical antihistamines and corticosteroids are also moderately recommended for CRS and allergic rhinitis patients with olfactory dysfunction [9]. Some antihistamines such as ketotifen, olopatadine, azelastine, bepotastine, and alcaftadine function as both H1 receptor antagonists and mast cell stabilizers [10, 11]. Receptor-independent effects are produced through mast cell stabilization, leading to inhibition of some inflammatory mediators [12]. Moreover, histamines also inhibit neutrophil activation, superoxide formation, and degranulation [13].

The first-generation antihistamines have anticholinergic properties, which increase the viscosity of nasal discharge and inhibit ciliary beats. In this context, these antihistamines are potentially more harmful than beneficial in treating rhinosinusitis. In contrast, although the second-generation antihistamines have minor sedative effects [14], these do not have anticholinergic properties [1]. In view of fewer potential adverse effects on cognition and being well tolerated, the second-generation H1 antihistamines (such as loratadine, cetirizine and fexofenadine) are also recommended as first-line therapy for pediatric AR patients [15].

42.1 Conclusions

The direct evidence for antihistamines in treating CRS is relatively scarce, especially for patients without comorbid allergic diseases. However, current evidence suggests that for CRS patients with comorbid AR, use of an antihistamine is a viable option for treatment strategy.

References

1. Seresirikachorn K, Khattiyawittayakun L, Chitsuthipakorn W, Snidvongs K. Antihistamines for treating rhinosinusitis: systematic review and meta-analysis of randomised controlled studies. J Laryngol Otol. 2018;132(2):105–10. https://doi.org/10.1017/s002221511700192x.
2. De Sutter AI, Saraswat A, van Driel ML. Antihistamines for the common cold. Cochrane Database Syst Rev. 2015;(11):CD009345. https://doi.org/10.1002/14651858.CD009345.pub2.
3. Braun JJ, Alabert JP, Michel FB, Quiniou M, Rat C, Cougnard J, et al. Adjunct effect of loratadine in the treatment of acute sinusitis in patients with allergic rhinitis. Allergy. 1997;52(6):650–5. https://doi.org/10.1111/j.1398-9995.1997.tb01044.x.
4. McCormick DP, John SD, Swischuk LE, Uchida T. A double-blind, placebo-controlled trial of decongestant-antihistamine for the treatment of sinusitis in children. Clin Pediatr. 1996;35(9):457–60. https://doi.org/10.1177/000992289603500905.
5. Kowalski ML, Lewandowska A, Wozniak J, Makowska J, Jankowski A, DuBuske L. Inhibition of nasal polyp mast cell and eosinophil activation by desloratadine. Allergy. 2005;60(1):80–5. https://doi.org/10.1111/j.1398-9995.2005.00642.x.
6. Mullol J, de Borja Callejas F, Martínez-Antón MA, Méndez-Arancibia E, Alobid I, Pujols L, et al. Mometasone and desloratadine additive effect on eosinophil survival and cytokine secretion from epithelial cells. Respir Res. 2011;12(1):23. https://doi.org/10.1186/1465-9921-12-23.
7. Haye R, Aanesen JP, Burtin B, Donnelly F, Duby C. The effect of cetirizine on symptoms and signs of nasal polyposis. J Laryngol Otol. 1998;112(11):1042–6. https://doi.org/10.1017/s0022215100142422.
8. Chipps BE, Harder JM. Antihistamine treatment for allergic rhinitis: different routes, different outcomes? Allergy Asthma Proc. 2009;30(6):589–94. https://doi.org/10.2500/aap.2009.30.3287.
9. Miwa T, Ikeda K, Ishibashi T, Kobayashi M, Kondo K, Matsuwaki Y, et al. Clinical practice guidelines for the management of olfactory dysfunction – secondary publication. Auris Nasus Larynx. 2019;46(5):653–62. https://doi.org/10.1016/j.anl.2019.04.002.
10. Mandhane SN, Shah JH, Thennati R. Allergic rhinitis: an update on disease, present treatments and future prospects. Int Immunopharmacol. 2011;11(11):1646–62. https://doi.org/10.1016/j.intimp.2011.07.005.
11. Holgate ST, Canonica GW, Simons FE, Taglialatela M, Tharp M, Timmerman H, et al. Consensus group on new-generation antihistamines (CONGA):

present status and recommendations. Clin Exp Allergy. 2003;33(9):1305–24. https://doi.org/10.1046/j.1365-2222.2003.01769.x.
12. Jutel M, Watanabe T, Akdis M, Blaser K, Akdis CA. Immune regulation by histamine. Curr Opin Immunol. 2002;14(6):735–40. https://doi.org/10.1016/s0952-7915(02)00395-3.
13. Seligmann BE, Fletcher MP, Gallin JI. Histamine modulation of human neutrophil oxidative metabolism, locomotion, degranulation, and membrane potential changes. J Immunol. 1983;130(4):1902–9.
14. Simons FE, Simons KJ. Histamine and H1-antihistamines: celebrating a century of progress. J Allergy Clin Immunol. 2011;128(6):1139–50.e4. https://doi.org/10.1016/j.jaci.2011.09.005.
15. Tang R, Sun JL, Yin J, Li Z. Artemisia allergy research in China. Biomed Res Int. 2015;2015:179426. https://doi.org/10.1155/2015/179426.

Antibiotics

43

Dawei Wu and Yongxiang Wei

Key Points

- Antibiotics have long been a mainstay of treatment in patients with chronic rhinosinusitis (CRS) mainly due to their antibacterial, anti-inflammatory, or immunomodulatory properties.
- The choice and duration of treatment with antibiotics is largely depended on the etiology, CRS phenotype, and disease activity.
- Despite the widespread use of short-term non-macrolide antibiotics to eliminate bacterial infections in patients with acute exacerbation of CRS, there is a paucity of evidence for their efficacy and double-blinded placebo-controlled study is warranted.
- Effective implementation of macrolide therapy in CRS patients depends on the appropriate patient selection and Th1-mediated non-eosinophilic CRS patients would achieve the most benefit when low-dose macrolide was used for durations of at least 3 months.
- The increasing prevalence of antibiotic resistance in patients with CRS underlines the importance of using culture-directed antibiotic therapy and the necessity to explore the optimal treatment duration.

43.1 Introduction

Although the exact role of the antibiotics in the treatment of chronic rhinosinusitis (CRS) remains unclear [1], antibiotics have long been a mainstay of treatment in patients with chronic rhinosinusitis mainly due to their antibacterial, anti-inflammatory, or immunomodulatory properties [2, 3]. The past decades have witnessed a remarkable change in the mechanism of CRS from the microbial infection in etiology to dysregulated immuno-inflammatory responses to exogenous or endogenous stimuli [4–7]. There are accumulating evidences supporting the critical role of sinonasal microbiome in the pathogenesis of CRS [8–12], either as a direct driver of chronic inflammation [4, 13, 14] or as being potentially involved in acute exacerbation of CRS [15, 16]. We are understanding the role of bacteria beyond what we understand as infection and dysbiosis of the sinus mucosal microbiome tends to be the key features of the CRS patients [10, 17]. In addition, CRS has been proved to be a heterogeneous and

D. Wu
Department of Otorhinolaryngology, Head and Neck Surgery, Beijing Anzhen Hospital, Capital Medical University, Beijing, China

Y. Wei (✉)
Department of Otorhinolaryngology, Head and Neck Surgery, Beijing Anzhen Hospital, Capital Medical University, Beijing, China

Department of Otorhinolaryngology, Head and Neck Surgery, Capital Institute of Pediatrics, Beijing, China

L. Zhang, C. Bachert (eds.), *Chronic Rhinosinusitis*, https://doi.org/10.1007/978-981-16-0784-4_43

refractory disease entity with distinct phenotypes and endotypes based on differentiation of inflammatory pathomechanisms [18–20]. These factors urge us to redefine the role of antibiotics for the treatment of CRS.

In order to assess the treatment outcome among CRS patients, the criterion of the clinical control has been put forward and the need of the antibiotics is an important evaluation indicator [21]. Recent studies have provided consistent evidence supporting the efficacy of antibiotics in CRS patients with certain characteristic [22–25], although there is insufficient scientific evidence to confirm the general benefit of the long-term macrolide antibiotics therapy for patients with CRS [26–29]. Hence, it is imperative to summarize the indication for antibiotic use among CRS patients with different subgroups, disease activity, and characteristics.

43.2 Antibiotics Treatment Strategies for Patients with CRS

The choice and duration of treatment with antibiotics is largely depended on the etiology, CRS phenotype, and disease activity [30]. CRS is characterized by persistent chronic sinonasal symptoms at baseline and a sudden temporary worsening of symptoms is defined as acute exacerbation of CRS (AECRS) [31]. Different antibiotics have been utilized for AECRS and CRS based on the distinct bacterial pathogenesis. Here we discuss the role of bacteria in patients with AECRS and CRS and then the general principle of the antibiotics selection (Fig. 43.1).

The triggers of AECRS are not well understood and both virus and bacteria are thought to be evolved during the acute exacerbation of CRS [3, 15]. Although viruses are responsible for most exacerbation episodes in CRS, the exact role of virus and whether there are secondary bacterial infections after viral infection is not clear [3, 32–34]. A study by Brook et al. showed that patients with AECRS showed unique microbial dynamics in which anaerobic and aerobic bacteria prevail and highlights the importance of obtaining cultures for guidance in selection of proper antibiotics. In addition, Brook compared the aerobic and anaerobic microbiology of maxillary between AECRS and CRS [35]. This study demonstrates that the organisms isolated from patients with AECRS were predominantly anaerobic and were similar to those generally recovered in CRS patients. However, aerobic bacteria that are usually found in acute rhinosinusitis (e.g., S pneumoniae, Haemophilus influenzae, and Moraxella catarrhalis) are also present in some of the episodes of AECRS [35]. A study by Merkley et al. showed that bacterial abundance is increased and diversity decreased during acute exacerbations of CRS and that antibiotic treatment led to the increased diversity [36]. This study supports the hypothesis of microbial overgrowth as a key driver of AECRS. In this review, we defined short-term antibiotic treatment as a treatment duration of no more than 4 weeks. Although it has been suggested that antibiotics may not change the clinical course [37], current consensus guidelines and expert opinion have favored the use of short-term antibiotics for AECRS in the setting of a positive culture [2, 3, 21, 31]. A recent study by Carol et al. showed that culture-directed antibiotics therapy in patients with AECRS could only yield an advantage in improving the long-term endoscopic scores compared with non-culture-directed antibiotics therapy [38]. Besides, culture-directed topical antibiotic treatment in recalcitrant CRS trended toward improvement in symptom severity and significantly improved endoscopic appearance [39].

The microbiomes of CRS patients are different from non-CRS patients with a relative enrichment of Corynebacterium, Diaphorobacter, and Peptoniphilus [40–42]. A series of studies have also supported the fact that the microbiome of CRS patients is characterized by reduced diversity, increased bacterial load, and to have less stable bacterial networks [43–45]. Furthermore, it has been demonstrated that CRS patients with particular phenotype have distinct compositions of resident bacterial communities and decreased diversity and the relative absence of commensals predict the worse outcomes following surgery [46]. Sinus cultures from patients with CRS usually

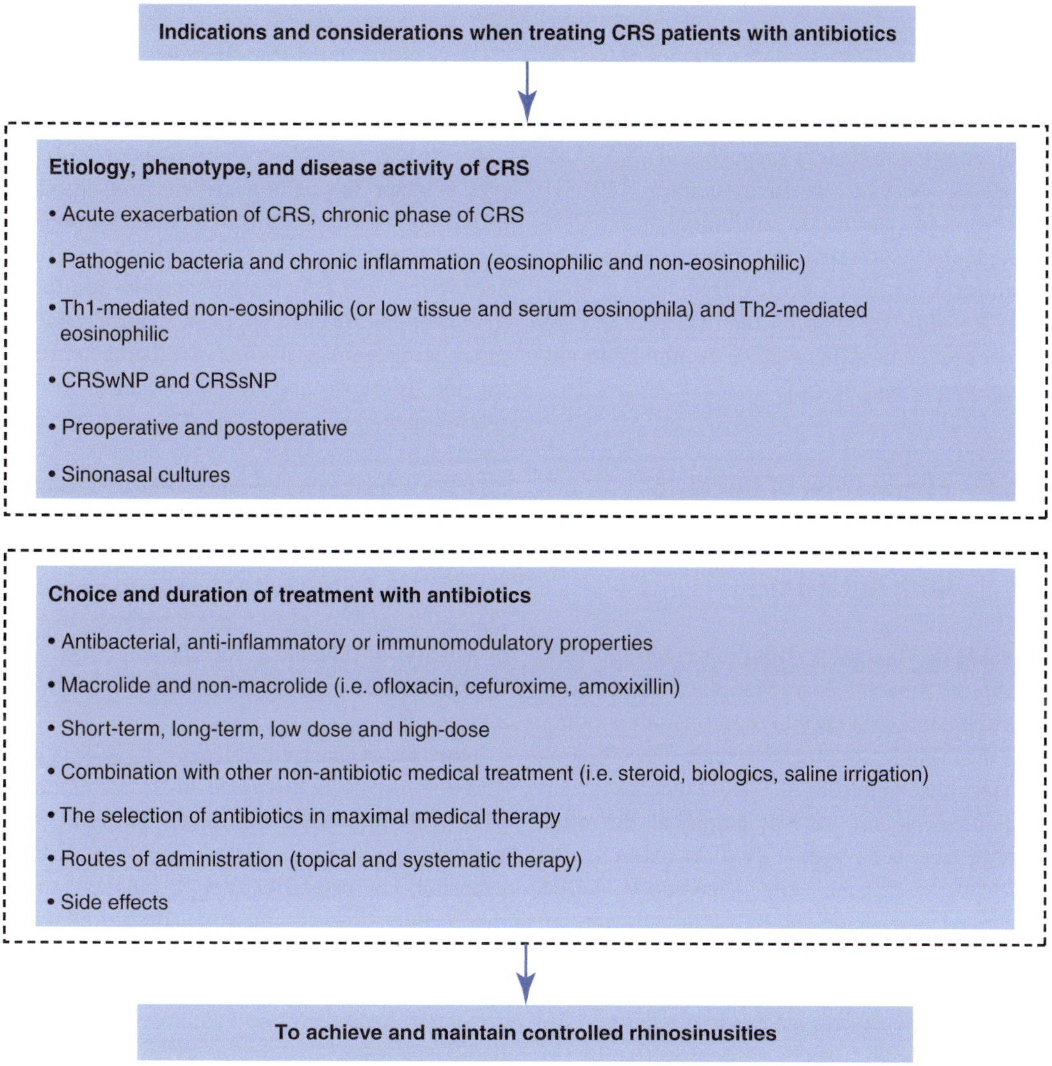

Fig. 43.1 Indications and considerations when treating CRS patients with antibiotics. CRS, chronic rhinosinusitis; CRSsNP, chronic rhinosinusitis without nasal polyps; CRSwNP, chronic rhinosinusitis with nasal polyps

present with a mixture of aerobes and anaerobes, with aerobes consisting of *Staphylococcus aureus* (*S. aureus*), methicillin-resistant *S. aureus* (MRSA), and/or Gram-negative bacilli [3, 12]. Besides, sinus cultures from up to two-thirds of patients with CRS showed anaerobes. Although several studies have attempted to identify the links between CRS and specific bacteria, it seems that only *Staphylococcus aureus* shows the confirmatory association with the pathogenesis of CRS [41, 47, 48]. Now, CRS is increasingly recognized as a chronic sinonasal inflammation partly caused by the imbalance or dysbiosis of the microbiome. So, the current therapy goal of CRS has been focused on the elimination of the chronic inflammation.

The current prescription of antibiotics routinely employed in the management of CRS can be divided into non-macrolide and macrolide antibiotics according to the International Consensus Statement on Allergy and Rhinology: Rhinosinusitis (ICAR:RS) [31] and European Position Paper on Rhinosinusitis and Nasal Polyps 2012 (EPOS2012) [21]. To be specific, non-macrolide antibiotics (i.e., ofloxacin, cefixime, cefuroxime, amoxicillin with or without clavulanic acid) comprises the mainstay of the short-term antibacterial therapy in CRS patients with the greatest benefit suspected in CRS exacerbations with a positive culture [49–53]. Furthermore, macrolide antibiotics (i.e., clarithromycin, azithromycin, roxithromycin, and erythromycin) have been utilized with a long-term low-dose regimen for the treatment of CRS for its exact anti-inflammatory or immunomodulatory properties [54–56].

43.3 Elimination of Bacterial Infections During Acute Exacerbations of CRS with Antibiotics

There is no consensus definition regarding what represents an acute exacerbation of CRS mainly due to the inconsistency in reporting of endpoints and the complex etiology of acute exacerbation. Instead, the diagnosis of CRS exacerbations is patient-driven and several empirical definition criteria have been widely used for research purpose [34, 57, 58]. An acute exacerbation of CRS is defined as an acute and transient worsening of preexisting symptoms in patients with CRS [21] and the frequency of CRS exacerbations is identified as an independent predictor of quality of life [57]. Patients with acute CRS exacerbation are mainly attributed to the bacterial infection and therefore recommended to be treated like acute rhinosinusitis with antibiotics or only observation [21, 58–60].

There is only one randomized controlled trial (RCT) about the treatment of CRS exacerbations [37]. This study concluded that amoxicillin-clavulanate for 2 weeks did not change the clinical course of AECRS compared with placebo and the addition of an oral antibiotic to ongoing topical intranasal steroid spray may not provide additional benefit during management of AECRS. Similarly, a recent RCT study of antibiotics for acute rhinosinusitis showed that although amoxicillin therapy accelerated the resolution of symptoms, both the amoxicillin and placebo groups had the same degree of improvement after 10 days of treatment [61]. It is therefore possible that antibiotics may accelerate the resolution of AECRS, but it remains unclear if they have any other benefit over observation alone. For example, whether the pathogenic bacteria are completed or partly eliminated after antibiotics therapy is not clear. The efficacy of non-macrolide antibiotics for CRS was presumably due to the therapeutic shift in the amount or proportion of microbes present on the mucosa, thereby correcting the dysbiosis and re-establishing a healthy microbiome [10, 17, 43]. The International Consensus Statement also notes that "There are no trials to endorse an evidence-based treatment of AECRS, though there is a tendency to treat AECRS like an episode of ARS or RARS" [31]. Despite the widespread use of short-term non-macrolide antibiotics in AECRS patients, there is a paucity of evidence for their efficacy and double-blinded placebo-controlled study is warranted.

The role of macrolide therapy in patients with AECRS has been discussed in a recent review [54]. The high-dose macrolide antibiotics are typically involved in the treatment of AECRS especially in penicillin-allergic patients and a therapeutic dose is usually administered for 10 days. A broad range of bacteria is susceptible to macrolide antibiotics. Macrolide antimicrobial coverage included the common respiratory pathogens such as *Streptococcus pneumoniae*, *Haemophilus influenzae*, *Streptococcus pyogenes*, *Staphylococcus aureus*, and *Moraxella catarrhalis* [55, 62, 63]. However, the current literature about the macrolide therapy that focused on the AECRS is still lacking and further studies are needed in the future.

43.4 Control of Persistent Inflammation During Chronic Phase of CRS with Antibiotics

CRS patients without an acute exacerbation typically present with a serial of sinonasal symptoms and abnormal nasal endoscopy or imaging findings consisting of inflammation or mucosal changes within the sinuses [31, 60]. CRS is now treated as persistent inflammatory disease process and the drivers of inflammation include allergens, microbial stimuli, or poorly understood exogenous or endogenous stimuli [4, 64]. The classification of CRS based on the presence of nasal polyps will not help to make a conclusion about the inflammatory subtypes. Recently, the differentiation of inflammatory pathomechanisms is increasingly necessary with the advent of biologics and the consequent endotyping of CRS according to the presence of type 2 immune response has been introduced into the management of CRS [65, 66]. These endotypes of CRS are also instructive for the antibiotics treatment of CRS and details would be discussed below.

Given the inflammatory nature of CRS, antibiotics with anti-inflammatory properties are frequently used to mitigate the inflammatory load systematically and locally. The majority of studies on antibiotics for CRS have examined the effect of oral macrolide antibiotics which are also known to possess anti-inflammatory properties [1, 3, 28, 54, 55]. In fact, there is little evidence for the use of systemic antibiotics in patients with CRS in general [1]. A recent meta-analysis of RCs supports the long-term low-dose macrolide in the management of CRSwNP patients during the postoperative period and this study also points out that it is necessary to determine which CRS subtype population benefits most from this regimen [29]. Factors associated with good macrolide effects have been recently identified. CRS patients with low IgE levels [67], persistent post-surgical rhinosinusitis with low serum and tissue eosinophilia [22], CRSwNP patients without comorbidity of asthma or non-steroidal-exacerbated respiratory disease or high serum IgE [68] benefit more from the long-term low-dose macrolide therapy. It is the level of eosinophil counts not the level of IgE or neutrophils that is highly associated with the degree of improvement after macrolide therapy [22, 69]. The recruited CRS patients in the previous studies which failed to consider these factors were heterogeneous and certainly showed different response to macrolide therapy. Thus, it is not a surprise to get a limited scientific evidence supporting the use of long-term low-dose macrolide therapy for CRS [27, 29, 70, 71]. Furthermore, long-term low-dose macrolides have been suggested as therapeutic option for CRSsNP [1, 21, 31], which is mainly due to the fact that most of the CRSsNP belong to the non-eosinophilic inflammatory phenotypes or non-type 2 immune response (approximately 7% in Europe) [65, 72]. It has also been proposed that the key to effective implementation of macrolide therapy in CRS is the appropriate patient selection [54] and Th1-mediated non-eosinophilic CRS patients would achieve the most benefit when low-dose macrolide was used for durations of at least 3 months [22, 73]. So, histopathologic analysis before treatment would help clinicians to identify patients most likely to benefit from the long-term low-dose macrolide therapy.

43.5 Combination with Other Non-antibiotic Medical Treatment: Add Treatment Benefit or Similar Efficacy

Medical treatment for CRS is routinely a combined therapy consisting of oral antibiotics, intranasal steroid spray, nasal saline irrigation, and other medicine (e.g., nasal antihistamine spray, mucus promoting agent). There are a series of clinical studies comparing the efficiency of macrolide antibiotics, alone or combined treatment with topical steroids. A Chinese study by Deng et al. concluded that the combination of long-term low-dose clarithromycin and nasal steroid spray for the treatment of first-time-diagnosed CRS did not show a better effect compared with a single nasal steroid spray regimen [74]. A recent meta-analysis study by Huang and Zhou showed that CRS patients with oral clarithromycin and nasal steroid spray with or without nasal saline irrigation may achieve better results compared with patients using nasal steroid spray with or without nasal saline irrigation [75]. But this study also pointed out that there was insufficient evidence to confirm the same efficacy of oral clarithromycin to nasal steroid spray. Similarly, Liu and colleagues found that the antibiotic, steroid, and combination therapy groups showed significant decrease of Lund-Mackay CT scores; however, no one regimen was superior to any other for treating CRSsNP [76].

What's more, antibiotics have traditionally been utilized as a component of maximal medical therapy (MMT) for the treatment of CRS [77, 78] and endoscopic sinus surgery (ESS) would be considered an option after failure of MMT. Currently, there is no consensus on the definition of MMT [79]. A prospective randomized cohort study by Sreenath and colleagues found that there was little difference in clinical outcomes between 3 weeks vs 6 weeks of antibiotic treatment as part of "maximal medical therapy" for CRS [80]. Similarly, a study by Ramakrishnan et al. showed that greater antibiotic therapy prior to ESS does not appear to be associated with better ESS outcomes and recommendations for antibiotic use as part of CRS-related medical therapy prior to ESS require further study [81]. Furthermore, the selection of antibiotics, in the regimen of MMT is also important. Günel et al. found that the use of antibiotics without independent anti-inflammatory properties (e.g., 4-week amoxicillin-clavulanic acid treatment) had limited efficacy in patients with eosinophilic CRS [82]. These studies indicate that MMT using antibiotics, with different properties should take the inflammatory phenotype of CRS into account and longer duration of antibiotic treatment in the setting of MMT is not recommended.

43.6 Antibiotics, After Endoscopic Sinus Surgery: Achieve Long-Term Surgical Outcome

ESS was recommended to medically refractory CRS patients who failed the initial medical treatment [83–85]. The goals of ESS for medically refractory CRS are to remove the inflammatory tissue, improve the ventilation of the paranasal sinuses by enlarging the natural drainage pathways, and improve access to the paranasal sinuses for topical medications [86]. Both topical and systematic antibiotics therapy play a crucial role in the management of postoperative CRS patients.

Topical antibiotics have been treated as adjunctive treatment of CRS because they offer the potential for high local concentration at the desired target site with minimization of systemic side effects [87]. A recent Cochrane review on the utility of topical antibiotics found that there are no RCTs of topical antibiotics available [1]. An evidence-based review by Rudmik and colleagues also concluded that current evidence recommended against the use of topical antibiotic therapy delivered using nebulized and spray techniques in routine cases of CRS [88]. A randomized, placebo-controlled, double-blind study by Jiang and colleagues proved that nasal irrigation with 200 μg/mL of AMB did not provide additional benefit compared with saline irrigation in the post-FESS care of CRS [89]. However, several studies demonstrated a beneficial effect of topical antibiotic therapy in recalcitrant chronic rhinosinusitis especially after ESS. Uren and colleagues found that nasal lavage with 0.05% Mupirocin may represent an effective and well-tolerated alternative treatment for post-surgical recalcitrant CRS [90]. Similarly, Ezzat and colleagues found that topical ofloxacin seems to be an effective and safe mode of treatment of refractory CRS after FESS due to biofilms' formation and recommend this modality of treatment postoperatively especially in refractory CRS [91]. Furthermore, a study by Lee and Davis also supported the use of high-volume culture-directed topical antibiotics in recalcitrant CRS [39]. Given the low-level evidence of the above studies, randomized, double-blinded, placebo-controlled trials are required to fully evaluate this modality of treatment in refractory CRS after ESS.

The role of oral antibiotics in the treatment of CRS after ESS has been thoroughly studied and postoperative antibiotics following ESS is thought to optimize the clinical outcomes [92, 93]. A recent national survey among Chinese otolaryngologists by Huang and colleagues showed that 72% of otolaryngologists prescribed oral antibiotics after ESS [94]. A randomized double-blind, placebo-controlled study by Haxel and colleagues evaluated the efficacy of macrolides in the postoperative period of CRS patients and concluded that general recommendation for long-term low-dose erythromycin treatment after surgery for CRS cannot be given [70]. However, a systematic review by Lasso and colleagues showed that only CRSwNP in postoperative period benefited from the long-term low-dose macrolides therapy [29]. It seems that macrolides treatment in the management of postoperative CRS patients suits to a certain group of CRS patients. Oakley et al. found that characteristics of macrolide responders in persistent post-surgical rhinosinusitis included low tissue and serum eosinophilia and absence of tissue squamous metaplasia [22]. The utility of long-term low-dose macrolides in the postoperative CRS patients is advocated to possibly improve the long-term surgical outcome. A study by Varvyanskaya and Lopatin showed that long-term low-dose macrolide antibiotics were able to control eosinophilic inflammation and to prevent early relapse of nasal polyps after ESS [95]. What's more, treatment with long-term low-dose azithromycin in combination with the conventional therapy could statistically reduce the recurrence rate of CRS symptoms after ESS [96]. As for the duration of macrolide treatment after ESS, a study by Nakamura and colleagues demonstrated that CRS patients with rhinorrhea or post-nasal drip should be treated for 6 months in order to improve the long-term ESS outcome [97].

In addition to the macrolide antibiotics, the role of oral non-macrolide antibiotics in the treatment of postoperative CRS patients has been studied. A randomized, double-blind, placebo-controlled study by Annys and colleagues evaluated efficiency of the 2-day course of cefuroxime axetil in CRS patients after ESS and demonstrated no significant effect on the sinonasal symptoms and endoscopic scores [98]. Similarly, a study by Jiang et al. showed that a 3-week course of amoxicillin/clavulanate in CRS patients after ESS did not improve the short-term outcome in terms of the sinonasal symptoms, endoscopic scores, rates of bacterial culture [99]. Another randomized, double-blind, placebo-controlled study by Albu and colleagues evaluated the efficiency of the 2-week course of amoxicillin-clavulanate in the postoperative care of CRS patients and demonstrated that postoperative antibiotics improved patient symptoms within the first 5 days and endoscopic appearance at the 12-day period [100]. These studies indicate that therapeutic benefits appear to be limited to early period after ESS and a longer course of non-macrolide antibiotics may provide a clinical response. However, further studies are needed to elucidate the exact function of non-macrolide antibiotics, in the setting of postoperative care of CRS patients.

43.7 Side Effects of Antibiotics

Side effects of antibiotics in the treatment of CRS have recently aroused increasing attention. It has been reported that the prevalence of side effect of short-term oral antibiotic treatment for CRS is 12–25% [51, 101, 102]. The most common side effect is gastrointestinal reaction which includes vomiting, nausea, diarrhea, and abdominal pain. Other side effects were urticaria medicamentosa, skin pruritus, vagal discomfort, facial edema, asthma, genital herpes, and allergic reaction. All of these side effects resolved after stopping the administered antibiotic. Side effects after the use of long-term low-dose oral macrolide antibiotics in CRS treatment were rare (0–3%) [67, 103–105]. The most significant issue is cardiovascular side effects [106]. Concerns about the risk of macrolides to induce arrhythmia have been raised. It has been reported that macrolide can lead to prolongation of the QT interval and the subsequent arrhythmia torsades de pointes [107]. Patients with risk factors such as QT-interval prolongation, bradycardia, hypomagnesemia, hypokalemia are not advised to use azithromycin by the American Food and Drug Administration [108]. Other side effects after the use of long-term low-dose oral macrolide antibiotics in CRS treatment include gastrointestinal side effects, hearing loss, and allergic reaction. All of these side effects resolved after ceasing the antibiotic.

The development of bacterial resistance, which is now a major public-health problem, is another important consequence of the use of antibiotics in the treatment of CRS patients. A study by Kingdom et al. found that there was increased antimicrobial resistance in CRS patients undergoing revision ESS when compared with CRS patients undergoing surgery for the first time [109]. Another study by Bhattacharyya et al. found that antibiotic resistance appeared to be emerging for erythromycin at a rate higher than for other antibiotics and MRSA (methicillin-resistant *Staphylococcus aureus*) maintained a significant presence in CRS patients with associated increased levels of antibiotic resistance [110]. Actually, acute exacerbations of CRS due to MRSA are routinely encountered [111]. In addition, Casey and colleagues identified a 9.22% incidence of MRSA-causing CRS [112]. The increasing prevalence of antibiotic resistance in patients with CRS underlines the importance of using culture-directed antibiotic therapy and the necessity to explore the optimal treatment duration.

43.8 Conclusions

Different antibiotics have been utilized for AECRS and CRS based on the distinct bacterial pathogenesis. Non-macrolide comprises the mainstay of the short-term antibacterial therapy in CRS patients with the greatest benefit suspected in CRS exacerbations with a positive culture. Furthermore, macrolide antibiotics have been utilized with a long-term low-dose regimen for the treatment of CRS for its exact anti-inflammatory or immunomodulatory properties. The key to effective implementation of macrolide therapy in CRS is the appropriate patient selection and Th1-mediated non-eosinophilic CRS patients would achieve the most benefit when low-dose macrolide was used for durations of at least 3 months. Whether there is additional benefit of antibiotics when combined with other medical treatment is not sure. MMT using antibiotics with different properties should take the inflammatory phenotype of CRS into account and longer duration of antibiotic treatment in the setting of MMT is not recommended. There is no clear evidence supporting the topical and systematic antibiotics therapy in the management of postoperative CRS patients.

43.9 Implications for Medical Practice

Antibiotics have been frequently prescribed for acute exacerbations in patients with CRS. There are more evidences supporting the fact that antibiotics with different properties should be tailored to CRS patients with different pathogenic bacteria, CRS phenotypes, and disease activity. Thus, the exact CRS patient selection together with culture-directed antibiotic therapy would certainly improve the efficacy of antibiotic treatment.

References

1. Head K, Chong LY, Piromchai P, Hopkins C, Philpott C, Schilder AG, et al. Systemic and topical antibiotics for chronic rhinosinusitis. Cochrane Database Syst Rev. 2016;(4):CD011994.
2. Bachert C, Hamilos DL. Are antibiotics useful for chronic rhinosinusitis? J Allergy Clin Immunol Pract. 2016;4(4):629–38.
3. Barshak MB, Durand ML. The role of infection and antibiotics in chronic rhinosinusitis. Laryngoscope Investig Otolaryngol. 2017;2(1):36–42.
4. Hamilos DL. Drivers of chronic rhinosinusitis: inflammation versus infection. J Allergy Clin Immunol. 2015;136(6):1454–9.
5. Stevens WW, Lee RJ, Schleimer RP, Cohen NA. Chronic rhinosinusitis pathogenesis. J Allergy Clin Immunol. 2015;136(6):1442–53.
6. Tan BK, Peters AT, Schleimer RP, Hulse KE. Pathogenic and protective roles of B cells and antibodies in patients with chronic rhinosinusitis. J Allergy Clin Immunol. 2018;141(5):1553–60.
7. Wu D, Wei Y, Bleier BS. Emerging role of proteases in the pathogenesis of chronic rhinosinusitis with nasal polyps. Front Cell Infect Microbiol. 2018;7:538.
8. Hamilos DL. Host-microbial interactions in patients with chronic rhinosinusitis. J Allergy Clin Immunol. 2014;133(3):640–53.e4.
9. Wagner BM, Waite DW, Hoggard M, Taylor MW, Biswas K, Douglas RG. Moving beyond descriptions of diversity: clinical and research implications of bacterial imbalance in chronic rhinosinusitis. Rhinology. 2017;55(4):291–7.

10. Mahdavinia M, Keshavarzian A, Tobin MC, Landay A, Schleimer RP. A comprehensive review of the nasal microbiome in chronic rhinosinusitis (CRS). Clin Exp Allergy. 2016;46(1):21–41.
11. Sivasubramaniam R, Douglas R. The microbiome and chronic rhinosinusitis. World J Otorhinolaryngol Head Neck Surg. 2018;4(3):216–21.
12. Brook I. Microbiology of chronic rhinosinusitis. Eur J Clin Microbiol Infect Dis. 2016;35(7):1059–68.
13. Lee K, Pletcher SD, Lynch SV, Goldberg AN, Cope EK. Heterogeneity of microbiota dysbiosis in chronic rhinosinusitis: potential clinical implications and microbial community mechanisms contributing to sinonasal inflammation. Front Cell Infect Microbiol. 2018;8:168.
14. Lan F, Zhang N, Holtappels G, Ruyck ND, Krysko O, Crombruggen KV, et al. Staphylococcus aureus induces mucosal type 2 immune response via epithelial cell derived cytokines. Am J Respir Crit Care Med. 2018;198(4):452–63.
15. Tan KS, Yan Y, Ong HH, Chow VT, Shi L, Wang D-Y. Impact of respiratory virus infections in exacerbation of acute and chronic rhinosinusitis. Curr Allergy Asthma Rep. 2017;17(4):24.
16. Wood AJ, Antoszewska H, Fraser J, Douglas RG, editors. Is chronic rhinosinusitis caused by persistent respiratory virus infection? International forum of allergy & rhinology. Hoboken, NJ: Wiley Online Library; 2011.
17. Choi EB, Hong SW, Kim DK, Jeon SG, Kim KR, Cho SH, et al. Decreased diversity of nasal microbiota and their secreted extracellular vesicles in patients with chronic rhinosinusitis based on a metagenomic analysis. Allergy. 2014;69(4):517–26. https://doi.org/10.1111/all.12374.
18. Cao PP, Wang ZC, Schleimer RP, Liu Z. Pathophysiologic mechanisms of chronic rhinosinusitis and their roles in emerging disease endotypes. Ann Allergy Asthma Immunol. 2019;122(1):33–40. https://doi.org/10.1016/j.anai.2018.10.014.
19. Bachert C, Akdis CA. Phenotypes and emerging endotypes of chronic rhinosinusitis. J Allergy Clin Immunol Pract. 2016;4(4):621–8. https://doi.org/10.1016/j.jaip.2016.05.004.
20. Gurrola J II, Borish L. Chronic rhinosinusitis: endotypes, biomarkers, and treatment response. J Allergy Clin Immunol. 2017;140(6):1499–508. https://doi.org/10.1016/j.jaci.2017.10.006.
21. Fokkens WJ, Lund VJ, Mullol J, Bachert C, Alobid I, Baroody F, et al. European position paper on rhinosinusitis and nasal polyps 2012. Rhinol Suppl. 2012;23:3 p preceding table of contents, 1–298.
22. Oakley GM, Christensen JM, Sacks R, Earls P, Harvey RJ. Characteristics of macrolide responders in persistent post-surgical rhinosinusitis. Rhinology. 2018;56(2):111–7.
23. Pinto ABS, Bezerra T, Pezato R, Teles TA, Pilan RM, Pinna FR, et al. Prospective open-label evaluation of long-term low-dose doxycycline for difficult-to-treat chronic rhinosinusitis with nasal polyps. Rhinology. 2017;55(2):175–80.
24. Božić DD, Pavlović B, Milovanović J, Jotić A, Čolović J, Ćirković I. Antibiofilm effects of amoxicillin–clavulanic acid and levofloxacin in patients with chronic rhinosinusitis with nasal polyposis. Eur Arch Otorhinolaryngol. 2018;275(8):2051–9.
25. de Bonnecaze G, Chaput B, Dupret-Bories A, Vergez S, Serrano E. Functional outcome after long-term low-dose trimethoprim/sulfamethoxazole in chronic rhinosinusitis with purulence: a prospective study. J Laryngol Otol. 2018;132(7):600–4.
26. Sreenath SB, Taylor RJ, Miller JD, Ambrose EC, Rawal RB, Ebert CS Jr, et al., editors. A prospective randomized cohort study evaluating 3 weeks vs 6 weeks of oral antibiotic treatment in the setting of "maximal medical therapy" for chronic rhinosinusitis. International forum of allergy & rhinology. Hoboken, NJ: Wiley Online Library; 2015.
27. Pynnonen MA, Venkatraman G, Davis GE. Macrolide therapy for chronic rhinosinusitis: a meta-analysis. Otolaryngol Head Neck Surg. 2013;148(3):366–73.
28. Russell PT, Bekeny JR. Oral antibiotics and the management of chronic sinusitis: what do we know? Curr Opin Otolaryngol Head Neck Surg. 2014;22(1):22–6.
29. Lasso A, Masoudian P, Quinn J, Cowan J, Labajian V, Bonaparte J, et al. Long-term low-dose macrolides for chronic rhinosinusitis in adults–a systematic review of the literature. Clin Otolaryngol. 2017;42(3):637–50.
30. Schwartz JS, Tajudeen BA, Cohen NA. Medical management of chronic rhinosinusitis – a review of traditional and novel medical therapies. Expert Opin Investig Drugs. 2017;26(10):1123–30. https://doi.org/10.1080/13543784.2017.1371699.
31. Orlandi RR, Kingdom TT, Hwang PH, Smith TL, Alt JA, Baroody FM, et al. International consensus statement on allergy and rhinology: rhinosinusitis. Int Forum Allergy Rhinol. 2016;6(Suppl 1):S22–209. https://doi.org/10.1002/alr.21695.
32. Rowan NR, Lee S, Sahu N, Kanaan A, Cox S, Phillips CD, et al. The role of viruses in the clinical presentation of chronic rhinosinusitis. Am J Rhinol Allergy. 2015;29(6):e197–200. https://doi.org/10.2500/ajra.2015.29.4242.
33. Liao B, Hu CY, Liu T, Liu Z. Respiratory viral infection in the chronic persistent phase of chronic rhinosinusitis. Laryngoscope. 2014;124(4):832–7. https://doi.org/10.1002/lary.24348.
34. Rank MA, Wollan P, Kita H, Yawn BP. Acute exacerbations of chronic rhinosinusitis occur in a distinct seasonal pattern. J Allergy Clin Immunol. 2010;126(1):168–9. https://doi.org/10.1016/j.jaci.2010.03.041.
35. Brook I. Bacteriology of chronic sinusitis and acute exacerbation of chronic sinusitis. Arch Otolaryngol Head Neck Surg. 2006;132(10):1099–101. https://doi.org/10.1001/archotol.132.10.1099.

36. Merkley MA, Bice TC, Grier A, Strohl AM, Man LX, Gill SR. The effect of antibiotics on the microbiome in acute exacerbations of chronic rhinosinusitis. Int Forum Allergy Rhinol. 2015;5(10):884–93. https://doi.org/10.1002/alr.21591.
37. Sabino HA, Valera FC, Aragon DC, Fantucci MZ, Titoneli CC, Martinez R, et al. Amoxicillin-clavulanate for patients with acute exacerbation of chronic rhinosinusitis: a prospective, double-blinded, placebo-controlled trial. Int Forum Allergy Rhinol. 2017;7(2):135–42. https://doi.org/10.1002/alr.21846.
38. Yan CH, Tangbumrungtham N, Maul XA, Ma Y, Nayak JV, Hwang PH, et al. Comparison of outcomes following culture-directed vs non-culture-directed antibiotics in treatment of acute exacerbations of chronic rhinosinusitis. Int Forum Allergy Rhinol. 2018;8(9):1028–33. https://doi.org/10.1002/alr.22147.
39. Lee VS, Davis GE. Culture-directed topical antibiotic treatment for chronic rhinosinusitis. Am J Rhinol Allergy. 2016;30(6):414–7. https://doi.org/10.2500/ajra.2016.30.4380.
40. Abreu NA, Nagalingam NA, Song Y, Roediger FC, Pletcher SD, Goldberg AN, et al. Sinus microbiome diversity depletion and Corynebacterium tuberculostearicum enrichment mediates rhinosinusitis. Sci Transl Med. 2012;4(151):151ra24. https://doi.org/10.1126/scitranslmed.3003783.
41. Feazel LM, Robertson CE, Ramakrishnan VR, Frank DN. Microbiome complexity and Staphylococcus aureus in chronic rhinosinusitis. Laryngoscope. 2012;122(2):467–72. https://doi.org/10.1002/lary.22398.
42. Stephenson MF, Mfuna L, Dowd SE, Wolcott RD, Barbeau J, Poisson M, et al. Molecular characterization of the polymicrobial flora in chronic rhinosinusitis. J Otolaryngol Head Neck Surg. 2010;39(2):182–7.
43. Hoggard M, Biswas K, Zoing M, Wagner Mackenzie B, Taylor MW, Douglas RG. Evidence of microbiota dysbiosis in chronic rhinosinusitis. Int Forum Allergy Rhinol. 2017;7(3):230–9. https://doi.org/10.1002/alr.21871.
44. Wagner Mackenzie B, Waite DW, Hoggard M, Douglas RG, Taylor MW, Biswas K. Bacterial community collapse: a meta-analysis of the sinonasal microbiota in chronic rhinosinusitis. Environ Microbiol. 2017;19(1):381–92. https://doi.org/10.1111/1462-2920.13632.
45. Psaltis AJ, Wormald PJ. Therapy of sinonasal microbiome in CRS: a critical approach. Curr Allergy Asthma Rep. 2017;17(9):59. https://doi.org/10.1007/s11882-017-0726-x.
46. Ramakrishnan VR, Hauser LJ, Feazel LM, Ir D, Robertson CE, Frank DN. Sinus microbiota varies among chronic rhinosinusitis phenotypes and predicts surgical outcome. J Allergy Clin Immunol. 2015;136(2):334–42.e1. https://doi.org/10.1016/j.jaci.2015.02.008.
47. Vickery TW, Ramakrishnan VR, Suh JD. The role of Staphylococcus aureus in patients with chronic sinusitis and nasal polyposis. Curr Allergy Asthma Rep. 2019;19(4):21. https://doi.org/10.1007/s11882-019-0853-7.
48. Lan F, Zhang N, Holtappels G, De Ruyck N, Krysko O, Van Crombruggen K, et al. Staphylococcus aureus induces a mucosal type 2 immune response via epithelial cell-derived cytokines. Am J Respir Crit Care Med. 2018;198(4):452–63. https://doi.org/10.1164/rccm.201710-2112OC.
49. Gehanno P, Cohen B. Effectiveness and safety of ofloxacin in chronic otitis media and chronic sinusitis in adult outpatients. Eur Arch Otorhinolaryngol. 1993;250(Suppl 1):S13–4.
50. Huck W, Reed BD, Nielsen RW, Ferguson RT, Gray DW, Lund GK, et al. Cefaclor vs amoxicillin in the treatment of acute, recurrent, and chronic sinusitis. Arch Fam Med. 1993;2(5):497–503.
51. Namyslowski G, Misiolek M, Czecior E, Malafiej E, Orecka B, Namyslowski P, et al. Comparison of the efficacy and tolerability of amoxycillin/clavulanic acid 875 mg b.i.d. with cefuroxime 500 mg b.i.d. in the treatment of chronic and acute exacerbation of chronic sinusitis in adults. J Chemother (Florence, Italy). 2002;14(5):508–17. https://doi.org/10.1179/joc.2002.14.5.508.
52. Hoza J, Salzman R, Starek I, Schalek P, Kellnerova R. Efficacy and safety of erdosteine in the treatment of chronic rhinosinusitis with nasal polyposis – a pilot study. Rhinology. 2013;51(4):323–7. https://doi.org/10.4193/Rhin13.039.
53. Adelson RT, Adappa ND. What is the proper role of oral antibiotics in the treatment of patients with chronic sinusitis? Curr Opin Otolaryngol Head Neck Surg. 2013;21(1):61–8. https://doi.org/10.1097/MOO.0b013e32835ac625.
54. Oakley GM, Harvey RJ, Lund VJ. The role of macrolides in chronic rhinosinusitis (CRSsNP and CRSwNP). Curr Allergy Asthma Rep. 2017;17(5):30. https://doi.org/10.1007/s11882-017-0696-z.
55. Harvey RJ, Wallwork BD, Lund VJ. Anti-inflammatory effects of macrolides: applications in chronic rhinosinusitis. Immunol Allergy Clin North Am. 2009;29(4):689–703. https://doi.org/10.1016/j.iac.2009.07.006.
56. Zimmermann P, Ziesenitz VC, Curtis N, Ritz N. The immunomodulatory effects of macrolides—a systematic review of the underlying mechanisms. Front Immunol. 2018;9:302. https://doi.org/10.3389/fimmu.2018.00302.
57. Phillips KM, Hoehle LP, Bergmark RW, Caradonna DS, Gray ST, Sedaghat AR. Acute exacerbations mediate quality of life impairment in chronic rhinosinusitis. J Allergy Clin Immunol Pract. 2017;5(2):422–6. https://doi.org/10.1016/j.jaip.2016.09.015.
58. Banoub RG, Phillips KM, Hoehle LP, Caradonna DS, Gray ST, Sedaghat AR. Relationship between chronic rhinosinusitis exacerbation frequency and

asthma control. Laryngoscope. 2018;128(5):1033–8. https://doi.org/10.1002/lary.26901.
59. Peters AT, Spector S, Hsu J, Hamilos DL, Baroody FM, Chandra RK, et al. Diagnosis and management of rhinosinusitis: a practice parameter update. Ann Allergy Asthma Immunol. 2014;113(4):347–85.
60. Rosenfeld RM, Piccirillo JF, Chandrasekhar SS, Brook I, Ashok Kumar K, Kramper M, et al. Clinical practice guideline (update): adult sinusitis. Otolaryngol Head Neck Surg. 2015;152(2 Suppl):S1–s39. https://doi.org/10.1177/0194599815572097.
61. Garbutt JM, Banister C, Spitznagel E, Piccirillo JF. Amoxicillin for acute rhinosinusitis: a randomized controlled trial. JAMA. 2012;307(7):685–92. https://doi.org/10.1001/jama.2012.138.
62. Blondeau JM, Shebelski SD, Hesje CK. Killing of Streptococcus pneumoniae by azithromycin, clarithromycin, erythromycin, telithromycin and gemifloxacin using drug minimum inhibitory concentrations and mutant prevention concentrations. Int J Antimicrob Agents. 2015;45(6):594–9. https://doi.org/10.1016/j.ijantimicag.2014.12.034.
63. Parnham MJ, Erakovic Haber V, Giamarellos-Bourboulis EJ, Perletti G, Verleden GM, Vos R. Azithromycin: mechanisms of action and their relevance for clinical applications. Pharmacol Ther. 2014;143(2):225–45. https://doi.org/10.1016/j.pharmthera.2014.03.003.
64. Kucuksezer UC, Ozdemir C, Akdis M, Akdis CA. Chronic rhinosinusitis: pathogenesis, therapy options, and more. Expert Opin Pharmacother. 2018;19(16):1805–15.
65. Bachert C, Zhang N, Hellings PW, Bousquet J. Endotype-driven care pathways in patients with chronic rhinosinusitis. J Allergy Clin Immunol. 2018;141(5):1543–51.
66. Yip J, Monteiro E, Chan Y. Endotypes of chronic rhinosinusitis. Curr Opin Otolaryngol Head Neck Surg. 2019;27(1):14–9.
67. Wallwork B, Coman W, Mackay-Sim A, Greiff L, Cervin A. A double-blind, randomized, placebo-controlled trial of macrolide in the treatment of chronic rhinosinusitis. Laryngoscope. 2006;116(2):189–93. https://doi.org/10.1097/01.mlg.0000191560.53555.08.
68. Pinto Bezerra Soter AC, Bezerra TF, Pezato R, Teles Abdo TR, Pilan RM, Pinna FR, et al. Prospective open-label evaluation of long-term low-dose doxycycline for difficult-to-treat chronic rhinosinusitis with nasal polyps. Rhinology. 2017;55(2):175–80. https://doi.org/10.4193/Rhin15.291.
69. Suzuki H, Ikeda K, Honma R, Gotoh S, Oshima T, Furukawa M, et al. Prognostic factors of chronic rhinosinusitis under long-term low-dose macrolide therapy. ORL J Otorhinolaryngol Relat Spec. 2000;62(3):121–7. https://doi.org/10.1159/000027731.
70. Haxel BR, Clemens M, Karaiskaki N, Dippold U, Kettern L, Mann WJ. Controlled trial for long-term low-dose erythromycin after sinus surgery for chronic rhinosinusitis. Laryngoscope. 2015;125(5):1048–55. https://doi.org/10.1002/lary.25052.
71. Videler WJ, Badia L, Harvey RJ, Gane S, Georgalas C, van der Meulen FW, et al. Lack of efficacy of long-term, low-dose azithromycin in chronic rhinosinusitis: a randomized controlled trial. Allergy. 2011;66(11):1457–68. https://doi.org/10.1111/j.1398-9995.2011.02693.x.
72. Cho SH, Kim DW, Gevaert P. Chronic rhinosinusitis without nasal polyps. J Allergy Clin Immunol Pract. 2016;4(4):575–82. https://doi.org/10.1016/j.jaip.2016.04.015.
73. Haruna S, Shimada C, Ozawa M, Fukami S, Moriyama H. A study of poor responders for long-term, low-dose macrolide administration for chronic sinusitis. Rhinology. 2009;47(1):66–71.
74. Deng J, Chen F, Lai Y, Luo Q, Xu R, Ou C, et al., editors. Lack of additional effects of long-term, low-dose clarithromycin combined treatment compared with topical steroids alone for chronic rhinosinusitis in China: a randomized, controlled trial. International forum of allergy & rhinology. Hoboken, NJ: Wiley Online Library; 2018.
75. Huang Z, Zhou B. Clarithromycin for the treatment of adult chronic rhinosinusitis: a systematic review and meta-analysis. Int Forum Allergy Rhinol. 2019; https://doi.org/10.1002/alr.22281.
76. Liu YF, Richardson CM, Bernard SH, Church CA, Seiberling KA. Antibiotics, steroids, and combination therapy in chronic rhinosinusitis without nasal polyps in adults. Ear Nose Throat J. 2018;97(6):167–72.
77. Dubin MG, Liu C, Lin SY, Senior BA. American Rhinologic Society member survey on "maximal medical therapy" for chronic rhinosinusitis. Am J Rhinol. 2007;21(4):483–8.
78. Sylvester DC, Carr S, Nix P. Maximal medical therapy for chronic rhinosinusitis: a survey of otolaryngology consultants in the United Kingdom. Int Forum Allergy Rhinol. 2013;3(2):129–32. https://doi.org/10.1002/alr.21084.
79. Dautremont JF, Rudmik L. When are we operating for chronic rhinosinusitis? A systematic review of maximal medical therapy protocols prior to endoscopic sinus surgery. Int Forum Allergy Rhinol. 2015;5(12):1095–103. https://doi.org/10.1002/alr.21601.
80. Sreenath SB, Taylor RJ, Miller JD, Ambrose EC, Rawal RB, Ebert CS Jr, et al. A prospective randomized cohort study evaluating 3 weeks vs 6 weeks of oral antibiotic treatment in the setting of "maximal medical therapy" for chronic rhinosinusitis. Int Forum Allergy Rhinol. 2015;5(9):820–8. https://doi.org/10.1002/alr.21542.
81. Ramakrishnan VR, Mace JC, Soler ZM, Smith TL. Is greater antibiotic therapy prior to ESS associated with differences in surgical outcomes in CRS? Laryngoscope. 2019;129(3):558–66. https://doi.org/10.1002/lary.27651.

82. Gunel C, Bleier BS, Meteoglu I. Antibiotics in eosinophilic chronic rhinosinusitis: rethinking maximal antimicrobial medical therapy. Laryngoscope. 2017;127(4):794–6. https://doi.org/10.1002/lary.26415.
83. Carr TF, Koterba AP, Chandra R, Grammer LC, Conley DB, Harris KE, et al. Characterization of specific antibody deficiency in adults with medically refractory chronic rhinosinusitis. Am J Rhinol Allergy. 2011;25(4):241–4. https://doi.org/10.2500/ajra.2011.25.3653.
84. Smith KA, Smith TL, Mace JC, Rudmik L. Endoscopic sinus surgery compared to continued medical therapy for patients with refractory chronic rhinosinusitis. Int Forum Allergy Rhinol. 2014;4(10):823–7. https://doi.org/10.1002/alr.21366.
85. Rudmik L, Soler ZM, Mace JC, Schlosser RJ, Smith TL. Economic evaluation of endoscopic sinus surgery versus continued medical therapy for refractory chronic rhinosinusitis. Laryngoscope. 2015;125(1):25–32. https://doi.org/10.1002/lary.24916.
86. Eloy JA, Marchiano E, Vazquez A. Extended endoscopic and open sinus surgery for refractory chronic rhinosinusitis. Otolaryngol Clin North Am. 2017;50(1):165–82. https://doi.org/10.1016/j.otc.2016.08.013.
87. Lim M, Citardi MJ, Leong JL. Topical antimicrobials in the management of chronic rhinosinusitis: a systematic review. Am J Rhinol. 2008;22(4):381–9. https://doi.org/10.2500/ajr.2008.22.3189.
88. Rudmik L, Hoy M, Schlosser RJ, Harvey RJ, Welch KC, Lund V, et al. Topical therapies in the management of chronic rhinosinusitis: an evidence-based review with recommendations. Int Forum Allergy Rhinol. 2013;3(4):281–98. https://doi.org/10.1002/alr.21096.
89. Jiang RS, Twu CW, Liang KL. Efficacy of nasal irrigation with 200 mug/mL amphotericin B after functional endoscopic sinus surgery: a randomized, placebo-controlled, double-blind study. Int Forum Allergy Rhinol. 2018;8(1):41–8. https://doi.org/10.1002/alr.22033.
90. Uren B, Psaltis A, Wormald PJ. Nasal lavage with mupirocin for the treatment of surgically recalcitrant chronic rhinosinusitis. Laryngoscope. 2008;118(9):1677–80. https://doi.org/10.1097/MLG.0b013e31817aec47.
91. Ezzat WF, Fawaz SA, Rabie H, Hamdy TA, Shokry YA. Effect of topical ofloxacin on bacterial biofilms in refractory post-sinus surgery rhino-sinusitis. Eur Arch Otorhinolaryngol. 2015;272(9):2355–61. https://doi.org/10.1007/s00405-014-3301-2.
92. Rudmik L, Smith TL. Evidence-based practice: postoperative care in endoscopic sinus surgery. Otolaryngol Clin North Am. 2012;45(5):1019–32.
93. Eloy P, Andrews P, Poirrier A-L. Postoperative care in endoscopic sinus surgery: a critical review. Curr Opin Otolaryngol Head Neck Surg. 2017;25(1):35–42.
94. Huang ZX, Li YX, Wu YB, Liu HC, Zhou B. Preoperative and postoperative medical therapies for chronic rhinosinusitis: national surveys among Chinese otolaryngologists. World J Otorhinolaryngol. 2018;4(4):258–62. https://doi.org/10.1016/j.wjorl.2018.06.001.
95. Varvyanskaya A, Lopatin A. Efficacy of long-term low-dose macrolide therapy in preventing early recurrence of nasal polyps after endoscopic sinus surgery. Int Forum Allergy Rhinol. 2014;4(7):533–41. https://doi.org/10.1002/alr.21318.
96. Amali A, Saedi B, Rahavi-Ezabadi S, Ghazavi H, Hassanpoor N. Long-term postoperative azithromycin in patients with chronic rhinosinusitis: a randomized clinical trial. Am J Rhinol Allergy. 2015;29(6):421–4. https://doi.org/10.2500/ajra.2015.29.4244.
97. Nakamura Y, Suzuki M, Yokota M, Ozaki S, Ohno N, Hamajima Y, et al. Optimal duration of macrolide treatment for chronic sinusitis after endoscopic sinus surgery. Auris Nasus Larynx. 2013;40(4):366–72. https://doi.org/10.1016/j.anl.2012.09.009.
98. Annys E, Jorissen M. Short term effects of antibiotics (Zinnat) after endoscopic sinus surgery. Acta Otorhinolaryngol Belg. 2000;54(1):23–8.
99. Jiang RS, Liang KL, Yang KY, Shiao JY, Su MC, Hsin CH, et al. Postoperative antibiotic care after functional endoscopic sinus surgery. Am J Rhinol. 2008;22(6):608–12. https://doi.org/10.2500/ajr.2008.22.3241.
100. Albu S, Lucaciu R. Prophylactic antibiotics in endoscopic sinus surgery: a short follow-up study. Am J Rhinol Allergy. 2010;24(4):306–9. https://doi.org/10.2500/ajra.2010.24.3475.
101. Fombeur JP, Barrault S, Koubbi G, Laurier JN, Ebbo D, Lecomte F, et al. Study of the efficacy and safety of ciprofloxacin in the treatment of chronic sinusitis. Chemotherapy. 1994;40(Suppl 1):24–8. https://doi.org/10.1159/000239313.
102. Legent F, Bordure P, Beauvillain C, Berche P. A double-blind comparison of ciprofloxacin and amoxycillin/clavulanic acid in the treatment of chronic sinusitis. Chemotherapy. 1994;40(Suppl 1):8–15. https://doi.org/10.1159/000239310.
103. Hashiba M, Baba S. Efficacy of long-term administration of clarithromycin in the treatment of intractable chronic sinusitis. Acta Otolaryngol Suppl. 1996;525:73–8.
104. Ichimura K, Shimazaki Y, Ishibashi T, Higo R. Effect of new macrolide roxithromycin upon nasal polyps associated with chronic sinusitis. Auris Nasus Larynx. 1996;23:48–56.
105. Ragab SM, Lund VJ, Scadding G. Evaluation of the medical and surgical treatment of chronic rhinosinusitis: a prospective, randomised, controlled trial. Laryngoscope. 2004;114(5):923–30. https://doi.org/10.1097/00005537-200405000-00027.

106. Ray WA, Murray KT, Hall K, Arbogast PG, Stein CM. Azithromycin and the risk of cardiovascular death. N Engl J Med. 2012;366(20):1881–90.
107. Li M, Ramos LG. Drug-induced QT prolongation and torsades de pointes. Pharm Ther. 2017;42(7):473.
108. Mosholder AD, Mathew J, Alexander JJ, Smith H, Nambiar S. Cardiovascular risks with azithromycin and other antibacterial drugs. N Engl J Med. 2013;368(18):1665–8.
109. Kingdom TT, Swain RE Jr. The microbiology and antimicrobial resistance patterns in chronic rhinosinusitis. Am J Otolaryngol. 2004;25(5):323–8.
110. Bhattacharyya N, Kepnes LJ. Assessment of trends in antimicrobial resistance in chronic rhinosinusitis. Ann Otol Rhinol Laryngol. 2008;117(6):448–52. https://doi.org/10.1177/000348940811700608.
111. Solares CA, Batra PS, Hall GS, Citardi MJ. Treatment of chronic rhinosinusitis exacerbations due to methicillin-resistant Staphylococcus aureus with mupirocin irrigations. Am J Otolaryngol. 2006;27(3):161–5. https://doi.org/10.1016/j.amjoto.2005.09.006.
112. Manarey CR, Anand VK, Huang C. Incidence of methicillin-resistant Staphylococcus aureus causing chronic rhinosinusitis. Laryngoscope. 2004;114(5):939–41. https://doi.org/10.1097/00005537-200405000-00029.

44 Decongestant and Nasal Irrigation

Xiaoping Lai and Gehua Zhang

Key Points

- Nasal decongestants conduce to the remission of nasal congestion but should not be used continuously for more than 1 week or repeatedly.
- Nasal irrigation performed with large volume is supposed to be more beneficial than other delivery modes. However, optimal solution is still controversial.
- Nasal irrigation is a crucial treatment in the postoperative period of FESS. It contributes to wound healing and the removal of blood and scars in the paranasal sinuses, preventing patients from wound infections.

44.1 Decongestant

Nasal decongestants can stimulate α-adrenergic receptors, and thereby constrict vascular smooth muscle, conducing to nasal mucosa shrinking in size and thus remission of nasal congestion. It is confirmed that decongestants have no effects on nasal polyp size, only reduce congestion of inferior and middle turbinates [1]. Therefore, decongestants are recommended prior to nasal endoscopy.

Nasal decongestants are divided into two groups:

- Sympathomimetic amines, including: phenolic (such as adrenaline, hydroxyamphetamine, phenylephrine, and tuaminoheptane) and non-phenolic (such as ephedrine, pseudoephedrine, and phenylpropanolamine).
- Imidazoline derivatives, such as naphazoline, oxymetazoline, tetryzoline, xylometazoline, clonazoline, and tramazoline.

These two groups vary in latency and duration of action (Table 44.1) [2]. They can be either used topically (as drops or sprays) or taken orally. Topical nasal decongestants should not be used continually for more than 1 week or repeatedly. Otherwise, patients will suffer from rebound congestion and rhinitis medicamentosa [3]. Some clinicians even found that topical nasal decongestants lead to hypertensive crisis and end-organ damage including retinopathy, irreversible renal damage, and left ventricular hypertrophy [4]. Topical nasal decongestants should be used with caution in pregnant woman because it might lead to fetal heart rate changes [5].

Up to now, there are no convincible randomized controlled trials to decide the efficacy of nasal decongestants in chronic rhinosinusitis (CRS). According to the European Position Paper

X. Lai · G. Zhang (✉)
Department of Otorhinolaryngology, The Third Affiliated Hospital of Sun Yat-sen University, Guangzhou, China
e-mail: zhanggeh@mail.sysu.edu.cn

L. Zhang, C. Bachert (eds.), *Chronic Rhinosinusitis*, https://doi.org/10.1007/978-981-16-0784-4_44

Table 44.1 Comparison of sympathomimetic amine and imidazoline derivative nasal decongestants [2]

	Sympathomimetic amines				Imidazoline derivatives					
Substance	Adrenaline	Ephedrine	Tuaminoheptane	Phenylephrine	Clonazoline	Tramazoline	Naphazoline	Tetryzoline	Xylometazoline	Oxymetazoline
Latency	5–6 s	10 min	15 min	15 min	5 min	5 min	15 min	15 min	20 min	20 min
Duration of action	20–30 min	3–4 h	1.5 h	1–2 h	8–12 h	11–12 h	2–6 h	4–6 h	10–11 h	10–12 h
Side effects	++++	+++	+++	+++	++	+	++	++	++	++

on Rhinosinusitis and Nasal Polyps 2020 (EPOS2020), nasal decongestants are not recommended to be used in CRS, only if in situations where the nose is very blocked [6]. Clinicians should weigh the benefits against the adverse effects while prescribing decongestants and remind the patients not to use them for more than 1 week.

44.2 Nasal Irrigation

Nasal irrigation is also utilized as an effective supplementary treatment of CRS. It is widely used in everyday clinical practice (Fig. 44.1). A Cochrane review of saline irrigations in patients with CRS concluded that the beneficial effects of saline irrigations outweigh the drawbacks for the majority of patients [7].

However, the exact mechanism of nasal irrigation remains unknown. Normative nasal irrigation is supposed to improve nasal mucosa function by direct cleaning of mucus; removing antigens, biofilms, or inflammatory mediators [8]; moisturizing the nasal mucosa and promoting mucociliary clearance function [9].

Nasal irrigation can be performed in different protocols. It varies in methods of delivery, compositions of solutions, and concentrations of solutions.

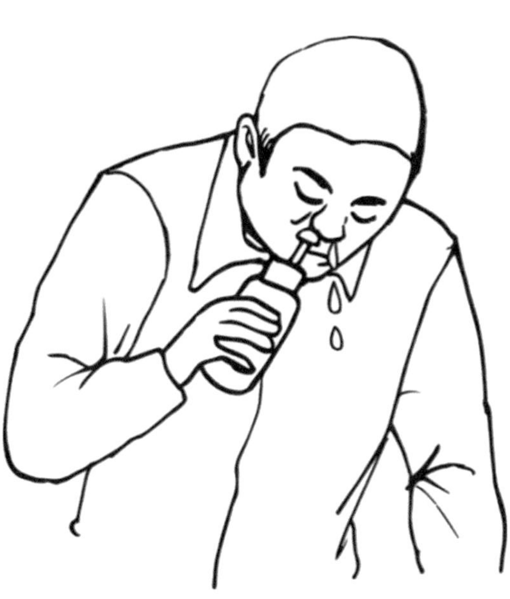

Fig. 44.1 Nasal irrigation technique

It is confirmed that high-volume is better for nasal irrigation than other delivery modes. The spray or nebulization method brings poorer intranasal distribution of saline solution than positive- or negative-pressure irrigation by nasal cavity douching [10, 11]. Likewise, Pynnonen et al. found that nasal irrigations performed with large volume and low positive pressure are more beneficial than saline sprays at improving quality of life and decreasing medication use [12].

Various compositions of solutions can be used for nasal irrigation and they are reported to bring benefits, such as hypertonic or isotonic saline, thermal water, sodium hyaluronate, xylitol, budesonide, and so on. It is controversial to decide which one to be optimal solution. The conclusions vary from study to study. Among the solutions mentioned above, saline is the most frequently used. A prospective, randomized, double-blind study including 70 patients found that a month of daily sulfurous-arsenical-ferruginous thermal water irrigation leads to lower nasal resistance and an increase in the number of ciliated cells [13]. Both endoscopic appearance and patient's subjective satisfaction after functional endoscopic sinus surgery (FESS) are improved by nasal douching with saline plus sodium hyaluronate [14]. Compared with placebo, budesonide transnasal nebulization improves symptom of eosinophilic CRS with nasal polyps, contributes to shrinkage of polyps, and helps to regulate cytokine expressions [15]. However, according to our previous study, no significant difference is found in terms of symptom scores and endoscopic scores between various solutions and normal saline for patients after FESS [16]. Three studies are included as a result of differences in outcome measures and insufficient data. More clinical trials are needed to draw a convincible conclusion and help guide clinical practice.

It is also important to choose the correct saline solution concentration with great attention. Hypertonic, isotonic, and hypotonic saline solutions were used in a large number of studies. Hypertonic saline is recommended because it can reduce mucosal edema and improve mucociliary clearance [9, 17]. The advantageous effects of isotonic saline are also proved by several researches [12, 18, 19]. Isotonic saline mainly works by mechanical cleaning. Kim et al. reported that isotonic saline is the most physiologic treatment because it brings no cellular damage to nasal mucosal morphology [19]. However, hypotonic saline seems to bring cellular edema and a moderate degree of ciliary damage in the same study [19].

Several studies have compared the effects of hypertonic versus isotonic solutions. Shoseyov et al. showed that treating with hypertonic saline relieves symptoms like cough, nasal secretion and improves radiology score when compared to normal saline in pediatric patients [20]. It is worth noting that the interference was undertaken by instillation of drops, not in the recommended form. A meta-analysis including nine studies (740 patients) found that hypertonic saline irrigation brings greater benefits over isotonic saline irrigation in reduction of symptoms [21], while a previous meta-analysis including three studies found no difference between two groups [22]. Overall, both concentrations can be employed in daily clinical practice. If one must be chosen, hypertonic solution seems to be more appropriate.

For those who are in the postoperative period of FESS, nasal irrigation is particularly beneficial. According to our previous study, nasal irrigation helps to improve the prognosis of CRS after endoscopic sinus surgery [23]. It contributes to wound healing and the removal of blood and scars in the paranasal sinuses, preventing patients from wound infections. According to EPOS2020, nasal irrigation helps to reduce symptom scores and endoscopic scores for CRS after FESS, indicating that it is a crucial treatment in the postoperative period of FESS [6]. FESS also improves the distribution of irrigation solutions in the paranasal sinuses, increasing the efficacy of this treatment [24]. Greater penetration of irrigation solutions is observed in postoperative and non-obstructed sinuses because of surgical ostial enlargement [25]. The authors propose a 3.95 mm ostial diameter to be the minimum size of sinus ostia for nasal irrigation penetration [25].

Nasal irrigation also brings some side effects, including epistaxis, local irritation, ear pain, headache, nasal burning, nasal drainage, bottle contamination, and hyposmia. Hypertonic saline is comparatively reported to cause more nasal discomfort [21]. Epistaxis and nasal burning are the most common adverse events. They might usually result from too heavy pressing or pressing the spout against the nasal septum. Despite adverse effects, the beneficial effects of saline irrigations outweigh the drawbacks, according to a Cochrane review [7].

In addition, the effect of nasal irrigation for CRS of children is unclear [26]. There are several studies reporting that children are benefitted from hypertonic saline [20]. Mild and limited side effects of nasal irrigation are found in children and the majority of children can tolerate it, regardless of age [27]. However, the current problem is lacking of convincible randomized controlled trials to weigh the advantages over adverse effects. High quality prospective studies are demanded to determine its exact impacts on pediatric patients.

In general, nasal irrigation is an effective, inexpensive, acceptable, well-tolerated convenient home-prepare supplement therapy for CRS. Patients can administrate nasal irrigation as directed by a physician and get guide technique online at https://www.fammed.wisc.edu/nasal-irrigation/.

44.3 For Future Daily Practice

Both decongestant and nasal irrigation help to improve symptoms of CRS. Considering the risks of rebound congestion and rhinitis medicamentosa, decongestant is recommended to be used temporarily when patient has a very stuffy nose. As for nasal irrigation, it can be easily administrated at home and benefits most patients, especially postoperative patients.

References

1. Johansson L, Oberg D, Melen I, Bende M. Do topical nasal decongestants affect polyps? Acta Otolaryngol. 2006;126(3):288–90. https://doi.org/10.1080/00016480500388877.
2. Passali D, Salerni L, Passali GC, Passali FM, Bellussi L. Nasal decongestants in the treatment of chronic nasal obstruction: efficacy and safety of use. Expert Opin Drug Saf. 2006;5(6):783–90. https://doi.org/10.1517/14740338.5.6.783.
3. Mortuaire G, de Gabory L, Francois M, Masse G, Bloch F, Brion N, et al. Rebound congestion and rhinitis medicamentosa: nasal decongestants in clinical practice. Critical review of the literature by a medical panel. Eur Ann Otorhinolaryngol Head Neck Dis. 2013;130(3):137–44. https://doi.org/10.1016/j.anorl.2012.09.005.
4. Buysschaert I, Van Dorpe J, Dujardin K. Hypertensive crisis and end-organ damage induced by over-the-counter nasal decongestant abuse. Eur Heart J. 2011;32(24):3114. https://doi.org/10.1093/eurheartj/ehr199.
5. Baxi LV, Gindoff PR, Pregenzer GJ, Parras MK. Fetal heart rate changes following maternal administration of a nasal decongestant. Am J Obstet Gynecol. 1985;153(7):799–800.
6. Fokkens WJ, Lund VJ, Hopkins C, Hellings PW, Kern R, Reitsma S, et al. European position paper on rhinosinusitis and nasal polyps 2020. Rhinology. 2020;58(Suppl S29):1–464. https://doi.org/10.4193/Rhin20.600.
7. Chong LY, Head K, Hopkins C, Philpott C, Glew S, Scadding G, et al. Saline irrigation for chronic rhinosinusitis. Cochrane Database Syst Rev. 2016;(4):Cd011995. https://doi.org/10.1002/14651858.CD011995.pub2.
8. Georgitis JW. Nasal hyperthermia and simple irrigation for perennial rhinitis. Changes in inflammatory mediators. Chest. 1994;106(5):1487–92.
9. Homer JJ, Dowley AC, Condon L, El-Jassar P, Sood S. The effect of hypertonicity on nasal mucociliary clearance. Clin Otolaryngol Allied Sci. 2000;25(6):558–60.
10. Wormald PJ, Cain T, Oates L, Hawke L, Wong I. A comparative study of three methods of nasal irrigation. Laryngoscope. 2004;114(12):2224–7. https://doi.org/10.1097/01.mlg.0000149463.95950.c5.
11. Olson DE, Rasgon BM, Hilsinger RL Jr. Radiographic comparison of three methods for nasal saline irrigation. Laryngoscope. 2002;112(8 Pt 1):1394–8. https://doi.org/10.1097/00005537-200208000-00013.
12. Pynnonen MA, Mukerji SS, Kim HM, Adams ME, Terrell JE. Nasal saline for chronic sinonasal symptoms: a randomized controlled trial. Arch Otolaryngol Head Neck Surg. 2007;133(11):1115–20. https://doi.org/10.1001/archotol.133.11.1115.
13. Ottaviano G, Marioni G, Giacomelli L, La Torre FB, Staffieri C, Marchese-Ragona R, et al. Smoking and chronic rhinitis: effects of nasal irrigations with sulfurous-arsenical-ferruginous thermal water: a prospective, randomized, double-blind study. Am J Otolaryngol. 2012;33(6):657–62. https://doi.org/10.1016/j.amjoto.2012.03.002.
14. Mozzanica F, Preti A, Gera R, Bulgheroni C, Cardella A, Albera A, et al. Double-blind, randomised controlled trial on the efficacy of saline nasal irrigation with sodium hyaluronate after endoscopic sinus surgery. J Laryngol Otol. 2019:1–9. https://doi.org/10.1017/s0022215119000446.
15. Wang C, Lou H, Wang X, Wang Y, Fan E, Li Y, et al. Effect of budesonide transnasal nebulization in patients with eosinophilic chronic rhinosinusitis with nasal polyps. J Allergy Clin Immunol. 2015;135(4):922–29.e6. https://doi.org/10.1016/j.jaci.2014.10.018.
16. Chen XZ, Feng SY, Chang LH, Lai XP, Chen XH, Li X, et al. The effects of nasal irrigation with various solutions after endoscopic sinus surgery: systematic review and meta-analysis. J Laryngol Otol. 2018;132(8):673–9. https://doi.org/10.1017/s0022215118000919.
17. Talbot AR, Herr TM, Parsons DS. Mucociliary clearance and buffered hypertonic saline solution. Laryngoscope. 1997;107(4):500–3.
18. Bachmann G, Hommel G, Michel O. Effect of irrigation of the nose with isotonic salt solution on adult patients with chronic paranasal sinus disease. Eur Arch Otorhinolaryngoloy. 2000;257(10):537–41.
19. Kim CH, Hyun Song M, Eun Ahn Y, Lee JG, Yoon JH. Effect of hypo-, iso- and hypertonic saline irrigation on secretory mucins and morphology of cultured human nasal epithelial cells. Acta Otolaryngol. 2005;125(12):1296–300. https://doi.org/10.1080/00016480510012381.
20. Shoseyov D, Bibi H, Shai P, Shoseyov N, Shazberg G, Hurvitz H. Treatment with hypertonic saline versus normal saline nasal wash of pediatric chronic sinusitis. J Allergy Clin Immunol. 1998;101(5):602–5. https://doi.org/10.1016/s0091-6749(98)70166-6.
21. Kanjanawasee D, Seresirikachorn K, Chitsuthipakorn W, Snidvongs K. Hypertonic saline versus isotonic saline nasal irrigation: systematic review and meta-analysis. Am J Rhinol Allergy. 2018;32(4):269–79. https://doi.org/10.1177/1945892418773566.
22. Harvey R, Hannan SA, Badia L, Scadding G. Nasal saline irrigations for the symptoms of chronic rhinosinusitis. Cochrane Database Syst Rev. 2007;(3):Cd006394. https://doi.org/10.1002/14651858.CD006394.pub2.
23. Huang ZZ, Chen XZ, Huang JC, Wang ZY, Li X, Chen XH, et al. Budesonide nasal irrigation improved Lund-Kennedy endoscopic score of chronic rhinosinusitis patients after endoscopic sinus surgery. Eur

Arch Otorhinolaryngol. 2019;276(5):1397–403. https://doi.org/10.1007/s00405-019-05327-6.

24. de Paiva Leite SH, Douglas RG. How does sinus surgery affect topical irrigation distribution? Curr Opin Otolaryngol Head Neck Surg. 2018;26(1):21–6. https://doi.org/10.1097/moo.0000000000000429.
25. Grobler A, Weitzel EK, Buele A, Jardeleza C, Cheong YC, Field J, et al. Pre- and postoperative sinus penetration of nasal irrigation. Laryngoscope. 2008;118(11):2078–81. https://doi.org/10.1097/MLG.0b013e31818208c1.
26. Hom J. Do decongestants, antihistamines, and nasal irrigation relieve the symptoms of sinusitis in children? Ann Emerg Med. 2013;61(1):35–6. https://doi.org/10.1016/j.annemergmed.2012.03.016.
27. Jeffe JS, Bhushan B, Schroeder JW Jr. Nasal saline irrigation in children: a study of compliance and tolerance. Int J Pediatr Otorhinolaryngol. 2012;76(3):409–13. https://doi.org/10.1016/j.ijporl.2011.12.022.

45 Probiotics, Bacterial Lysates, and Proton Pump Inhibitors

Luping Zhu and Lei Cheng

Key Points

- Patients with CRS exhibit an imbalance in microbial community in the sinus, usually higher abundance of pathogenic bacteria and lower diversity of microbiota.
- Probiotics may maintain a healthy sinus ecosystem by directly manipulating the microbiome, or countering inflammation.
- Bacterial lysates may induce non-specific or specific immune response, thereby relieving symptoms of CRS.
- Antireflux medications used for GERD may mitigate CRS symptoms, which suggests a therapeutic potential of PPIs for CRS.

45.1 Introduction

Chronic rhinosinusitis (CRS) is a disorder of the nose and paranasal sinuses characterized by chronic inflammation of over 12 weeks. According to the European Position Paper on Rhinosinusitis and Nasal Polyps (EPOS) 2012, CRS presents with at least two of the following symptoms: nasal obstruction, nasal discharge, facial pain or pressure, and reduction or loss of smell [1]. These symptoms, if existing for over 12 weeks without complete anesis, may be used to distinguish CRS from acute sinusitis. Epidemiological surveys show that CRS, as one of the most prevalent chronic diseases worldwide, attacks approximately 8% of Chinese [2] and 4.5–12% of North Americans and Europeans [3]. CRS patients often display bad mood, fatigue, and decline in sleep, productivity, and cognition, all worsening their quality of life.

CRS is a heterogeneous disease characterized by persistent sinonasal inflammation. The pathogenesis of CRS is only partially understood. The pathophysiology of CRS involves bacteria, viruses, fungi, and many other infectious agents [4–7]. Besides, non-infectious factors, including anatomic abnormalities and genetic defects, innate immune deficiencies, allergy, aspirin sensitivity, and biofilm formation, have all been considered as etiological factors of CRS. Related treatments are always designed to enhance sinus drainage, reduce mucosal edema, and eradicate infections. A combination of medicine is recommended, including topical and oral corticosteroids, oral antibiotics, and nasal saline irrigations. Functional endoscopic surgery (FESS) is effective for patients showing high symptom scores and poor adaptation to medication. The surgical

L. Zhu
Department of Otorhinolaryngology, The Second Affiliated Hospital, Nanjing Medical University, Nanjing, China

L. Cheng (✉)
Department of Otorhinolaryngology and Clinical Allergy Center, The First Affiliated Hospital, Nanjing Medical University, Nanjing, China
e-mail: chenglei@jsph.org.cn

L. Zhang, C. Bachert (eds.), *Chronic Rhinosinusitis*, https://doi.org/10.1007/978-981-16-0784-4_45

procedure aims to restore sinus ventilation by widening the ostia of sinus cavity and reducing inflammatory load [8]. However, the medication and surgery recommended by the guidelines of EPOS 2012 cannot control the disease completely, since 30% of CRS sufferers continue to demonstrate signs and symptoms [8].

Over the past decade, the pathophysiology of CRS has been furthered. Various hypotheses on the pathogenesis have been proposed, pertaining to superantigen, fungi, immune barrier, and dysfunctional eicosanoid [1]. For instance, it was hypothesized that an impaired sinonasal epithelial barrier could increase the exposure to inhaled pathogens, antigens, and particulates in the setting of a disordered host immune response, consequently promoting the chronic inflammation. New understanding of the pathogenesis paves the way for the creation of effective treatment strategies. Though the knowledge about CRS etiology is still limited, mounting evidence, like that from well-controlled studies, demonstrates the contribution of microbiota dysbiosis to the pathophysiology of CRS. In addition, gastric acid reflux is also potentially implicated in CRS pathogenesis. Restoring the microbial composition by probiotics, bacterial lysates, or antireflux medications may be beneficial for CRS. Here, we propose some potential treatment strategies for CRS based on recent theoretical fruits.

45.2 Microbiota Dysbiosis in the Pathogenesis of CRS

The mechanisms underlying chronic sinonasal inflammation are not completely defined. Bacteria have been considered as the primary causative factors of CRS [9, 10]. Numerous previous studies sought to identify a single causative organism for CRS, but none in the sinonasal microbiota has been determined [6].

The sinonasal microbiome is a large population mixed with pathogenic and commensal bacteria. A systematic review demonstrated that the total bacterial burden in CRS was similar to that in the controls among the heterogeneous studies [6]. *Firmicutes*, *Actinobacteria,* and *Bacteroides phyla* were identified in every sample of controls and patients with CRS [6]. Diverse microbiomes, including *Pseudomonas, Staphylococcus,* and *Streptococcus* that are classically considered as causative agents of respiratory disease, also present in healthy subjects [11–13].

Emerging evidence indicates that local mucosal microbial composition and function are related to the immune response in the host airway. In some cases, CRS results from an immune hyperresponsiveness to commensal microbiome [14]. Disrupted microbiome is associated with increased disease severity and poor postoperative outcomes.

CRS exerts a wide spectrum of influences on microorganisms, inflammatory effector cells, tissue repair and remodeling, and perturbation of immunoglobulins, chemokines, and even eicosanoids [15, 16]. Moreover, a variety of innate and adaptive immune molecules participate in inflammatory processes. Patients with CRS showed increased levels of IL-4, IL-5, IL-8, IL-13, eosinophils, and basophils in the nasal lavage [14].

Recently, focus has been put on the role of the entire microbial community residing in the sinuses [17]. "Dysbiosis" has been proposed as a mechanism modulating inflammation in the sinuses [18]. This hypothesis suggests that external factors (such as antibiotic, fungi, diet) can trigger dysbiosis in microbial community, thus reducing diversity and increasing bacterial load responsible for the initiation or maintenance of CRS. Aberrant bacterial assemblages are more common in subjects with comorbidities, such as asthma and cystic fibrosis [19].

Samples from patients with CRS showed greater bacterial abundance and lower diversity. *Bacteroidetes* decreased while *Proteobacteria* increased in the CRS group at the phylum level [20]. Dysbiosis of bacterial community may drive the pathogenesis or influence the severity of CRS [19]. A reduction in commensal bacterial diversity, combined with an increase in the growth of pathogenic bacteria, can elicit an inflammatory response. *Staphylococcus aureus*

(*S. aureus*) is a key pathogenic factor for CRS. The *S. aureus* abundance increased in CRSwNP patients [20]. *S. aureus* disrupted the epithelial barrier by secreting extracellular proteases in cultured human nasal epithelial cells [21]. Once the barrier is impaired, exposure to pathogens increases and bacterial colonization accelerates. In addition, dysbiotic microbiota is dominated by various genera, including *Staphylococcus*, *Streptococcus*, *Haemophilus*, *Pseudomonas*, *Moraxella*, or *Fusobacterium* [19]. The heterogeneity of CRS may be associated with the diversity of sinus bacterial microbiota and host immune responses [22].

Understanding the role of the microbiota in CRS helps develop new therapeutics regulating microbiota composition or activity. Increasing research is digging into the potential of translational microbiome in altering microbiota composition or function. New treatments could potentially reduce the use of antibiotics.

45.3 Probiotics in the Treatment of CRS

Probiotics can maintain a healthy sinus ecosystem by directly manipulating the microbiome. Probiotics are defined as live and host-benefiting bacteria [23]. They can be used either as living antibiotics or immune-modulatory intervention. *Lactobacillus*, or *Bifidobacterium* spp., is the primary species used in traditional probiotic supplements. In the treatment of CRS, supplementing probiotics may help restore the balance between beneficial commensals and pathogenic species.

Literature describes that commensal bacteria may alleviate intestinal inflammation and hypersensitivity reaction. In the gut, the commensal microbiome directly acts on epithelial cells, stabilizing tight junctions and enhancing the gut epithelial barrier through their "colonization resistance" [24]. *Bacteroides fragilis*, a microbiome in the healthy gut, could produce anti-inflammatory cytokine IL-10 and polysaccharide A (PSA) that regulated the development of Foxp3$^+$ Treg cells [25]. Microbial-derived butyrate, a common short-chain fatty acid (SCFA), exerted anti-inflammatory effects on the GI epithelium through regulating NF-κB activation [26] and also influenced the differentiation and expression of colonic Treg cells [27]. The gut commensal *Clostridia* could induce CD4$^+$ Foxp3$^+$ Treg differentiation, a process driven by production of microbial SCFAs [28].

The development and function of multiple populations of intestinal immune cells can only be realized in the presence of microbiota. Gut-colonizing bacteria react with TLRs embedded in the intestinal epithelium, stimulate nucleotide-binding oligomerization domain receptors (NODs) or lectins signaling pathways, modulate the maturation of DCs and their cytokine pattern [24], activate immune effector cells, such as macrophages, B cells, NK cells, Th1 cells and Th2 cells, cytotoxic T cells, and Treg cells [29].

CRS consists of many phenotypes and endotypes, like CRSwNP/CRSsNP defined according to the presence/absence of nasal polyps. The chronic mucosal inflammation matches the responses of Th1 and Th2 cells [30]. Atopy plays multiple functions in CRSwNP [31, 32] that is associated with asthma and allergic rhinitis [33, 34]. Increased numbers of basophils [35], innate type 2 lymphoid cells, and mast cells may be involved in non-allergic and allergic chronic nasal inflammation [36].

The use of probiotics in the prevention of pediatric allergy has been extensively investigated in many randomized controlled trials and systematic meta-analyses [37–39]. Some results show that probiotic supplement was effective for eczema prevention in pregnancy and infancy [38, 39], suggesting that probiotics may be anti-inflammatory when administered orally or topically in the sinonasal tract. However, the interaction between microbiome and probiotics in the host immune system is expected to be revealed.

Encouraging finding has been made in a mouse model of sinusitis that confirmed *Staphylococcus epidermidis* could protect the mice against *S. aureus*-induced sinusitis [40]. In malnourished mice, nasal instillation of

Lactobacillus casei could confer protection against *Streptococcus pneumoniae* by enhancing host innate immune response [41]. Intranasal administration of *Lactobacillus rhamnosus* GG protected the mice from H1N1 influenza by activating lung natural killer cells [42].

However, these results from animal models and *in vitro* experiments have not been examined clinically. Laboratory research to identify probiotics is still relatively nascent. To date, published evidence does not support the use of probiotics for CRS. Rare studies have been conducted to explore the efficacy of topical or orally probiotics on recurrent infections in the rhinosinusitis patients. One placebo-controlled trial showed that compared with the placebo, oral use of *Lactobacillus rhamnosus R0011* did not improve quality of life scores in patients with chronic inflammatory rhinosinusitis [43]. Another clinical study showed that after 2 weeks' nasal administration of honeybee LAB microbiome, CRSsNP patients were well tolerated, but no change was observed in their symptom severity, microbiological flora, and local inflammatory activity [44]. More data are required to address whether probiotics are beneficial for CRS patients. Well-designed research has to be established based on small homogenous cohorts of CRS patients.

Future studies should resolve the following puzzles, such as live or dead probiotics, local or oral administration, and single use or adjuvant to antibiotics [45]. Other questions are pertaining to probiotics strain, optimal dosage, duration of treatment, synergistic effects of multiple strains, especially safety. Laboratory test should be performed prior to make sure multiple strains do not counteract with each other.

Probiotics-based intervention for CRS is an emerging field [46], but there is little doubt that probiotics can exert indirect or direct immunomodulatory effects. Teasing out the mechanism through which microbial dysbiosis drives the chronic sinusitis disease will facilitate the strategies of using probiotics for microbiome manipulation. Well-designed studies on specific individuals or sub-populations of CRS are needed to explore the interaction between probiotics and microbiomes.

45.4 Bacterial Lysates in the Treatment of CRS

Bacterial lysates are microbial-derived immunostimulants that can induce a non-specific response, in combination with cellular and humoral immune responses [47]. Bacterial lysates target specific immunocompetent cells through activating pathogen-recognizing receptors [48]. Bacterial lysates can also induce innate immunity dependent on TLR2 or TLR6, and TLR9, facilitate the synthesis of polyclonal immunoglobulins (IgA and IgG classes), and activate immunocompetent cells (including $CD4^+$ lymphocytes, natural killer cells, and B lymphocytes) [48, 49]. Treg cells induced by bacterial lysates might attenuate Th2 allergic responses [48].

Working with TLRs, bacterial lysates can initiate Th1-skewed immune response, thereby relieving symptoms of CRS [50, 51]. OM-85 is one commercially available bacterial lysate (brand name is Broncho-Vaxom), containing lysates from bacteria responsible for common respiratory infections: *S. aureus*, *Haemophilus influenzae*, *Streptococcus pneumoniae*, *Klebsiella pneumoniae*, *Klebsiella ozaenae*, *Streptococcus pyogenes*, *Streptococcus sanguinis*, and *Moraxella catarrhalis*. A multicenter randomized double-blind study showed that Broncho-Vaxom treated patients with chronic purulent sinusitis showed significantly relieved symptoms, including headache, purulent nasal discharge, cough, and expectoration [52]. Several randomized controlled trials demonstrated the efficacy of bacterial lysates in children with respiratory tract infection [53]. Bacterial lysates can effectively reduce the frequency of rhinosinusitis attacks and ameliorate related symptoms [54]. However, no changes in laboratory tests (hematology and clinical chemistry) were observed in patients with recurrent CRS [55]. Bacterial lysates stimulate the immune system to enhance the body's natural defenses against a wide spectrum of respiratory infections, rhinosinusitis in particular [47, 56]. The EPOS 2012 and the Pan-American Association of Otorhinolaryngology and Head and Neck Surgery guidelines recommend bacterial lysates (like OM-85) as an option for CRS, though only in adults [1, 57].

45.5 Proton Pump Inhibitors (PPIs) in the Treatment of CRS

CRS and gastroesophageal reflux disease (GERD) are two common clinical entities. The connection between CRS and gastroesophageal reflux (GER) was first reported in the early 1990s [58]. Gastric acid may flow back to the nose and nasopharynx, a process involved in CRS pathophysiology [58, 59]. Laryngopharyngeal reflux (LPR) has been found as a potential contributor to CRS. But a causative connection between reflux and CRS progression remains to be debated. Recent studies have revealed the epidemiologic association between CRS and GERD. In a large cohort of children with and without GERD, a higher prevalence of sinusitis was observed in the GERD group [60]. In a cohort of patients with CRS, especially, who were refractory to medical [61] or surgical therapy [62, 63], higher incidences of GER [63], LPR [64], or nasopharyngeal reflux (NPR) [63] were found. However, these studies are sample-size-limited and lack standardized diagnostic criteria (like pH value) of GER, which brings bias to their reliability.

A high-power research evaluated the National Ambulatory Medical Care Survey and the National Hospital Ambulatory Medical Care Survey of the United States between 2005 and 2010. The research found no association between the use of PPIs and CRS diagnosis, based on 590,772 observations at outpatient, emergency, and otolaryngology departments. Therefore, PPIs should not be recommended for CRS [65].

Till now, the American Academy of Otolaryngology-Head and Neck Surgery (AAO-HNS) expert panel and Canadian Practice Guideline have never supported the use of anti-reflux medication in the management of CRS. The EPOS 2012 guidelines reported that PPIs do not benefit CRS adults, but CRS children [1]. Yet, strong evidence supporting the use of PPI was deduced from a randomized controlled study on the treatment of postnasal drainage (PND), but not CRS [66]. This study answered the question whether treating reflux could relieve patients' PND symptoms. The patients with NPR ($pH < 5$) were treated with lansoprazole (twice, daily), and the symptoms were assessed at baseline and 8 and 16 weeks. Significant improvement was observed in the outcomes of SNOT-20, Sinus Disease Questionnaires, and the Quality of Life in Reflux and Dyspepsia (QoLRAD) Questionnaires [66]. However, it is a trial of empirical PPIs, and does not support that reflux could cause PND symptoms. Other studies had assessed the effect PPIs on CRS symptoms, but the results were conflicting. A study showed that reflux treatment achieved a 79% reduction in sinusitis symptom severity in adults refractory to drug therapy [61].

Another study evaluated the extra-gastroesophageal symptoms response to antireflux interventions. PPI therapy for GERD children significantly reduced chronic nasal obstruction (83.87%) and nasal secretion (80%), respectively [67]. Unfortunately, the patients also received antihistamine therapy, which confounded the results.

A double-blind randomized placebo-controlled trial showed that after 8 weeks of omeprazole (20 mg, once daily), the signs and symptoms of comorbid CRS were significantly reduced [68]. CRSwNP often features tissue eosinophilia that is associated with poor prognosis. Recent findings showed that PPIs directly modulated the expression of eotaxin-3 in patients with eosinophilic diseases, suggestive of the therapeutic potential of PPIs for CRSwNP [69]. Though encouraging, these studies are limited by their small sizes. Further randomized controlled studies should be organized to better understand the role of PPIs in CRS.

45.6 Conclusions

To date, we are not in a position to fully understand the pathogenesis of CRS, and only limited evidence has demonstrated the beneficial effect of above treatment strategies for CRS. Many questions remain to be answered. In this new field, however, the etiological mechanisms of CRS need further exploration. More evidence-based and well-designed researches will speed up the pace of novel treatment invention.

References

1. Fokkens WJ, Lund VJ, Mullol J, Bachert C, Alobid I, Baroody F, et al. European position paper on rhinosinusitis and nasal polyps 2012. Rhinol Suppl. 2012;23:3 p preceding table of contents, 1–298.
2. [Chinese guidelines for diagnosis and treatment of chronic rhinosinusitis (2018)]. Zhonghua Er Bi Yan Hou Tou Jing Wai Ke Za Zhi = Chinese J Otorhinolaryngol Head Neck Surg. 2019;54(2):81–100. https://doi.org/10.3760/cma.j.issn.1673-0860.2019.02.001
3. DeConde AS, Soler ZM. Chronic rhinosinusitis: epidemiology and burden of disease. Am J Rhinol Allergy. 2016;30(2):134–9. https://doi.org/10.2500/ajra.2016.30.4297.
4. Hoggard M, Wagner Mackenzie B, Jain R, Taylor MW, Biswas K, Douglas RG. Chronic rhinosinusitis and the evolving understanding of microbial ecology in chronic inflammatory mucosal disease. Clin Microbiol Rev. 2017;30(1):321–48. https://doi.org/10.1128/cmr.00060-16.
5. Hamilos DL. Host-microbial interactions in patients with chronic rhinosinusitis. J Allergy Clin Immunol. 2014;133(3):640–53.e4.
6. Anderson M, Stokken J, Sanford T, Aurora R, Sindwani R. A systematic review of the sinonasal microbiome in chronic rhinosinusitis. Am J Rhinol Allergy. 2016;30(3):161–6. https://doi.org/10.2500/ajra.2016.30.4320.
7. Ramakrishnan VR, Hauser LJ, Feazel LM, Ir D, Robertson CE, Frank DN. Sinus microbiota varies among chronic rhinosinusitis phenotypes and predicts surgical outcome. J Allergy Clin Immunol. 2015;136(2):334–42.e1. https://doi.org/10.1016/j.jaci.2015.02.008.
8. Desrosiers M. Refractory chronic rhinosinusitis: pathophysiology and management of chronic rhinosinusitis persisting after endoscopic sinus surgery. Curr Allergy Asthma Rep. 2004;4(3):200–7. https://doi.org/10.1007/s11882-004-0027-z.
9. Araujo E, Palombini BC, Cantarelli V, Pereira A, Mariante A. Microbiology of middle meatus in chronic rhinosinusitis. Am J Rhinol. 2003;17(1):9–15.
10. Benninger MS, Ferguson BJ, Hadley JA, Hamilos DL, Jacobs M, Kennedy DW, et al. Adult chronic rhinosinusitis: definitions, diagnosis, epidemiology, and pathophysiology. Otolaryngol Head Neck Surg. 2003;129(3 Suppl):S1–32. https://doi.org/10.1016/s0194-5998(03)01397-4.
11. Stressmann FA, Rogers GB, Chan SW, Howarth PH, Harries PG, Bruce KD, et al. Characterization of bacterial community diversity in chronic rhinosinusitis infections using novel culture-independent techniques. Am J Rhinol Allergy. 2011;25(4):e133–40. https://doi.org/10.2500/ajra.2011.25.3628.
12. Ramakrishnan VR, Feazel LM, Gitomer SA, Ir D, Robertson CE, Frank DN. The microbiome of the middle meatus in healthy adults. PLoS One. 2013;8(12):e85507. https://doi.org/10.1371/journal.pone.0085507.
13. Abreu NA, Nagalingam NA, Song Y, Roediger FC, Pletcher SD, Goldberg AN, et al. Sinus microbiome diversity depletion and Corynebacterium tuberculostearicum enrichment mediates rhinosinusitis. Sci Transl Med. 2012;4(151):151ra24. https://doi.org/10.1126/scitranslmed.3003783.
14. Aurora R, Chatterjee D, Hentzleman J, Prasad G, Sindwani R, Sanford T. Contrasting the microbiomes from healthy volunteers and patients with chronic rhinosinusitis. JAMA Otolaryngol Head Neck Surg. 2013;139(12):1328–38. https://doi.org/10.1001/jamaoto.2013.5465.
15. Kato A. Immunopathology of chronic rhinosinusitis. Allergol Int. 2015;64(2):121–30. https://doi.org/10.1016/j.alit.2014.12.006.
16. Yan Y, Gordon WM, Wang DY. Nasal epithelial repair and remodeling in physical injury, infection, and inflammatory diseases. Curr Opin Otolaryngol Head Neck Surg. 2013;21(3):263–70. https://doi.org/10.1097/MOO.0b013e32835f80a0.
17. Cleland EJ, Bassiouni A, Vreugde S, Wormald PJ. The bacterial microbiome in chronic rhinosinusitis: richness, diversity, postoperative changes, and patient outcomes. Am J Rhinol Allergy. 2016;30(1):37–43. https://doi.org/10.2500/ajra.2016.30.4261.
18. Lee JT, Frank DN, Ramakrishnan V. Microbiome of the paranasal sinuses: update and literature review. Am J Rhinol Allergy. 2016;30(1):3–16. https://doi.org/10.2500/ajra.2016.30.4255.
19. Hoggard M, Biswas K, Zoing M, Wagner Mackenzie B, Taylor MW, Douglas RG. Evidence of microbiota dysbiosis in chronic rhinosinusitis. Int Forum Allergy Rhinol. 2017;7(3):230–9. https://doi.org/10.1002/alr.21871.
20. Choi EB, Hong SW, Kim DK, Jeon SG, Kim KR, Cho SH, et al. Decreased diversity of nasal microbiota and their secreted extracellular vesicles in patients with chronic rhinosinusitis based on a metagenomic analysis. Allergy. 2014;69(4):517–26. https://doi.org/10.1111/all.12374.
21. Murphy J, Ramezanpour M, Stach N, Dubin G, Psaltis AJ, Wormald PJ, et al. *Staphylococcus Aureus* V8 protease disrupts the integrity of the airway epithelial barrier and impairs IL-6 production in vitro. Laryngoscope. 2018;128(1):E8–e15. https://doi.org/10.1002/lary.26949.
22. Cope EK, Goldberg AN, Pletcher SD, Lynch SV. Compositionally and functionally distinct sinus microbiota in chronic rhinosinusitis patients have immunological and clinically divergent consequences. Microbiome. 2017;5(1):53. https://doi.org/10.1186/s40168-017-0266-6.
23. Fiocchi A, Pawankar R, Cuello-Garcia C, Ahn K, Al-Hammadi S, Agarwal A, et al. World Allergy Organization—McMaster University guidelines for allergic disease prevention (GLAD-P): probiotics. World Allergy Org J. 2015;8(1):4. https://doi.org/10.1186/s40413-015-0055-2.

24. Schabussova I, Wiedermann U. Lactic acid bacteria as novel adjuvant systems for prevention and treatment of atopic diseases. Curr Opin Allergy Clin Immunol. 2008;8(6):557–64. https://doi.org/10.1097/ACI.0b013e328317b88b.
25. Round JL, Mazmanian SK. Inducible Foxp3+ regulatory T-cell development by a commensal bacterium of the intestinal microbiota. Proc Natl Acad Sci U S A. 2010;107(27):12204–9. https://doi.org/10.1073/pnas.0909122107.
26. Inan MS, Rasoulpour RJ, Yin L, Hubbard AK, Rosenberg DW, Giardina C. The luminal short-chain fatty acid butyrate modulates NF-kappaB activity in a human colonic epithelial cell line. Gastroenterology. 2000;118(4):724–34. https://doi.org/10.1016/s0016-5085(00)70142-9.
27. Furusawa Y, Obata Y, Fukuda S, Endo TA, Nakato G, Takahashi D, et al. Commensal microbe-derived butyrate induces the differentiation of colonic regulatory T cells. Nature. 2013;504(7480):446–50. https://doi.org/10.1038/nature12721.
28. Atarashi K, Tanoue T, Oshima K, Suda W, Nagano Y, Nishikawa H, et al. Treg induction by a rationally selected mixture of clostridia strains from the human microbiota. Nature. 2013;500(7461):232–6. https://doi.org/10.1038/nature12331.
29. Gareau MG, Sherman PM, Walker WA. Probiotics and the gut microbiota in intestinal health and disease. Nat Rev Gastroenterol Hepatol. 2010;7(9):503–14. https://doi.org/10.1038/nrgastro.2010.117.
30. Kramer MF, Burow G, Pfrogner E, Rasp G. In vitro diagnosis of chronic nasal inflammation. Clin Exp Allergy. 2004;34(7):1086–92. https://doi.org/10.1111/j.1365-2222.2004.01989.x.
31. Pearlman AN, Chandra RK, Chang D, Conley DB, Tripathi-Peters A, Grammer LC, et al. Relationships between severity of chronic rhinosinusitis and nasal polyposis, asthma, and atopy. Am J Rhinol Allergy. 2009;23(2):145–8. https://doi.org/10.2500/ajra.2009.23.3284.
32. Robinson S, Douglas R, Wormald PJ. The relationship between atopy and chronic rhinosinusitis. Am J Rhinol. 2006;20(6):625–8. https://doi.org/10.2500/ajr.2006.20.2907.
33. Promsopa C, Kansara S, Citardi MJ, Fakhri S, Porter P, Luong A. Prevalence of confirmed asthma varies in chronic rhinosinusitis subtypes. Int Forum Allergy Rhinol. 2016;6(4):373–7. https://doi.org/10.1002/alr.21674.
34. Marcus S, Roland LT, DelGaudio JM, Wise SK. The relationship between allergy and chronic rhinosinusitis. Laryngoscope Investig Otolaryngol. 2019;4(1):13–7. https://doi.org/10.1002/lio2.236.
35. Mahdavinia M, Carter RG, Ocampo CJ, Stevens W, Kato A, Tan BK, et al. Basophils are elevated in nasal polyps of patients with chronic rhinosinusitis without aspirin sensitivity. J Allergy Clin Immunol. 2014;133(6):1759–63. https://doi.org/10.1016/j.jaci.2013.12.1092.
36. Takabayashi T, Kato A, Peters AT, Suh LA, Carter R, Norton J, et al. Glandular mast cells with distinct phenotype are highly elevated in chronic rhinosinusitis with nasal polyps. J Allergy Clin Immunol. 2012;130(2):410–20.e5. https://doi.org/10.1016/j.jaci.2012.02.046.
37. West CE. Probiotics for allergy prevention. Benefic Microbes. 2016;7(2):171–9. https://doi.org/10.3920/bm2015.0073.
38. Kalliomäki M, Salminen S, Arvilommi H, Kero P, Koskinen P, Isolauri E. Probiotics in primary prevention of atopic disease: a randomised placebo-controlled trial. Lancet. 2001;357(9262):1076–9. https://doi.org/10.1016/S0140-6736(00)04259-8.
39. Zuccotti G, Meneghin F, Aceti A, Barone G, Callegari ML, Di Mauro A, et al. Probiotics for prevention of atopic diseases in infants: systematic review and meta-analysis. Allergy. 2015;70(11):1356–71. https://doi.org/10.1111/all.12700.
40. Cleland EJ, Drilling A, Bassiouni A, James C, Vreugde S, Wormald PJ. Probiotic manipulation of the chronic rhinosinusitis microbiome. Int Forum Allergy Rhinol. 2014;4(4):309–14. https://doi.org/10.1002/alr.21279.
41. Villena J, Barbieri N, Salva S, Herrera M, Alvarez S. Enhanced immune response to pneumococcal infection in malnourished mice nasally treated with heat-killed *Lactobacillus casei*. Microbiol Immunol. 2009;53(11):636–46. https://doi.org/10.1111/j.1348-0421.2009.00171.x.
42. Harata G, He F, Hiruta N, Kawase M, Kubota A, Hiramatsu M, et al. Intranasal administration of *Lactobacillus rhamnosus* GG protects mice from H1N1 influenza virus infection by regulating respiratory immune responses. Lett Appl Microbiol. 2010;50(6):597–602. https://doi.org/10.1111/j.1472-765X.2010.02844.x.
43. Mukerji SS, Pynnonen MA, Kim HM, Singer A, Tabor M, Terrell JE. Probiotics as adjunctive treatment for chronic rhinosinusitis: a randomized controlled trial. Otolaryngol Head Neck Surg. 2009;140(2):202–8. https://doi.org/10.1016/j.otohns.2008.11.020.
44. Mårtensson A, Abolhalaj M, Lindstedt M, Mårtensson A, Olofsson TC, Vásquez A, et al. Clinical efficacy of a topical lactic acid bacterial microbiome in chronic rhinosinusitis: a randomized controlled trial. Laryngoscope Investig Otolaryngol. 2017;2(6):410–6. https://doi.org/10.1002/lio2.93.
45. Kramer MF, Heath MD. Probiotics in the treatment of chronic rhinoconjunctivitis and chronic rhinosinusitis. J Allergy. 2014;2014:983635. https://doi.org/10.1155/2014/983635.
46. Cope EK, Lynch SV. Novel microbiome-based therapeutics for chronic rhinosinusitis. Curr Allergy Asthma Rep. 2015;15(3):504. https://doi.org/10.1007/s11882-014-0504-y.
47. Rozy A, Chorostowska-Wynimko J. Bacterial immunostimulants--mechanism of action and clinical application in respiratory diseases. Pneumonol Alergol Pol. 2008;76(5):353–9.

48. Kearney SC, Dziekiewicz M, Feleszko W. Immunoregulatory and immunostimulatory responses of bacterial lysates in respiratory infections and asthma. Ann Allergy Asthma Immunol. 2015;114(5):364–9. https://doi.org/10.1016/j.anai.2015.02.008.
49. Alecsandru D, Valor L, Sánchez-Ramón S, Gil J, Carbone J, Navarro J, et al. Sublingual therapeutic immunization with a polyvalent bacterial preparation in patients with recurrent respiratory infections: immunomodulatory effect on antigen-specific memory CD4+ T cells and impact on clinical outcome. Clin Exp Immunol. 2011;164(1):100–7. https://doi.org/10.1111/j.1365-2249.2011.04320.x.
50. Zagar S, Löfler-Badzek D. Broncho-Vaxom in children with rhinosinusitis: a double-blind clinical trial. ORL J Otorhinolaryngol Related Spec. 1988;50(6):397–404. https://doi.org/10.1159/000276020.
51. Razi CH, Harmancı K, Abacı A, Özdemir O, Hızlı S, Renda R, et al. The immunostimulant OM-85 BV prevents wheezing attacks in preschool children. J Allergy Clin Immunol. 2010;126(4):763–9. https://doi.org/10.1016/j.jaci.2010.07.038.
52. Heintz B, Schlenter WW, Kirsten R, Nelson K. Clinical efficacy of Broncho-Vaxom in adult patients with chronic purulent sinusitis—a multicentric, placebo-controlled, double-blind study. Int J Clin Pharmacol Ther Toxicol. 1989;27(11):530–4.
53. Yin J, Xu B, Zeng X, Shen K. Broncho-Vaxom in pediatric recurrent respiratory tract infections: a systematic review and meta-analysis. Int Immunopharmacol. 2018;54:198–209. https://doi.org/10.1016/j.intimp.2017.10.032.
54. Chen J, Zhou Y, Nie J, Wang Y, Zhang L, Shi Q, et al. Bacterial lysate for the prevention of chronic rhinosinusitis recurrence in children. J Laryngol Otol. 2017;131(6):523–8. https://doi.org/10.1017/S0022215117000524.
55. Habermann W, Zimmermann K, Skarabis H, Kunze R, Rusch V. Reduction of acute recurrence in patients with chronic recurrent hypertrophic sinusitis by treatment with a bacterial immunostimulant (*Enterococcus faecalis*) Bacteriae of human origin. Arzneimittelforschung. 2002;52(8):622–7. https://doi.org/10.1055/s-0031-1299941.
56. De Benedetto F, Sevieri G. Prevention of respiratory tract infections with bacterial lysate OM-85 bronchomunal in children and adults: a state of the art. Multidiscip Respir Med. 2013;8(1):33. https://doi.org/10.1186/2049-6958-8-33.
57. Dibildox-Martinez J, Mayorga Butron JL, Macías Fernández LA, Casiano RR, Carrau RL, Javer AR. Pan-American clinical guideline on rhinosinusitis. Otolaryngol Head Neck Surg. 2012;147(2 Suppl):253. https://doi.org/10.1177/0194599812451426a408.
58. Ulualp SO, Toohill RJ, Hoffmann R, Shaker R. Possible relationship of gastroesophagopharyngeal acid reflux with pathogenesis of chronic sinusitis. Am J Rhinol. 1999;13(3):197–202. https://doi.org/10.2500/105065899781389777.
59. Loehrl TA, Samuels TL, Poetker DM, Toohill RJ, Blumin JH, Johnston N. The role of extraesophageal reflux in medically and surgically refractory rhinosinusitis. Laryngoscope. 2012;122(7):1425–30. https://doi.org/10.1002/lary.23283.
60. El-Serag HB, Gilger M, Kuebeler M, Rabeneck L. Extraesophageal associations of gastroesophageal reflux disease in children without neurologic defects. Gastroenterology. 2001;121(6):1294–9. https://doi.org/10.1053/gast.2001.29545.
61. Ozmen S, Yücel OT, Sinici I, Ozmen OA, Süslü AE, Oğretmenoğlu O, et al. Nasal pepsin assay and pH monitoring in chronic rhinosinusitis. Laryngoscope. 2008;118(5):890–4. https://doi.org/10.1097/MLG.0b013e318165e324.
62. Ulualp SO, Toohill RJ, Shaker R. Pharyngeal acid reflux in patients with single and multiple otolaryngologic disorders. Otolaryngol Head Neck Surg. 1999;121(6):725–30. https://doi.org/10.1053/hn.1999.v121.a98010.
63. DelGaudio JM. Direct nasopharyngeal reflux of gastric acid is a contributing factor in refractory chronic rhinosinusitis. Laryngoscope. 2005;115(6):946–57. https://doi.org/10.1097/01.Mlg.0000163751.00885.63.
64. Phipps CD, Wood WE, Gibson WS, Cochran WJ. Gastroesophageal reflux contributing to chronic sinus disease in children: a prospective analysis. Arch Otolaryngol Head Neck Surg. 2000;126(7):831–6. https://doi.org/10.1001/archotol.126.7.831.
65. Gilani S, Pynnonen MA, Shin JJ. National practice patterns of antireflux medication for chronic rhinosinusitis. JAMA Otolaryngol Head Neck Surg. 2016;142(7):627–33. https://doi.org/10.1001/jamaoto.2016.0937.
66. Vaezi MF, Hagaman DD, Slaughter JC, Tanner SB, Duncavage JA, Allocco CT, et al. Proton pump inhibitor therapy improves symptoms in postnasal drainage. Gastroenterology. 2010;139(6):1887–93.e1; quiz e11. https://doi.org/10.1053/j.gastro.2010.08.039.
67. Megale SR, Scanavini AB, Andrade EC, Fernandes MI, Anselmo-Lima WT. Gastroesophageal reflux disease: its importance in ear, nose, and throat practice. Int J Pediatr Otorhinolaryngol. 2006;70(1):81–8. https://doi.org/10.1016/j.ijporl.2005.05.021.
68. Anzić SA, Turkalj M, Župan A, Labor M, Plavec D, Baudoin T. Eight weeks of omeprazole 20 mg significantly reduces both laryngopharyngeal reflux and comorbid chronic rhinosinusitis signs and symptoms: randomised, double-blind, placebo-controlled trial. Clin Otolaryngol. 2018;43(2):496–501. https://doi.org/10.1111/coa.13005.
69. Min JY, Ocampo CJ, Stevens WW, Price CPE, Thompson CF, Homma T, et al. Proton pump inhibitors decrease eotaxin-3/CCL26 expression in patients with chronic rhinosinusitis with nasal polyps: possible role of the nongastric H,K-ATPase. J Allergy Clin Immunol. 2017;139(1):130–41.e11. https://doi.org/10.1016/j.jaci.2016.07.020.

46 Impact of Endotyping on the Indication for Surgery

Claus Bachert

Key Points

- Surgery today is considered a standard part of the patient's management. However, the surgical approaches are not standardized, and recurrence after conventional endoscopic sinus surgery is reportedly high.
- The decision of the surgical approach should be based on the risk of recurrence of the underlying inflammation and thus on mucosal endotyping. The spectrum currently spreads over the mucosa-sparing approach to the complete mucosal removal (reboot) approach.

Surgery today often is summarized as "FESS", functional endoscopic sinus surgery; however, this technique was developed in the 1980s and revolutionized the sinus surgery, but was primarily aimed at CRS without nasal polyps [1]. The principle was based on observations on the mucociliary clearance from the sinuses into the nose, which should be restored. Another physical approach was the "narrow passage," resulting in the lack of ventilation and drainage of sinus areas behind it [2]. It is only now that the focus changes to the sinus mucosa itself, which needs another approach, which we call "reboot." Reboot stands for complete removal of the diseased sinus mucosa, and regrowth from the nasal cavity mucosa into the sinuses to "reboot" sinus mucosal functionality.

Nowadays, with the acceptance of mucosal endotypes, also surgical approaches should appreciate the variation in management which is necessary to repair sinus pathology; the old principle "one fits all" is not valid anymore. The majority of patients suffer from a type 1 CRS, possibly limited to a single or few sinuses, with little risk of recurrence, when properly approached by the principles of Messerklinger and Stammberger; no mucosal immunology would justify the removal of this mucosa. The restoration of ventilation and drainage, although not completely understood in terms of pathophysiology, will reduce symptoms, and restore sinus physiology on the long term. However, at the other end of the spectrum, a severe type 2 immune reaction often occupying all sinuses will definitely not be managed by the same approach, which leaves the sinus mucosa in place. The argument that the opening of the sinuses would facilitate the administration of topical drugs, mostly corticosteroids, may be partially correct;

C. Bachert (✉)
Upper Airways Research Laboratory and Department of Oto-Rhino-Laryngology, Ghent University, Ghent, Belgium

Division of ENT Diseases, CLINTEC, Karolinska Institute, University of Stockholm, Stockholm, Sweden

First Affiliated Hospital, Sun Yat-sen University, International Upper Airway Research Centre, Guangzhou, China
e-mail: claus.bachert@ugent.be

L. Zhang, C. Bachert (eds.), *Chronic Rhinosinusitis*, https://doi.org/10.1007/978-981-16-0784-4_46

however, based on the fact that the same topical drugs often cannot control the nasal polyps (see Chap. 52—Biologics; here they serve as controls!), and the distribution of topical drugs into all sinuses is difficult if not impossible to achieve, the management of severe nasal polyps clearly asks for another solution. Thus, in severe nasal polyps, a disease which worldwide is associated with type 2 immune reactions, the removal of the diseased sinus mucosa is an alternative, which we established recently [3]. The nasal mucosa overgrows the sinuses and covers the period and bone within 4–6 weeks; the expanding nasal mucosa has a lower risk of polyp growth, and shows much less inflammation compared to the sinus mucosa. This technique is aimed at severe CRSwNP, involving the ethmoidal and maxillary sinuses, but also sphenoid and frontal sinuses.

It is a challenge in the coming years to define surgical approaches tailored to mucosal endotypes, and include those into integrated care pathway concepts tailored from uncomplicated CRS to recurrent and severe CRSwNP. This will need also appreciating severe persistent disease asking for long-term management to control disease over decades.

References

1. Stammberger H, Posawetz W. Functional endoscopic sinus surgery. Concept, indications and results of the Messerklinger technique. Eur Arch Otorhinolaryngol. 1990;247(2):63–76. https://doi.org/10.1007/bf00183169.
2. Jankowski R, Pigret D, Decroocq F. Comparison of functional results after ethmoidectomy and nasalization for diffuse and severe nasal polyposis. Acta Otolaryngol. 1997;117(4):601–8. https://doi.org/10.3109/00016489709113445.
3. Alsharif S, Jonstam K, van Zele T, Gevaert P, Holtappels G, Bachert C. Endoscopic sinus surgery for type-2 CRS wNP: an endotype-based retrospective study. Laryngoscope. 2019;129(6):1286–92. https://doi.org/10.1002/lary.27815.

Surgical Procedures

47

Ashleigh Halderman and Bradley F. Marple

Key Points

- Endoscopic sinus surgery (ESS) is safe and effective at improving quality of life in patients with chronic sinusitis, however, it is technically challenging due to the complex anatomy of the paranasal sinuses.
- Preoperative evaluation and review of multiplanar computed tomography scans are essential for selecting patients who will benefit from surgery and for performing safe and effective surgery.
- A consistent method to each ESS and a stepwise approach is recommended to provide the safest and most effective surgical dissection.

47.1 Introduction

Since the introduction of endoscopic sinus surgery (ESS) in the 1980s, the field of rhinology has experienced a renaissance in the surgical management of sinonasal disease [1]. The introduction of the endoscope enabled the field of rhinology to evolve surgically from the macroscopic external and endonasal approaches of that era to the functional and less invasive sinonasal procedures in use today. The development of high-resolution, thin-cut, tri-planar computed tomography (CT) scans further served to advance our understanding of sinonasal pathology and its treatment. Modern ESS is significantly safer and more successful than in the past, however, it remains technically challenging in large part due to the complex anatomy of the paranasal sinuses.

A. Halderman · B. F. Marple (✉)
Southwestern Medical Center, Department of Otolaryngology, Head and Neck Surgery, University of Texas, Dallas, TX, USA
e-mail: ashleigh.halderman@utsouthwestern.edu; bradley.marple@utsouthwestern.edu

47.2 Preoperative Evaluation

Preoperative CT imaging is a critical initial step in surgical planning, and helps the surgeon to understand each patient's unique anatomy. Multiplanar CT reconstruction optimizes assessment of anatomy and has been shown to impact surgical planning in more than 50% of cases [2]. Additionally, preoperative CT imaging allows identification of anatomic variants potentially placing patients at risk for complications during ESS.

A standard approach, or "check list," for reviewing CT imaging allows for consistent assessment of information within each patient's exam. The term "CLOSE" can be used as mnemonic device to direct such systematic review [3, 4]. "CLOSE" stands for cribriform plate, lamina papyracea, onodi cell, sphenoid sinus pneumatization, and (anterior) ethmoidal artery (AEA) [3, 4]. Table 47.1 further details the "CLOSE"

L. Zhang, C. Bachert (eds.), *Chronic Rhinosinusitis*, https://doi.org/10.1007/978-981-16-0784-4_47

Table 47.1 The "CLOSE" Mnemonic for evaluation of preoperative CT scans [3, 4]

Anatomic structure	Evaluate	Recommended imaging plane
Cribriform plate	Height and symmetry, bony dehiscence	Coronal
Lamina papyracea	Haller cell, relationship of uncinate to orbital wall, evidence of prior medial or inferior orbital fracture	Coronal and axial
Onodi cell	Presence, relationship with OCR, dehiscence of the optic nerve	Coronal
Sphenoid sinus pneumatization	Intrasinus septum attachment point, pneumatization of the OCR, dehiscence of optic nerve or ICA, pneumatization pattern	Axial, sagittal, coronal
Ethmoidal artery (anterior)	Location within or below the skull base, dehiscence of the bony canal	Coronal

Key: *OCR* opticocarotid recess, *ICA* internal carotid artery

method for reviewing CT scans. From this, a surgical plan can be constructed taking patient anatomy into consideration for the most complete and safe surgery possible.

47.3 Endoscopic Sinus Surgery: Surgical Approach

A consistent method to each ESS through the use of a stepwise approach is recommended. Each step, in turn, exposes landmarks critical for the progressive surgical dissection. Understandably, some variability in the sequence of these steps may be necessary in revision cases as the typical anatomic landmarks may be altered beyond recognition or missing entirely.

47.3.1 Initial Assessment and Exposure

47.3.1.1 Nasal Endoscopy

As an initial step, nasal endoscopy is routinely performed, which provides for assessment of the septum, turbinates, middle meatus, sphenoethmoid recess, and nasopharynx. In selected cases a septoplasty may be required to provide access necessary for surgery.

47.3.1.2 Septoplasty

The choice of an open versus endoscopic septoplasty depends upon the surgeon's experience; however, the principles that underlie each technique are essentially the same. 1% Lidocaine with 1:100,000 epinephrine injected deep to the mucoperichondrium of the bilateral septum can provide for improved hemostasis during the procedure. Using a #15 scalpel, an incision in made through the mucoperichondrium of the septum. The location of the incision can be tailored to the region of the septum of interest. An elevator is used to elevate the mucoperichondrium from the underlying septal cartilage and bone until the junction between the bony and cartilaginous septum is identified. This can be bluntly separated using an elevator. Working through the opening in the bony-cartilaginous junction, the contralateral mucoperichondrium can be elevated in a fashion similar to that described above. Once adequate bilateral elevation is accomplished the deviated sections of septum are resected or modified, taking care to maintain adequate dorsal and caudal support along of the quadrangular cartilage [5].

47.3.1.3 Concha Bullosa Resection

In some cases, pneumatization of the middle turbinate (concha bullosa) can limit access to the middle meatus. The presence of a concha bullosa can be confirmed on preoperative imaging (Fig. 47.1). In such cases, resection of the lateral lamella of the concha bullosa can provide surgical access to the middle meatus while maintaining the anatomic integrity of the middle turbinate (Fig. 47.1).

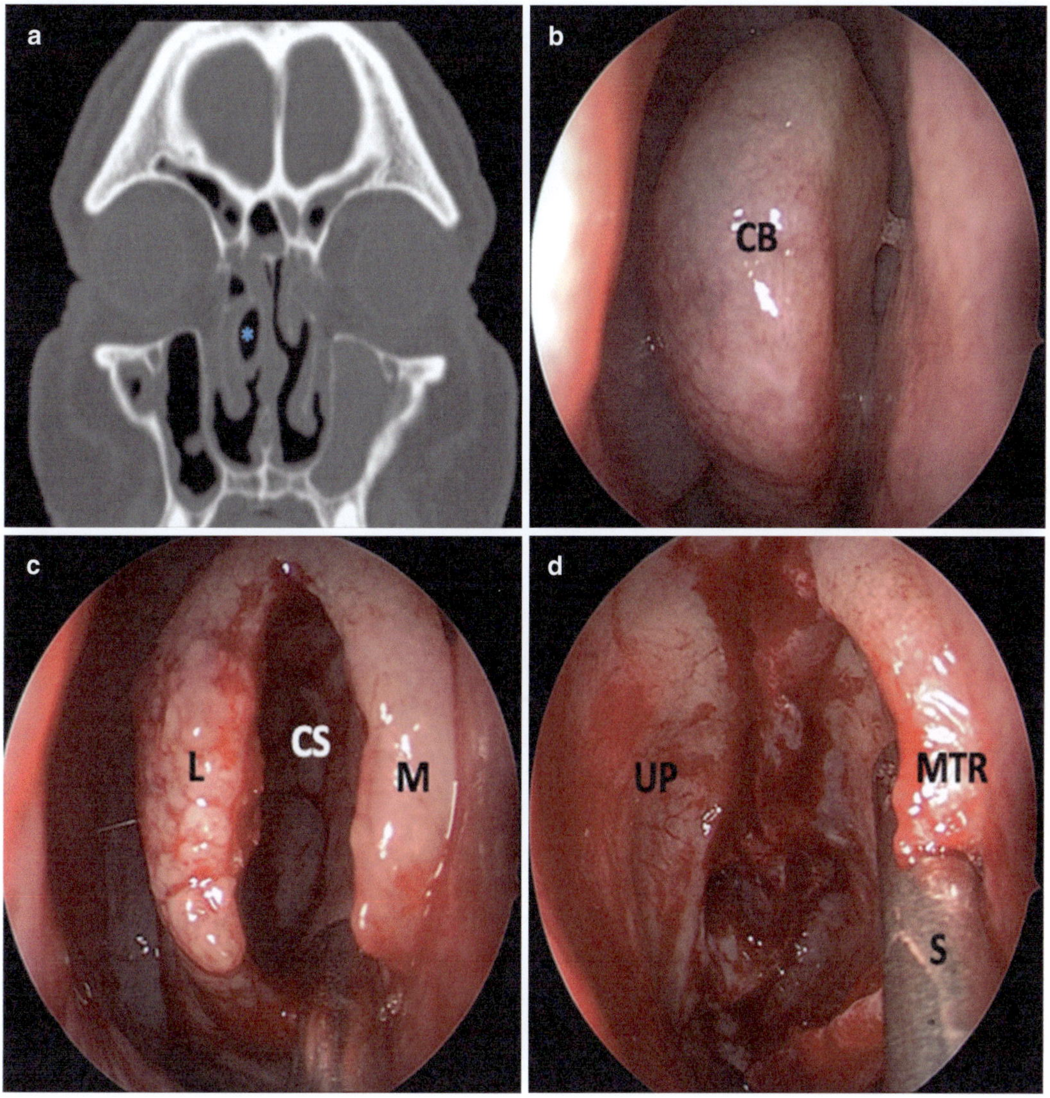

Fig. 47.1 (**a**) Right concha bullosa on coronal CT marked with an asterisk. (**b**) Endoscopic image of the concha bullosa (CB). (**c**) Dissection of the CB showing the lateral wall (L), medial wall (M), and the conchal space (CS). (**d**) Following resection of the L showing the uncinate process (UP) and the middle turbinate remnant (MTR) being retracted by the suction (S)

47.3.2 Performing ESS

47.3.2.1 Uncinectomy

The uncinate process is identified as a stable initial landmark within the lateral middle meatus. Arising from the ethmoid bone, the uncinate process extends posteromedially from its insertion on the lateral wall of the middle meatus, and serves as the medial limit of the ethmoid infundibulum. Resection of this structure provides exposure to the natural ostium of the maxillary sinus, the bulla ethmoidalis, and the lamina papyracea. Incomplete resection of the uncinate increases the risk of middle turbinate lateralization, middle meatal stenosis, recirculation, and can act as a nidus of inflammation [6, 7].

Several methods for uncinectomy have been described. In cases of limited infundibular space, retrograde resection of the uncinate can be useful. The posterior edge of the uncinate is identified anterior to the bulla ethmoidalis. A back-biting instrument is then used to transect the uncinate from its posterior edge to its point of insertion. Care must be taken to avoid injury of the bone of the maxillary line as this could result in damage to the nasolacrimal apparatus. The portion of the uncinate superior to this initial cut is then resected completely.

In instances where there is a clear infundibular space between the uncinate and the lamina, an anterior-to-posterior approach can be utilized. The insertion of the uncinate process and the lateral nasal wall is identified, representing the anterior extent of the infundibulum. A sickle knife is then used to make an incision through the uncinate process into the infundibulum. This incision is then extended along the insertion of the uncinate in a superior direction. Through cuts can then be used to separate the superior and inferior attachments of the uncinate resulting in complete removal.

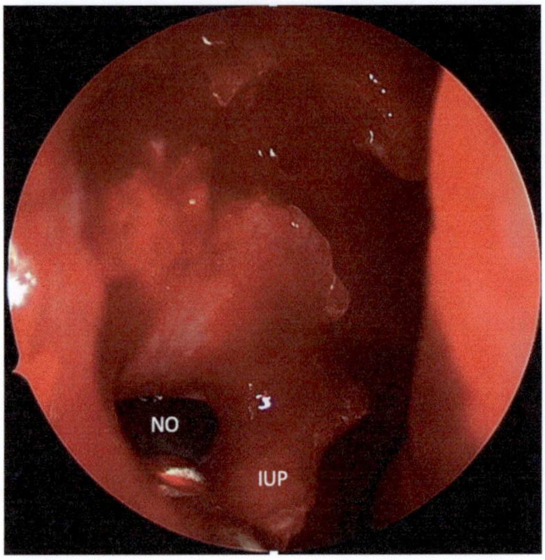

Fig. 47.2 Intraoperative photo following resection of the uncinate process on the right demonstrating the natural os (NO) of the maxillary sinus and residual inferior uncinate process (IUP)

47.3.2.2 Maxillary Antrostomy

With the uncinate resected, the medial maxillary wall can be fully visualized. The natural ostium of the maxillary sinus can be identified using an angled endoscope (30°, 45°, or 70°) immediately posterior to the cut inferior edge of the uncinate process posterior to the maxillary line [6] (Fig. 47.2). A middle meatal antrostomy (MMA) is created by widening the natural ostium in a posterior/inferior direction using either cutting instrumentation or dilation. The size of the resulting MMA remains a matter of debate [6, 7], with the ultimate size typically dictated by the severity and nature of disease within the maxillary sinus. In many cases, postoperative care will help to determine the size of the MMA, recognizing that maxillary antrum size has been correlated with rate of air flow into the maxillary sinuses and effectiveness of topical medication delivery [8–10].

Along the line of attachment of the uncinate lay the anterior and posterior fontanelles; areas of bony dehiscence of the medial maxillary wall. As many as 23% of patients may demonstrate a defect in the posterior fontanelle that gives rise to an accessory ostium. It is critical that the surgeon recognizes an accessory ostium in this location as separate and distinct from the natural ostium to avoid performance of an incorrectly positioned middle meatal antrostomy. This creates a phenomenon, known as a dual ostial configuration, which can lead to "recirculation" between the natural ostium and the misplaced MMA, and interruption of effective maxillary sinus outflow [11, 12] (Fig. 47.3). Recirculation caused by a dual ostial configuration is one of the most common causes of persistent maxillary sinusitis after ESS [11, 12].

Creation of an MMA can be accomplished through a variety of methods. The intent of these procedures is to provide access to the maxillary antrum and/or encouraging appropriate mucociliary clearance. Balloon catheter dilation (BCD) serves to dilate the natural ostium of the maxillary sinus and can be considered when tissue removal is not necessary. BCD is typically best suited for recurrent acute rhinosinusitis (RARS) and mild chronic sinusitis without nasal polyps (CRSsNP) [13].

MMA should be performed when access to the maxillary sinus is required to facilitate removal of inflammatory tissue, debris, or neoplasm, or when it is anticipated that topical medications will be necessary [6, 7, 14, 15]. The maximum size of the MMA is determined by the following anatomic boundaries: nasolacrimal

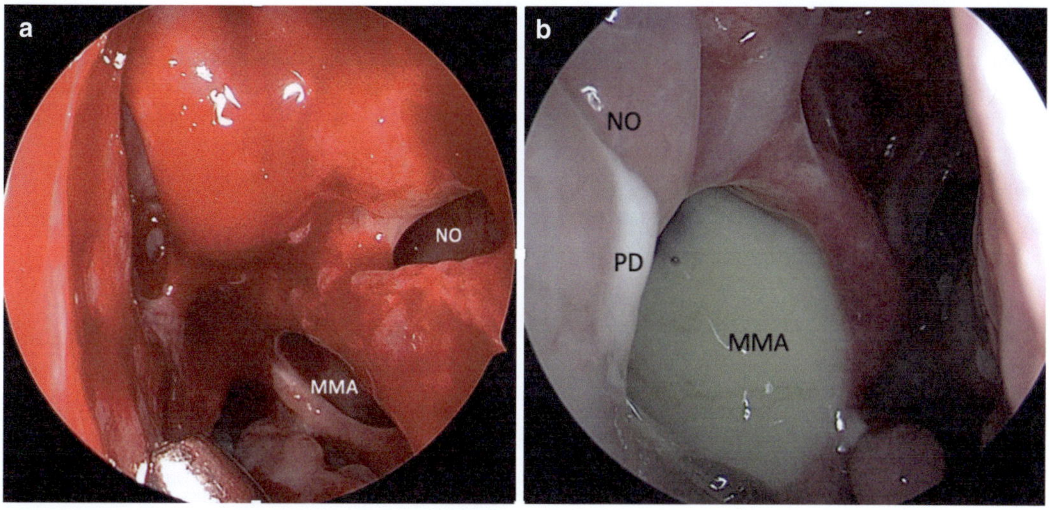

Fig. 47.3 Two examples of recirculation or dual ostial configuration. (**a**) The natural os (NO) is separate from the middle meatal maxillary antrostomy (MMA). (**b**) Again the NO is separate from the MMA and purulent drainage (PD) can be seen recirculating from the NO and back into the MMA

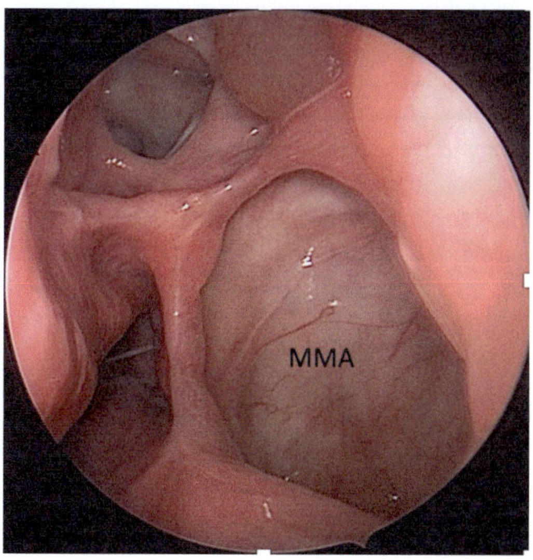

Fig. 47.4 Example of a middle meatal maxillary antrostomy (MMA) into which the natural os was incorporated

duct anteriorly, inferior turbinate attachment inferiorly, posterior wall of the maxillary sinus posteriorly, and the orbital floor superiorly. When complete, the ideal shape of the MMA will appear "pear-shaped," indicating that the natural ostium is in continuity with the antrostomy, thus preventing recirculation [6] (Fig. 47.4).

Techniques used to widen the existing natural ostium of the maxillary sinus fundamentally rely upon intact and effective mucociliary clearance. In disease processes that involve disruption of mucociliary function (e.g., cystic fibrosis, primary ciliary dyskinesia, scarring, etc.), gravity-dependent drainage may be necessary [7, 16, 17]. This can be accomplished via extension of the MMA inferiorly into the inferior meatus through performance of an endoscopic megamaxillary antrostomy (EMMA) or the modified endoscopic medial maxillectomy (MEMM). Thus far, EMMA for recalcitrant chronic maxillary sinus has been shown to effectively reduce sinonasal symptoms, corticosteroid and antibiotic use, and improve both endoscopic and radiographic findings [16, 18].

47.3.2.3 Ethmoidectomy

Given the complexity and individual variation within the ethmoid, a thorough understanding of its anatomy is essential. The ethmoid exists as an unpaired bone positioned along the anterior skull base and interposed between the two orbits. The anterior and posterior ethmoid sinuses are located along the lateral aspect of this bone bilaterally. These cells are limited medially by the middle and superior turbinates, laterally by the lamina papyracea (orbit), and posteriorly by the face of the sphenoid. Given the ethmoid roof is "open" along its lateral aspect, the superior limits of the ethmoid cells are made up of a medial projection of the frontal bone, which articulates with the lateral lamella of the cribriform (central portion of the superior ethmoid bone).

The ethmoid sinuses are separated anatomically into an anterior and posterior group of cells by the vertical portion of the middle turbinate basal lamella. The basal lamella lies in a coronal plane and attaches superior to the skull base and laterally to the lamina papyracea. There are typically 10–15 air cells within the entire ethmoid complex. The posterior compartment has between 1–5 separate air cells and the anterior compartment accounts for the remainder [19].

At a conceptual level, the goal of an ethmoidectomy is complete removal of the partitions separating the individual cells. Performance of a complete ethmoidectomy is fundamental to the success of ESS. Incomplete ethmoidectomy is observed in 31–74% of cases following surgery, and is the most common clinical finding present in patients requiring revision surgery [20]. Residual ethmoid partitions contribute to persistent inflammation by trapping secretions, impeding delivery of saline and topical medications, and obstructing nearby outflow tracts [21, 22].

Ethmoidectomy is most frequently a progressive dissection performed in an anterior-to-posterior direction, allowing the surgeon to sequentially provide increased access to more posterior cells. Given that the ethmoid skull base and location of the orbits are obscured by the anatomic location of intact ethmoid cells, it is generally considered safest to initiate dissection within the inferomedial aspect of the ethmoids to avoid inadvertent injury to these critical boundaries. The lamina papyracea and skull base are identified in the early phases of the procedure to serve as reliable landmarks critical for intraoperative orientation, as well as to ensure the safety of these structures. Additionally, early identification of the skull base and lamina papyracea helps to define the limits of the surgical field and facilitates creation of a wider working space.

The bulla ethmoidalis serves as the typical starting point for the anterior portion of an ethmoidectomy. The ethmoid bulla is a consistent and recognizable feature of the anterior ethmoid cells

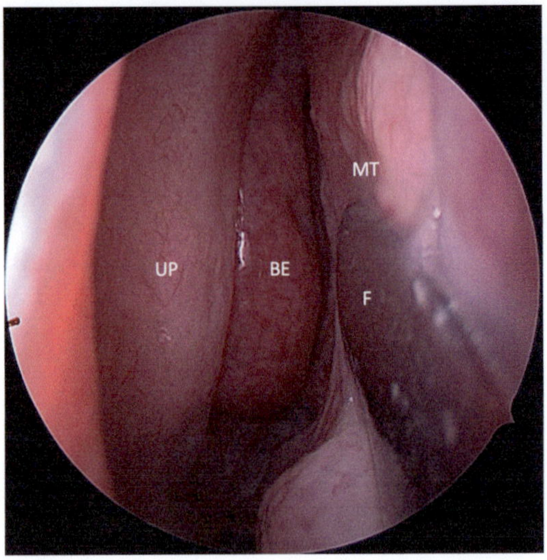

Fig. 47.5 Endoscopic view of an undissected right anterior ethmoid cavity. The middle turbinate (MT) is being medialized with the freer (F) to show the uncinate process (UP) and the bulla ethmoidalis (BE)

and is the first encountered cell after removal of the uncinate process (Fig. 47.5). The lamellae of the ethmoid bulla insert onto the medial orbital wall and thus represent an early opportunity to identify the lamina papyracea (orbit). Starting along its medial border, the bulla is entered and its lamella are resected laterally to their insertion on the lamina papyracea. Care is taken to ensure complete removal of both the floor and the roof of the bulla.

Complete resection of the ethmoid bulla creates a space within the anterior ethmoid system that is bound laterally by the lamina papyracea, medially by the parasagittal plane of the middle turbinate, and posteriorly by the basal lamella of the middle turbinate. As is the case with the ethmoid bulla, the basal lamella is a consistent anatomic landmark and should be identified during the performance of an ethmoidectomy. The vertical plane of the basal lamella serves to differentiate the anterior ethmoid cells from those of the posterior ethmoid system. An anterior ethmoidectomy, for example, would address those cells located anterior to the basal lamella, while a posterior ethmoidectomy would encompass the cells posterior to this landmark.

The basal lamella is transgressed to facilitate transition from the anterior ethmoid cells into the posterior ethmoid cells. Given that this maneuver will often be "blind," it is critical to penetrate the basal lamella in a location that prevents injury to the skull base or orbit. The roof of the maxillary sinus serves as good landmark identifying the level of the floor of the orbit. Penetration of the basal lamella inferior to the horizontal plane that corresponds to the roof of the maxillary antrum ensures protection of the ethmoid skull base. Likewise, identification of the lamina papyracea prevents inadvertent orbital entry. Once penetrated, the basal lamella can be resected under direct visualization. Care should be taken to protect the inferolateral attachment of the basal lamella along the lateral nasal wall, as this provides structural support for the middle turbinate. Posterior ethmoidectomy is accomplished by sequentially removing ethmoid lamella to the level of the skull base superiorly and the posterior lamina papyracea laterally.

Significant variability in the anatomy of the sinuses occurs as the natural result of ethmoid pneumatization. In fact, no two sets of sinuses are the same. This variability, however, has some consistency, leading to several well-recognized patterns of ethmoid development. One such important ethmoid variant is known as a sphenoethmoid cell (Onodi cell). In up to 28% of patients [23], a sphenoethmoid cell will occur as a result of a posterior ethmoid cell that pneumatized posteriorly over the superolateral aspect of the sphenoid sinus. This pattern causes displacement of the true sphenoid sinus medially and inferiorly [24]. The clinical relevance of this variant is that the location of the ethmoid pneumatization is into the region of the sphenoid body adjacent to the optic nerve and internal carotid artery (ICA) (Fig. 47.6). In theory, failure to recognize this altered anatomic relationship can lead to disorientation and inadvertent injury to these structures.

Another example of variability influenced by ethmoid pneumatization is that of the position of the anterior ethmoidal artery relative to the skull base. Located along the anterior ethmoid skull base approximately 1 cm posterior to the frontal infundibulum, the anterior ethmoidal artery courses in a posterolateral to anteromedial direction as it travels from the ophthalmic artery to the middle cranial fossa [25]. The anterior ethmoid artery extends below the skull base in a bony mesentery in up to 40% of patients, rendering it vulnerable to injury during removal of anterior ethmoid partitions if not recognized [26].

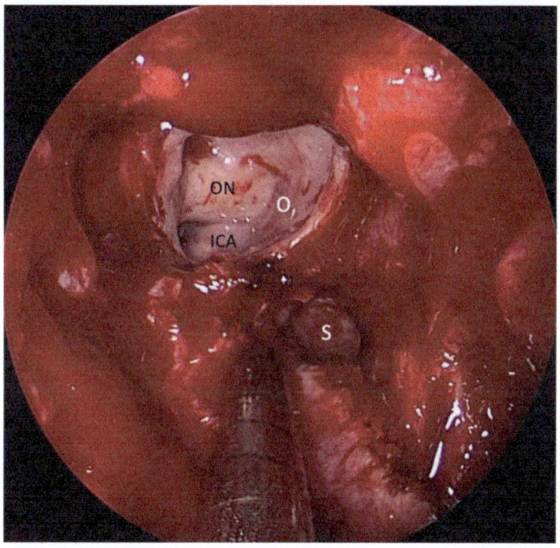

Fig. 47.6 Endoscopic, intraoperative view of a right sphenoid sinus (S). Superior and lateral to the S is an onodi (O) cell where the optic nerve (ON) and internal carotid artery (ICA) can be seen

47.3.2.4 Sphenoid Sinusotomy

Safe access to the sphenoid sinus can be achieved via several approaches and is best described relative to the position of the superior turbinate. The "transnasal approach" can be performed either with or without a posterior ethmoidectomy. The key feature of this approach is identification of the natural ostium of the sphenoid sinus medial to the inferior 1/3 of the superior turbinate [27, 28]. Identification of the sphenoid ostium is facilitated by lateralization or resection of the inferior portion of the superior turbinate. Once identified, the sphenoid ostium is extended superiorly and laterally under direct visualization using cutting instrumentation. Care should be taken to limit dissection inferior to the natural ostium of the sinus to avoid injury to the nasal septal branches of the sphenopalatine artery.

The "transethmoid approach" requires prior completion of a posterior ethmoidectomy. The anterior wall of the sphenoid sinus is penetrated lateral to the superior turbinate at the approximate level of the natural ostium of the sinus. It is important to note that this approach relies upon a "blind" transition from the posterior ethmoid system into the sphenoid sinus, and therefore can increase risk of injury to the posterior ethmoid skull base, carotid artery, and/or optic nerve. These risks can be minimized by ensuring sphenoid penetration along the inferior medial aspect of the poster ethmoid sinuses. Once an opening is made into the sphenoid sinus, it can be opened in a manner similar to that of the "transnasal" approach.

Once in the sphenoid sinus, care must be taken to protect critical surrounding structures. The position of the intrasinus septum is variable and should be studied on preoperative CT scan. This partition within the sphenoid inserts directly onto the optic canal in 30% of sphenoid sinuses and on the carotid canal in 37% [23, 29], therefore removal is best accomplished using cutting instrumentation.

47.3.2.5 Frontal Sinusotomy

At a conceptual level, frontal sinusotomy is a relatively simple procedure. The goal of the surgery is to simply remove all ethmoid cells present within the frontal outflow tract (FOT). In reality, however, the frontal sinus (FS) is frequently the most challenging aspect of ESS. Variable ethmoid anatomy, anatomic location, and need for angled instruments can render surgery in this region technically challenging.

The frontal outflow tract is made up of the frontal infundibulum, the frontal ostium, and the frontal recess. In the majority of cases it is the frontal recess that is the primary site of intervention during surgery. The frontal recess is bound laterally by the lamina papyracea, medially by the middle turbinate, anteriorly by the agger nasi, and posteriorly by the ethmoid bulla or suprabullar cells. While the middle turbinate and lamina papyracea are fairly consistent landmarks, the agger nasi cell and suprabullar cells show significant variability. Two classification systems have been devised to name these cells. The first was introduced by Bent et al. [30] and is shown in Table 47.2. The International Frontal Sinus Anatomy Classification (IFAC) [33] is a more recently described system and is also shown in Table 47.2.

Table 47.2 Frontal cell classification systems [31, 32]

Bent and Kuhn		IFAC		
Cell name	Description	Cell name	Description	Abbreviation
Type I	Single cell located above the agger nasi	Agger nasi cell	Located anterior to the origin of the MT, or above the anterior insertion of MT into lateral nasal wall	ANC
Type II	Two or more cells above the agger nasi but inferior to nasal beak	Supra agger nasi cell	Located above the ANC, does not pneumatize into the frontal sinus	SAC
Type III	Cell above the agger nasi that pneumatizes into the frontal sinus	Supra agger frontal cell	Located above the ANC with pneumatization into the frontal sinus	SAFC
Type IV	Isolated frontal cell contained entirely within the frontal sinus	Supra bulla cell	Located above the bulla, does not pneumatize into the frontal sinus	SBC
		Supra frontal bulla cell	Located above the bulla with pneumatization into the frontal sinus	SBFC
		Supraorbital ethmoid cell	Anterior ethmoid cell that pneumatizes over the roof of the orbit around, anterior to or posterior to the AEA	SOEC
		Frontal septal cell	Located in the interfrontal sinus septum along the medial aspect of the FOT	FSC

Key: *IFAC* International Frontal Sinus Anatomy Classification, *MT* middle turbinate, *AEA* anterior ethmoid artery, *FOT* frontal outflow tract

Table 47.3 Extent of frontal surgery classification [32, 34–36]

IFAC grade	Description	Draf equivalent
0	Balloon dilation	N/a
1	Clearance of cells in the FR that are not obstructing the ostium	Draf I
2	Clearance of cells directly obstructing the ostium	
3	Clearance of cells pneumatizing through the ostium without enlargement of ostium	
4	Clearance of cells pneumatizing through ostium into sinus with enlargement of ostium	Draf IIa
5	Enlargement of ostium from lamina papyracea to nasal septum	Draf IIb
6	Removal of the entire floor of the frontal sinus joining the left and right ostia into a common ostium with a septal window	Draf III

Key: *FR* frontal recess

The most common classification for the extent of FS surgery is the Draf classification (Table 47.3) [37–39]. However, a more recent international classification for endoscopic frontal sinus surgery (EFSS) has been proposed (Table 47.3) [33].

FS surgery can range from balloon dilation (Grade 0) to complete removal of the floor of the frontal sinuses, joining the two sinuses into a single common cavity (Grade 6 or Draf III). Several factors must be considered when deciding upon the degree to which the FOT will be dissected. The underlying disease process, patient symptoms, extent of disease, patient anatomic features, surgeon experience, and resulting size of the surgical opening all influence the extent of dissection. Several studies have demonstrated significantly higher patency rates when the surgical opening measures >4.5 cm [31, 32, 40]. Generally, the least invasive procedure possible to achieve an adequately sized opening is recommended. A stepwise approach, such as moving from IFAC Grade 0 up to Grade 6, is typically employed with the most advanced procedures rarely being done in primary surgery but reserved for revision cases or tumor resection.

The extent of dissection appears to have important implications on both patency rates and delivery of saline/topical medications. The patency of Draf IIa sinusotomies ranges between 67.6–92% compared to 88–96% for Draf III's [34, 40, 41]. Comparing distribution of saline and rate of lavage, Draf III sinusotomy was superior to both Draf IIb and Draf IIa in a cadaveric study [35]. For these reasons, some authors have begun to advocate for upfront Draf III sinusotomies in recalcitrant forms of sinusitis such as massive polyposis or Aspirin Exacerbated Respiratory Disease (AERD) [36, 42].

47.4 Conclusion

The field of ESS and rhinology has seen tremendous growth in the form of technological advancements and improved knowledge and understanding of the disease processes involving the paranasal sinuses. The mastery of ESS, however, remains firmly rooted in a foundational understanding of anatomy. While the management of sinus disease, technology/tools with which surgery is performed, and indications for surgery will continue to evolve, the concepts of ESS based upon anatomy will remain the same.

References

1. Kennedy DW. Technical innovations and the evolution of endoscopic sinus surgery. Ann Otol Rhinol Laryngol Suppl. 2006;196:3–12. https://doi.org/10.1177/00034894061150s902.
2. Kew J, Rees GL, Close D, Sdralis T, Sebben RA, Wormald PJ. Multiplanar reconstructed computed tomography images improves depiction and understanding of the anatomy of the frontal sinus and recess. Am J Rhinol. 2002;16(2):119–23.
3. Weitzel EK, Floreani S, Wormald PJ. Otolaryngologic heuristics: a rhinologic perspective. ANZ J Surg. 2008;78(12):1096–9. https://doi.org/10.1111/j.1445-2197.2008.04757.x.
4. O'Brien WT Sr, Hamelin S, Weitzel EK. The preoperative sinus CT: avoiding a "CLOSE" call with surgical complications. Radiology. 2016;281(1):10–21. https://doi.org/10.1148/radiol.2016152230.

5. Seth R, Haffey T, McBride JM, Sindwani R. Intranasal landmarks for adequate L-strut preservation during endoscopic septoplasty. Am J Rhinol Allergy. 2014;28(3):265–8. https://doi.org/10.2500/ajra.2014.28.4042.
6. Kennedy DW, Adappa ND. Endoscopic maxillary antrostomy: not just a simple procedure. Laryngoscope. 2011;121(10):2142–5. https://doi.org/10.1002/lary.22169.
7. Thompson CF, Conley DB. What is the optimal maxillary antrostomy size during sinus surgery? Curr Opin Otolaryngol Head Neck Surg. 2015;23(1):34–8. https://doi.org/10.1097/MOO.0000000000000128.
8. Frank DO, Zanation AM, Dhandha VH, McKinney KA, Fleischman GM, Ebert CS Jr, et al. Quantification of airflow into the maxillary sinuses before and after functional endoscopic sinus surgery. Int Forum Allergy Rhinol. 2013;3(10):834–40. https://doi.org/10.1002/alr.21203.
9. Harvey RJ, Goddard JC, Wise SK, Schlosser RJ. Effects of endoscopic sinus surgery and delivery device on cadaver sinus irrigation. Otolaryngol Head Neck Surg. 2008;139(1):137–42. https://doi.org/10.1016/j.otohns.2008.04.020.
10. Hyo N, Takano H, Hyo Y. Particle deposition efficiency of therapeutic aerosols in the human maxillary sinus. Rhinology. 1989;27(1):17–26.
11. Kane KJ. Recirculation of mucus as a cause of persistent sinusitis. Am J Rhinol. 1997;11(5):361–9. https://doi.org/10.2500/105065897781286034.
12. Parsons DS, Stivers FE, Talbot AR. The missed ostium sequence and the surgical approach to revision functional endoscopic sinus surgery. Otolaryngol Clin North Am. 1996;29(1):169–83.
13. Cingi C, Bayar Muluk N, Lee JT. Current indications for balloon sinuplasty. Curr Opin Otolaryngol Head Neck Surg. 2019;27(1):7–13. https://doi.org/10.1097/MOO.0000000000000506.
14. Snidvongs K, Pratt E, Chin D, Sacks R, Earls P, Harvey RJ. Corticosteroid nasal irrigations after endoscopic sinus surgery in the management of chronic rhinosinusitis. Int Forum Allergy Rhinol. 2012;2(5):415–21. https://doi.org/10.1002/alr.21047.
15. Thomas WW 3rd, Harvey RJ, Rudmik L, Hwang PH, Schlosser RJ. Distribution of topical agents to the paranasal sinuses: an evidence-based review with recommendations. Int Forum Allergy Rhinol. 2013;3(9):691–703. https://doi.org/10.1002/alr.21172.
16. Cho DY, Hwang PH. Results of endoscopic maxillary mega-antrostomy in recalcitrant maxillary sinusitis. Am J Rhinol. 2008;22(6):658–62. https://doi.org/10.2500/ajr.2008.22.3248.
17. Wang EW, Gullung JL, Schlosser RJ. Modified endoscopic medial maxillectomy for recalcitrant chronic maxillary sinusitis. Int Forum Allergy Rhinol. 2011;1(6):493–7. https://doi.org/10.1002/alr.20070.
18. Costa ML, Psaltis AJ, Nayak JV, Hwang PH. Long-term outcomes of endoscopic maxillary mega-antrostomy for refractory chronic maxillary sinusitis. Int Forum Allergy Rhinol. 2015;5(1):60–5. https://doi.org/10.1002/alr.21407.
19. Bolger WE. Anatomy of the paranasal sinuses. In: Kennedy DW, Bolger W, Zinreich S, editors. Diseases of the sinuses: diagnosis and management. Hamilton, ON/Lewiston, NY: B.C. Decker, Inc.; 2001. p. xvii, 430 p.
20. Levine CG, Casiano RR. Revision functional endoscopic sinus surgery. Otolaryngol Clin North Am. 2017;50(1):143–64. https://doi.org/10.1016/j.otc.2016.08.012.
21. Kennedy DW, Ramakrishnan VR. Functional endoscopic sinus surgery: concepts, surgical indications, and techniques. In: Kennedy DW, Hwang PH, editors. Rhinology: diseases of the nose, sinuses, and skull base. New York, NY: Thieme; 2012. p. 306–35.
22. Ling FTK, Kountakis SE. Revision functional endoscopic sinus surgery. In: Kennedy DW, Hwang PH, editor. Rhinology: diseases of the nose, sinuses and skull base. New York, NY: Thieme; 2012. p. 336–46.
23. Batra PS, Citardi MJ, Gallivan RP, Roh HJ, Lanza DC. Software-enabled CT analysis of optic nerve position and paranasal sinus pneumatization patterns. Otolaryngol Head Neck Surg. 2004;131(6):940–5. https://doi.org/10.1016/j.otohns.2004.07.013.
24. Stammberger HR, Kennedy DW, Anatomic TG. Paranasal sinuses: anatomic terminology and nomenclature. Ann Otol Rhinol Laryngol Suppl. 1995;167:7–16.
25. Lee WC, Ming Ku PK, van Hasselt CA. New guidelines for endoscopic localization of the anterior ethmoidal artery: a cadaveric study. Laryngoscope. 2000;110(7):1173–8. https://doi.org/10.1097/00005537-200007000-00020.
26. Moon HJ, Kim HU, Lee JG, Chung IH, Yoon JH. Surgical anatomy of the anterior ethmoidal canal in ethmoid roof. Laryngoscope. 2001;111(5):900–4. https://doi.org/10.1097/00005537-200105000-00027.
27. Wise SK, Orlandi RR, DelGaudio JM. Sinonasal development and anatomy. In: Kennedy DW, Hwang PH, editors. Rhinology: diseases of the nose, sinuses, and skull base. New York, NY: Thieme; 2012. p. 1–19.
28. Yanagisawa E, Yanagisawa K, Christmas DA. Endoscopic localization of the sphenoid sinus ostium. Ear Nose Throat J. 1998;77(2):88–9.
29. Batra PS, Citardi MJ, Gallivan RP, Roh HJ, Lanza DC. Software-enabled computed tomography analysis of the carotid artery and sphenoid sinus pneumatization patterns. Am J Rhinol. 2004;18(4):203–8.
30. Bent JP, Cuilty-Siller C, Kuhn FA. The frontal cell as a cause of frontal sinus obstruction. Am J Rhinol. 1994;8:185–91.
31. Chandra RK, Palmer JN, Tangsujarittham T, Kennedy DW. Factors associated with failure of frontal sinusotomy in the early follow-up period. Otolaryngol Head Neck Surg. 2004;131(4):514–8. https://doi.org/10.1016/j.otohns.2004.03.022.
32. Naidoo Y, Bassiouni A, Keen M, Wormald PJ. Long-term outcomes for the endoscopic modified Lothrop/Draf III procedure: a 10-year review. Laryngoscope.

2014;124(1):43–9. https://doi.org/10.1002/lary.24258.
33. Wormald PJ, Hoseman W, Callejas C, Weber RK, Kennedy DW, Citardi MJ, et al. The international frontal sinus anatomy classification (IFAC) and classification of the extent of endoscopic frontal sinus surgery (EFSS). Int Forum Allergy Rhinol. 2016;6(7):677–96. https://doi.org/10.1002/alr.21738.
34. Anderson P, Sindwani R. Safety and efficacy of the endoscopic modified Lothrop procedure: a systematic review and meta-analysis. Laryngoscope. 2009;119(9):1828–33. https://doi.org/10.1002/lary.20565.
35. Barham HP, Ramakrishnan VR, Knisely A, Do TQ, Chan LS, Gunaratne DA, et al. Frontal sinus surgery and sinus distribution of nasal irrigation. Int Forum Allergy Rhinol. 2016;6(3):238–42. https://doi.org/10.1002/alr.21686.
36. Morrissey DK, Bassiouni A, Psaltis AJ, Naidoo Y, Wormald PJ. Outcomes of modified endoscopic Lothrop in aspirin-exacerbated respiratory disease with nasal polyposis. Int Forum Allergy Rhinol. 2016;6(8):820–5. https://doi.org/10.1002/alr.21739.
37. Weber RK, Hosemann W. Comprehensive review on endonasal endoscopic sinus surgery. GMS Curr Top Otorhinolaryngol Head Neck Surg. 2015;14:Doc08. https://doi.org/10.3205/cto000123.
38. Draf W. Endonasal microendoscopic frontal sinus surgery, the Fulda concept. Oper Tech Otolaryngol Head Neck Surg. 1991;2:234–40. https://doi.org/10.1016/S1043-1810(10)80087-9.
39. Weber R, Draf W, Kratzsch B, Hosemann W, Schaefer SD. Modern concepts of frontal sinus surgery. Laryngoscope. 2001;111(1):137–46. https://doi.org/10.1097/00005537-200101000-00024.
40. DeConde AS, Smith TL. Outcomes after frontal sinus surgery: an evidence-based review. Otolaryngol Clin North Am. 2016;49(4):1019–33. https://doi.org/10.1016/j.otc.2016.03.024.
41. Kikawada T, Fujigaki M, Kikura M, Matsumoto M, Kikawada K. Extended endoscopic frontal sinus surgery to interrupted nasofrontal communication caused by scarring of the anterior ethmoid: long-term results. Arch Otolaryngol Head Neck Surg. 1999;125(1):92–6. https://doi.org/10.1001/archotol.125.1.92.
42. Orgain CA, Harvey RJ. The role of frontal sinus drillouts in nasal polyposis. Curr Opin Otolaryngol Head Neck Surg. 2018;26(1):34–40. https://doi.org/10.1097/MOO.0000000000000425.

48 Reboot Surgery

Claus Bachert

Key Points

- For severe CRSwNP, the reboot approach has been developed, aiming at complete removal of the sinus mucosa, but not touching the nasal mucosa. From the nasal mucosa, the coverage of the sinuses takes place, allowing a mucosal reboot with low polyp recurrence risk.
- The reboot approach also considerably reduces inflammatory biomarkers in the mucosa.

Nasal polyps with type 2 inflammation are classically characterized by asthma comorbidity in up to 70% of patients and disease recurrence, with figures ranging from 38% to 60% at 12 months follow-up [1–4]. Clinical signs for treatment failure risk and disease recurrence are bronchial asthma, Aspirin or NSAID-Exacerbated Respiratory Disease (AERD, N-ERD), and atopy [5, 6]; peripheral blood, mucus, and mucosal eosinophilia and elevated blood and tissue IgE values—patterns of type 2T-cell inflammation—are biomarkers for more severe disease and nasal polyp recurrence [7]. Severe, difficult-to-treat CRSwNP subjects are therefore often repeatedly exposed to surgical management of various kinds. Surgical approaches have varied over the years, ranging from less extended "polyp extraction" to more extended "nasalization" procedures [8–10]. For CRSwNP, because of the high recurrence rates, more extended approaches have been proposed "to widely access the sinuses, open them for local treatment, and reduce the inflammatory load" [11]. Performing randomized controlled studies to compare different surgical techniques is demanding to perform, and reliable studies comparing different approaches including sufficient patients are lacking. Removal or "stripping of the mucosa" was not recommended due to fear of scarring, inflammation of the denuded bone, and non-functional mucosa [12], derived from single surgeons observations.

In patients with severe nasal polyps, scheduled for reboot surgery at Ghent University Hospital, with asthma comorbidity in >50% and former surgery in >70% of the patients, we could demonstrate that the mucosa in all sinuses to a similar degree as in the nasal polyps shows type 2 immune disease characterized by elevated levels of IgE, ECP, and IL-5. Furthermore, the inflammation was not different between the polyps and the non-polyp tissue next to them. These observa-

C. Bachert (✉)
Upper Airways Research Laboratory and Department of Oto-Rhino-Laryngology, Ghent University, Ghent, Belgium

Division of ENT Diseases, CLINTEC, Karolinska Institute, University of Stockholm, Stockholm, Sweden

First Affiliated Hospital, Sun Yat-sen University, International Upper Airway Research Centre, Guangzhou, China
e-mail: claus.bachert@ugent.be

L. Zhang, C. Bachert (eds.), *Chronic Rhinosinusitis*, https://doi.org/10.1007/978-981-16-0784-4_48

tions supported the reboot approach and underlined the need for removal of all sinus mucosa (publication submitted). In fact, as type 2 immune reactions are associated with a deficit in wound healing, the removal of this condition thus is a prerequisite for normal wound healing.

Sinus surgery for CRSwNP should be performed in an attempt to control disease long-term and to improve the patients' symptoms, overall quality of life, and possibly reduce the risk of asthma development. In the process of understanding the disease at its molecular level, appreciating the type 2 inflammation and its associated deficiencies in defense against bacteria and viruses as well as epithelial repair, we have introduced the concept of "reboot" surgery, based on the removal of all inflamed sinus mucosa and allowing the regrowth of functional nasal mucosa, growing from the preserved nasal mucosa into the sinuses within weeks after surgery [13]. This approach has been developed after primarily unsuccessful conventional mucosa-sparing endoscopic sinus surgery (ESS) approaches, but may also be indicated in severe cases as primary surgery.

We hypothesized that the complete removal of the sinus mucosa together with the microbiota, the intramucosal germs, and the significant immune dysfunction would present a possibility to impact on the natural course of the disease. According to the above discussed approach to select the surgical technique to match the pheno- and endotype of CRS, the reboot approach only is indicated in severe type 2 nasal polyps, involving at least the ethmoidal and maxillary sinuses and visible in the nasal cavity with a polyp score of 4 or more out of 8, with or without comorbid asthma, and with or without prior surgery. The aim is the removal of the ethmoidal cells and the wide opening of the maxillary sinuses, in order to completely remove the mucosa from the orbital lamina, the skull base, and the maxillary sinus walls including the alveolar recesses. If the frontal sinuses are involved, as indicated by at least a partial opacification of the frontal sinuses, a Draf 3 procedure should be considered, certainly if the patient suffers from frontal pressure or pain or has undergone more than one former surgery. The Draf 3 procedure in this case is not the aim, but only the access way to remove the sinus mucosa of the frontal sinuses. If the procedure includes the frontal sinuses, we call it "full reboot," otherwise "partial reboot."

The reboot technique aims to accomplish a total removal of all mucosa from all affected sinuses, leaving the periosteum where possible. The procedure starts with a wide antrostomy and a complete removal of all the mucosa from the maxillary sinus, including the alveolar recess mucosa, using 30° and 70° endoscopes. Furthermore, the anterior and posterior ethmoids including the lamina orbitalis, skull base, and the lateral aspects of the middle turbinate are cleared from mucosa. The sphenoid sinus of course needs specific attention for the major structures passing along its lateral walls and roof, the internal carotid arteries, and the optic nerves. The experienced surgeon should aim to remove the diseased mucosa from the floor and medial parts of the sphenoid under endoscopic view, and to also create a wide access through reduction of the anterior sphenoid sinus wall up to the skull base. Then, the frontal recess is approached, completing the removal of the anterior skull base mucosa into the frontal sinus as wide as possible. The middle turbinate is preserved as much as possible as a landmark, except for the parts that are destroyed or occupied by the disease, or for the anterior parts that need to be taken during the Draf III procedure. The superior turbinate mostly needs to be removed when approaching the sphenoid and clearing the central skull base. Finally, for a full reboot surgery, a Draf III procedure is performed, giving maximal access to both frontal sinuses by partially removing the interfrontal septum. The frontal sinus mucosa is then completely removed from the posterior and anterior walls, using specific instruments (e.g., a curved frontal sinus curette, frontal sinus punches); creating a wide access will allow the surgeon to remove the whole mucosa of the frontal sinus walls. After controlling the area for bleeding and irrigating the sinuses, two packs of Merocel® are placed bilaterally into the middle meatus and nasal cavities and removed the next morning.

It was the intention to remove all "sinus mucosa"; however, we are aware of the fact that this may not be achieved, specifically from the lateral frontal and sphenoid sinuses and the alveolar recess of the maxillary sinus due to limitations in viewing and instrumentation. The incomplete removal of mucosa from the sphenoid sinuses seems less critical than from the frontal or maxillary sinuses. At the end of the reboot surgery, the sinus mucosa is removed as complete as possible, with only the periosteum partially left over, and the nasal mucosa has been left untouched as much as possible (Fig. 48.1). It is, therefore, reasonable to assume that the nasal mucosa growth over the sinus walls from the edges of the inferior turbinate, anterior nasal cavity, and middle turbinate and septum, as there is no sinus mucosa left to form new mucosa (Fig. 48.2a). The time for reepithelialization is 4–6 weeks (Fig. 48.2b), with a healthy and moisturized mucosa of normal thickness without edema or scar formation, but may be delayed in case of infections, which consequently should be avoided. As type 2 cytokines such as IL-4 and IL-13 impair epithelial tight junction expression and barrier formation [14], the eradication of the type 2 inflammation may allow better wound healing post-operatively, starting from the nasal mucosa of the inferior and middle turbinates as well as the septum over the sinus walls under non-inflamed conditions.

All patients should follow a thorough post-op care and follow-up, consisting of saline irrigation, doxycycline 100 mg per day for 6 weeks, and topical GCS drops (Fluticasone propionate) once daily in head-down position for long-term. The use of post-op long-term (6–8 weeks) doxycycline has shown to improve mucosal healing in different studies [15, 16]. Our current data indicate that compared with the classical ESS approach, recurrence rates over 3 years after surgery can be reduced from 40–50% to below 15% using the reboot approach (Fig. 48.3). The reboot approach results in a major reduction in inflammatory mediators and cytokines in the nasal mucosa and secretions, and in the formation of a functional ciliated mucosal layer with goblet cells over all sinuses, as shown by biopsy about 2 years after surgery (Fig. 48.4). Well known to ENT surgeons, the resection of larger areas of the sinus mucosa often is needed in cases of inverted papilloma or malignant sinus tumors, with an appropriate wound healing and closure of the mucosal lining thereafter [17, 18].

The complication rate is identical to the rate of conventional ESS, as the borders for both operations are alike; however, special care should be taken when working with cutting instruments in the area of the lamina orbitalis or the skull base. Extensive surgery might potentially lead to increased complication rates and more severe

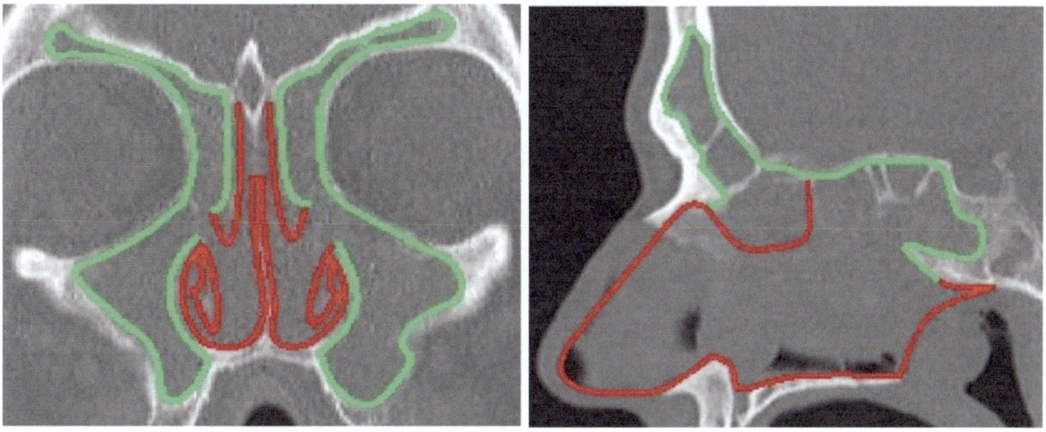

Fig. 48.1 Green lines show the mucosal areas completely removed during the reboot surgery, red lines show the mucosal areas that are kept untouched. (**a**) Coronal view, notice the untouched parts of the middle turbinate kept as important suppliers for epithelial regrowth and surgical landmarks. (**b**) Sagittal view (Alsharif et al. Laryngoscope 2019)

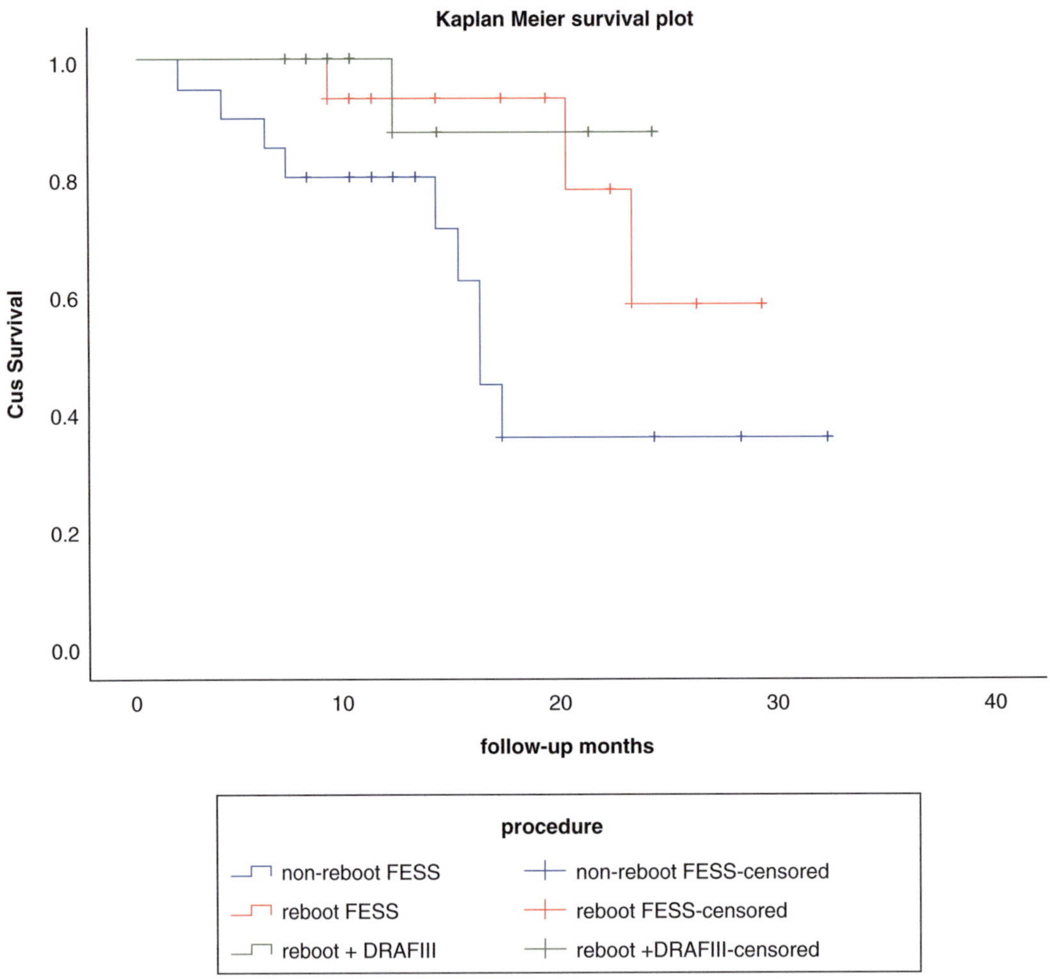

Fig. 48.2 Kaplan Meier survival plot for the three groups of patients. Relapse rates were 13% for the reboot group vs 45% for the non-reboot group ($p = 0.02$). Notice the lower number of relapses ($n = 1$) and the later time of recurrence (12 months) for the full reboot group followed by the partial reboot with ($n = 3$) relapses and 4 months for the earliest recurrence, while the non-reboot group demonstrated more ($n = 9$) relapses and 2 months for the earliest recurrence ($p = 0.038$) of at least one polyp (Alsharif et al. Laryngoscope 2019)

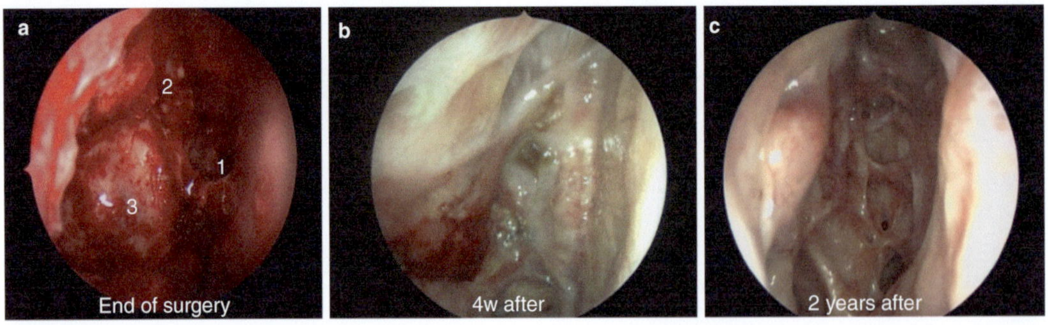

Fig. 48.3 (**a**) Endoscopic view of the sphenoidal (1) and ethmoidal skull base (2) and lamina orbitalis (3) at end of surgery and (**b**) 4 weeks after surgery; nearly complete closure of the mucosal layer with reepithelialisation from the septum; in this case, there was a complete destruction of the middle turbinate by nasal polyps with consecutive removal. (**c**) 2 years after surgery

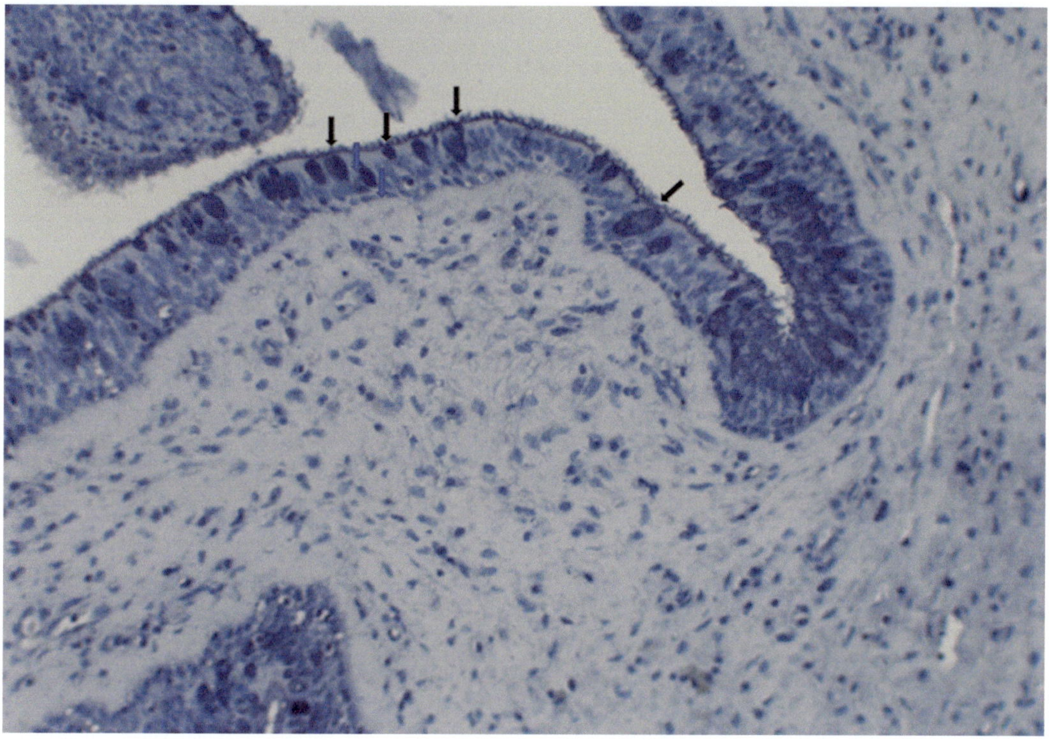

Fig. 48.4 Ciliated and goblet cell (arrows) expressing newly formed mucosa covering the posterior lamina orbitalis 2 years after reboot surgery

complications. A previous study on a more extensive form of surgery compared to a minimal approach did not show any severe complications, with no differences in complication rates between the groups [19, 20]. We, however, advocate that this procedure should only be performed by a surgeon with excellent knowledge and experience of endoscopic sinus surgery including Draf III procedures to minimize the risk of complications.

Concentrations of IgE, SE-IgE, ECP, and IL-5 confirmed moderate to severe mucosal type 2 inflammation in the mucosal samples during surgery. In line with this, significantly increased concentrations of these cytokines and mediators were also found in nasal secretions; although still different from controls, there was a significant and clinically meaningful decrease of nsIgE ($p = 0.03$), nsECP ($p = 0.04$), and nsIL-5 ($p = 0.04$) 12 months after reboot surgery compared to baseline. These observations underline that part of the success is based on a profound reduction of inflammation. However, different from therapy with biologics, after which nasal polyps again develop after cessation of treatment, nasal polyps after reboot surgery recur in less than 10% over 3 years, indicating that reboot surgery induces additional changes to the newly formed sinus mucosa, derived from the nasal cavity, which suppresses polyp regrowth.

As demonstrated by postoperative SNOT-22 scoring, patients show improved sinusitis-related quality of life, and suffer from minimal symptom burden. However, the recovery of smell may take several weeks or months, and cannot be promised to individual patients, as the risk of losing smell increases with the number of surgeries performed.

References

1. DeConde AS, Soler ZM. Chronic rhinosinusitis: epidemiology and burden of disease. Am J Rhinol Allergy. 2016;30(2):134–9. https://doi.org/10.2500/ajra.2016.30.4297.

2. Halawi AM, Smith SS, Chandra RK. Chronic rhinosinusitis: epidemiology and cost. Allergy Asthma Proc. 2013;34(4):328–34. https://doi.org/10.2500/aap.2013.34.3675.
3. Wynn R, Har-El G. Recurrence rates after endoscopic sinus surgery for massive sinus polyposis. Laryngoscope. 2004;114(5):811–3. https://doi.org/10.1097/00005537-200405000-00004.
4. Mendelsohn D, Jeremic G, Wright ED, Rotenberg BW. Revision rates after endoscopic sinus surgery: a recurrence analysis. Ann Otol Rhinol Laryngol. 2011;120(3):162–6. https://doi.org/10.1177/000348941112000304.
5. Matsuwaki Y, Ookushi T, Asaka D, Mori E, Nakajima T, Yoshida T, et al. Chronic rhinosinusitis: risk factors for the recurrence of chronic rhinosinusitis based on 5-year follow-up after endoscopic sinus surgery. Int Arch Allergy Immunol. 2008;146(Suppl 1):77–81. https://doi.org/10.1159/000126066.
6. Hoover GE, Newman LJ, Platts-Mills TA, Phillips CD, Gross CW, Wheatley LM. Chronic sinusitis: risk factors for extensive disease. J Allergy Clin Immunol. 1997;100(2):185–91. https://doi.org/10.1016/s0091-6749(97)70223-9.
7. Van Zele T, Holtappels G, Gevaert P, Bachert C. Differences in initial immunoprofiles between recurrent and nonrecurrent chronic rhinosinusitis with nasal polyps. Am J Rhinol Allergy. 2014;28(3):192–8. https://doi.org/10.2500/ajra.2014.28.4033.
8. Stammberger H, Posawetz W. Functional endoscopic sinus surgery. Concept, indications and results of the Messerklinger technique. Eur Arch Otorhinolaryngol. 1990;247(2):63–76. https://doi.org/10.1007/bf00183169.
9. Jankowski R, Pigret D, Decroocq F. Comparison of functional results after ethmoidectomy and nasalization for diffuse and severe nasal polyposis. Acta Otolaryngol. 1997;117(4):601–8. https://doi.org/10.3109/00016489709113445.
10. Hoseini SM, Saedi B, Aghazadeh K. Meticulous endoscopic sinus surgery to prevent recurrence of massive nasal polyposis. J Laryngol Otol. 2012;126(8):789–94. https://doi.org/10.1017/s0022215112001193.
11. Wigand ME, Steiner W, Jaumann MP. Endonasal sinus surgery with endoscopical control: from radical operation to rehabilitation of the mucosa. Endoscopy. 1978;10(4):255–60. https://doi.org/10.1055/s-0028-1098304.
12. Bassiouni A, Wormald PJ. Role of frontal sinus surgery in nasal polyp recurrence. Laryngoscope. 2013;123(1):36–41. https://doi.org/10.1002/lary.23610.
13. Alsharif S, Jonstam K, van Zele T, Gevaert P, Holtappels G, Bachert C. Endoscopic sinus surgery for type-2 CRS wNP: an endotype-based retrospective study. Laryngoscope. 2019;129(6):1286–92. https://doi.org/10.1002/lary.27815.
14. Soyka MB, Wawrzyniak P, Eiwegger T, Holzmann D, Treis A, Wanke K, et al. Defective epithelial barrier in chronic rhinosinusitis: the regulation of tight junctions by IFN-γ and IL-4. J Allergy Clin Immunol. 2012;130(5):1087–96.e10. https://doi.org/10.1016/j.jaci.2012.05.052.
15. Van Zele T, Gevaert P, Holtappels G, Beule A, Wormald PJ, Mayr S, et al. Oral steroids and doxycycline: two different approaches to treat nasal polyps. J Allergy Clin Immunol. 2010;125(5):1069–76.e4. https://doi.org/10.1016/j.jaci.2010.02.020.
16. Pinto Bezerra Soter AC, Bezerra TF, Pezato R, Teles Abdo TR, Pilan RM, Pinna FR, et al. Prospective open-label evaluation of long-term low-dose doxycycline for difficult-to-treat chronic rhinosinusitis with nasal polyps. Rhinology. 2017;55(2):175–80. https://doi.org/10.4193/Rhin15.291.
17. Wolfe SG, Schlosser RJ, Bolger WE, Lanza DC, Kennedy DW. Endoscopic and endoscope-assisted resections of inverted sinonasal papillomas. Otolaryngol Head Neck Surg. 2004;131(3):174–9. https://doi.org/10.1016/j.otohns.2004.05.011.
18. Miglani A, Patel SH, Kosiorek HE, Hinni ML, Hayden RE, Lal D. Endoscopic resection of sinonasal mucosal melanoma has comparable outcomes to open approaches. Am J Rhinol Allergy. 2017;31(3):200–4. https://doi.org/10.2500/ajra.2017.31.4435.
19. Hopkins C, Slack R, Lund V, Brown P, Copley L, Browne J. Long-term outcomes from the English national comparative audit of surgery for nasal polyposis and chronic rhinosinusitis. Laryngoscope. 2009;119(12):2459–65. https://doi.org/10.1002/lary.20653.
20. Chen FH, Deng J, Hong HY, Xu R, Guo JB, Hou WJ, et al. Extensive versus functional endoscopic sinus surgery for chronic rhinosinusitis with nasal polyps and asthma: a 1-year study. Am J Rhinol Allergy. 2016;30(2):143–8. https://doi.org/10.2500/ajra.2016.30.4271.

49 Complications of Endoscopic Sinus Surgery

Yi Dong and Bing Zhou

Key Points

- Although endoscopic sinus surgery benefits both patients and doctors, the complications of this surgery still present a challenge to rhinologists.
- A thorough understanding and familiarity with the anatomy and anatomical variations, lesions, necessary surgical skills, and instrumentation involved in endoscopic sinus surgery will be helpful to reduce or avoid complications.
- Timely and appropriate management may reduce and eliminate the damage caused by complications.

In 1987, Stankiewicz [1] reported the first large series describing complications related to endoscopic sinus surgery (ESS). The description included 90 patients who underwent intranasal ethmoidectomy, with an overall complication rate of 29%. With the development of nasal endoscopic surgery techniques and instruments, the incidence of complications has substantially decreased [2–9]. However, because of the rise of endoscopic transnasal cranial base surgery in recent years, serious complications such as cranial base injury, intracranial infection and hemorrhage, and internal carotid artery injury are receiving increasingly more attention [10–16]. Despite surgeons' best efforts, complications still occur.

Y. Dong · B. Zhou (✉)
Department of Otolaryngology, Head and Neck Surgery, Beijing Tongren Hospital, Capital Medical University, Beijing, China
e-mail: entzhou@263.net

49.1 Causes of Complications in ESS

No rhinologist wishes to encounter complications of ESS, but such complications are impossible to avoid. ESS is performed in a narrow space adjacent to the orbital cavity, skull base, internal carotid artery, and other extremely important anatomical structures. Accidental damage to any of these structures may have very serious consequences, even endangering the lives of patients. The reported incidence of complications associated with ESS ranges from 0.3% to 22.4% (median, 7.0%) [3, 17–19]. Understanding the anatomy of sinuses, using skilled surgical techniques, being patient during the operation, and performing a careful surgical procedure are the key factors of avoiding intraoperative and postoperative complications.

L. Zhang, C. Bachert (eds.), *Chronic Rhinosinusitis*, https://doi.org/10.1007/978-981-16-0784-4_49

Table 49.1 Classification of complications based on anatomic area

Anatomic area	Complications
Orbital	Lamina papyracea injury and fat exposure
	Intraorbital hematoma
	Muscle injury
	Optic nerve injury
Intracranial	Cerebrospinal fluid (CSF) leakage
	Carotid injury
	Intracranial infection
Nasal	Epistaxis
	Synechiae
	Secondary lacrimal duct obstruction
	Secondary sinusitis
	Bone remodeling

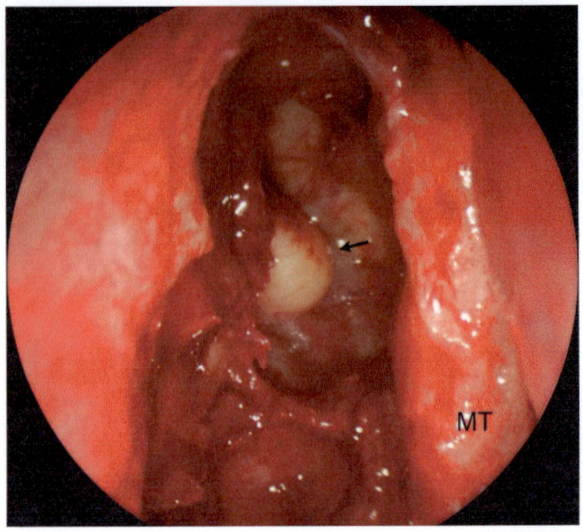

Fig. 49.1 Endoscopic view of small of amount of orbital fat (*black arrow*) that herniated into the posterior ethmoid area. *MT* middle turbinate

49.2 Classification of Complications in ESS

This chapter mainly introduces the classification and treatment of complications of ESS. A classification of complications based on anatomic area is provided in Table 49.1. The severity of these complications varies widely. Some scholars divide the complications into severe and minor complications [19]. Severe complications refer to those more harmful and difficult to recover and require active treatment, including intraorbital hematoma, muscle injury, optic nerve injury, secondary lacrimal duct obstruction , cerebrospinal fluid leakage, intracranial complications, carotid injury, and epistaxis requiring blood transfusion. Fat exposure, orbital congestion, orbital emphysema, minor epistaxis, and secondary sinusitis are regarded as minor complications.

49.2.1 Orbital Complications

49.2.1.1 Lamina Papyracea Injury and Orbital Fat Exposure

Injury to the lamina papyracea that forms the medial orbital wall may occur during uncinectomy near the start of sinus surgery or ethmoidotomy. An incision in the uncinate process that is directed too far lateral or posterior can enter the orbit through the lamina papyracea. Inadvertent injury or removal of the lamina papyracea with exposure of the periorbita usually has no adverse consequences if it is quickly recognized and the periorbita has not been injured. Although this complication does not cause significant dysfunction, it is a common surgical complication, particularly for beginning surgeons.

Nasal packing is usually avoided in such cases because placement of packing over the orbital defect causes air or blood to enter the orbital tissues. Fat removal should not be attempted, and the surgical cavity should not be packed too tightly to avoid intraorbital infection and increased intraorbital pressure.

Although a small degree of untraceable orbital fat prolapse is not dangerous (Fig. 49.1), it becomes dangerous if more bleeding occurs in the surgical cavity and the lamina papyracea injury is very close to the orbital apex. Once blood enters the orbital apex, sometimes even very little blood, an orbital apex hematoma can develop and cause visual impairment or blindness. More seriously, it can lead to orbital apex syndrome. Therefore, intraoperative bleeding must be managed with no packing or minimal packing according to the condition of the operative cavity.

49.2.1.2 Intraorbital Hematoma

Bleeding into the orbit secondary to vessel injury or bleeding from the anterior or posterior ethmoid artery can cause an intraorbital hematoma and increased intraorbital pressure with retinal ischemia. This is a potentially severe complication of ESS [20].

Medical management of a slowly expanding orbital hematoma without visual loss includes removal of the nasal packing and eye massage. Administration of systemic steroids and mannitol can reduce edema and aqueous humor production. If these measures do not lead to clinical improvement, medial orbital decompression may be necessary.Orbital congestion usually dissipates within 1 week after surgery. Otherwise, if the intraorbital hematoma continues to progress, orbital decompression surgery should be performed to prevent the intraorbital pressure from increasing and oppressing the optic nerve.

49.2.1.3 Eye Muscle Injury

During ESS, the medial rectal muscle is the most endangered among all of the eye muscles, there is little chance of damage to other eye muscles. Damage to the medial rectal muscle is more frequently caused by injury to the lamina papyracea and periorbita during ESS involving the middle and posterior parts of ethmoid sinus than that involving the anterior parts; this is because the extraconal layer of fatty tissue is thinner beyond the insertion location of the medial rectal muscle at the bulb. The medial rectal muscle could be injured either by a surgical instrument, such as ethmoid forceps, directly or by the blood or nerve supply injury indirectly. In 1994, Setliff and Parsons introduced a revolutionary powered cutting instrument termed the "hummer" (also known as the shaver, microresector, or microdebrider) that allows precise surgical control, constant and clear visualization, minimal intraoperative bleeding, and reduced surgical time [21]. Powered cutting instruments are effective and efficient tools in ESS. However, they are also associated with many severe orbital complications (Fig. 49.2). Their use should be tempered with the knowledge that iatrogenic defects or natural dehiscences of the thin bones of the orbit may result in injuries to the orbital contents, particularly the extraocular muscles and their surrounding fascial attachments. When operating near the lamina papyracea, the tip of the power instrument must not be pressed too hard on the lamina papyracea.

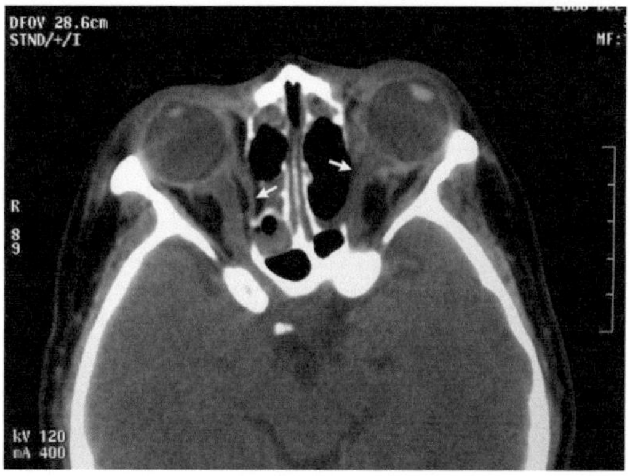

Fig. 49.2 Axial paranasal sinus CT scan of bilateral medial rectal muscle injuries due to the use of a microdebrider in ESS (soft tissue window). This 45-year-old woman presented with right lateral strabismus and left orbital apex syndrome. CT showed a discontinuous left medial rectal muscle and a right continuous but thinner medial rectal muscle (*arrows*)

Misinterpreting a fat hernia bulging into the ethmoid sinus as a nasal polyp can also result in complications. During the removal of this "polyp," the eye muscle is caught and injured. Injury to the contents of the orbit occur in patients with anatomical variants of the ethmoid such as Onodi cells and infraorbital cells; injury may also occur when the lamina papyracea is missing because of previous operations, trauma, or severe polyposis of the ethmoid. The optic nerve can be injured in the apex of the orbit or in the optic nerve canal if it is bulging medially into the posterior parts of the ethmoid sinuses or the superolateral part of the sphenoidal sinus, or if it is without bony layers (Onodi cell).

The main symptom of eye muscle injury is double vision. Examination reveals varying degrees of eye movement disturbance. Direct eye muscle injury requires surgical correction, but surgery can only restore the eye position, not the function of the damaged muscle. Therefore, the operator should be highly alert to the overflow of orbital fat to avoid further damaging the eye muscle. If a muscle contusion has occurred, anti-infection treatment is usually followed by recovery; however, if the internal rectus muscle damage is severe, the function cannot be restored, and surgical repair by an ophthalmologist is required.

49.2.1.4 Optic Nerve Injury

The optic nerve may be damaged by direct and indirect trauma, and its potential for recovery is very low, particularly when direct injury has occurred. Direct injury to the optic nerve usually occurs with use of a high-speed drill or electrocoagulation. In some cases, the injury is directly caused by the suction applied by an assistant during ESS, which can lead to fracture of the optic canal (Fig. 49.3). In rare cases, direct damage to the optic nerve is caused by a power instrument. Indirect injury often results from an intraorbital hematoma. Occasionally, very tight packing can also lead to optic ischemia and vision loss. Therefore, intensive care should be taken not only to avoid direct injury to the nerve but also to avoid indirect damage, such as that induced by excessive heating during drilling of the optic canal or by the drill itself. Once the function of the optic nerve appears to have been reduced or lost, recovery is very difficult. It is crucial to avoid the occurrence of this complication.

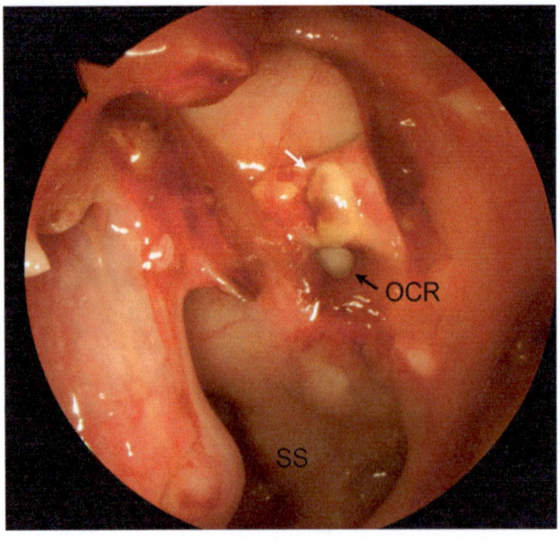

Fig. 49.3 Endoscopic view of an optic nerve canal fracture (*white arrow*) in a left Onodi cell. The surgeon used a curette to dissect the floor of the Onodi cell, and the optic nerve canal fracture was caused by excessive force. *SS* sphenoid sinus, *OCR* optic nerve canal–internal carotid artery recess

Prevention of optic nerve injury during ESS is critical because such injury lacks treatment. Optic nerve injury usually presents as partial loss of vision or blindness. If injury to the optic nerve is suspected during surgery, high-dose systemic corticosteroids should be administered and an ophthalmologic consultation should be performed. A postoperative magnetic resonance imaging scan is necessary to evaluate the location and extent of this injury. Immediate optic nerve canal decompression can be an option in this situation.

49.2.2 Intracranial Complications

49.2.2.1 Cerebrospinal Fluid (CSF) Leakage

Intraoperative CSF leakage often occurs when the skull base has been damaged during ESS [22]. Such complications often occur during severe intraoperative bleeding, which can obscure intranasal anatomical landmarks and lead to surgical disorientation. The surgeon cannot rely solely on the image navigation system for identification of such a critical structure. During revision surgery, the lack of normal or clear landmarks can also result in confusion, particularly for beginning surgeons. In such cases, the disease along the skull base should be left untreated and the operation terminated.

The thinnest area of the skull base, and the area most susceptible to injury, is at the junction of the anterior ethmoid artery and the middle turbinate along the anterior ethmoid roof [23] (Fig. 49.4). The incidence of CSF leakage after pituitary surgery is reportedly 2–3%, but a higher incidence is reported after extended transsphenoidal approaches [24].

For most intraoperative CSF leaks, repair with a single layer consisting of a free intranasal mucosal flap harvested from the septum, turbinate, or nasal cavity is necessary to repair the defect. Occasionally, larger defects require an additional structural layer, such as a perpendicu-

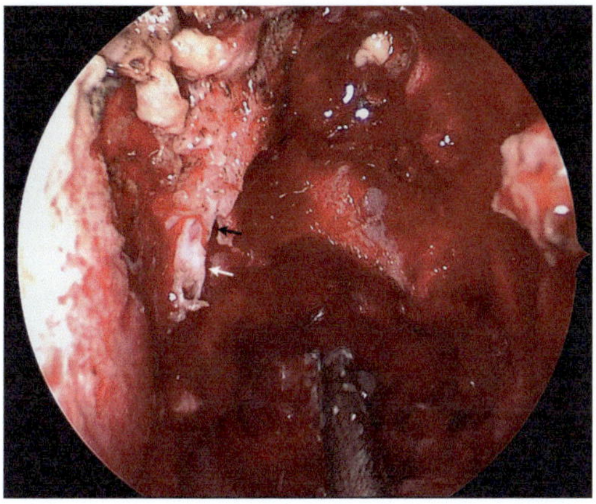

Fig. 49.4 Intraoperative CSF leakage in the anterior part of the cribriform plate of a patient with a nasal inverting papilloma. The surgeon became confused after the middle turbinectomy and used the Kerrison punch to directly bite the cribriform. The skull base defect (*black arrow*) and the broken dura mater (*white arrow*) are located in the center of the endoscopic field

lar plate of ethmoid placed on the intracranial side of the defect. For such cases, the CSF leakage repair procedure should be performed intraoperatively, and nasal packing should not be used with an expectation that self-healing will occur because the risk of postoperative intracranial infection may be increased. After the operation, sensitive antibiotics that can cross the blood–brain barrier should be administered to prevent intracranial infection.

49.2.2.2 Carotid Injury

Injury to the internal carotid artery is a life-threatening complication that can occur during ESS. Although this complication occurs in less than 0.1% of patients who undergo sinus surgery [19], its consequences can be devastating and may include intracranial injury with stroke. Because of the importance of avoiding this complication, protection of the internal carotid artery is well established in ESS. However, with the recent advancements in endoscopic skull base surgery, the topic of internal carotid artery injury has become an area of focus again. The causes of internal carotid artery injury are related to anatomic, pathological and surgical factors [25]. Among the anatomical factors, the internal carotid artery (ICA) can be damaged intraoperatively due to the dehiscent ICA canal, bulging of the vessel, and ICA displaced by the lesion. Previous surgical procedure, postradiotherapy, tumor encircling ICA > 120° may contribute to the pathologic vulnerability of the ICA. Finally, when the ICA needs for wide exposure intraoperatively, it is easy to be injured in surgical resection.

The ICA courses along the lateral wall of the sphenoid sinus immediately inferior to the optic carotid recess and forms a specific anatomical structure (Fig. 49.5). Preoperative imaging often provides the surgeon with a map that can guide the adoption of the most appropriate surgical strategy. Injury to the carotid artery may occur when the sphenoid sinus is entered too far laterally or when surgical dissection is performed along the lateral sphenoid wall and the carotid canal is penetrated. If the lesion is only located around the internal carotid artery and is adhered to it, precise dissection should be performed. If the resection is much more difficult, other approaches should be considered. Carotid injury can be avoided simply by entering the sphenoid sinus medially through the natural sphenoid ostium and enlarging this opening in an inferior and medial direction away from the laterally positioned carotid artery. Instrumentation within the lateral sphenoid sinus is not usually necessary during routine sinus surgery; when such instrumentation is performed, such as with a high-speed bur, extreme caution is needed. The intersphenoidal septum can insert onto the bony canal overlying the carotid artery, and arterial injury has been reported with removal of this partition. When injury to the carotid artery occurs, profuse bleeding will rapidly fill the nasal cavity. The surgeon must gain control of the bleeding by packing the sphenoid sinus with iodoform gauze or muscle, if possible. Aggressive fluid resuscitation should be begun immediately, and hemodynamic control must be achieved to maintain cerebral perfusion. A blood sample should also be typed and cross-matched for transfusion of blood products. Once the patient has been stabilized, definitive treatment should be performed by the interven-

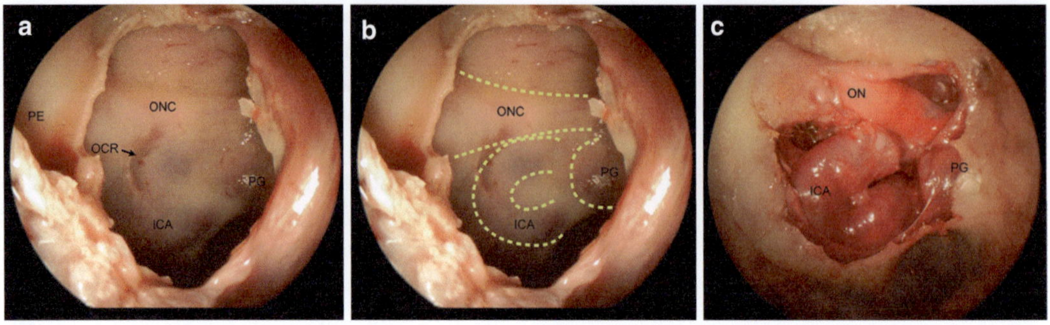

Fig. 49.5 Endoscopic anatomic characteristics of the relationship among the internal carotid artery (ICA), optic nerve canal (ONC), and pituitary gland (PG) in the sphenoid sinus. (**a**) Lateral wall of sphenoid sinus. (**b**) Dashed lines show the projections of the ONC, ICA, and PG. (**c**) The optic nerve (ON), ICA, and PG can be seen after dissecting the bony wall of the sphenoid sinus. *PE* posterior ethmoid sinus, *OCR* optic nerve canal–internal carotid artery recess

tional radiologist using angiography to identify the site and extent of vascular injury. A balloon occlusion test to verify adequate cross-perfusion may be performed by the interventional neuroradiologist prior to permanent occlusion of the internal carotid artery. Cross-cranial vascular bypass may be performed to prevent brain ischemia and stroke only when internal carotid artery occlusion is not a viable option.

49.2.3 Postoperative Complications

49.2.3.1 Intracranial Infection

With respect to intracranial infections, both meningitis and intracranial abscesses have been reported following ESS. Meningitis is usually the result of CSF leakage, which may either not be obvious during the operation or not managed quickly and properly. Direct bacterial spread may occur from the sinonasal cavity through a skull base defect. When a patient complains of severe headache, high fever, and nuchal rigidity after sinus surgery, this complication should be considered. Emergency evaluation with a CT scan, lumbar puncture, and neurologic consultation is indicated. Intravenous antibiotics are the preferred method of treatment for meningitis. The diagnosis of an intracranial abscess is confirmed by magnetic resonance imaging. Intravenous antibiotics should be administered under the care of infectious disease and neurology consultants. The operation cavity may need to be cleaned and debrided when there is definite evidence of infection.

49.2.3.2 Epistaxis

Epistaxis is a common complication, occurring in 2% of patients after ESS. It usually occurs on the day of surgery; it may also occur 5–7 days after surgery, but this is relatively rare [17]. Bleeding from the nasal septum, which may lead to a septal hematoma, is also rare. The most common sites of postoperative bleeding are the middle turbinates, posterior fontanelle of the middle antrostomy, and inferior margin of the ostium of the sphenoid sinus. The blood vessels responsible for bleeding arise from different branches of the sphenopalatine artery, including the branch of the middle turbinate located in the posterior part of the root of the middle turbinate, branch of the posterior fontanelle arising from the branch of the inferior turbinate, posterior nasoseptal artery traversing the lower margin of the sphenoidal ostium, and one of the main branches of the sphenopalatine artery. Thus, the site most prone to bleeding after maxillary sinus surgery is the posterior lower part of the maxillary sinus opening window, while that after sphenoidal sinus surgery is the external lower part of the sphenoidal sinus opening window.

A large amount of bleeding the day after surgery is usually due to a small rupture. Delayed bleeding is often associated with hard blowing of the nose or a dry nose. In such cases, adding a local filler is usually ineffective. If necessary, the bleeding site should be carefully identified under general anesthesia in the operating room. Bipolar coagulation is optimal for rapid hemostasis. Because the patient already experienced bleeding during the first operation, the surgeon should consider the possibility of anemia or even hemorrhagic shock. Maintenance of the patient's vital signs and adequate blood volume is essential. Even during surgery, good communication should be maintained with the anesthesiologist, the vital signs monitored, and blood transfusions performed if necessary.

If severe (≥800 mL) and recurrent bleeding occurs several weeks after sinus surgery, the past treatment experiences and history of internal carotid artery injury should be reviewed. This information may indicate the formation of a pseudoaneurysm, one of the most catastrophic complications. Immediate interventional radiotherapy is the most effective treatment option.

49.2.3.3 Cavity Synechiae

Adhesions or synechiae usually develop 2–3 weeks after surgery. Minor adhesions within the surgical cavity generally do not cause symptoms and do not require management (Fig. 49.6). However, severe adhesions or synechiae secondary to mucosal scarring can be a source of postoperative anosmia, recurrent sinusitis, and mucocele formation (Fig. 49.7). Although a silicone spacer or packing material placed at the time of surgery may decrease the incidence of adhesion formation, a partial middle turbinectomy, outfracture of the inferior turbinate, or septoplasty should be performed prospectively. If adhesions are noted at the time of outpatient endoscopy examination during the first postoperative week, they can usually be divided with minimal patient discomfort. However, resection of synechiae in the outpatient department is more difficult when it is severe or when the nasal cavity has become very narrow. Even for mild adhesion, revision surgery is definitely required under general anesthesia.

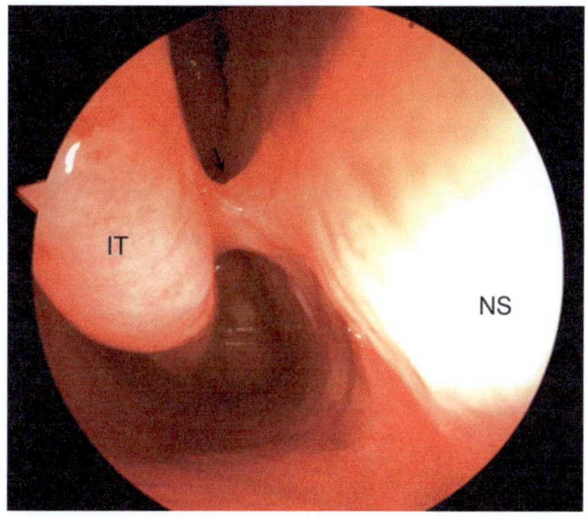

Fig. 49.6 Endoscopic view of a minor inferior turbinate (IT)–nasal septum (NS) adhesion

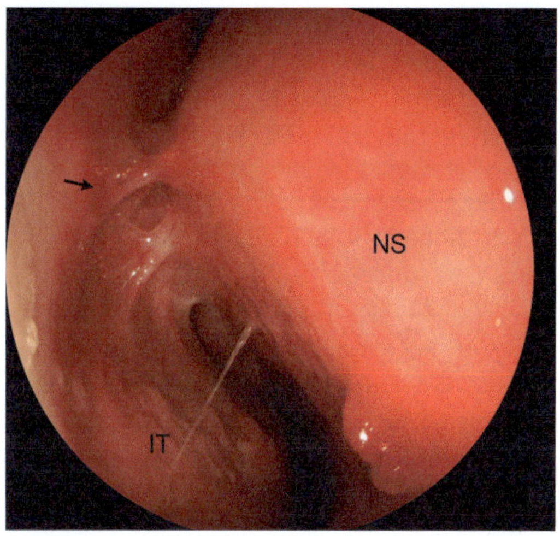

Fig. 49.7 Endoscopic view of obvious adhesion (*arrow*) between lateral wall of nasal cavity and nasal septum (NS), which should be managed by septoplasty. *IT* inferior turbinate

49.2.3.4 Secondary Lacrimal Duct Obstruction

Persistent epiphora after transnasal ESS indicates that the lacrimal sac or nasolacrimal duct was damaged during the operation. It is more common to damage the lacrimal sac when removing the uncinate process or to damage the nasolacrimal duct when performing the middle meatal antrostomy or sometimes the inferior meatal antrostomy. The average distance between the lacrimal duct and anterior margin of

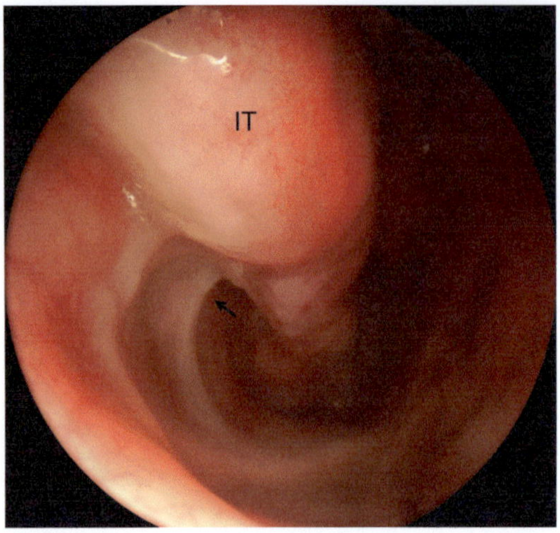

Fig. 49.8 Endoscopic view of inferior meatal mucosal scarring (arrow) that led to chronic dacryocystitis following endoscopic inferior meatal antrostomy. *IT* inferior turbinate

the ostium of the maxillary sinus is 9 mm. Attention should be paid to the opening of the maxillary sinus with use of a backward bite punch. If hard bone is touched, the operation should be stopped to prevent damage to the nasolacrimal duct. If obvious nasolacrimal duct injury occurs during the operation, scar-induced stricture of the lacrimal duct and dacryocystitis is expected to occur after the operation; thus, dacryocystorhinostomy should be performed simultaneously. If inferior meatal antrostomy is performed, the mucosa around the window should be preserved, especially Hasner's membrane, the natural orifice of the lacrimal duct in the nasal cavity (Fig. 49.8).

49.2.3.5 Secondary Sinusitis

It is commonly believed that secondary sinusitis mainly appears following use of the endoscopic endonasal approach to treat anterior-middle cranial fossa diseases. In fact, postoperative secondary sinusitis is common after routine ESS. As described above, synechiae due to mucosal scarring can lead to recurrent sinusitis. Clinically, frontal sinusitis is the most common type of sinusitis, followed by maxillary sinusitis and sphenoidal sinusitis, respectively. Because of the complicated anatomy of the frontal recess, precise entry into the frontal sinus is still challenging for surgeons. The remnant frontal recess cells or mucosal scar formation often blocks the outflow of the frontal sinus, resulting in recalcitrant frontal sinusitis. Secondary maxillary sinusitis is often associated with severe mucosal injury during the operation. Alternatively, the natural ostium of the maxillary sinus was not protected during the ethmoidectomy and the ostium became narrow or closed after surgery. Similarly, secondary sphenoidal sinusitis usually results from damage to the mucosa of the anterior wall of the sinus or the presence of a narrow opening.

Poor sinus ventilation and drainage or obstruction of a nasal sinus, which are important factors leading to secondary sinusitis, will certainly cause infection of the sinuses and a series of clinical symptoms such as facial pressure, purulent nasal discharge, and nasal block. Endoscopic and imaging evaluations are very important in such patients. Once the diagnosis has been established, medical therapy is the first option, and the inflammatory granulation tissue, cysts, and purulent secretion must be removed. A nasal douche comprising saline mixed with corticosteroids is also beneficial. If the symptoms cannot be relieved after appropriate medical treatment, revision sinus surgery is indicated. Endoscopic intervention is required to fully open the sinuses and remove the irreversible inflammatory lesions.

49.2.3.6 Bone Remodeling

Bone remodeling is often thought to be a histopathologic phenomenon, not a complication of sinus surgery. Due to intensive research on the etiology of chronic rhinosinusitis, rhinologists have paid more attention to the effects of bone remodeling in patients with this condition. The phenomena that occur in the pathogenesis of chronic rhinosinusitis are well known. Normally, the bone system is constantly formed and resorbed, maintaining a state of balance. Bone remodeling is a state in which the system is out of balance. During nasal endoscopic surgery, excessive avulsion of the nasal mucosa and injury to the periosteum and even bone may lead

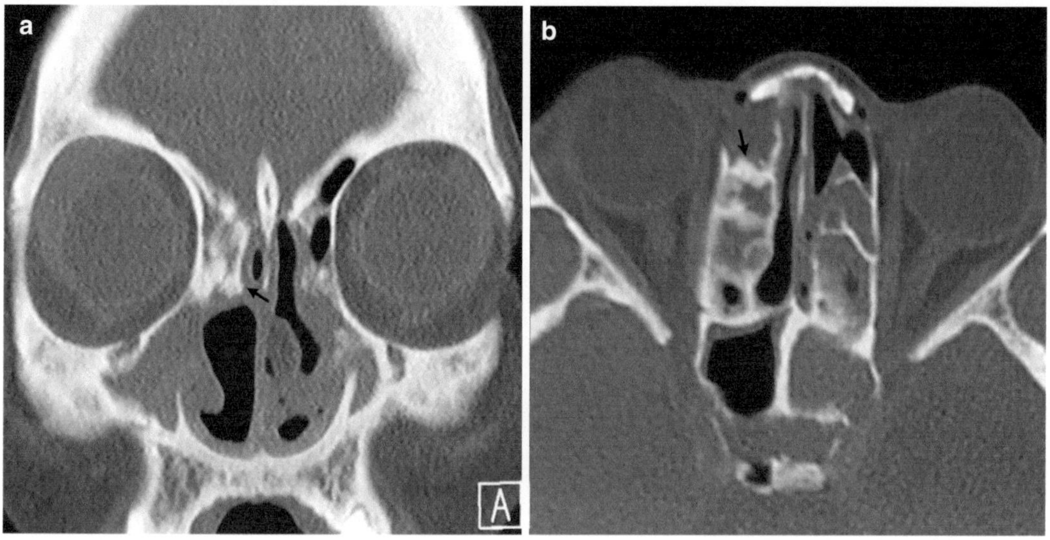

Fig. 49.9 Sinus CT images (left: coronal view; right: axis view) of bone remodeling after an inappropriate nasal endoscopic sinus surgery. A 58-year-old female patient, who has bilateral headache for 10 years after a nasal endoscopic surgery for 20 years. The CT scans showed bone thickened in both ethmoid sinuses and the right frontal recess (*black arrows*)

to bone remodeling. Bone remodeling may lead to prolonged and unhealed sinusitis and affect the outcome of endoscopic surgery (Fig. 49.9). The most common presentation of bone remodeling is bony hyperplasia that can be observed on both a CT scan and by nasal endoscopy. Unreasonable or inappropriate surgical management is a risk factor for bone remodeling (i.e., bony hyperplasia), which can become the main cause of persistent sinusitis and symptoms after surgery. Moreover, the proliferous bone can make the revision surgery much more difficult. Therefore, physicians must protect the sinus mucosa as much as possible during the operation and avoid unnecessary mucosal avulsion. If removal of the lesion inevitably results in bone exposure, a nasal mucosa flap can be used for repair, or additional bone resection can be performed to reduce the area of bare bone. A vascularized pedicle septal mucosal flap, which can inhibit mucosal scarring and new bone formation is recommended to cover the tough bone in some sinus surgeries, such as the Draf IIb or III procedure. During the revision sinus surgery, bone resection is needed for patients with marked bone hyperplasia.

49.3 Conclusions

Complications of ESS are often associated with a poor understanding of the sinonasal anatomy and inadequate preparation. Preoperatively focusing on the features of the lesions, potential surgical pitfalls, variations or malformations of the sinonasal anatomy, operating technique, surgical instruments, and intraoperative hemostasis methods can help to avoid or decrease the incidence of complications. Prompt recognition and appropriate management are needed when complications occur, and this usually results in good patient outcomes.

References

1. Stankiewicz JA. Complications of endoscopic intranasal ethmoidectomy. Laryngoscope. 1987;97(11):1270–3. https://doi.org/10.1288/00005537-198711000-00004.
2. Kimmelman C, Weisman R, Osguthorpe J, et al. The efficacy and safety of transnasal ethmoidectomy. Laryngoscope. 1988:1178–82.
3. Stankiewicz JA. Complications in endoscopic intranasal ethmoidectomy: an update. Laryngoscope. 1989;99(7 Pt 1):686–90. https://doi.org/10.1288/00005537-198907000-00004.

4. Krings JG, Kallogjeri D, Wineland A, Nepple KG, Piccirillo JF, Getz AE. Complications of primary and revision functional endoscopic sinus surgery for chronic rhinosinusitis. Laryngoscope. 2014;124(4):838–45. https://doi.org/10.1002/lary.24401.
5. Thacker NM, Velez FG, Demer JL, Rosenbaum AL. Strabismic complications following endoscopic sinus surgery: diagnosis and surgical management. J AAPOS. 2004;8(5):488–94. https://doi.org/10.1016/j.jaapos.2003.09.001.
6. Eloy JA, Svider PF, Setzen M. Clinical pearls in endoscopic sinus surgery: key steps in preventing and dealing with complications. Am J Otolaryngol. 2014;35(3):324–8. https://doi.org/10.1016/j.amjoto.2014.01.013.
7. Cottrill E, Becker SS, DeLaurentis D. Pearls and pitfalls: medico-legal considerations for sinus surgery. Curr Opin Otolaryngol Head Neck Surg. 2014;22(1):75–9. https://doi.org/10.1097/moo.0000000000000024.
8. Hosemann W, Draf C. Danger points, complications and medico-legal aspects in endoscopic sinus surgery. GMS Curr Top Otorhinolaryngol Head Neck Surg. 2013;12:Doc06. https://doi.org/10.3205/cto000098.
9. Soyka MB, Holzmann D. Correlation of complications during endoscopic sinus surgery with surgeon skill level and extent of surgery. Am J Rhinol. 2005;19(3):274–81.
10. Cappabianca P, Cavallo LM, Esposito F, De Divitiis O, Messina A, De Divitiis E. Extended endoscopic endonasal approach to the midline skull base: the evolving role of transsphenoidal surgery. Adv Tech Stand Neurosurg. 2008;33:151–99. https://doi.org/10.1007/978-3-211-72283-1_4.
11. Snyderman C, Kassam A, Carrau R, Mintz A, Gardner P, Prevedello DM. Acquisition of surgical skills for endonasal skull base surgery: a training program. Laryngoscope. 2007;117(4):699–705. https://doi.org/10.1097/MLG.0b013e318031c817.
12. Kassam A, Snyderman CH, Mintz A, Gardner P, Carrau RL. Expanded endonasal approach: the rostrocaudal axis. Part I. Crista galli to the sella turcica. Neurosurg Focus. 2005;19(1):E3.
13. Kassam A, Snyderman CH, Mintz A, Gardner P, Carrau RL. Expanded endonasal approach: the rostrocaudal axis. Part II. Posterior clinoids to the foramen magnum. Neurosurg Focus. 2005;19(1):E4.
14. Kassam AB, Gardner P, Snyderman C, Mintz A, Carrau R. Expanded endonasal approach: fully endoscopic, completely transnasal approach to the middle third of the clivus, petrous bone, middle cranial fossa, and infratemporal fossa. Neurosurg Focus. 2005;19(1):E6.
15. Kassam A, Snyderman CH, Carrau RL, Gardner P, Mintz A. Endoneurosurgical hemostasis techniques: lessons learned from 400 cases. Neurosurg Focus. 2005;19(1):E7.
16. Brown SM, Anand VK, Tabaee A, Schwartz TH. Role of perioperative antibiotics in endoscopic skull base surgery. Laryngoscope. 2007;117(9):1528–32. https://doi.org/10.1097/MLG.0b013e3180caa177.
17. Dalziel K, Stein K, Round A, Garside R, Royle P. Endoscopic sinus surgery for the excision of nasal polyps: a systematic review of safety and effectiveness. Am J Rhinol. 2006;20(5):506–19. https://doi.org/10.2500/ajr.2006.20.2923.
18. Kennedy DW, Shaman P, Han W, Selman H, Deems DA, Lanza DC. Complications of ethmoidectomy: a survey of fellows of the American Academy of Otolaryngology-Head and Neck Surgery. Otolaryngol Head Neck Surg. 1994;111(5):589–99. https://doi.org/10.1177/019459989411100509.
19. May M, Levine HL, Mester SJ, Schaitkin B. Complications of endoscopic sinus surgery: analysis of 2108 patients—incidence and prevention. Laryngoscope. 1994;104(9):1080–3. https://doi.org/10.1288/00005537-199409000-00006.
20. Stankiewicz JA. Blindness and intranasal endoscopic ethmoidectomy: prevention and management. Otolaryngol Head Neck Surg. 1989;101(3):320–9. https://doi.org/10.1177/019459988910100305.
21. Setliff R, Parsons P. The "Hummer": new instrumentation for functional endoscopic sinus surgery. Am J Rhinol allergy. 1994;8:275–8.
22. Kennedy DW, Hwang PH. Rhinology: diseases of the nose, sinuses, and skull base. New York: Thieme; 2012.
23. Kainz J, Stammberger H. The roof of the anterior ethmoid: a place of least resistance in the skull base. Am J Rhinol Allergy. 1989;3:191–9.
24. Cappabianca P, Cavallo LM, Esposito F, Valente V, De Divitiis E. Sellar repair in endoscopic endonasal transsphenoidal surgery: results of 170 cases. Neurosurgery. 2002;51(6):1365–71; discussion 71–2.
25. AlQahtani A, London NR Jr, Castelnuovo P, Locatelli D, Stamm A, Cohen-Gadol AA, et al. Assessment of factors associated with internal carotid injury in expanded endoscopic endonasal skull base surgery. JAMA Otolaryngol Head Neck Surg. 2020;146(4):364–72. https://doi.org/10.1001/jamaoto.2019.4864.

Peri-operative Management

50

Jian Li and Weiping Wen

Key Points

- Peri-operative management is the critical factor in the potential success or failure of endoscopic sinus surgery.
- Peri-operative assessment and follow-up continuously help improving surgery quality and the life quality of patients.

50.1 Introduction

Endoscopic sinus surgery (ESS) is accepted as the surgical management of the choice for chronic sinusitis or polyps. Recently the instruments and techniques have improved. The quality of the ESS has developed better than before. Even though, the primary goal of the surgery is to achieve and maintain clinical control in CRS. Peri-operative management is either important for improving surgery quality or for improving the life quality and disease control after surgery [1]. So from the preoperative assessment and to the postoperative management, standardized procedures and treatments are needed for disease control [2–4]. Here we describe the popular and regular clinical management in peri-operative stage. In the future, high quality studies are still needed for the standardization of peri-operative management.

J. Li · W. Wen (✉)
Otorhinolaryngology Department, The First Affiliated Hospital of Sun Yat-sen University, Guangzhou, China
e-mail: wenwp@mail.sysu.edu.cn

50.2 Preoperative Objective Assessment by Endoscopy and CT Scan

Endoscopy examination can define the phenotype CRSsNP or CRSwNP. The presence of mucopurulent secretions is usually seen in the nasal cavity and meatus. The CT scan can be used as the diagnosis of CRS following endoscopy, which can show positive signs such as osteomeatal complex obstruction, mucosal thickening, soft tissue masses (details in Chap. 24—Radiological imaging chapter). For CRS, the endoscopic findings can confirm the diagnosis without CT scan. The CT scan may be reserved until the point at which the operation is being contemplated or just before surgery intervention [5–7]. The CT scan is mandatory to confirm the CRS severity and the anatomy of the patient prior to surgery [8]. There are a number of systems published to facilitate preoperative interpretation of the images; the CLOSE mnemonic is widely used (C: cribriform niche; L: lamina papyracea; O: Onodi spheno-ethmoidal cells; S: Sphenoid sinus; E: Ethmoidal arteries.). Wormald reported a new international frontal sinus anatomy classification and classification of the extent of endo-

L. Zhang, C. Bachert (eds.), *Chronic Rhinosinusitis*, https://doi.org/10.1007/978-981-16-0784-4_50

scopic frontal sinus surgery, which provided a practical method to confirm the anatomy of the frontal sinus including the drainage pathway of the frontal sinus before surgery. The new classification helps young surgeons to make a virtual surgery in his or her head before the surgery on patients. According to this new method, preoperative assessment of the CT scan can be standardized [9].

50.3 Preoperative Control of General Conditions Such as Hypertension, Diabetes, Coagulation Dysfunction, and Asthma

The control of general conditions before surgery is to improve the surgical field and surgery quality. Better conditions means better safety of patients during surgery and less complications after surgery. Anti-coagulants and/or aspirin/NSAIDS can cause excess bleeding during sinus surgery. The surgeon should set up the timing of the preoperative stopping of these drugs [10]. Lower airway inflammation often co-exists in CRS, with up to two thirds of patients with CRS affected by comorbid asthma. Pulmonary function in CRS patients is significantly reduced compared to non-CRS individuals, which should be tested before surgery, even in patients that do not report bronchial symptoms [11–13].

50.4 Bacteriology Before Surgery

Microbiome composition can be highly variable among individuals with CRS. The imbalance within the nasal microbiome is associated with various allergic and inflammatory diseases of the airways. Bacterial cultures can be performed under endoscopy if purulent secretions can be seen in the nasal cavity or meatus [10]. Bacteria can be isolated if needed. Antibiotic sensitivity can be simultaneously performed [14, 15] (Details in Chap. 13—Microbiology of chronic rhinosinusitis chapter).

50.5 Biopsy Before Surgery

If differential diagnosis is needed, especially for single-side CRS, biopsy can be performed under endoscopy to differentiate polyps to some tumors. At the same time, eosinophils in polyp tissue can be counted under microscopy. Recently, some studies assessing nasal epithelia from brushing or nasal epithelial cultures showed significant epigenetic changes in polyps tissue [16]. For the future, the brushing epithelia could be a regular "cell" biopsy, which can help make individual treatment strategies for every patient [17].

50.6 Postoperative Management of Nasal Packs

If nasal packs can be avoided, it is best to do so. Bleeding needs to be dealt with before the end of the surgery, and it is usually due to one of the branches of the sphenopalatine artery. Suction diathermy is usually needed to stop bleeding. If more than moderate bleeding is still going on at the end of the surgery, some kinds of nasal packs are usually needed [5, 10, 18]. But it is better to remove the packs as soon as possible after surgery. The packing time should be less than 48–72 h. Actually, to reduce bleeding during surgery, the preoperative stopping of medication that can cause bleeding like anti-coagulants and/or aspirin/NSAIDS, and the stopping of special foods containing vasodilator effects in Asia area, are also important [19]. Preoperative management cannot only reduce bleeding during surgery, but reduce the opportunity of nasal packs at the end of surgery [10]. The packing materials can be divided into non-absorbable and absorbable materials. And absorbable materials include gels and other hemostats that may be instilled into nasal and/or sinus cavities. A meta-analysis comparing absorbable and non-absorbable dressings found no differences in terms of symptoms after surgery [20].

50.7 Postoperative Douching

The patients need to learn how to douche with saline. Fibrinous exudates or crusts usually exist in the first several weeks after surgery. The postoperative recovery period can be plagued by the repeated crusts. Most patients are recommended to douche at least twice daily for 2 weeks. After 2 weeks, douching frequency could be once to twice daily until 8–12 weeks after surgery [5, 18, 21]. Postoperative douching with saline can improve symptom-based and endoscopic outcomes with low risk of harm. A recent meta-analysis found three trials reported that nasal irrigation using normal saline and various solutions was found to be effective in reducing symptom scores and endoscopic scores for CRS after FESS [22]. For patients with type 2 inflammation, saline with topical steroid can be recommended [17]. Topical steroid can either inhibit the inflammation of the nasal mucosa or inhibit the bacterial infection in the nasal cavity according to some recent studies [22]. For patients with purulent infectious condition, some topical antibiotics such as tobramycin can be recommended. Douching can help patients relieve the symptoms and the endoscopic appearance of mucosa [15].

50.8 Follow-Up and Postoperative Endoscopic Reexamination

In the first few days after surgery, debridement is usually advocated. In several months after surgery, endoscopic reexamination is needed to remove crusts and fibrinous exudates. After sinus surgery patients should be aware that it is so important to continuously look after the lining of their paranasal sinuses. The first endoscopic reexamination should be at 1 week after surgery. Then outpatient visit is needed once every 2 weeks, which can continue for 3 until 2 months after surgery. After 2 months, the patients can be asked to come back every 1 month for reexamination [7, 10, 23]. During the course, douching and topical steroid should be continuously used to control the inflammation and help recovery of cilia and mucosa [21]. Some patients with the type 2 polyps or suffering from asthma should follow-up for a long term, even for the whole life [17]. Long follow-up is needed to confirm the high percentage of uncontrolled patients after surgery. From a clinical as well as from a research perspective, a gold standard to assess disease control in CRS still remains needed. So the follow-up plan maybe changed in time as the research progresses.

50.9 Follow-Up and Postoperative Evaluation

Efficacy evaluation should be performed via subjective and objective methods. The SNOT-22 and VAS for total as well as individual symptoms are validated tools that are widely known in the field of CRS and used for assessing Quality of Life and symptom severity. VAS of total symptoms and the single symptom, Lund–Mackay CT score, and Lund–Kennedy endoscopy score are recommended for CRS patients after surgery. SF-36 life quality score and SNOT-20 sinusitis life quality score are also suggested, and can provide more comprehensive and scientific information [2, 3]. Recently many new questionnaires have been used to evaluate CRS symptoms. These include the Sinus Control Test (SCT), the 31-Item Rhinosinusitis Outcome Measure (RSOM-31), the Sinonasal questionnaire (SNAQ-11), and the Rhinosinusitis Disability Index (RSDI) 15. In addition, some questionnaires for the impact on QoL and general health status including the 36-item Short Form (SF-36), the 12-item Short Form (SF-12), and the EuroQol-5Dimension-5Level (EQ-5D-5L).

References

1. Simmen D, Jones N. Manual of endoscopic sinus and skull base surgery. New York: Stuttgart Georg Thieme Verlag; 2014.
2. Dietz de Loos DA, Segboer CL, Gevorgyan A, Fokkens WJ. Disease-specific quality-of-life questionnaires in rhinitis and rhinosinusitis: review and evaluation. Curr Allergy Asthma Rep. 2013;13(2):162–70. https://doi.org/10.1007/s11882-012-0334-8.
3. Piccirillo JF, Merritt MG Jr, Richards ML. Psychometric and clinimetric validity of the 20-item sino-nasal outcome test (SNOT-20). Otolaryngol Head Neck Surg. 2002;126(1):41–7. https://doi.org/10.1067/mhn.2002.121022.
4. Xu G, Zhao CX. Clinical effecacies of chronic rhinosinusitis. Zhonghua er bi yan hou tou jing wai ke za zhi = Chinese J Otorhinolaryngol Head Neck Surg. 2013:115–6.
5. Li HB, Shi JB, Xu G. [Comment on the European position paper on rhinosinusitis and nasal polyps 2012]. Zhonghua er bi yan hou tou jing wai ke za zhi = Chinese J Otorhinolaryngol Head Neck Surg. 2012;47(10):877–9.
6. Knai C, Brusamento S, Legido-Quigley H, Saliba V, Panteli D, Turk E, et al. Systematic review of the methodological quality of clinical guideline development for the management of chronic disease in Europe. Health Policy (Amsterdam, Netherlands). 2012;107(2–3):157–67. https://doi.org/10.1016/j.healthpol.2012.06.004.
7. Rosenfeld RM, Piccirillo JF, Chandrasekhar SS, Brook I, Ashok Kumar K, Kramper M, et al. Clinical practice guideline (update): adult sinusitis. Otolaryngol Head Neck Surg. 2015;152(2 Suppl):S1–s39. https://doi.org/10.1177/0194599815572097.
8. Wormald PJ, Hoseman W, Callejas C, Weber RK, Kennedy DW, Citardi MJ, et al. The international frontal sinus anatomy classification (IFAC) and classification of the extent of endoscopic frontal sinus surgery (EFSS). Int Forum Allergy Rhinol. 2016;6(7):677–96. https://doi.org/10.1002/alr.21738.
9. Error M, Ashby S, Orlandi RR, Alt JA. Single-blinded prospective implementation of a preoperative imaging checklist for endoscopic sinus surgery. Otolaryngol Head Neck Surg. 2018;158(1):177–80. https://doi.org/10.1177/0194599817731740.
10. Shi JB, Xu G. [Perioperative treatment of chronic rhinosinusitis]. Zhonghua er bi yan hou tou jing wai ke za zhi = Chinese J Otorhinolaryngol Head Neck Surg. 2013;48(2):111–3.
11. Chen L. Application of antiallergic drugs in the treatment of chronic rhinosinusitis. Zhonghua Er Bi Yan Hou Tou Jing Wai Ke Za Zhi. 2013:107–8.
12. Philpott CM, Erskine S, Hopkins C, Kumar N, Anari S, Kara N, et al. Prevalence of asthma, aspirin sensitivity and allergy in chronic rhinosinusitis: data from the UK National Chronic Rhinosinusitis Epidemiology Study. Respir Res. 2018;19(1):129. https://doi.org/10.1186/s12931-018-0823-y.
13. Massoth L, Anderson C, McKinney KA. Asthma and chronic rhinosinusitis: diagnosis and medical management. Med Sci (Basel, Switzerland). 2019;7(4) https://doi.org/10.3390/medsci7040053.
14. Jiang RS, Liang KL, Yang KY, Shiao JY, Su MC, Hsin CH, et al. Postoperative antibiotic care after functional endoscopic sinus surgery. Am J Rhinol. 2008;22(6):608–12. https://doi.org/10.2500/ajr.2008.22.3241.
15. Cherian LM, Cooksley C, Richter K, Ramezanpour M, Paramasivan S, Wormald PJ, et al. Effect of commercial nasal steroid preparation on bacterial growth. Int Forum Allergy Rhinol. 2019;9(7):766–75. https://doi.org/10.1002/alr.22312.
16. DeConde AS, Smith TL. Classification of chronic rhinosinusitis-working toward personalized diagnosis. Otolaryngol Clin North Am. 2017;50(1):1–12. https://doi.org/10.1016/j.otc.2016.08.003.
17. Bayar Muluk N, Cingi C, Scadding GK, Scadding G. Chronic rhinosinusitis-could phenotyping or endotyping aid therapy? Am J Rhinol Allergy. 2019;33(1):83–93. https://doi.org/10.1177/1945892418807590.
18. Fokkens WJ, Lund VJ, Mullol J, Bachert C, Alobid I, Baroody F, et al. EPOS 2012: European position paper on rhinosinusitis and nasal polyps 2012. A summary for otorhinolaryngologists. Rhinology. 2012;50(1):1–12. https://doi.org/10.4193/Rhino50E2.
19. Valentine R, Wormald PJ. Nasal dressings after endoscopic sinus surgery: what and why? Curr Opin Otolaryngol Head Neck Surg. 2010;18(1):44–8. https://doi.org/10.1097/MOO.0b013e3283346f36.
20. Yan M, Zheng D, Li Y, Zheng Q, Chen J, Yang B. Biodegradable nasal packings for endoscopic sinonasal surgery: a systematic review and meta-analysis. PLoS One. 2014;9(12):e115458. https://doi.org/10.1371/journal.pone.0115458.
21. Adappa ND, Wei CC, Palmer JN. Nasal irrigation with or without drugs: the evidence. Curr Opin Otolaryngol Head Neck Surg. 2012;20(1):53–7. https://doi.org/10.1097/MOO.0b013e32834dfa80.
22. Chen XZ, Feng SY, Chang LH, Lai XP, Chen XH, Li X, et al. The effects of nasal irrigation with various solutions after endoscopic sinus surgery: systematic review and meta-analysis. J Laryngol Otol. 2018;132(8):673–9. https://doi.org/10.1017/s0022215118000919.
23. Rosenfeld RM, Piccirillo JF, Chandrasekhar SS, Brook I, Kumar KA, Kramper M, et al. Clinical practice guideline (update): Adult Sinusitis Executive Summary. Otolaryngol Head Neck Surg. 2015;152(4):598–609. https://doi.org/10.1177/0194599815574247.

Surgery Outcome and Predictors

51

Fenghong Chen and Jianbo Shi

Key Points

- Endoscopic Sinus Surgery (ESS) may be considered relatively safe and appropriate for CRS with/without NP.
- However, recurrence rates may vary and are related to type 2 immune markers.
- Predictors for recurrence after ESS are tissue and blood eosinophils, IL-5, comorbid asthma, allergic sensitization, and ethmoid sinus disease detected by CT scan.

A number of prospective studies have shown that endoscopic sinus surgery (ESS) is relatively effective for managing CRS patients without NP rather than with NP, but robust prospective studies are lacking. Multiple predictors were found for the outcome after ESS. The outcome of ESS can be assessed in multiple dimensions, such as symptoms and quality of life improvement, polyp recurrence, and disease control level [1]; see Chap. 53. However, due to the high recurrence rate especially in ECRS, the goal of the management of CRS currently is shifting from cure to achieve and maintain clinical disease control; patients should not have symptoms, or the symptoms are not bothersome. Long-term control of the sinus mucosa often remains an unmet need; this implies that new surgical techniques and/or biologics are urgently needed to possibly ameliorate this situation.

F. Chen · J. Shi (✉)
Otorhinolaryngology Hospital, The First Affiliated Hospital of Sun Yat-sen University, Guangzhou, China

51.1 Symptoms and Quality of Life Improvement and Prediction

ESS has become a standard surgical choice for CRS and often also is used in refractory ESS. There are numerous published studies documenting significant symptomatic improvement following ESS, as well as improvement in disease-specific and generic QOL. However, most of these studies are non-randomized and uncontrolled (level III), and only few randomized controlled trials are available [2, 3].

Stein and et al. [4] identified CRS patients who underwent ESS using the State Ambulatory Surgery Database for the state of California between 2005 and 2011. Of 61,339 patients who underwent ESS, 4078 (6.65%) returned for revision ESS within relatively short time. They found positive predictors of revision to be a diagnosis of nasal polyps (AOR: 1.20, 95% CI: 1.11–1.29, $p < 0.001$) and female gender (AOR: 1.20, 95% CI: 1.11–1.29, $p < 0.001$). A total of 1459 patients of CRS were followed until 5 years after ESS [5]. The mean SNOT-22 score for all patients was 28.2 (standard deviation

L. Zhang, C. Bachert (eds.), *Chronic Rhinosinusitis*, https://doi.org/10.1007/978-981-16-0784-4_51

[SD] = 22.4) at 5 years after surgery. This is remarkably similar to the results observed at 3 months (25.5), 12 months (27.7), and 36 months (27.7), and represents a 14-point improvement over the baseline score. In a smaller long-term prospective study, 59 adult patients were followed for 10.9 years (±13.8 months), on average. Mean QOL significantly improved between baseline and 6 months and remained durable to 10 years. A 17% revision surgery rate within the 10-year follow-up period was observed with a 25% revision rate in CRS with polyposis [6]. Calus et al. [7] report the long-term outcome of FESS for 47 patients with CRSwNP, who underwent primary or revision extended ESS in a prospective study. They followed patients before and 6 years and 12 years after surgery. There still was a significantly better symptom score and total nasal endoscopic polyp score compared to before surgery; however, within the 12-year follow-up period, 30 out of 38 patients developed recurrent nasal polyps, of which 14 patients underwent additional revision surgery. Comorbid allergic sensitization and tissue IL-5 levels were found to be significant predictors for the need of revision surgery. Hopkins C et al. [8] and Alakärppä et al. [9], respectively, found the preoperative 22-item Sinonasal Outcome Test (SNOT-22) could predict the surgical improvement. Patients with a preoperative score of <20 failed to achieve a mean improvement greater than the minimal clinically important difference (MCID). Patients with a SNOT-22 score greater than 30 had more than 70% chance to achieve the MCID. Patients with CRSwNP had greater temporary improvement than patients with CRSsNP [8].

51.2 Polyp Recurrence and Revision Surgery and Prediction

The poly recurrence rates are ranging from 8% to 55% [10–14]. Mucosal eosinophilia is widely accepted as a risk factor for polyp recurrence. However, there is no unanimous histopathologic criterion to diagnosis eosinophilic CRS currently. Studies focusing on the ability of eosinophil predicting polyp recurrence are summarized in Table 51.1. Some studies defined eosinophilic CRS depended on eosinophil count/HPF (400× magnification), while others based criteria on the proportion of eosinophil cells as a percentage of the total inflammatory cell count in the sample. Researchers have suggested "5" [18, 34], "10" [10, 13, 19, 35], "20" [20],"55" [11], "70" [12], "100" [17], "120" [15] eosinophils absolute count/HPF as appropriate cutoff points; others have suggested "5%" [22], "10%" [23], "20%" [21], or "27%" [11] eosinophils percentage count as relevant cutoff values. Also, the methods to measure the eosinophils and inflammatory cells varied. Some used one single dense infiltrated field, and some counted the cells with a 10 × 10-mm reticulate present in the eyepiece, and others counted five or ten random HPF fields. McHugh et al. [24] studied whether high tissue eosinophilia could be used to define ECRS based on likelihood of recurrence by meta-analysis. After identifying 11 articles (n = 3138), they found a cutoff value of >55 eos/HPF to show the highest sensitivity and specificity. Meta-regression analysis performed showed that the Quality Assessment of Diagnostic Accuracy Studies score, geographic location, follow-up time, and study design did not affect the test accuracy.

Eosinophilic inflammation markers, Charcot–Leyden crystal (CLC) [25, 26], eosinophil cationic protein (ECP) [27], eotaxin-3 [28], periostin [29], and IL-5 [20] also showed some value to predict polyp recurrence. Wu et al. [25] illustrated the predictive value of CLC protein level in nasal secretions for polyp recurrence. They reported that 62.96% (68/108) of patients developed recurrence during a 12- to 33-month postoperative follow-up. A CLC concentration of 34.24 ng/mL can predict postoperative polyp recurrence with 92.6% sensitivity and 87.5% specificity. Qi et al. [26] also found the relative CLC mRNA levels in nasal brushings may serve as a reliable non-invasive biomarker to predict CRSwNP recurrence.

Nakayama et al. [16] conducted a prospective study to investigate the effect of mucosal

Table 51.1 Studies summarized recurrence rate in ECRS and NECRS

Study First author, year	Study design, subject number	Country	ECRS criteria	Author's reason for defining ECRS	Biopsy location	Author's definition of recurrence	Mean time to recurrence (months)	Follow-up (months)	Percentage of ECRS	Recurrence % (*n*) Total, ECRS, NECRS
Matsuwaki, 2008 [15]	R, $n = 56$	Japan	>120	Highest odds ratio for recurrence (OR, 3.2; $p < 0.001$)	NP or sinus mucosa	Need for revision ESS	NR	60	12.5%	16.1%, 85.7%, 6.1%
Nakayama, 2011 [16]	P, $n = 175$	Japan	>70	Showed the minimum p value ($p = 0.001$) and highest AUC (0.673)	NP or ethmoid mucosa	Grade ≥ 1 NP	NR	17.5	50.8%	22.8%, 34.8%, 10.5%
Ikeda, 2013 [17]	P, $n = 130$	Japan	>100	ROC curve and cox proportional hazard model showed the minimum p value	NP	Presence of NP middle meatus	28 ± 12	48	32.3%	36.2%, 47.6%, 25.0%
Vlaminck, 2014 [18]	P, $n = 221$	Belgium	>5	Based on Soler et al. 2009 [35]	Sinus mucosa	Recurrent diseased mucosa with ≥3 sinus symptoms ≥1 month with systemic steroids	NR	36	57.9%	22.2%, 32.0%, 8.6%
Brescia, 2016 [19]	P, $n = 179$	Italy	>10	No specific reason provided	NP	Grade ≥ 1 NP	22.3 ± 10.7	32.8 ± 14.7	41.3%	13.4%, 21.6%, 7.6%
Grgic, 2015 [20]	P, $n = 30$	Croatia	>20	Highest RR for polyp recurrence (RR, 41%; $p < 0.05$)	NP	Grade ≥ 1 NP	NR	24	73.3%	36.6%, 40.9%, 25.0%
Lou, 2015 [11]	R, $n = 387$	China	>55	Youden index: optimal sensitivity, specificity, and AUC (0.969; $p < 0.001$)	NP	Recurrent NP, 1 year postsurgery with symptoms >1 month	NR	34 ± 5	49.6%	55.2%, 97.4%, 13.8%

(continued)

Table 51.1 (continued)

Study First author, year	Study design, subject number	Country	ECRS criteria	Author's reason for defining ECRS	Biopsy location	Author's definition of recurrence	Mean time to recurrence (months)	Follow-up (months)	Percentage of ECRS	Recurrence % (*n*) Total, ECRS, NECRS
Tokunaga, 2015 [12]	R, $n = 1716$	Japan	>70	Most significant value for Kaplan–Meier curve recurrence free rate	NP	Grade ≥ 1 NP	NR	22.6	39.1%	23.1%, 33.0%, 16.7%
Brescia, 2016 [13]	P, $n = 143$	Italy	>10	No specific reason provided	NP	Grade ≥ 1 NP	19 ± 10	17 ± 10	41.3%	13.4%, 21.6%, 7.6%
Do, 2016 [10]	P, $n = 110$	Australia	>10	Based on Snidvongs et al. [36]	Ethmoid mucosa	Requirement of long-term oral steroids	NR	>12	55.4%	8.1%, 13.1%, 2.0%
Rosati, 2020 [21]	P, $n = 44$	Italy	>20%	Based on literature	NP	Polypoid mucosa with bothersome symptoms (>1 month)	NR	8–10 years	47.7%	40.9%, 66.7%, 17.4%

AUC area under the curve, *ECRS* eosinophilic chronic rhinosinusitis, *ESS* endoscopic sinus surgery; *HPF* high-power field, *HTE* high tissue eosinophilia, *NECRS* non-eosinophilic chronic rhinosinusitis, *NP* nasal polyps, *NR* not reported, *NRD* non-recurrent disease, *OR* odds ratio, *P* prospective, *R* retrospective, *RD* recurrent disease, *ROC* receiver operating characteristic, *RR* relative risk eosinophilia on the recurrence of nasal polyps. The recurrence rate was 22.9% (40/175) in a mean 17.5 months follow-up period. The recurrence rate in ECRS was 34.8% and 10.5% in NECRS. Patients with mucosal eosinophilia (70/HPF and over) had a poor prognosis. Asthma, polyp score, CT score, and allergic rhinitis were also predictors of recurrence. Brescia et al. [13] conducted a prospective study in 143 patients. The mean follow-up was 17 months. In their study, mucosal eosinophilia was the only independent prognostic factor for poly recurrence, using 10 ≥ eosinophils per field as the diagnostic criterion for ECRS. The relative risk for polyp recurrence was 2.92 in ECRS (NECRS as 1.0). In another study [14], the authors recruited 240 patients who underwent ESS for CRSwNP and had a postoperative follow-up longer than 12 months. They compared the prognostic role of the neutrophil-to-lymphocyte ratio (NLR) and eosinophil-to-lymphocyte ratio (ELR) and the basophil-to-lymphocyte ratio (BLR). The polyp recurrence rate in this study was 14.7%. The mean NLR, ELR, and BLR were significantly higher in patients whose disease recurred than in those remaining recurrence-free, but the discriminatory power of the NLR, ELR, or BLR in terms of disease recurrence was disappointingly low. Grgic et al. [20] included 30 patients operated for nasal polyps and follow-up at least 2 years. High IL-5 concentrations positively correlated to greater risk for poly recurrence, but did not reach significance. Local IgE immunohistochemical reactivity in polyp specimens did not have any effect on polyp recurrence.

Clinical characteristics of CRS are also used to predict polyp recurrence. T. Tokunaga et al. [12] found blood eosinophilia (>5%), ethmoid sinus disease detected by CT scan, bronchial asthma, aspirin, and nonsteroidal anti-inflammatory drug intolerance were associated significantly with recurrence. Meng et al. reported the ratio of total ethmoid sinus scores and maxillary sinus scores for both sides (E/M ratio) taken from the Lund–Mackay score predicted CRSwNP recurrence [30]. Amali et al. [31] found that polypoid changes of the middle turbinate are associated with risk of polyp recurrence after surgery.

51.3 Difficult-to-Treat CRS and Uncontrolled Disease and Prediction

Patients who do not achieve an acceptable level of disease control despite intranasal corticosteroid treatment, up to two short courses of antibiotics or systemic corticosteroids in the last year and former adequate surgery are considered to have uncontrolled severe CRS (see Chap. 53). Based on this definition, the study from Liao and colleagues [32] revealed that up to 30% of Chinese CRS patients demonstrated uncontrolled severe CRS [33]. Tao and colleagues [34] report 47.8% of patients to have controlled, 22.1% partially controlled, and 30.1% uncontrolled CRS over 1-year follow-up after surgery. Multiple regression models found tissue eosinophils, blood eosinophils, a Lund–Mackay (LM) score ≥ 15, and a CT ethmoid (E) ≥ maxillary (M) score as independent risk factors.

References

1. Fokkens WJ, Lund VJ, Hopkins C, Hellings PW, Kern R, Reitsma S, et al. European position paper on rhinosinusitis and nasal polyps 2020. Rhinology. 2020;58(Suppl S29):1–464.
2. Rimmer J, Fokkens W, Chong LY, Hopkins C. Surgical versus medical interventions for chronic rhinosinusitis with nasal polyps. Cochrane Database Syst Rev. 2014;(12):CD006991.
3. Ragab SM, Lund VJ, Scadding G. Evaluation of the medical and surgical treatment of chronic rhinosinusitis: a prospective, randomised, controlled trial. Laryngoscope. 2004;114(5):923–30.
4. Stein NR, Jafari A, DeConde AS. Revision rates and time to revision following endoscopic sinus surgery: a large database analysis. Laryngoscope. 2018;128(1):31–6.
5. Hopkins C, Slack R, Lund V, Brown P, Copley L, Browne J. Long-term outcomes from the English national comparative audit of surgery for nasal polyposis and chronic rhinosinusitis. Laryngoscope. 2009;119(12):2459–65. https://doi.org/10.1002/lary.20653.
6. Smith TL, Schlosser RJ, Mace JC, Alt JA, Beswick DM, DeConde AS, et al. Long-term outcomes of

endoscopic sinus surgery in the management of adult chronic rhinosinusitis. Int Forum Allergy Rhinol. 2019;9(8):831–41.
7. Calus L, Van Bruaene N, Bosteels C, Dejonckheere S, Van Zele T, Holtappels G, et al. Twelve-year follow-up study after endoscopic sinus surgery in patients with chronic rhinosinusitis with nasal polyposis. Clin Transl Allergy. 2019;9:30.
8. Hopkins C, Rudmik L, Lund VJ. The predictive value of the preoperative Sinonasal Outcome Test-22 score in patients undergoing endoscopic sinus surgery for chronic rhinosinusitis. Laryngoscope. 2015;125(8):1779–84.
9. Alakarppa AI, Koskenkorva TJ, Koivunen PT, Alho OP. Predictive factors of a beneficial quality of life outcome in patients undergoing primary sinonasal surgery: a population-based prospective cohort study. Eur Arch Otorhinolaryngol. 2018;275(5): 1139–47.
10. Do TQ, Barham HP, Earls P, Sacks R, Christensen JM, Rimmer J, et al. Clinical implications of mucosal remodeling from chronic rhinosinusitis. Int Forum Allergy Rhinol. 2016;6(8):835–40.
11. Lou H, Meng Y, Piao Y, Wang C, Zhang L, Bachert C. Predictive significance of tissue eosinophilia for nasal polyp recurrence in the Chinese population. Am J Rhinol Allergy. 2015;29(5):350–6.
12. Tokunaga T, Sakashita M, Haruna T, Asaka D, Takeno S, Ikeda H, et al. Novel scoring system and algorithm for classifying chronic rhinosinusitis: the JESREC Study. Allergy. 2015;70(8):995–1003.
13. Brescia G, Marioni G, Franchella S, Ramacciotti G, Giacomelli L, Marino F, et al. A prospective investigation of predictive parameters for post-surgical recurrences in sinonasal polyposis. Eur Arch Otorhinolaryngol. 2016;273(3):655–60.
14. Brescia G, Pedruzzi B, Barion U, Cinetto F, Giacomelli L, Martini A, et al. Are neutrophil-, eosinophil-, and basophil-to-lymphocyte ratios useful markers for pinpointing patients at higher risk of recurrent sinonasal polyps? Am J Otolaryngol. 2016;37(4):339–45.
15. Matsuwaki Y, Ookushi T, Asaka D, Mori E, Nakajima T, Yoshida T, et al. Chronic rhinosinusitis: risk factors for the recurrence of chronic rhinosinusitis based on 5-year follow-up after endoscopic sinus surgery. Int Arch Allergy Immunol. 2008;146(Suppl 1):77–81. https://doi.org/10.1159/000126066.
16. Nakayama T, Yoshikawa M, Asaka D, Okushi T, Matsuwaki Y, Otori N, et al. Mucosal eosinophilia and recurrence of nasal polyps – new classification of chronic rhinosinusitis. Rhinology. 2011;49(4):392–6.
17. Ikeda K, Shiozawa A, Ono N, Kusunoki T, Hirotsu M, Homma H, et al. Subclassification of chronic rhinosinusitis with nasal polyp based on eosinophil and neutrophil. Laryngoscope. 2013;123(11):E1–9.
18. Vlaminck S, Vauterin T, Hellings PW, Jorissen M, Acke F, Van Cauwenberge P, et al. The importance of local eosinophilia in the surgical outcome of chronic rhinosinusitis: a 3-year prospective observational study. Am J Rhinol Allergy. 2014;28(3):260–4.
19. Brescia G, Marioni G, Franchella S, Ramacciotti G, Velardita C, Giacomelli L, et al. Can a panel of clinical, laboratory, and pathological variables pinpoint patients with sinonasal polyposis at higher risk of recurrence after surgery? Am J Otolaryngol. 2015;36(4):554–58.
20. Grgic MV, Cupic H, Kalogjera L, Baudoin T. Surgical treatment for nasal polyposis: predictors of outcome. Eur Arch Otorhinolaryngol. 2015;272(12):3735–43.
21. Rosati D, Rosato C, Pagliuca G, Cerbelli B, Della Rocca C, Di Cristofano C, et al. Predictive markers of long-term recurrence in chronic rhinosinusitis with nasal polyps. Am J Otolaryngol. 2020;41(1):102286.
22. Kim JW, Hong SL, Kim YK, Lee CH, Min YG, Rhee CS. Histological and immunological features of non-eosinophilic nasal polyps. Otolaryngol Head Neck Surg. 2007;137(6):925–30.
23. Cao PP, Li HB, Wang BF, Wang SB, You XJ, Cui YH, et al. Distinct immunopathologic characteristics of various types of chronic rhinosinusitis in adult Chinese. J Allergy Clin Immunol. 2009;124(3):478–84, 84.e1–2.
24. McHugh T, Snidvongs K, Xie M, Banglawala S, Sommer D. High tissue eosinophilia as a marker to predict recurrence for eosinophilic chronic rhinosinusitis: a systematic review and meta-analysis. Int Forum Allergy Rhinol. 2018;8(12):1421–9.
25. Wu D, Yan B, Wang Y, Zhang L, Wang C. Predictive significance of Charcot-Leyden crystal protein in nasal secretions in recurrent chronic rhinosinusitis with nasal polyps. Int Arch Allergy Immunol. 2020:1–11.
26. Qi S, Yan B, Liu C, Wang C, Zhang L. Predictive significance of Charcot-Leyden crystal mRNA levels in nasal brushing for nasal polyp recurrence. Rhinology. 2020;58(2):166–74.
27. Lu PC, Lee TJ, Huang CC, Chang PH, Chen YW, Fu CH. Serum eosinophil cationic protein: a prognostic factor for early postoperative recurrence of nasal polyps. Int Forum Allergy Rhinol. 2020; https://doi.org/10.1002/alr.22664.
28. Yamada T, Miyabe Y, Ueki S, Fujieda S, Tokunaga T, Sakashita M, et al. Eotaxin-3 as a plasma biomarker for mucosal eosinophil infiltration in chronic rhinosinusitis. Front Immunol. 2019;10:74.
29. Ninomiya T, Noguchi E, Haruna T, Hasegawa M, Yoshida T, Yamashita Y, et al. Periostin as a novel biomarker for postoperative recurrence of chronic rhinosinitis with nasal polyps. Sci Rep. 2018;8(1):11450.
30. Meng Y, Zhang L, Lou H, Wang C. Predictive value of computed tomography in the recurrence of chronic rhinosinusitis with nasal polyps. Int Forum Allergy Rhinol. 2019;9(11):1236–43.
31. Amali A, Bidar Z, Rahavi-Ezabadi S, Mikaniki N, Sadrehosseini SM. Polypoid change of middle turbinate is associated to an increased risk of polyp recurrence after surgery in patients with chronic rhinosinusitis with nasal polyps. Eur Arch Otorhinolaryngol. 2018;275(8):2021–5.

32. Liao B, Liu JX, Li ZY, Zhen Z, Cao PP, Yao Y, et al. Multidimensional endotypes of chronic rhinosinusitis and their association with treatment outcomes. Allergy. 2018;73(7):1459–69.
33. Liao B, Liu JX, Guo CL, Li ZY, Pan L, Liu Z. A panel of clinical and biological markers predict difficult-to-treat chronic rhinosinusitis. Allergy. 2020;75(4):946–9.
34. Tao X, Chen F, Sun Y, Wu S, Hong H, Shi J, et al. Prediction models for postoperative uncontrolled chronic rhinosinusitis in daily practice. Laryngoscope. 2018;128(12):2673–80.
35. Soler ZM, Sauer DA, Mace J, Smith TL. Relationship between clinical measures and histopathologic findings in chronic rhinosinusitis. Otolaryngol Head Neck Surg. 2009;141(4):454–61.
36. Snidvons K, Lam M, Sacks R, Earls P, Kalish L, Phillips PS, et al. Structured histopathology profiling of chronic rhinosinusitis in routine practice. Int Forum Allergy Rhinol.2012;2(5):376–85.

Biologics in Chronic Rhinosinusitis with Nasal Polyps

52

Claus Bachert

Key Points

- Clinically severe CRSwNP is associated with type 2 immune reactions within the sinus mucosa, characterized by increased concentrations of the cytokines IL-4, IL-5, and IL-13, elevated IgE and numbers of eosinophils.
- As in other type 2 diseases such as asthma, atopic dermatitis, these cytokines and mediators can be specifically targeted by monoclonal antibodies, the so-called biologics.
- For CRSwNP, several antibodies have been successfully applied in studies, with Dupilumab leading the development and approved in the USA and Europe.
- Dupilumab reduces the patients polyp burden to a great deal, sparing oral corticosteroid use and surgery, and is well tolerated.

Based on the pathomechanisms described in Chaps. 5–17 and the endotyping approach as introduced in Chaps. 20 and 21, it is evident that specific innovative approaches in severe uncontrolled CRSwNP would target at type 2 immune reactions. Appropriate patients suffer from uncontrolled severe CRSwNP, defined as bilateral nasal polyps of Davos grade 4 out of 8, despite continuous twice daily nasal glucocorticosteroids (GCS) and eventually oral courses of GCS, and/or despite adequate former sinus surgery, and/or asthma comorbidity, eventually with N-ERD [1]. In daily clinic, these patients nearly always have used topical GCS twice daily for many years, and two out of three patients had at least one former surgery and/or oral GCS within the last 2 years; furthermore, more than 60% suffer from comorbid late-onset asthma. This actually states that current treatment possibilities have not lead to a control of the disease, and any further oral GCS use or further conventional surgery is associated with an increased risk for the patient without promising long-term benefit. In these patients, an innovative approach is clearly needed.

After pivotal studies in asthma, atopic dermatitis, and other type 2 diseases, the possibility of treating nasal polyps was finally evaluated (Table 52.1). Omalizumab, which targets free IgE and complexes it preventing the binding to IgE receptors, was introduced in 2003 for the treatment of severe asthma in the USA, and then in Europe. 10 years later, the first study in CRSwNP was published [2]. Proof-of-concept studies with biologics directed against IL5 (Reslizumab and Mepolizumab) in CRSwNP were published in 2006 and 2011, but registered

C. Bachert (✉)
Upper Airways Research Laboratory and Department of Oto-Rhino-Laryngology, Ghent University, Ghent, Belgium

Division of ENT Diseases, CLINTEC, Karolinska Institute, University of Stockholm, Stockholm, Sweden
e-mail: claus.bachert@ugent.be

L. Zhang, C. Bachert (eds.), *Chronic Rhinosinusitis*, https://doi.org/10.1007/978-981-16-0784-4_52

Table 52.1 Reported studies with biologics in nasal polyposis and therapeutic effect

	Mepolizumab	Omalizumab	Dupilumab	Mepolizumab
Year	2011[9]	2013[2]	2016[3] 2019[4]	2017[10]
Target molecule	IL-5	IgE	IL-4 receptor alpha	IL-5
Study design[a]	Single centre	Two centres	Multicentre (13 sites)	Multicenter (six sites)
NO. (verum/placebo)	30 (20/10)	23 (15/8)	60 (30/30)	105 (54/51)
Asthma % (verum/placebo)	43% (50%/30%)	100% (100%/100%)	58% (63%/53%)	78% (81%/75%)
Former surgery % (verum/placebo)	77% (75%/80%)	83% (87%/75%)	58% (63%/53%)	100% (100%/100%)
End point and last visit (weeks)	8w/48w	16w/20w	16w/16w	25w/25w
Therapeutic effects	Significant reduction of polyp scores; reduction of blood eosinophil counts, serum ECP, and IL-5Rα, IL-6, MPO in nasal secretion	Significant reduction of polyp and CT scores, improvement of symptoms of upper and lower airway and AQLQ	Significant reduction of polyp and CT scores, improvement of smelling, symptoms, and quality of life (SNOT-22); improvement of FEV1 and ACQ5. Reduced plasma eotaxin-3, serum and nasal secretion tIgE, and nasal tissue tIgE, IL13, ECP, PARK, Eotaxin 1,2,3	Significant reduction of polyp score, improvement of smelling, symptoms, and quality of life (SNOT-22)

[a]All these studies were randomized, double-blind, placebo-controlled studies. tIgE, total serum immunoglobulin E. *AQLQ* Asthma Quality of Life Questionnaire, *ACQ5* 5-item Asthma Control Questionnaire, *PnIF* Peak Nasal Inspiratory Flow, *FEV1* forced expiratory volume, *SNOT-22* Sino-nasal Outcome Test, *ECP*, eosinophil cationic protein, *IL-5Rα* IL-5 receptor α subunit, *TARC* Thymus and Activation-Regulated Chemokine, *PARK* pulmonary and activation-regulated chemokine, *MPO* myeloperoxidase

for asthma prior to nasal polyps; registration of Mepolizumab likely is achievable, but the Phase 3 trial has not been terminated yet. Benralizumab, an anti-IL5 receptor antagonist, also currently is in Phase 3. Finally, the first biologic for the indication of CRSwNP most likely will be Dupilumab, an anti-IL4 receptor antagonist, with Phase 2 study results published in 2016 [3] and Phase 3 trial results just published now [4]. Dupilumab has been registered in 2019 for CRSwNP in the USA, and possibly will be registered also in Europe in the same year.

From Phase 2 studies, it was obvious that biologics such as Mepolizumab, Omalizumab, and Dupilumab all would significantly reduce the nasal polyp score to a clinically relevant extent (nasal polyp score (NPS) at baseline about 6 points, reduction of 1–2 points average at end of treatment over placebo). With this effect, other observations were repeatedly made, such as the reduction of the Lund–Mackay CT score, the reduction of the nasal and sinus symptoms, an increase in smell and smell testing, and an increase in quality of life measured by SNOT-22 and RSOM-31, indicating clinically relevant effects on the disease [5] (Table 52.2). Furthermore, in patients with asthma, Dupilumab and Omalizumab increased lung function and asthma control in patients with CRSwNP and comorbid asthma. Finally, dependent on the mechanism of the biologic, reductions in blood and tissue eosinophils or serum IgE levels were noticed [5]. Also local effects were recorded: Dupilumab treatment reduced multiple biomarkers of type 2 inflammation in polyp tissues and nasal secretions of

Table 52.2 What to expect from biologics in the treatment of CRSwNP?

Clinically	
Reduction of endoscopic nasal polyp score	Dupilumab, mepolizumab, omalizumab
Lund-Mackay CT scan score	Dupilumab, omalizumab
Reduction of relevant nasal symptoms	Dupilumab, mepolizumab, omalizumab
Increase in smell (UPSIT and VAS)	Dupilumab, mepolizumab, omalizumab
Increase in quality of life (SNOT-22 and RSOM-31)	Dupilumab, mepolizumab, omalizumab
In asthmatic patients	
Increase in lung function (FEV1 percent predicted)	Dupilumab, omalizumab
Asthma control (ACQ and AQLQ)	Dupilumab, omalizumab
Biomarker	
Reduction in blood eosinophil numbers	Mepolizumab
Reduction in serum IgE levels	Dupilumab, omalizumab
Reduction in tissue eosinophil numbers	Dupilumab, mepolizumab

Source: Bachert C et al., J Allergy Clin Immunol. 2018;141:1543–1551

patients with CRSwNP, demonstrating that antagonism of IL-4Rα signalling suppresses type 2 cytokine dependent processes, such as mucosal IgE formation, as well as the expression of chemokines attracting inflammatory cells to the nasal mucosa [6] (Fig. 52.1).

52.1 Anti-IL5 Strategies

The mode of action is different for the mentioned biologics; Reslizumab and Mepolizumab are anti-IL-5 antibodies, capturing interleukin-5 in serum, bone marrow, and mucosal tissues, which are essential for the migration, chemotaxis and recruitment, activation, proliferation, maturation, and survival of eosinophil granulocytes [7]. IL-5 is produced by lymphoid cells, specifically Th2 cells, but also innate lymphoid cells (ILC2), mast cells, γδ-T cells, and eosinophils. IL-5 binds to the α subunit of the IL-5 receptor (IL-5Rα), expressed on eosinophils and to a lesser extent on basophils in its transmembrane form; the receptor also exists in a soluble form, possibly interfering with anti-IL-5 receptor approaches within the mucosal tissue. The stimulation of the receptor complex subsequently activates multiple signalling pathways. Benralizumab, a humanized mAb that binds with high affinity to the α-chain of the human IL-5R, blocks its activation and signal transduction. Benralizumab, due to its afucosylation, also binds to the main activating receptor (FcgR) expressed on NK cells, macrophages, and neutrophils, which enhance the antibody-dependent cell-mediated cytotoxicity (ADCC) function [8]. The activation of ADCC is unique to benralizumab, enabling it to rapidly reduce the number of circulating and tissue eosinophils. Blood eosinophils and basophils and their precursors are profoundly reduced. Biologics targeting IL-5 or its receptor can possibly interfere with the eosinophils at different levels, from the bone marrow to the blood and airway mucosal tissue.

A first study with Reslizumab showed efficacy; however, this antibody was not further developed in this indication. In a proof-of-concept double-blind randomized study in severe nasal polyps, mostly recurrent after surgery and refractory to glucocorticosteroids, 20 patients received 2 single intravenous injections (28 days apart) of 750 mg of mepolizumab and 10 patients placebo. Twelve of 20 patients receiving mepolizumab had a significant improvement in the nasal polyp score and CT scan evaluation vs. 1 out of 10 patients receiving placebo at 8 weeks [9]. In a later randomized, double-blind, placebo-controlled trial, recruiting 105 patients with recurrent nasal polyps requiring surgery, 750 mg of intravenous mepolizumab or placebo every 4 weeks for a total of 6 doses in addition to daily topical corticosteroid treatment was applied. The primary end point was the number of patients no longer requiring surgery at week 25 of treatment, based on a composite end point of endoscopic nasal polyp score and nasal polyposis severity visual analogue scale (VAS) score. A significantly greater proportion of patients in the mepolizumab group compared with the placebo group no longer required surgery at week 25 (30% vs.

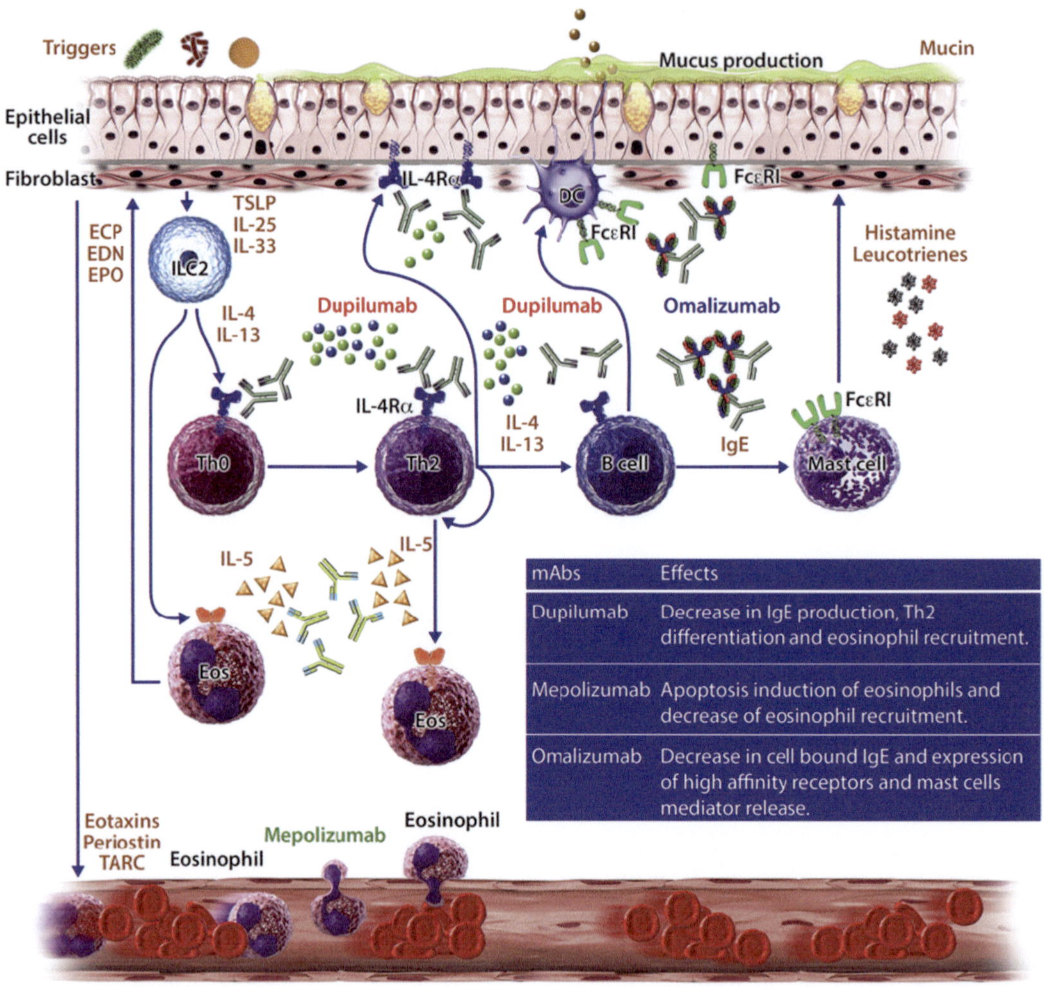

Fig. 52.1 Biologics targeting type 2 immune reactions. *DC* dendritic cell, *ECP* eosinophil cationic protein, *EDN* eosinophil-derived neurotoxin, *Eos* eosinophils, *EPO* eosinophil peroxidase, *IL-4Rα* IL-4 receptor α, *TSLP* thymic stromal lymphopoietin. (Source: Bachert et al. J Allergy Clin Immunol. 2018)

10%, $p < .006$). There was a significant improvement in nasal polyp severity VAS score, endoscopic nasal polyp score, all individual VAS symptom scores, and the SNOT-22 score in the mepolizumab compared to the placebo group. Mepolizumab's safety profile was comparable with that of placebo [10]. There is currently a Phase 3 study ongoing, the results of which will further help to evaluate the effects of this drug. A major point is the possibly lower responder rate, and means to preselect patients based on biomarkers.

52.2 Anti-IgE

Immunoglobulin E (IgE) antibodies are well recognized for their role in mediating allergic reactions, and their powerful effector functions activated through binding to Fc receptors FcεRI on mast cells, basophils, and dendritic cells, and FcεRII/CD23 on B cells. Upon stimulation of the receptors through cross-linking of IgE, mast cells and basophils release a plethora of mediators, among which leukotrienes, prostaglandins, and cytokines such as IL-4, IL-5, and IL-13. These cytokines impact on eosinophils, T cells, and epithelial cells and perpetuate the type 2 immune reaction. Omalizumab, therefore, most likely interferes with IgE at several levels, from the dendritic cell to the mast cell and basophil, as well as the B cell [11]. As described before, IgE also plays a role in non-allergic diseases such as nasal polyposis and non-allergic late-onset asthma, diseases which are characterized by massive polyclonal IgE formation locally in the airway mucosal tissue [12]. This IgE is functional and releases mast cell mediators, which in turn further maintain the inflammatory reaction [13].

As a proof-of-concept study, a randomized, double-blind, placebo-controlled trial of allergic and non-allergic patients with nasal polyps and comorbid asthma, was conducted. Subjects received 4–8 subcutaneous doses of omalizumab ($n = 16$) or placebo ($n = 8$). The primary end point was the reduction in total nasal endoscopic polyp scores at week 16. Secondary end points included a change in sinus opacification, nasal and asthma symptoms, results of validated life quality questionnaires for upper and lower airways, and serum/nasal secretion biomarker levels. There was a significant decrease in the total nasal endoscopic polyp scores after 16 weeks in the omalizumab treated group, which was confirmed by the Lund–Mackay score of the CT changes. Omalizumab had a beneficial effect on upper and lower airway symptoms (nasal congestion, anterior rhinorrhoea, loss of sense of smell, wheezing, and dyspnoea) and on quality-of-life scores, independent of the presence of allergy [2]. This study demonstrated with small numbers of patients that the response to Omalizumab was clinically significant, reaching a reduction of the nasal polyp score of app. 2.5 points, and of symptoms related to the disease, and confirmed the role of locally produced polyclonal IgE.

First results of two Phase 3 studies recently became available, demonstrating that omalizumab was more effective compared with placebo in patients with inadequate response to intranasal corticosteroids, added to an intranasal mometasone therapy. Omalizumab significantly reduced the nasal polyp score and the average daily nasal congestion score compared with placebo at week 24, with improvements seen as early as week 4. Furthermore, the average daily sense of smell score, the average daily posterior and anterior rhinorrhoea scores, and the SNOT-22 scores were significantly better with treatment. Reductions in systemic glucocorticosteroids over the 6 months or nasal surgery, but also ameliorations for AQLQ, did not reach significance, probably due to the limited duration and number of patients in the study. Further, the UPSIT showed improvement after 24 weeks. Although these studies were performed in a relatively small population and over 6 months only, preliminary data demonstrate the effectiveness of Omalizumab in nasal polyp disease added to nasal glucocorticosteroid treatment. The reduction in nasal polyp score was smaller compared to the proof-of-concept study, which may indicate the difference between study populations in these studies.

52.3 Anti-IL-4 Receptor Alpha Antagonism

A first randomized [3], double-blind, placebo-controlled parallel-group study with Dupilumab was conducted in the United States and Europe in the years 2013/2014. Sixty adults with chronic sinusitis and nasal polyposis refractory to intranasal corticosteroids received subcutaneous dupilumab (a 600 mg loading dose followed by 300 mg weekly; $n = 30$) or placebo ($n = 30$); all patients received mometasone furoate nasal spray twice daily for 16 weeks. Among the patients, 35 had comorbid asthma, 51 completed the study. The primary endpoint was the bilateral nasal polyp score, which demonstrated a significant difference in the verum treated versus the placebo-treated patients, indicating a clinically relevant effect. Least squares (LS) mean change in nasal polyp score was −0.3 (95% CI, −1.0 to 0.4) with placebo and −1.9 (95% CI, −2.5 to −1.2) with dupilumab, resulting in a LS mean difference of −1.6 [95% CI, −2.4 to −0.7];

$p < .001$). Furthermore, CT scan evaluation using the Lund–Mackay CT total score was highly significant between groups, as well as the 22-item SinoNasal Outcome Test and sense of smell assessed by UPSIT. The most common adverse events were nasopharyngitis (33% with placebo, 47% with dupilumab), injection site reactions (7% vs. 40%), and headache (17% vs. 20%). Thus, the principle of antagonizing IL-4 and IL-13 in addition to topical glucocorticosteroid treatment proved to be highly effective in nasal polyp disease, and further studies with longer treatment duration were justified.

Dupilumab Phase 3 results from 2 studies including more than 700 patients have recently been published [4]. About two out of three patients had former surgery and/or oral GCS use within 2 years, and about 60% suffered from mostly non-severe asthma. The recommended dose of dupilumab (300 mg every 2 weeks) significantly improved the co-primary endpoints nasal polyp score (NPS) and nasal congestion score (NCS). At 24 weeks, the mean difference in NPS of dupilumab treatment versus placebo was −2.06 (95% CI −2.43 to −1.69; $p < 0.0001$) and −1.80 (−2.10 to −1.51; $p < 0.0001$) in the two studies, the difference in NCS was −0.89 (−1.07 to −0.71; $p < 0.0001$) and −0.87 (−1.03 to −0.71; $p < 0.0001$). Furthermore, all monitored secondary endpoints including total symptom score, daily loss of smell, sinus opacification (CT) score, the smell test (UPSIT), and disease-specific quality of life SNOT-22 score were significantly reduced vs. placebo. Within 4 weeks, the percentage of subjects with anosmia was reduced from 75% to impressive 30%, approximately, with dupilumab, but without a relevant change in the placebo group; this effect was maintained over the study period, interestingly, the nasal polyp score changed at a slower speed compared to the smell, indication an anti-inflammatory rather than an anti-obstructive effect of the drug being related to this effect. Also lung function and asthma control significantly improved in those patients with asthma. The reductions in type 2 biomarkers in serum (total IgE, TARC, eotaxin-3, and periostin) and in nasal secretions (ECP, eotaxin-3, and total IgE) paralleled the effects described earlier [6]. Interestingly, the drug was well tolerated, with the most common adverse events (nasopharyngitis, worsening of nasal polyps and asthma, headache, epistaxis) observed more frequently with placebo than with Dupilumab. Also the number of viral infections was reduced, as it has been observed in former studies in inner city asthma [14].

Termination of the treatment after 24 weeks resulted in the partial recurrence of disease, with increase in nasal polyp score and symptoms, whereas the continuation of treatment provided further relief over the next 28 weeks, reducing the nasal polyp score by nearly 2.5 scores from start of treatment (Figs. 52.2 and 52.3). In contrast, the NPS in the placebo group showed a slight increase over the year of treatment, albeit the mometasone twice daily application. It is likely that the further treatment in the second year would have a further benefit, with more patients reaching a low polyp score and clinical burden. The clinical effects were observed in patients with and without asthma or AERD, and also were independent from former surgery.

For the first time, the effect of a biologic on oral glucocorticosteroid (OCS) use and "real/planned" surgeries was monitored; the numbers of patients receiving systemic GCSs were reduced by >70%, and those receiving surgery by >80% in the dupilumab vs. placebo groups. However, not everybody reacts profoundly to the treatment; depending on the parameter chosen, non-responders represent 20–35% of treated patients at week 24 of treatment. However, only 12.5% of subjects in the verum group needed at least one further course of oral glucocorticosteroids or surgery over 1 year of treatment, indicating that Dupilumab drastically reduced the need for any further additional measures.

52.4 Biologics in Clinical Practice

Although only scarcely used today, the studies using biologics in nasal polyps give a clear view on how powerful this medication may be, once it is approved and conditions for their use have been defined. Of course, pricing issues will play

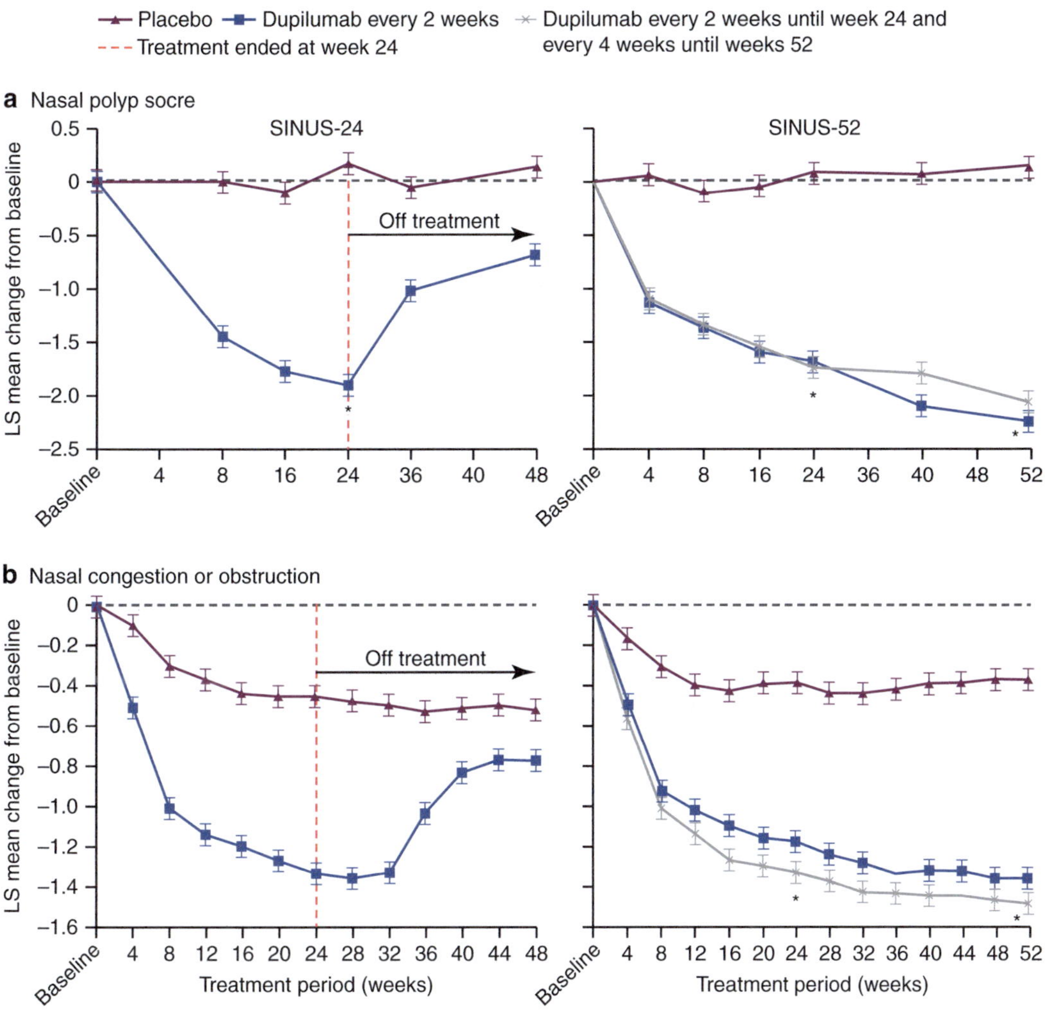

Fig. 52.2 Effect of Dupilumab applied over 24 and 52 weeks on nasal polyp (**a**) and nasal congestion scores (**b**) in a Phase 3 clinical trial. (Source: Bachert et al. Lancet 2019)

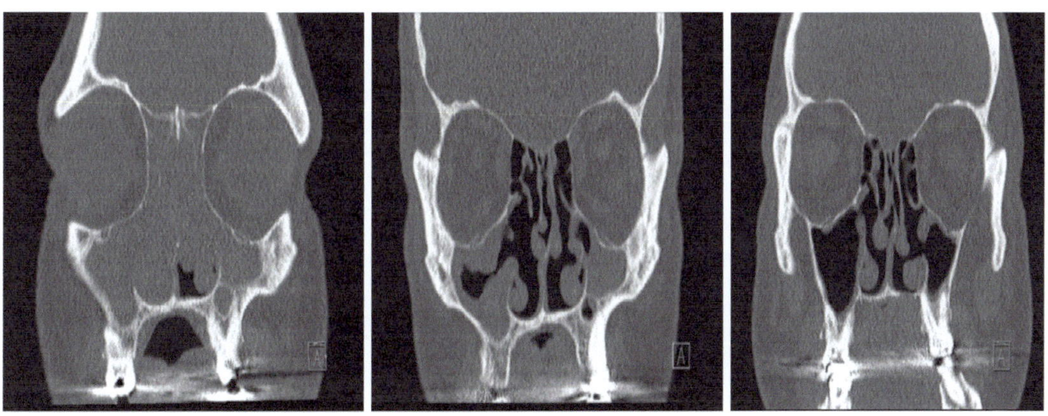

Fig. 52.3 Sinus CT scans over 1 year (left to right) of a CRSwNP subject under the treatment with Dupilumab

an important role, but also the selection of patients, the definition of severe disease, the evaluation of former treatments including surgical techniques and approaches, the recognition of type 2 immune disease in the individual patient, and eventually biomarkers to predict the response to the treatment with highest possible likelihood. The response likelihood very much will depend on the percentage of type 2 immune responses in a specific region or continent (see Chap. 21), with type 2 immune reactions being prevalent in less than 40 to more than 80% of cases depending on the continent. It, therefore, is of utmost importance to at least identify patients with type 2 immune reactions and exclude those with non-type 2 disease, as long as we do not have any specific approaches for this immune reaction [15].

Unfortunately, no markers to predict treatment responses for individual biologics have been identified. Specifically, there is no predictive value in increased blood eosinophils for anti-IL5 treatment, or in patients with allergy or high serum IgE concentrations for anti-IgE treatment. Furthermore, none of these parameters predicts the response to Dupilumab. Further research will hopefully identify useful serum or nasal secretion markers in the near future.

Current dosing schemes, applications, and adverse events are given in Tables 52.3 and 52.4. These may have impact on the decision of the physician and the patient on the biologic to choose, together with the responder rate, the speed of action, and the mean achievable effect size. With the development of this innovative therapeutic area, more possibilities will arise, that cannot be predicted today; therefore, a consistent learning process will characterize the translation of clinical immunology into daily practice. The care pathways currently applicable are discussed in the next chapter.

Table 52.3 Biologics used for CRSwNP

mAbs	Mechanism of action	Dose adult >12 years	Mode of application
Omalizumab	Binds free IgE	75–600 mg (1–4 doses) every 2 or 4 weeks Determined by basal IgE levels (IU/ml), measured before starting treatment, and body weight (kg)	Subcutaneous: upper arm, thigh, or abdomen 75 mg or 150 mg powder and solvent for solution for injection. The reconstituted solution must be used immediately
Mepolizumab	Inhibits IL-5	100 mg every 4 weeks	Subcutaneous: upper arm, thigh, or abdomen 100 mg powder to be reconstituted with 1.2 ml of water for injections. The reconstituted solution must be used immediately
Benralizumab	Inhibits binding of IL-5 to IL-5Rα receptor Direct eosinophil cytotoxic effects	30 mg every 4 weeks for three times, then 30 mg every 8 weeks	Subcutaneous: upper arm, thigh, or abdomen 30 mg pre-filled syringe Store in a refrigerator (2–8 °C). Do not freeze. Do not shake
Dupilumab	Blocks Il-4Rα receptor	300 mg every 2 weeks	Subcutaneous: upper arm, thigh, or abdomen 300 mg pre-filled syringe Store in a refrigerator (2–8 °C). Do not freeze. Do not shake
Reslizumab	Inhibits IL-5	3 mg/kg every 4 weeks	Intravenous infusion of 20–50 min through a sterile, non-pyrogenic, single use, low protein binding infusion filter (0.2 μm) 2.5 ml or 10 ml vial 1 ml contains 10 mg of Reslizumab Store in a refrigerator (2–8 °C). Do not freeze

Table 52.4 Side effects of biologics

	Very common	Common	Uncommon	Rare	Very rare[§]/Not known
Omalizumab[a]	Pyrexia[**]	Headache[*]	Allergic bronchospasm	Anaphylactic reaction	Allergic granulomatous vasculitis (i.e. Churg–Strauss syndrome)
		Injection site reactions	Coughing	Angioedema	Alopecia
		Upper abdominal pain[**]	Dizziness	Laryngoedema	Arthralgia
			Diarrhoea	Parasitic infection	Idiopathic thrombocytopenia
			Dyspeptic signs and symptoms	Systemic lupus erythematosus (SLE)	Joint swelling
			Fatigue		Myalgia
			Flushing		Serum sickness (fever and lymphadenopathy)
			Influenza-like illness		
			Nausea		
			Paraesthesia		
			Pharyngitis		
			Photosensitivity		
			Postural hypotension		
			Pruritus		
			Rash		
			Somnolence		
			Syncope		
			Swelling arms		
			Urticaria		
			Weight increase		
Mepolizumab[b]	Headache	Administration-related reactions (systemic non-allergic)[****]		Anaphylactic reaction	
		Back pain			
		Eczema			
		Hypersensitivity reactions (systemic allergic)[***]			
		Injection site reactions			
		Lower respiratory tract infection			

(continued)

Table 52.4 (continued)

	Very common	Common	Uncommon	Rare	Very rare[§]/Not known
		Nasal congestion			
		Pharyngitis			
		Pyrexia			
		Upper abdominal pain			
		Urinary tract infection			
Benralizumab[c]		Headache			Anaphylactic reaction
		Hypersensitivity reactions*****			
		Injection site reactions			
		Pharyngitis			
		Pyrexia			
Dupilumab[d]	Injection site reactions	Blepharitis			Anaphylactic reaction[§]
		Conjunctivitis			Serum sickness[§]
		Eosinophilia			
		Eye pruritus			
		Headache			
		Oral herpes			
Reslizumab[e]		Blood creatine phosphokinase increased	Anaphylactic reaction		
			Myalgia		

Sources: [a]https://www.ema.europa.eu/en/documents/product-information/xolair-epar-product-information_en.pdf last update 25/07/2019; [b]https://www.ema.europa.eu/en/documents/product-information/nucala-epar-product-information_en.pdf last update 20/09/2019; [c]https://www.ema.europa.eu/en/documents/product-information/fasenra-epar-product-information_en.pdf last update 27/08/2019; [d]https://www.ema.europa.eu/en/documents/product-information/dupixent-epar-product-information_en.pdf last update 28/06/2019; [e]https://www.ema.europa.eu/en/documents/product-information/cinqaero-epar-product-information_en.pdf last update 21/03/2019

*Very common in children 6 to <12 years of age, **in children 6 to <12 years of age, ***systemic reactions including hypersensitivity (e.g. anaphylaxis, urticaria, angioedema, rash, bronchospasm, hypotension) have been reported at an overall incidence comparable to that of placebo, ****the most common manifestations associated with reports of systemic non-allergic administration-related reactions were rash, flushing, and myalgia; these manifestations were reported infrequently and in <1% of subjects receiving mepolizumab 100 mg subcutaneously, *****hypersensitivity reactions were defined by the following grouped preferred terms: "Urticaria", "Papular urticaria", and "Rash". Very common (≥1/10), common (≥1/100 to <1/10), uncommon (≥1/1000 to <1/100), rare (≥1/10,000 to <1/1000), [§]very rare (<1/10,000), not known (cannot be estimated from the available data)

References

1. Bachert C, Zhang N, Cavaliere C, Weiping W, Gevaert E, Krysko O. Biologics for chronic rhinosinusitis with nasal polyps. J Allergy Clin Immunol. 2020;145(3):725–39. https://doi.org/10.1016/j.jaci.2020.01.020.
2. Gevaert P, Calus L, Van Zele T, Blomme K, De Ruyck N, Bauters W, et al. Omalizumab is effective in allergic and nonallergic patients with nasal polyps and asthma. J Allergy Clin Immunol. 2013;131(1):110–6.e1. https://doi.org/10.1016/j.jaci.2012.07.047.
3. Bachert C, Mannent L, Naclerio RM, Mullol J, Ferguson BJ, Gevaert P, et al. Effect of subcutaneous dupilumab on nasal polyp burden in patients with chronic sinusitis and nasal polyposis: a randomized clinical trial. JAMA. 2016;315(5):469–79. https://doi.org/10.1001/jama.2015.19330.
4. Bachert C, Han JK, Desrosiers M, Hellings PW, Amin N, Lee SE, et al. Efficacy and safety of dupilumab in patients with severe chronic rhinosinusitis with nasal polyps (LIBERTY NP SINUS-24 and LIBERTY NP SINUS-52): results from two multicentre, randomised, double-blind, placebo-controlled, parallel-group phase 3 trials. Lancet (London). 2019;394(10209):1638–50. https://doi.org/10.1016/s0140-6736(19)31881-1.
5. Ren L, Zhang N, Zhang L, Bachert C. Biologics for the treatment of chronic rhinosinusitis with nasal polyps – state of the art. World Allergy Org J. 2019;12(8):100050. https://doi.org/10.1016/j.waojou.2019.100050.
6. Jonstam K, Swanson BN, Mannent LP, Cardell LO, Tian N, Wang Y, et al. Dupilumab reduces local type 2 pro-inflammatory biomarkers in chronic rhinosinusitis with nasal polyposis. Allergy. 2019;74(4):743–52. https://doi.org/10.1111/all.13685.
7. Corren J. New targeted therapies for uncontrolled asthma. J Allergy Clin Immunol Pract. 2019;7(5):1394–403. https://doi.org/10.1016/j.jaip.2019.03.022.
8. Dávila González I, Moreno Benítez F, Quirce S. Benralizumab: a new approach for the treatment of severe eosinophilic asthma. J Investig Allergol Clin Immunol. 2019;29(2):84–93. https://doi.org/10.18176/jiaci.0385.
9. Gevaert P, Van Bruaene N, Cattaert T, Van Steen K, Van Zele T, Acke F, et al. Mepolizumab, a humanized anti-IL-5 mAb, as a treatment option for severe nasal polyposis. J Allergy Clin Immunol. 2011;128(5):989–95.e1–8. https://doi.org/10.1016/j.jaci.2011.07.056.
10. Bachert C, Sousa AR, Lund VJ, Scadding GK, Gevaert P, Nasser S, et al. Reduced need for surgery in severe nasal polyposis with mepolizumab: randomized trial. J Allergy Clin Immunol. 2017;140(4):1024–31.e14. https://doi.org/10.1016/j.jaci.2017.05.044.
11. Humbert M, Bousquet J, Bachert C, Palomares O, Pfister P, Kottakis I, et al. IgE-mediated multimorbidities in allergic asthma and the potential for omalizumab therapy. J Allergy Clin Immunol. 2019;7(5):1418–29. https://doi.org/10.1016/j.jaip.2019.02.030.
12. Bachert C, Humbert M, Hanania NA, Zhang N, Holgate S, Buhl R, et al. Staphylococcus aureus and its IgE-inducing enterotoxins in asthma: current knowledge. Eur Respir J. 2020;55(4) https://doi.org/10.1183/13993003.01592-2019.
13. Zhang N, Holtappels G, Gevaert P, Patou J, Dhaliwal B, Gould H, et al. Mucosal tissue polyclonal IgE is functional in response to allergen and SEB. Allergy. 2011;66(1):141–8. https://doi.org/10.1111/j.1398-9995.2010.02448.x.
14. Busse WW, Maspero JF, Rabe KF, Papi A, Wenzel SE, Ford LB, et al. Liberty asthma QUEST: phase 3 randomized, double-blind, placebo-controlled, parallel-group study to evaluate dupilumab efficacy/safety in patients with uncontrolled, moderate-to-severe asthma. Adv Ther. 2018;35(5):737–48. https://doi.org/10.1007/s12325-018-0702-4.
15. Cardell LO, Stjärne P, Jonstam K, Bachert C. Endotypes of chronic rhinosinusitis: impact on management. J Allergy Clin Immunol. 2020;145(3):752–6. https://doi.org/10.1016/j.jaci.2020.01.019.

53 Integrated Care Pathways

Claus Bachert and Nan Zhang

Key Points

- Definitions are provided that allow precise descriptions of conditions.
- The decision-making process for surgery, a biologic, or a combination of both approaches is described based on an analysis of efficacy data and side effects or risks.
- Criteria for patient selection and drug selection are provided.
- The patient's perspective is of great importance; an informed patient should join the decision-making process.
- Guidance is provided for the evaluation of the biologic after 6 and 12 months, and consequences if expectations are not met.

To elaborate integrated care pathways, we first need to exactly define what we mean by what expression. These definitions and management consequences are modified from a recent article published as a consensus of the EUFOREA group (Bachert et al., Uncontrolled Severe Chronic Rhinosinusitis with Nasal Polyps (CRSwNP): EUFOREA Definitions and Management).

C. Bachert (✉)
Upper Airways Research Laboratory and Department of Oto-Rhino-Laryngology, Ghent University, Ghent, Belgium

Division of ENT Diseases, CLINTEC, Karolinska Institute, University of Stockholm, Stockholm, Sweden
e-mail: claus.bachert@ugent.be

N. Zhang (✉)
Upper Airways Research Laboratory and Department of Oto-Rhino-Laryngology, Ghent University, Ghent, Belgium
e-mail: nan.zhang@ugent.be

53.1 Definitions: How to Define Uncontrolled Severe Type 2 CRSwNP with Comorbid Disease?

53.1.1 The EUFOREA Group Agreed on the Following Definitions

Severe CRSwNP is defined as bilateral chronic rhinosinusitis with nasal polyps (CRSwNP) with a nasal polyp score (NPS) of ≥4 out of 8 points, <u>and</u> persistent symptoms including loss of smell and/or taste, nasal obstruction, secretion and/or post-nasal drip, and facial pain or pressure, with the need for add-on treatment to intranasal corticosteroids (INCS).

Comments: The diagnosis of CRSwNPs, therefore, demands a nasal endoscopy, best performed with a rigid 0° or 30° nasal endoscope. The nasal polyp score (NPS) has been defined previously [1] and used in all Phase 3 studies using biologic drugs in CRSwNP [2–8], resulting in a maximum bilateral score of 8. A NPS ≥4 can be assumed if NPs are visible below the inferior border of the middle turbinate on both sides (or

L. Zhang, C. Bachert (eds.), *Chronic Rhinosinusitis*, https://doi.org/10.1007/978-981-16-0784-4_53

below the dorsal attachment of the inferior turbinate, should the middle turbinate be partially or fully resected after surgery).

The presence of bilateral nasal polyps alone is not sufficient to define severe CRSwNP; the disease also needs to be symptomatic. The following PROs can be used to define the severe phenotype: a nasal congestion score (NCS, 0–3 points) of ≥2 points, a SNOT-22 of >35 or a total Visual Analogue Scale (VAS) of 5 cm out of 10 cm or more.

The presence of bilateral nasal polyps visualized by nasal endoscopy in nearly all cases implies the involvement of the sinuses, at least the ethmoid sinuses, which can be confirmed by CT scan. Nasal polyps are a manifestation of CRSwNP, the terms are considered interchangeable for clinical use.

Uncontrolled CRSwNP is defined as "persistent or recurring despite long-term INCS, and having received at least one course of systemic corticosteroids in the preceding 2 years (or having a medical contraindication or intolerance to systemic corticosteroids) and/or previous sinonasal surgery" (unless having a medical contraindication or being unwilling to undergo surgery).

Comments: One course of systemic corticosteroids refers to a minimum of 5 days of systemic corticosteroids at a dose of 0.5–1 mg/kg/day or more. The use of long-term low dose corticosteroids is not recommended, but would be accepted to fulfil the criteria. Previous sinonasal surgery refers to any surgical procedure from the resection of polyps from the nose and sinuses to conventional sinus surgery (endoscopic sinus surgery, ESS) or extended approaches (often described as "Draf III procedure", "nasalization", or complete sinus mucosa removal ("reboot") [9–13].

CRSwNP with comorbid disease is defined as "nasal polyp disease with other co-existing type 2 inflammatory diseases such as asthma, N-ERD, atopic dermatitis/eczema, allergic rhinitis, urticaria, food allergy or eosinophil esophagitis".

Comments: Asthma here refers to any asthma severity, early- or adult-onset asthma, allergic or non-allergic. In uncontrolled severe CRSwNP subjects, >80% of asthma patients report adult-onset asthma. Other type 2 diseases are often associated with type 2 airway disease and increase the likelihood of this immune reaction also in the upper airways/sinuses.

53.1.2 Endotyping in Uncontrolled Severe CRSwNP Based on Clinical Signs and Biomarkers

Endotyping refers to the identification of type 2 or non-type 2 immune reactions, as currently only this differentiation is clinically relevant in determining treatment with a biologic therapy. It may be assumed that in the coming years, a further differentiation into type 1/type 3 immune reactions may become relevant, and further biologics targeting other cytokines become available.

Depending on the geographical region and ethnicity of the patient, CRSwNP is characterized by type 2 mucosal inflammation in approximately 15–85% of the patients [14–19]. Type 2 inflammation is clearly associated with more severe sinus disease and symptoms, asthma comorbidity, and recurrence of disease after surgery [20, 21]. It is, therefore, of importance to differentiate type 2 from non-type 2 CRSwNP for the prediction of the natural course of disease, response to medical and surgical interventions, and consecutively the long-term management and selection of therapeutic measures. For the indication of recently available type 2 biologics including anti-IL4 receptor alpha (Dupilumab), anti-IgE (Omalizumab), and anti-IL5/R (Mepolizumab, Benralizumab), an underlying type 2 inflammation should be highly likely (>90%).

Comments: Non-type 2 CRSwNP and CRSsNP are common in cystic fibrosis, primary ciliary dyskinesia, chronic obstructive pulmonary disease, but also in a large number of subjects without underlying disease, specifically in some Asian regions. However, the percentage of CRSwNP patients with type 2 disease is increasing in Asia [14, 22–24].

Blood eosinophils of >300 cells/µl and total serum IgE of 150 kU/L will most likely represent

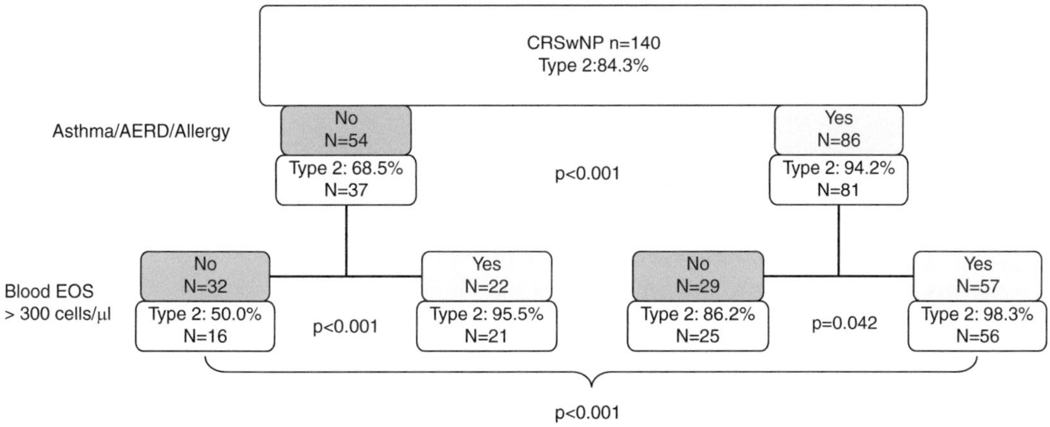

Fig. 53.1 Identification of type 2 immune reactions within CRSwNP tissue (IL-5 positivity) based on clinical signs and blood eosinophils (original material from 323 CRSwNP patients from Ghent). Although 84% of tissue can be recognized as type 2 (IL-5 positive), this percentage increases to 94%, if subjects with comorbid asthma and/or AERD and/or allergy are considered. In asthma/AERD/allergy positive subjects with blood eosinophils above 300 cells/μl, this percentage increases to 98%. In those subjects without any of these type 2 diseases, blood eosinophil counts should be considered; if blood eosinophils are above 300 cells/μl, the percentage of type 2 immune reaction within the polyp tissue increases to 95%, whereas the patients with eosinophil counts below 300 cells/μl are only type 2 positive in 50%. Using this algorithm, we do not recognize about 14% of CRSwNP subjects with type 2, but retain high specificity (97%) [20]

strong indicators for type 2 CRSwNP, but data are lacking to proof the latter at the moment. Blood eosinophils of 150 cells/μl and total serum IgE of 100 kU/L can be used as moderate indicators for type 2 CRSwNP. The GINA guidelines define blood eosinophils ≥150 cells/μl once during the last year as indicative for type 2 inflammation in severe asthma [25]. As most uncontrolled severe CRSwNP patients (>70%) also suffer from asthma comorbidity, the number of blood eosinophils may be due to both, upper and/or lower airway disease. SE-IgE (IgE to *Staphylococcus aureus* enterotoxins) is commonly associated with IgE polyclonality (high total IgE compared to no or low specific IgEs to various allergens). Skin prick testing is not advised for the testing of SE-IgE or polyclonality. However, a positive skin prick test (SPT) to one or more inhalant allergens is a modest indicator for type 2 inflammatory CRSwNP.

Where surgery was undertaken for CRSwNP, and polyps were sent for histological evaluation to determine tissue eosinophils, this finding is pointing to a type 2 inflammation. In case no former surgery or biopsy was performed, but endotyping is considered necessary, a biopsy of nasal polyp tissue in an office procedure under local anaesthesia may be discussed. However, this is unnecessary when the patient suffers from comorbid asthma and/or has blood eosinophil levels above 300 cells/μl (see later). Further, relying on staining eosinophils in the harvested tissue only may fail to secure or exclude type 2 inflammation [14, 26], as numbers may vary at different regions within the tissue [27]. In contrast, measurements of mediators such as IL-5, IgE, and ECP have been established and successfully used to differentiate type 2 from non-type 2 CRSwNP [15, 28–30] (Fig. 53.1).

53.1.3 Sinus Surgery or a Biologic Approach, or a Combination of Both?

In a patient with uncontrolled severe type 2 CRSwNP, at a time point in the patient's "disease carrier" when the patient has experienced non-effective systemic GCS therapy or surgery, a long-term plan should be elaborated together with an informed patient. This plan needs to consider the endotype, the comorbidities, and other possible treatment approaches for those comorbidities, and the former treatment history (surgeries, systemic GCS and their efficacy, duration of effect, and adverse events).

According to current patient rights, the patient must be informed about the aims, reasonable expectations, and possible side effects and complications of all authorized treatments available for the disease. Furthermore, the physician is obliged to inform the patient also about available alternatives—in case of proposed surgery, this includes pharmacologic drugs and biologics depending on the national availability. The aim is to have an informed patient to share the decision making in this situation; this gains importance with the complexity of the interventions available and the history of former therapeutic approaches.

The American Rhinologic Society and American College of Allergy, Asthma, and Immunology are working together on creating a patient oriented tool (Shared Decision Making Tool) that physicians can use to help navigate informed patients [31] to the various choices for nasal polyp treatment (Personal communication JK Han).

Surgical approaches can be differentiated into functional endoscopic sinus surgery (ESS) [32–34] with the aim of opening all sinuses ("full house") and removing all nasal and sinus polyps but preserving the sinus mucosa, and the nasalization and reboot approaches [12, 35, 36] aiming at the complete removal of polyp and sinus mucosa from all sinuses involved. This again always includes the maxillary and ethmoidal sinuses, but may also include the frontal and sphenoidal sinuses, including the creation of wide openings (mostly the Draf III frontal sinus approach and the sphenoid drill-out) [37, 38] to completely remove the sinus mucosa. It has been demonstrated that these approaches in severe CRSwNP lead to less recurrence compared to conventional approaches [12, 39, 40] and are followed by an effective healing process with functional mucosa [12, 41].

Should the patient and the physician choose for a biologic drug approach, the physician should decide on the possible choices among the biologics and make a choice with the informed patient, also considering drug availability and patient-relevant questions such as practical issues with drug application. Before a surgical procedure should be planned, a period of 6 months—and eventually 12 months, if the patient's response to the treatment is as expected or better—should be considered to enable the physician to recognize the suitability of/the response to the drug in an individual patient. A surgical procedure may not be considered necessary any more in up to two thirds of the patients under biologic treatment.

Has a surgical approach been chosen aiming at long-term disease suppression, no biologic drug should be considered for at least 6 months and would only be indicated in case of recurrence. A fixed combination plan with surgery and biologic treatment starting in parallel or within short time is not advised, as the response of the individual patient to the surgery or to the biologic is impossible to evaluate. Approaches such as a limited surgery combined with application of a biologic drug are not recommended as such approaches would lead to maximal costs and risks of adverse events/complications in all patients. However, if a surgery has been performed and shows to be insufficient to long-term suppress nasal polyp growth and symptoms even with continuation of INCS, a lower than four NPS may be considered sufficient to indicate a biologic treatment.

53.2 Evaluation of Efficacy vs. Adverse Events/ Complications for Surgery and Biologics

53.2.1 Efficacy of Biologics in Phase 3 Trials

There are currently three biologics which already finalized Phase 3 trials (two parallel DBPCR studies with anti-IL4 receptor alpha, Dupilumab, NCT02912468 and NCT02898454; two parallel DBPCR studies with anti-IgE, Omalizumab, NCT03280550 and NCT03280537; one DBPCR trial with anti-IL5, Mepolizumab, NCT03085797) and one drug still ongoing (Benralizumab, NCT03401229). These studies were all based on a similar study design and included a high number of participants (n = 265–724). In all studies the effect of the biologic was compared to placebo added to a continuous treatment with intranasal corticosteroids throughout the whole study period. Dupilumab is the first biologic registered in the EU and USA as an add-on treatment of severe CRSwNP, not sufficiently controlled by systemic corticosteroids and/or surgery. The patients recruited into the finalized studies had bilateral nasal polyps with a NPS (score) ≥5/8, had asthma in 48–71%, and prior surgery in 54–100% of subjects, and were symptomatic with impairment of smell and nasal obstruction as major symptoms.

In all Phase 3 trials, the primary endpoints (reduction in NPS and nasal congestion/obstruction score) were met with changes in the NPS between 0.7 (median, Mepolizumab) and 2.4 (mean, Dupilumab, Liberty 52w) over placebo after 52 weeks. NPS reductions at 24 weeks were from 0.7 (mean, Omalizumab, mean of Polyp 1 and 2 studies) to 2.06 (mean, Dupilumab, Liberty 24w). Of importance, smell was significantly improved with all drugs, however at different speed and magnitude; Dupilumab demonstrated a strong and fast effect on smell, reducing the percentage of anosmic subjects from 76% at baseline to 26% after 24 weeks of treatment [2]. SNOT-22 reflecting disease-specific quality of life also improved significantly by 14–21 score points, clearly surpassing the MCID of >8.9. Dupilumab also showed a significant reduction in the CT-based Lund–Mackay-Score by 5–7.5 points. Dupilumab and Mepolizumab, in addition to the reduction in NPS and symptoms as well as quality of life, demonstrated a reduction in the need of systemic corticosteroids and surgery over 1 year of treatment vs. placebo. A reduction of at least one NPS point or more was achieved in 50–65% of the verum-treated subjects over the trials.

Thus, these biologics offer a new treatment approach to many patients with type 2 CRSwNP insufficiently controlled by intranasal corticosteroids; asthma or N-ERD comorbidity also needs to be taken into consideration then. When surgery is considered, biologics should also be mentioned to the patient as an alternative, or a combination of biologic and surgical approaches has to be discussed, with the biologic treatment first for reasons discussed above. As there are no head to head comparisons between these biologics at the moment, the choice of drug should be based on availability, potential specific limitations such as eosinophil numbers or IgE levels (for Mepolizumab and Omalizumab), responder rates, and expected size of effects in responders.

53.2.2 Efficacy of Surgery from Available Literature

The efficacy of sinus surgery is difficult to evaluate as there are various forms of sinus surgery as well as opinions on the extent of sinus surgery. For example, the term "sinus surgery" is used for balloon dilation of a sinus ostium, a minimally invasive sinus surgery just aiming to open the sinus drainage pathway, (functional) endoscopic sinus surgery to remove polyps from the nasal cavity and sinuses, or following the mucosal concept approach removing all sinus mucosal tissue. Experts agree that for CRSwNP, at least an endoscopic sinus surgery with opening of the ostiomeatal complex, the maxillary and ethmoid sinuses with removal of nasal polyps and thickened sinus mucosa should be performed. However, some recommend creating large sinus openings to all sinuses including the frontal sinus such as described as "modified Lothrop" [42], and the complete removal of the sinus mucosa described as "reboot surgery" [12]. Finally, there is variability in the extent of sinus surgery, but also the quality of sinus surgery may vary substantially.

Due to these factors, the evidence for efficacy of endoscopic sinus surgery is and will remain low. Most of the evidence will be retrospective, with only a few prospective cohort studies using a common standardized surgical approach. Most evidence is based on one or few centres, possibly one prominent surgeon, and therefore not transferable to other centres, let alone "all surgeons or surgeries". Data from the UK National Sinonasal

Table 53.1 Long-term recurrence of polyps following ESS for CRSwNP

Author	Year	No. of patients	Study Design	Follow-up (mo)	Mean time to recurrence (mo)	Polyp Recurrence (%)
Nakayama [44]	2011	175	Prospective	17.5	NA	22.9
Ikeda [45]	2013	130	Prospective	48	28	36.2
Brescia [46]	2015	179	Prospective	18–47	23	13.4
Grgic [47]	2015	30	Prospective	24	NA	36.7
Lou [48]	2015	387	Retrospective	29–39	NA	55.3
Tokunaga [49]	2015	1716	Retrospective	22.6	NA	23.1
Brescia [50]	2016	143	Prospective	9–29	17	14.7
DeConde [51]	2017	129	Prospective	18	NA	40
Calus [52]	2019	47	Prospective	148	NA	78.9

Audit involving national centres demonstrated a surgical revision rate of 21% over 5 years [43]. As it will remain difficult to perform prospective multicentre randomized trials of high quality for the efficacy of sinus surgery, international registries could be of some help to evaluate real life evidence.

Sinus surgery for nasal polyposis most often debulks and removes nasal polyps, but recurrence is likely after surgery (Table 53.1). Therefore is it imperative to post-operatively guide the patient and maintain postoperative medical treatment to prevent polyp recurrence. Even with postoperative topical corticosteroid medical therapy, the recurrence rate may be high. In a prospective cohort study of 244 patients with endoscopic sinus surgery, 40% of nasal polyps recurred within 18 months despite postoperative medical treatment [51]. Therefore there is a clear unmet need for other approaches to better manage patients with nasal polyposis.

53.2.3 AEs in Phase 3 Trials with Biologics

We here discuss adverse events related to recent Phase 3 trials of Dupilumab [2], Omalizumab [3–5], and Mepolizumab [6], reflecting the dosing schemes that will be relevant after registration. The proportion of patients who experienced ≥1 treatment-emergent AE was lower in the verum-treated compared to the placebo-treated patients. The majority of events across all studies were of mild-to-moderate intensity. AEs occurring in ≥3% of patients include headache, dizziness, abdominal pain, nasopharyngitis, and injection site reactions, being slightly more frequent in the Omalizumab treated vs. the placebo group; on the other hand, asthma exacerbations, nasal polyps, and congestion occurred less frequent, without significant differences between groups. Similarly, headache and nasopharyngitis, nasal polyps with need for treatment, upper respiratory tract infections, and worsening of asthma were more frequent with placebo than with Dupilumab, whereas cough, bronchitis, arthralgia, and injection site reactions were slightly more frequent in the two Dupilumab groups than in placebo. None of the observations were significant. Conjunctivitis was reported in seven patients receiving Dupilumab and in one patient receiving placebo; none of these cases were serious, severe, or associated with treatment discontinuation. In summary, biologics show a good tolerability without major AEs.

53.2.4 Complications of Sinus Surgery

About 50/100000 persons are subjected to endoscopic-endonasal sinus surgery (ESS) every year in Europe, irrespective to the fact, that formal and comparative evidence of the long-term effectiveness of surgical procedures still is limited. ESS for CRS is technically demanding due to the narrow anatomical spaces, the individual and puzzling microanatomy in close proximity to delicate structures like the eye and brain.

Table 53.2 Complications of ESS [53–56]

Grade	Definition	Substrate and Type of Complication
I	Minor complication (resolving/manageable, low risk)	• Mucosa: synechia (no functional deficit), local infection • Minor vessels: bleeding (transfusion not necessary) • Orbita: minor lesion of lamina papyracea (emphysema, ecchymosis) • Afferent nerves: laceration (minor facial hypaesthesia/dental numbness)
II	Relevant complication (specific measures needed)	• Mucosa: synechia (need of revision surgery), atrophic rhinitis, toxic shock syndrome • Paranasal vessels: damage to sphenopalatine/ethmoidal artery (major bleeding ± transfusion) • Naso-lacrimal duct: lesion (tearing) • Afferent nerves: laceration (major hypaesthesia, hyperaesthesia/neuralgia) • Skull base: minor CSF leak with intact intracranial structures (meningitis)
III	Serious complication (risk of major persistent deficit)	• Orbita: haematoma (need of emergency intervention); muscular lesion (diplopia); volume change (enophthalmos) • Olfactory mucosa: destruction (severe hyposmia/anosmia) • Optic nerve: trauma (functional deficit) • Skull base: major CSF leak (meningitis/brain abscess; major pneumocephalus ± intracranial tension; secondary encephalocele) • Endocranium: direct trauma of brain/vessels (intracranial bleeding; neurologic deficits) • Internal carotid artery: laceration (critical bleeding)
IV	Lethal complication	(Death)

Surgeons performing ESS are faced with excusable and sometimes also avoidable mistakes and complications. These complications may be rated as "minor" or "major complication" (Table 53.2)—not to mention exceptional reports about absurd complications [57]. Some less severe adverse events may resolve spontaneously (e.g. mild orbital ecchymosis), others may cause persisting decrease in quality of life (e.g. dry nose feeling, crusting). Emergency revisional surgery may also be necessary (e.g. in case of dural defects or major orbital haematoma) and irreversible damage (e.g. blindness, death) may occur in rare cases. Referring to numerical data in literature, routine EES interventions are generally associated with minor complications in about 5% and major complications in 0.5–1% [53]. The number of endoscopic-endonasal interventions is increasing in recent years revealing significant regional differences and also individual technical as well as conceptual preferences [58]. Regardless of the fact that complication rates of endoscopic sinus surgery have generally decreased in the years after international adoption of modern minimum-invasive techniques, the increased number and complexity of today's interventions is still mirrored in actual reports on patient injuries [59, 60].

53.2.5 The Patient Perspective on Biologics

Patients, who have reached the limits of what current licensed treatment and techniques including surgery can offer, often feel like they may never gain control of this difficult condition. For these patients, biologics will represent an important new dimension in the way their condition is managed and offer some hope that a level of disease control could be attainable.

It is important to understand that self-administering a subcutaneous injection may be a new and possibly daunting prospect for a patient; however, most patients might be treated with home injection. To give their full consent, an important part of both medical ethics and international human rights law, to receiving a biologic, patients need to be informed and educated on a number of factors relating to this treatment [31].

A patient would expect and the physician must present information regarding risks, alternatives, and success rates in a language the patient can understand, and typically should include the following:

- A description of the recommended treatment or procedure;
- Any known side effects/risks and how they compare to other treatment options;
- Efficacy of the treatment in relation to available alternative treatments including surgery;
- The probable results if no treatment is undertaken;
- How to practically administer and manage the treatment, e.g. self-injection, expected treatment duration, any lifestyle modifications that will be required;
- Potential impact on smell/taste—normally the most important symptom for CRSwNP patients.

Once in possession of these facts the patient can then enter into a considered discussion with their physician—understanding the chronicity of the disease—as to whether a biologic is the right course of treatment for them.

53.3 Specific Considerations for Biologics

Selection of patients and predicting the response to a specific biologic drug.

There are currently no parameters that could be used to predict the individual response of a patient to any of the biologics, specifically in uncontrolled severe CRSwNP following the definitions specified in this article. However, drug-specific rules need to be applied (see below) (Fig. 53.2a, b).

53.4 Limitations for the Selection of a Biologic Drug

Specific indications and limitations for the indication of individual biologics should be followed when provided. For the moment, the following limitations are taken from the asthma indication:

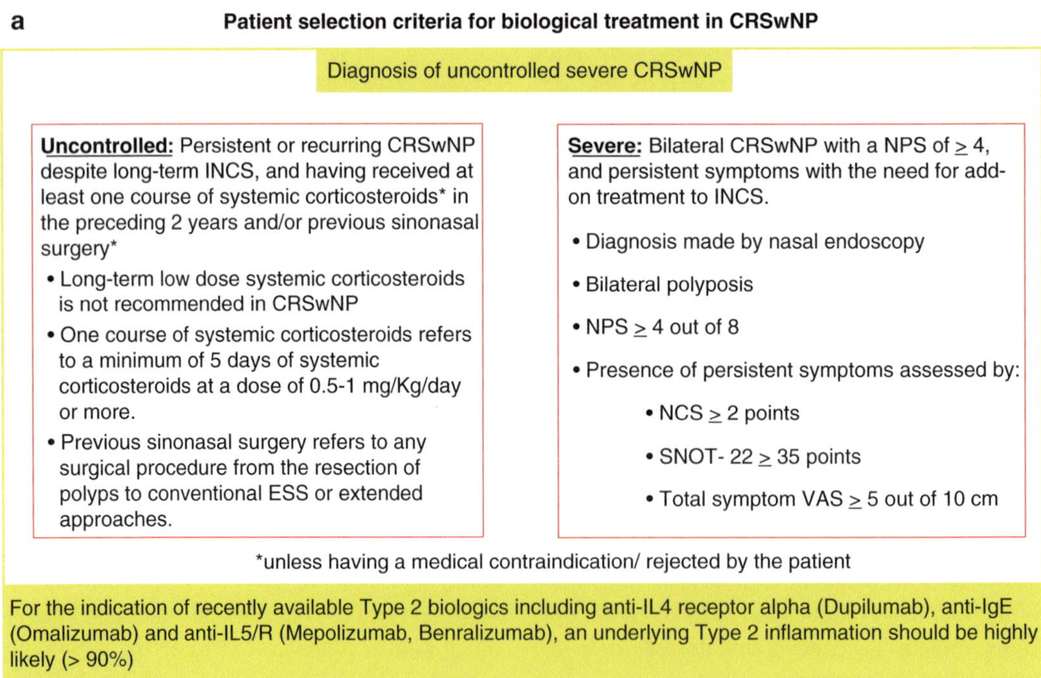

Fig. 53.2 (**a**) Patient selection criteria. (**b**) Selection and monitoring of biologics

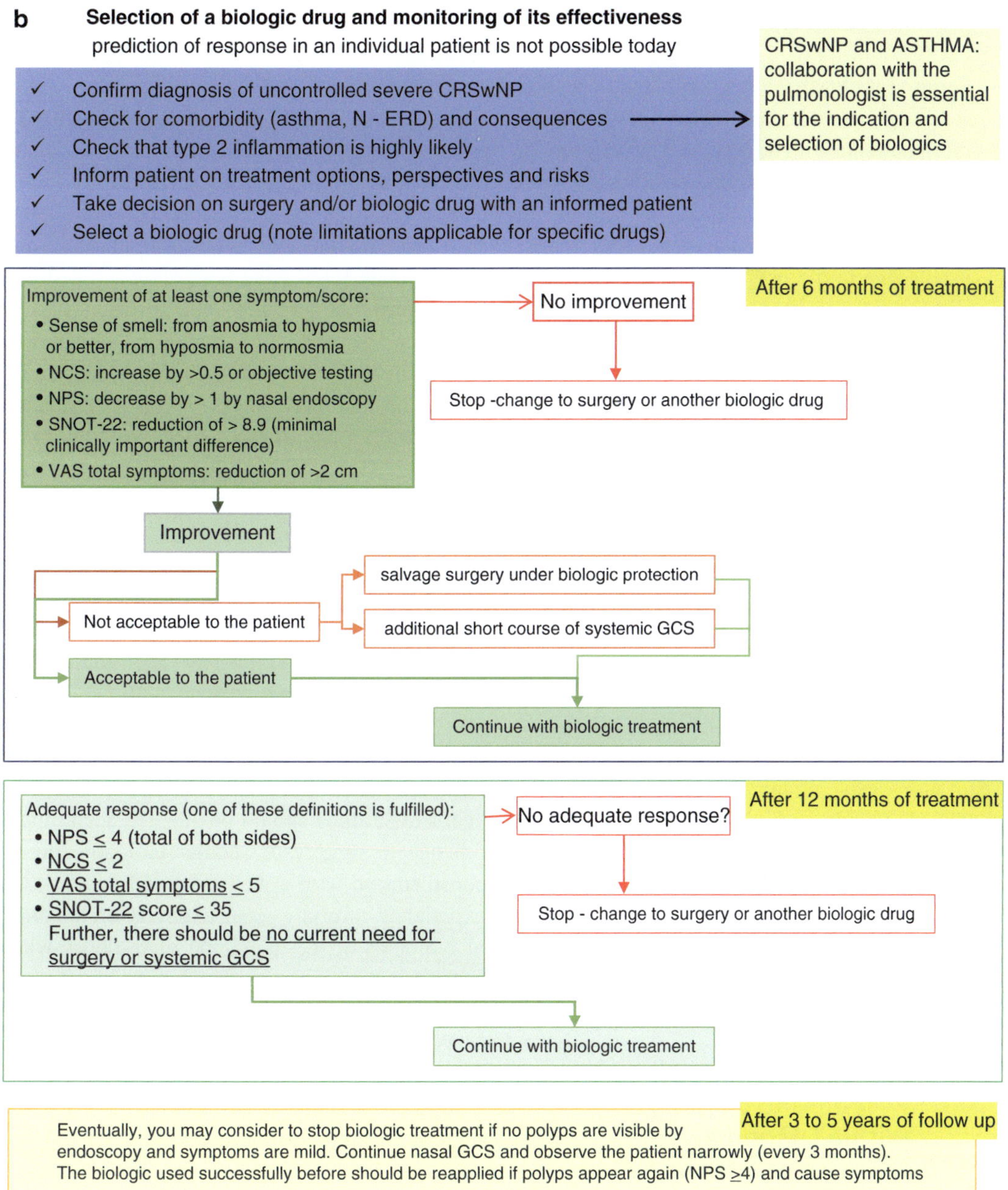

Fig. 53.2 (continued)

- Age 12 years and older: not relevant in CRSwNP, as very few patients with the disease younger than 12 years will be observed.
- Eosinophil counts: For Mepolizumab and Benralizumab, blood eosinophil counts ≥300 cells/μl ($\geq 0.3 \times 10^9$ cells/L) in the last 12 months have been associated with greater efficacy in asthma [61–65]. However, efficacy has also been demonstrated in patients with blood eosinophils between 150 and 300 cells/μl for Mepolizumab [66]. No data is available for CRSwNP; however, blood eosinophil numbers are already integrated into the algo-

rithm to identify type 2 immune responses in CRSwNP (see Fig. 53.1).

- Serum IgE levels: For Omalizumab, a total serum IgE of 30 IU/ml ≤basal IgE ≤1500 IU/ml in patients with a body weight between 20 and 150 kg and at least one positive allergen-specific IgE is recommended in Europe. In CRSwNP, the allergen-specific IgE is not usable due to the polyclonality of the IgE; it has been shown that allergen-specific IgE is frequently expressed in tissue, but not measurable in the serum of patients. Furthermore, Omalizumab was effective in allergic and non-allergic patients with CRSwNP [4, 21]. Under treatment, serum IgE will increase due to complex formation with the drug, but dosing should be maintained.
- For Dupilumab, there are no known limitations for blood or serum parameters.

As prediction of response in an individual patient is not possible today, other criteria may be applied for selecting the first drug to start with. These may consist of availability and reimbursement in a specific country, maximum efficacy on major parameters, onset of action, responder rates, and lower airway efficacy. There is no experience on the optimal choice of a second biologic drug, if the first one fails, and no head to head comparisons between biologics have been performed.

53.5 Evaluation of the Clinical Response to a Biologic Within 6 Months of Treatment: "Continue or Stop" Rules

EUFOREA has previously defined criteria to support patient selection for biologics and monitoring the clinical response to treatment [67], however, due to the developments in this fast evolving field, those criteria can now be replaced and detailed. When a biologic drug has been selected to treat uncontrolled severe CRSwNP, it is important to monitor the response of the patient to the drug; depending on the biologic drug and outcome measure used, non-responders may be expected in 25–50% of cases. To avoid inadequate treatment and associated unnecessary costs, a response to the treatment should be expected within 6 months; there only is a small chance that drugs begin meaningfully reducing disease burden after that time point.

Phase 3 studies with Dupilumab and Omalizumab [2–5] have both demonstrated that the majority of patients—but not all—reach a reduction of NPS and symptoms (including smell) of 75% or more of the 24 week values within the first 8–12 weeks. A further reduction of disease burden after week 24, building up on the achieved reduction at that moment, has been demonstrated with Dupilumab at 52 weeks of treatment. The group, therefore, decided on a 6 month period to evaluate the response of an individual patient to a biologic and to define the "continue or stop" rules. When a clear change for at least one symptom has been met, the therapy with the biologic drug may be continued. In the other case, the patient does not show adequate response to the treatment within 6 months, and the chance for a later response is small. The management strategy should be adapted accordingly (change to surgery or another biologic drug in consideration with a well-informed patient). No experience currently exists to advice on the order of biologics or the likelihood of response when using a second biologic, which also may depend on the primary biologic used.

Within these first 6 months, no drugs other than topical GCS should be administered together with the biologic to be able to differentiate response from no response.

53.6 "Continue or Stop" Rules

The "continue or stop" rules make use of several symptom-based and endoscopy-based outcomes; at least one has to be met compared to baseline for continuation of the biologic treatment.

- Improvement of *sense of smell*: from anosmia to hyposmia or better, from hyposmia to normosmia (e.g. UPSIT test >18, and/or ≥4 points better, and/or loss of smell score (0–3) ≥0.5 points better);

- Improvement of *nasal congestion/blockage*: NCS (0–3) decrease by ≥0.5 or objective testing (e.g. peak nasal inspiratory flow increase by ≥20 L/min);
- Reduction in *NPS* (0–8) ≥1 (or equivalent) by nasal endoscopy compared to baseline;
- Reduction in *SNOT-22* score (0–110) of ≥8.9 (minimal clinically important difference);
- Reduction in *VAS total symptoms (0–9)* of ≥2 cm.

If the biologic treatment does not achieve at least one outcome criterion, the treatment should be discontinued as the chance for a clinically meaningful response at 12 months is rather small. Another biologic drug, if available and indicated, may be applied instead, or a surgical approach.

53.7 The Treatment Response Has Been Verified Within 6 Months

There are several options in this situation, depending on the remaining burden of disease:

If the degree of partial response is considered acceptable to the patient, continuation of the drug over another 6 month is advised and follow-up at 12 months planned. It is expected that a further reduction of the nasal polyp burden and relief of the patient's symptoms can be achieved.

If control of the disease is not acceptable to the patient, an additional short course of systemic GCS may be considered with the patient immediately reducing burden of disease under continuation of drug application. It has been determined that the drug is effective in this patient, and its continuation can be justified.

As an alternative, "salvage surgery under biologic protection" may be considered to reduce the remaining mass of polyps and burden of disease under continuation of the biologic. Again, the drug's effectiveness in this patient has been demonstrated and its continuation can be justified. However, the long-term benefit of surgery in this situation has only anecdotally been demonstrated.

53.8 Treatment Evaluation After 12 Months

After 12 months of treatment, with or without additional systemic corticosteroids or removal of polyp mass by surgery, a low disease burden should be reached, which can be maintained over the following years.

Definition of an adequate response after 12 month treatment with a biologic drug:

Nasal polyp score (NPS) equal or smaller than 4 (total of both sides) or maintaining the result at 6 months, if smaller;
Nasal congestion score (NCS) ≤2 (Nasal passage allows nearly normal breathing in resting conditions);
All symptoms are moderate or less (except smell, which may not recover due to former damage);
VAS total symptoms ≤5;
SNOT-22 score <30.

Further, there should be *no current need for surgery or systemic GCS.*

When one of these definitions is fulfilled, and no current need for surgery or systemic GCS exists, the biologic should be continued; it is currently unclear whether the use of biologics can be discontinued under optimal conditions (no polyps visible anymore by endoscopy and symptoms mild or none) after several (e.g. 3–5) years. In that case, the patient has to be observed closely (every 3 months), and the biologic used successfully before should be restarted if polyps (NPS ≥5) appear again and cause increased symptoms. As the risk of neutralizing antibodies formed by the patient is small, this approach is reasonable.

Phase 3 trials of these biologics were conducted in conjunction with maintenance topical steroid therapy. However, patients tend to show low adherence to nasal medication once symptoms are reduced. Treatment with the biologic, once correctly indicated, should be continued even after discontinuation of the INCS.

Real life studies and registries will be helpful to further refine these recommendations.

53.9 Approach in Patients with CRSwNP and Asthma/N-ERD

The collaboration with the pulmonologist is essential in patients with severe CRSwNP and asthma, and a multidisciplinary approach for treatment decisions including selection of biologics would help improve patient outcome for both conditions. Furthermore, patients with moderate to severe asthma need to be optimized and monitored after sinus surgery. During treatment with a biologic drug for CRSwNP, asthma should be monitored, and vice versa; patients are expected to also profit from the treatment of their comorbidity. This also includes N-ERD, which is considered an indication for biologics [54].

References

1. Gevaert P, Lang-Loidolt D, Lackner A, Stammberger H, Staudinger H, Van Zele T, et al. Bachert***Nasal IL-5 levels determine the response to anti-IL-5 treatment in patients with nasal polyps. J Allergy Clin Immunol. 2006;118(5):1133–41. https://doi.org/10.1016/j.jaci.2006.05.031.
2. Bachert C, Han JK, Desrosiers M, Hellings PW, Amin N, Lee SE, et al. Efficacy and safety of dupilumab in patients with severe chronic rhinosinusitis with nasal polyps (LIBERTY NP SINUS-24 and LIBERTY NP SINUS-52): results from two multicentre, randomised, double-blind, placebo-controlled, parallel-group phase 3 trials. Lancet (London). 2019;394(10209):1638–50. https://doi.org/10.1016/s0140-6736(19)31881-1.
3. A clinical trial of omalizumab in participants with chronic rhinosinusitis with nasal polyps—Full text view—ClinicalTrials.gov. Retrieved April 19, 2020, from https://clinicaltrials.gov/ct2/show/NCT03280550.
4. Gevaert PO, Omachi TA, Corren J, Mullol J, Han J, Lee SE, Kaufman D, Ligueros-Saylan M, Howard M, Zhu R, Owen R, Wong K, Islam L, Bachert C. Efficacy and safety of omalizumab in patients with chronic rhinosinusitis with nasal polyposis: results from two, multicenter, randomized, double-blind, placebo-controlled phase III trials (POLYP 1 and POLYP 2). J Allergy Clin Immunol Pract. 2020;146(3):595–605.
5. An extension study of omalizumab in participants with chronic rhinosinusitis with nasal polyps—Full text view—ClinicalTrials.gov. Retrieved April 19, 2020, from https://clinicaltrials.gov/ct2/show/NCT03478930.
6. Effect of mepolizumab in severe bilateral nasal polyps—Full text view—ClinicalTrials.gov. Retrieved April 19, 2020, from https://clinicaltrials.gov/ct2/show/NCT03085797.
7. Efficacy and safety study of benralizumab for patients with severe nasal polyposis—Full text view—ClinicalTrials.gov. Retrieved April 19, 2020, from https://clinicaltrials.gov/ct2/show/NCT03401229.
8. Efficacy and safety study of benralizumab in patient with eosinophilic chronic rhinosinusitis with nasal polyps (ORCHID)—Full text view—ClinicalTrials.gov. Retrieved April 19, 2020, from https://clinicaltrials.gov/ct2/show/NCT04157335.
9. Hox V, Lourijsen E, Jordens A, Aasbjerg K, Agache I, Alobid I, et al. Benefits and harm of systemic steroids for short- and long-term use in rhinitis and rhinosinusitis: an EAACI position paper. Clin Transl Allergy. 2020;10(1) https://doi.org/10.1186/s13601-019-0303-6.
10. Bassiouni A, Wormald PJ. Role of frontal sinus surgery in nasal polyp recurrence. Laryngoscope. 2013;123(1): 36–41. https://doi.org/10.1002/lary.23610.
11. Sharma R, Lakhani R, Rimmer J, Hopkins C. Surgical interventions for chronic rhinosinusitis with nasal polyps. Cochrane Database Syst Rev. 2014;(11):Cd006990. https://doi.org/10.1002/14651858.CD006990.pub2.
12. Alsharif S, Jonstam K, van Zele T, Gevaert P, Holtappels G, Bachert C. Endoscopic sinus surgery for type-2 CRS wNP: an endotype-based retrospective study. Laryngoscope. 2019;129(6):1286–92. https://doi.org/10.1002/lary.27815.
13. Bachert C, Marple B, Hosemann W, Cavaliere C, Wen W, Zhang N. Endotypes of chronic rhinosinusitis with nasal polyps: pathology and possible therapeutic implications. J Allergy Clin Immunol Pract. 2020;8(5):1514–9. https://doi.org/10.1016/j.jaip.2020.03.007.
14. Wang X, Zhang N, Bo M, Holtappels G, Zheng M, Lou H, et al. Diversity of T(H) cytokine profiles in patients with chronic rhinosinusitis: a multicenter study in Europe, Asia, and Oceania. J Allergy Clin Immunol. 2016;138(5):1344–53. https://doi.org/10.1016/j.jaci.2016.05.041.
15. Tomassen P, Vandeplas G, Van Zele T, Cardell LO, Arebro J, Olze H, et al. Inflammatory endotypes of chronic rhinosinusitis based on cluster analysis of biomarkers. J Allergy Clin Immunol. 2016;137(5):1449–56.e4. https://doi.org/10.1016/j.jaci.2015.12.1324.
16. Zhang Y, Gevaert E, Lou H, Wang X, Zhang L, Bachert C, et al. Chronic rhinosinusitis in Asia. J Allergy Clin Immunol. 2017;140(5):1230–9. https://doi.org/10.1016/j.jaci.2017.09.009.
17. Wang ET, Zheng Y, Liu PF, Guo LJ. Eosinophilic chronic rhinosinusitis in East Asians. World J Clin Cases. 2014;2(12):873–82. https://doi.org/10.12998/wjcc.v2.i12.873.
18. Cao PP, Li HB, Wang BF, Wang SB, You XJ, Cui YH, et al. Distinct immunopathologic characteristics of various types of chronic rhinosinusitis in adult Chinese.

J Allergy Clin Immunol. 2009;124(3):478–84, 84.e1–2. https://doi.org/10.1016/j.jaci.2009.05.017.
19. Zhang N, Van Zele T, Perez-Novo C, Van Bruaene N, Holtappels G, DeRuyck N, et al. Different types of T-effector cells orchestrate mucosal inflammation in chronic sinus disease. J Allergy Clin Immunol. 2008;122(5):961–8. https://doi.org/10.1016/j.jaci.2008.07.008.
20. Bachert C, Zhang N, Cavaliere C, Weiping W, Gevaert E, Krysko O. Biologics for chronic rhinosinusitis with nasal polyps. J Allergy Clin Immunol. 2020;145(3):725–39. https://doi.org/10.1016/j.jaci.2020.01.020.
21. Bachert C, Zhang L, Gevaert P. Current and future treatment options for adult chronic rhinosinusitis: focus on nasal polyposis. J Allergy Clin Immunol. 2015;136(6):1431–40. https://doi.org/10.1016/j.jaci.2015.10.010.
22. Kim SJ, Lee KH, Kim SW, Cho JS, Park YK, Shin SY. Changes in histological features of nasal polyps in a Korean population over a 17-year period. Otolaryngol Head Neck Surg. 2013;149(3):431–7. https://doi.org/10.1177/0194599813495363.
23. Katotomichelakis M, Tantilipikorn P, Holtappels G, De Ruyck N, Feng L, Van Zele T, et al. Inflammatory patterns in upper airway disease in the same geographical area may change over time. Am J Rhinol Allergy. 2013;27(5):354–60. https://doi.org/10.2500/ajra.2013.27.3922.
24. Wang W, Gao Y, Zhu Z, Zha Y, Wang X, Qi F, et al. Changes in the clinical and histological characteristics of Chinese chronic rhinosinusitis with nasal polyps over 11 years. Int Forum Allergy Rhinol. 2019;9(2):149–57. https://doi.org/10.1002/alr.22234.
25. Diagnosis and management of difficult-to-treat and severe asthma—Global initiative for asthma—GINA. Retrieved April 19, 2020, from https://ginasthma.org/severeasthma/.
26. Bachert C, Sousa AR, Lund VJ, Scadding GK, Gevaert P, Nasser S, et al. Reduced need for surgery in severe nasal polyposis with mepolizumab: randomized trial. J Allergy Clin Immunol. 2017;140(4):1024–31.e14. https://doi.org/10.1016/j.jaci.2017.05.044.
27. Weibman AR, Huang JH, Stevens WW, Suh LA, Price CPE, Lidder AK, et al. A prospective analysis evaluating tissue biopsy location and its clinical relevance in chronic rhinosinusitis with nasal polyps. Int Forum Allergy Rhinol. 2017;7(11):1058–64. https://doi.org/10.1002/alr.22005.
28. Bachert C, Zhang N, Holtappels G, De Lobel L, van Cauwenberge P, Liu S, et al. Presence of IL-5 protein and IgE antibodies to staphylococcal enterotoxins in nasal polyps is associated with comorbid asthma. J Allergy Clin Immunol. 2010;126(5):962–8, 8.e1–6. https://doi.org/10.1016/j.jaci.2010.07.007.
29. Mygind N, Dahl R, Bachert C. Nasal polyposis, eosinophil dominated inflammation, and allergy. Thorax. 2000;55(Suppl 2):S79–83. https://doi.org/10.1136/thorax.55.suppl_2.s79.
30. Van Zele T, Claeys S, Gevaert P, Van Maele G, Holtappels G, Van Cauwenberge P, et al. Differentiation of chronic sinus diseases by measurement of inflammatory mediators. Allergy. 2006;61(11):1280–9. https://doi.org/10.1111/j.1398-9995.2006.01225.x.
31. Satyanarayana Rao KH. Informed consent: an ethical obligation or legal compulsion? J Cutan Aesthet Surg. 2008;1(1):33–5. https://doi.org/10.4103/0974-2077.41159.
32. Orlandi RR, Kingdom TT, Hwang PH, Smith TL, Alt JA, Baroody FM, et al. International consensus statement on allergy and rhinology: rhinosinusitis. Int Forum Allergy Rhinol. 2016;6(Suppl 1):S22–209. https://doi.org/10.1002/alr.21695.
33. Stammberger H, Posawetz W. Functional endoscopic sinus surgery. Concept, indications and results of the Messerklinger technique. Eur Arch Otorhinolaryngol. 1990;247(2):63–76. https://doi.org/10.1007/bf00183169.
34. Wigand ME. Transnasal, endoscopical sinus surgery for chronic sinusitis. I. A biomechanical concept of the endonasal mucosa surgery (author's transl). HNO. 1981;29(7):215–21.
35. Jankowski R, Rumeau C, Nguyen DT, Gallet P. Updating nasalisation: from concept to technique and results. Eur Ann Otorhinolaryngol Head Neck Dis. 2018;135(5):327–34. https://doi.org/10.1016/j.anorl.2018.05.006.
36. Jankowski R. Nasalisation: technique chirurgicale. J Fr d'OtoRhino-Laryngologie. 1995;44:221–6.
37. Van Zele T, Pauwels B, Dewaele F, Gevaert P, Bachert C. Prospective study on the outcome of the sphenoid drill out procedure. Rhinology. 2018;56(2):178–82. https://doi.org/10.4193/Rhin17.078.
38. Schick B, Draf W. The frontal sinus. In: Rhinology and facial plastic surgery. Berlin, Heidelberg: Springer; 2009. p. 567–73.
39. Shirazi MA, Silver AL, Stankiewicz JA. Surgical outcomes following the endoscopic modified Lothrop procedure. Laryngoscope. 2007;117(5):765–9. https://doi.org/10.1097/MLG.0b013e3180337d7b.
40. Anderson P, Sindwani R. Safety and efficacy of the endoscopic modified Lothrop procedure: a systematic review and meta-analysis. Laryngoscope. 2009;119(9):1828–33. https://doi.org/10.1002/lary.20565.
41. Georgalas C, Hansen F, Videler WJM, Fokkens WJ. Long terms results of Draf type III (modified endoscopic Lothrop) frontal sinus drainage procedure in 122 patients: a single centre experience. Rhinology. 2011;49(2):195–201. https://doi.org/10.4193/Rhin10.153.
42. Draf W. Endonasal micro-endoscopic frontal sinus surgery: the Fulda concept. Oper Tech Otolaryngol Head Neck Surg. 1991;2:234–40.
43. Hopkins C, Slack R, Lund V, Brown P, Copley L, Browne J. Long-term outcomes from the English national comparative audit of surgery for nasal polyposis and chronic rhinosinusitis. Laryngoscope. 2009;119(12):2459–65. https://doi.org/10.1002/lary.20653.
44. Nakayama T, Yoshikawa M, Asaka D, Okushi T, Matsuwaki Y, Otori N, et al. Mucosal eosinophilia

and recurrence of nasal polyps – new classification of chronic rhinosinusitis. Rhinology. 2011;49(4):392–6. https://doi.org/10.4193/Rhino10.261.
45. Ikeda K, Shiozawa A, Ono N, Kusunoki T, Hirotsu M, Homma H, et al. Subclassification of chronic rhinosinusitis with nasal polyp based on eosinophil and neutrophil. Laryngoscope. 2013;123(11):E1–9. https://doi.org/10.1002/lary.24154.
46. Brescia G, Marioni G, Franchella S, Ramacciotti G, Velardita C, Giacomelli L, et al. Can a panel of clinical, laboratory, and pathological variables pinpoint patients with sinonasal polyposis at higher risk of recurrence after surgery? Am J Otolaryngol. 2015;36(4):554–8. https://doi.org/10.1016/j.amjoto.2015.01.019.
47. Grgić MV, Ćupić H, Kalogjera L, Baudoin T. Surgical treatment for nasal polyposis: predictors of outcome. Eur Arch Otorhinolaryngol. 2015;272(12):3735–43. https://doi.org/10.1007/s00405-015-3519-7.
48. Lou H, Meng Y, Piao Y, Wang C, Zhang L, Bachert C. Predictive significance of tissue eosinophilia for nasal polyp recurrence in the Chinese population. Am J Rhinol Allergy. 2015;29(5):350–6. https://doi.org/10.2500/ajra.2015.29.4231.
49. Tokunaga T, Sakashita M, Haruna T, Asaka D, Takeno S, Ikeda H, et al. Novel scoring system and algorithm for classifying chronic rhinosinusitis: the JESREC study. Allergy. 2015;70(8):995–1003. https://doi.org/10.1111/all.12644.
50. Brescia G, Marioni G, Franchella S, Ramacciotti G, Giacomelli L, Marino F, et al. A prospective investigation of predictive parameters for post-surgical recurrences in sinonasal polyposis. Eur Arch Otorhinolaryngol. 2016;273(3):655–60. https://doi.org/10.1007/s00405-015-3598-5.
51. DeConde AS, Mace JC, Levy JM, Rudmik L, Alt JA, Smith TL. Prevalence of polyp recurrence after endoscopic sinus surgery for chronic rhinosinusitis with nasal polyposis. Laryngoscope. 2017;127(3):550–5. https://doi.org/10.1002/lary.26391.
52. Calus L, Van Bruaene N, Bosteels C, Dejonckheere S, Van Zele T, Holtappels G, et al. Twelve-year follow-up study after endoscopic sinus surgery in patients with chronic rhinosinusitis with nasal polyposis. Clin Transl Allergy. 2019;9:30. https://doi.org/10.1186/s13601-019-0269-4.
53. Hosemann W, Draf C. Danger points, complications and medico-legal aspects in endoscopic sinus surgery. GMS Curr Top Otorhinolaryngol Head Neck Surg. 2013;12:Doc06. https://doi.org/10.3205/cto000098.
54. Kowalski ML, Agache I, Bavbek S, Bakirtas A, Blanca M, Bochenek G, et al. Diagnosis and management of NSAID-exacerbated respiratory disease (N-ERD)—a EAACI position paper. Allergy. 2019;74(1):28–39. https://doi.org/10.1111/all.13599.
55. Fokkens WJ, Lund VJ, Hopkins C, Hellings PW, Kern R, Reitsma S, et al. European position paper on rhinosinusitis and nasal polyps 2020. Rhinology. 2020;58(Suppl S29):1–464. https://doi.org/10.4193/Rhin20.600.
56. Siedek V, Pilzweger E, Betz C, Berghaus A, Leunig A. Complications in endonasal sinus surgery: a 5-year retrospective study of 2,596 patients. Eur Arch Otorhinolaryngol. 2013;270(1):141–8. https://doi.org/10.1007/s00405-012-1973-z.
57. Chang JR, Grant MP, Merbs SL. Enucleation as endoscopic sinus surgery complication. JAMA Ophthalmol. 2015;133(7):850–2. https://doi.org/10.1001/jamaophthalmol.2015.0706.
58. Toppila-Salmi S, Rihkanen H, Arffman M, Manderbacka K, Keskimaki I, Hytönen ML. Regional differences in endoscopic sinus surgery in Finland: a nationwide register-based study. BMJ Open. 2018;8(10):e022173. https://doi.org/10.1136/bmjopen-2018-022173.
59. Blomgren K, Aaltonen LM, Lehtonen L, Helmiö P. Patient injuries in operative rhinology during a ten-year period: review of national patient insurance charts. Clin Otolaryngol. 2018;43(1):7–12. https://doi.org/10.1111/coa.12894.
60. Ramakrishnan VR, Kingdom TT, Nayak JV, Hwang PH, Orlandi RR. Nationwide incidence of major complications in endoscopic sinus surgery. Int Forum Allergy Rhinol. 2012;2(1):34–9. https://doi.org/10.1002/alr.20101.
61. Pavord ID, Korn S, Howarth P, Bleecker ER, Buhl R, Keene ON, et al. Mepolizumab for severe eosinophilic asthma (DREAM): a multicentre, double-blind, placebo-controlled trial. Lancet (London, England). 2012;380(9842):651–9. https://doi.org/10.1016/s0140-6736(12)60988-x.
62. Bel EH, Wenzel SE, Thompson PJ, Prazma CM, Keene ON, Yancey SW, et al. Oral glucocorticoid-sparing effect of mepolizumab in eosinophilic asthma. N Engl J Med. 2014;371(13):1189–97. https://doi.org/10.1056/NEJMoa1403291.
63. Ortega HG, Liu MC, Pavord ID, Brusselle GG, FitzGerald JM, Chetta A, et al. Mepolizumab treatment in patients with severe eosinophilic asthma. N Engl J Med. 2014;371(13):1198–207. https://doi.org/10.1056/NEJMoa1403290.
64. Farne HA, Wilson A, Powell C, Bax L, Milan SJ. Anti-IL5 therapies for asthma. Cochrane Database Syst Rev. 2017;9(9):Cd010834. https://doi.org/10.1002/14651858.CD010834.pub3.
65. Bleecker ER, Wechsler ME, JM FG, Menzies-Gow A, Wu Y, Hirsch I, et al. Baseline patient factors impact on the clinical efficacy of benralizumab for severe asthma. Eur Respir J. 2018;52(4) https://doi.org/10.1183/13993003.00936-2018.
66. Ortega HG, Yancey SW, Mayer B, Gunsoy NB, Keene ON, Bleecker ER, et al. Severe eosinophilic asthma treated with mepolizumab stratified by baseline eosinophil thresholds: a secondary analysis of the DREAM and MENSA studies. Lancet Respir Med. 2016;4(7):549–56. https://doi.org/10.1016/s2213-2600(16)30031-5.
67. Fokkens WJ, Lund V, Bachert C, Mullol J, Bjermer L, Bousquet J, et al. EUFOREA consensus on biologics for CRSwNP with or without asthma. Allergy. 2019;74(12):2312–9. https://doi.org/10.1111/all.13875.

54 Unmet Needs

Luo Zhang and Claus Bachert

As a heterogeneous disease entity, CRS is a global issue that affects up to 12% of the population in Europe and the USA, and 8% in China, brings ponderous clinical, social, and economic burden. The clinical and immune characteristics of CRS in different regions vary, including recurrence rate, remodeling, cellular and molecular pathomechanisms. Traditionally, the disease is classified based on clinical phenotypes, CRSwNP and CRSsNP, which could not elaborately discriminate between subgroups, and further efforts are necessary to establish endotypes in the daily clinical practice. Clinically, although adequate surgeries and medication have been applied, 30–50% of the patients with CRS appear to be uncontrolled, continuously suffering from severe symptoms, especially for those with Type 2, highly eosinophilic CRSwNP. It is essential to develop further understanding for the varieties of the endotypes, to develop biomarkers and point-of-care therapies, so that the principles of precision medicine could then be applied. The final aim is to reveal the underlying mechanisms offering various targets for treatment despite the similar clinical manifestations, in order to provide individualized treatment in both areas, surgery and pharmacotherapy.

Topical and systemic corticosteroids are essential in the treatment of CRS. Still, we do have incomplete knowledge on responsiveness to corticosteroids, including glucocorticoid resistance, and side effects over long term. It is an unmet need to also investigate the traditional treatments in order to not only lower the risk of relevant adverse effects, but also develop possible individualized treatment pathways.

Apart from pharmacotherapy, surgical options, from functional to extensive approaches should also be investigated thoroughly in particular endotypes of disease, rather than the clinical picture only, developing a better option for surgeons to select the optimal approach for each individual patient.

Thanks to endeavors contributed by scientists all over the world, recently, possible variations of endotypes in CRS were discovered, which are affected by the region, the environment, but also

L. Zhang
Department of Otolaryngology, Head and Neck Surgery, Beijing Tongren Hospital, Capital Medical University, Beijing, China

Beijing Key Laboratory of Nasal Diseases, Beijing Institute of Otolaryngology, Beijing, China

C. Bachert (✉)
Upper Airways Research Laboratory and Department of Oto-Rhino-Laryngology, Ghent University, Ghent, Belgium

Division of ENT Diseases, CLINTEC, Karolinska Institute, University of Stockholm, Stockholm, Sweden

First Affiliated Hospital, Sun Yat-sen University, International Upper Airway Research Centre, Guangzhou, China
e-mail: claus.bachert@ugent.be

L. Zhang, C. Bachert (eds.), *Chronic Rhinosinusitis*, https://doi.org/10.1007/978-981-16-0784-4_54

genetic background and bacterial impact. Therefore, large-scaled multicenter trials are needed to elaborate targeted diagnostic and therapeutic tools in the future. Targeting the endotype of dominant type 2 inflammation and the relevant pathways, biologics such as anti-IgE, anti-IL4Ra, anti-IL5, and anti-IL5Ra have been introduced using large trials and will be further applied into clinical practice. Head-to-head clinical trials should be performed to compare the efficacies between biologics, and real life studies will be necessary to establish care pathways combining standard of care today with those innovative treatments. Patient's stratification, identification of promising biologics, balance of economic costs, and patient's satisfaction should be further investigated for optimizing treatment strategies and maximizing treating efficiency.

Correction to: Staphylococcus aureus and Its Proteins

Goran Abdurrahman and Barbara M. Bröker

Correction to: Chapter 14 in: L. Zhang, C. Bachert (eds.), *Chronic Rhinosinusitis*, https://doi.org/10.1007/978-981-16-0784-4_14

The book was inadvertently published with the error in the name and affiliation of Goran Abdurrahman and has been updated as below:

The author name Goran Abdurrahmanm has been changed to Goran Abdurrahman.

In the affiliation of Goran Abdurrahman, the "Department of Immunology" has been changed to "Institute of Immunology".

The updated version of the chapter can be found at
https://doi.org/10.1007/978-981-16-0784-4_14

L. Zhang, C. Bachert (eds.), *Chronic Rhinosinusitis*, https://doi.org/10.1007/978-981-16-0784-4_55

Index

A
Acquired immune system, 147–149
Acute exacerbation of CRS (AECRS), 341, 342, 344, 348
Adenocarcinoma, 261, 262
Adenoid cystic carcinoma (ACC), 260, 261
Adenoidectomy, 269, 273–274, 281–284
Adoptive immunity, 1, 31, 32, 34, 72
Allergic fungal rhinosinusitis (AFRS), 21, 115, 141, 158, 188, 273
Allergic fungal sinusitis, 62, 160, 167–173, 279
Allergic rhinitis (AR), 98, 101, 102, 107, 142, 152, 159, 161, 178, 187–189, 192, 194, 203, 230, 271, 273, 277, 278, 281, 282, 284, 299, 300, 333, 337, 338, 363, 407, 422
Antibacterial defense, 61, 73–74
Antibiotics, 140, 147, 151, 162, 172, 205, 206, 272–274, 280–282, 304, 315, 318, 322, 341–348, 361, 363, 364, 393, 394, 400, 401, 407
Anti-IL5 strategies, 411–412
Aspirin-exacerbated respiratory disease(AERD), 24, 42, 160, 161, 164, 178, 201–202, 207, 243, 334, 379, 383, 414, 423
Asthma, 21, 143, 160, 189–191, 194, 202, 271, 300, 407, 410, 422, 424

B
Bacterial lysates, 361–365
Barcelona smell test-24 (BAST-24), 229, 232, 233
Benign tumors, 247–250, 253
Biologics, 2, 14, 39, 76, 103, 173, 177, 178, 202, 239, 242–244, 345, 370, 387, 403, 409–419, 422, 424–432, 436
Biomarkers, 25, 34, 57, 58, 76, 142, 175, 176, 178, 182, 239–245, 383, 410, 412, 414, 416, 435
Blood eosinophils, 59, 178, 243, 244, 407, 411, 416, 422, 423, 429
Bronchiectasis, 12, 194, 271

C
Chronic pulmonary obstructive disease, 193–194
Chronic rhinosinusitis (CRS), 1, 3, 4, 9, 10, 12, 19, 21, 22, 32, 37, 38, 47, 57–58, 81, 89, 90, 98, 103, 107, 109–113, 121, 133, 134, 139, 140, 147, 157–164, 167, 176, 178, 181, 183, 187, 189, 202, 207, 239, 248, 267, 277, 291, 303, 313, 317, 319, 327, 329, 333, 338, 341, 355, 361, 369, 384, 399, 403, 435
Chronic rhinosinusitis with nasal polyps (CRSwNP), 22, 75, 121, 134, 135, 140, 164, 183, 188, 303–305, 343, 409–419, 421
Colonization, 20, 40, 58, 59, 61, 72, 94, 98, 103, 108, 121–124, 127, 128, 141, 143, 148, 163, 173, 188, 193, 363
Complications of endoscopic sinus surgery, 389–397
Computerized X-ray tomography (CT), 4, 6, 13, 14, 58, 142, 158–160, 169, 171, 189, 190, 192, 202, 203, 205, 212–213, 215, 224, 225, 239, 247–249, 255, 256, 260, 261, 263, 267–271, 280, 282, 283, 292, 327, 346, 371, 372, 378, 391, 394, 397, 399–401, 407, 410, 411, 413–415, 422
Concha bullosa resection, 372–373
Congenital immune system, 147–148, 153
Connecticut chemosensory clinical re-search Center (CCCRC), 229, 230, 232, 234
Coronavirus (CorV), 114, 133, 141
Corticosteroids resistance, 329, 330
CRSsNP, Asian CRSwNP, 69
Cysteinyl leukotrienes (CysLTs), 59, 152, 191–193, 201, 333, 334
Cystic fibrosis (CF), 19, 69, 71, 90, 97, 159, 160, 204–205, 270–274, 278, 283, 284, 362, 375, 422

D
Decongestant, 269, 273, 355–358
DNA methylation, 23, 90, 141

L. Zhang, C. Bachert (eds.), *Chronic Rhinosinusitis*, https://doi.org/10.1007/978-981-16-0784-4

E

Endoscopic sinus surgery (ESS), 13–15, 190, 193, 204, 205, 207, 211, 212, 274, 284, 304–306, 310, 317, 319, 320, 322, 325–327, 346–348, 358, 371–379, 384, 385, 387, 389–397, 399, 403–407, 422, 424–427
Endotypes, 33, 34, 38–39, 70, 71, 74–76, 93, 98, 102, 142, 158, 160, 161, 175–178, 182, 183, 187, 239, 240, 242, 243, 342, 345, 363, 369–370, 435
Environmental triggers, 139–141
Eosinophilic, 22, 24, 25, 33, 38, 40, 41, 52, 57–58, 60–62, 69, 70, 72, 74, 75, 82–85, 101–103, 127, 140–143, 150–152, 158, 160, 162–164, 169, 173, 175, 181–183, 190, 191, 203, 204, 243, 244, 254, 272, 293, 300, 306, 314, 315, 329, 330, 333, 334, 346, 347, 357, 365, 404, 435
Eosinophilic cationic protein (ECP), 23, 58, 60–62, 84, 101, 161, 176, 177, 181, 183, 240, 241, 272, 300, 304, 314, 383, 387, 404, 410, 412, 414, 423
Eosinophilic extracellular traps (EETs), 61, 62, 74, 175
Eosinophilic granulomatosis with polyangiitis (EGPA), 143, 203–204, 207, 299–301
Eosinophilic mucin, 62, 167–170, 172, 203
Epithelial cilia, 98–100
Epstein-Barr virus, 51, 254, 261
Ethmoidectomy, 211, 216–218, 274, 283, 375–377, 389, 396

F

Frontal sinusotomy, 213, 378–379
Functional endoscopic surgery (FESS), 188, 193, 211–225, 273, 274, 282–284, 317–319, 346, 357, 358, 361, 369, 401, 404

G

Gastroesophageal reflux (GER), 193, 278, 365
Genome-wide association studies (GWAS), 20–22
Glucocorticoid receptor (GR), 303, 330
Granulomatosis with polyangiitis (GPA), 287, 292
Group 2 innate lymphoid cells 2, 38–41, 43

H

Health-related quality of life (HRQoL), 9, 11–15, 193
Histone modificationsin, 23–24
Human rhinovirus (HRV), 103, 114, 133–136

I

Immune dysregulation, 150–152, 299, 300
Immune regulation, 74–75, 149–153
Immune regulatory system, 147–153
Immunodeficiency, 160, 205–206, 278, 279, 282
Immunoglobulin (Ig)G4-related disease (IgG4-RD), 291–296
Immunoglobulin E (IgE) antibodies, 2, 21, 22, 33, 34, 39, 40, 48, 52, 58, 108, 115, 123–128, 142, 143, 150–152, 160–162, 164, 168, 169, 172, 175–178, 182, 188, 190, 191, 193, 202, 203, 241–244, 269, 272, 293, 300, 304, 345, 383, 387, 407, 409–414, 416, 422, 423, 425, 430
Influenza virus (IFV), 93, 133, 134, 136, 141
Innate immunity, 31, 62, 115, 148, 272, 364
Integrated care pathways, 421–432

J

Junctional proteins, 100–102
Juvenile angiofibroma (JA), 248–249

L

Leukotriene receptor antagonists (LTRAs), 172, 299, 333, 334

M

Malignant tumors, 260–263, 280
Maxillary antrostomy, 274, 374–375
Merocel®, 241, 325, 327, 384
Microbiology, 107–116, 168, 240, 400
Mucociliary clearance, 31, 89–94, 141, 148, 152, 170, 193, 204, 206, 207, 213, 269, 271, 272, 281, 284, 357–358, 369, 374, 375
Mucosal barrier, 98
Multi-omics, 240, 244–245

N

Nasal endoscopy, 4, 5, 14, 159, 161, 168–169, 187, 205, 239, 269, 284, 344, 355, 372, 397, 421, 422
Nasal irrigation, 192, 273, 282, 296, 310, 346, 356–358, 401
Nasal spray corticosteroid, 296, 310, 311, 314, 315, 318, 413
NasoPore®, 325–327
Nebulization corticosteroids, 306, 313–316, 357
Neutrophils, 2, 23, 31–33, 62, 69–76, 83, 84, 123, 149, 152, 175, 240, 287, 314, 330, 345, 411
Non-steroidal anti-inflammatory drug (NSAID)-exacerbated respiratory disease (N-ERD), 97, 178, 187, 188, 191–193, 201, 202, 400

O

Odontogenic rhinosinusitis, 205
Olfactory event-related potentials (OERPs), 235
Olfactory neuroblastoma (ON), 261, 262
Osteoma, 247–248

P

Paediatric Barcelona Olfactory Test (pBOT-6), 231, 234
Paediatric CRS, 271–273
Patient reported outcomes (PRO), 9, 11–15, 319

Peri-operative management, 399–401
Phenotypes of CRS, 24, 25, 142, 143, 160–161, 203, 204
Prevalence, 4–6, 39, 134, 136, 140–143, 150, 158, 161, 168, 176, 188, 189, 193, 194, 201, 202, 206, 227, 254, 256, 267–269, 271, 274, 277, 299, 306, 347, 348, 365
Primary ciliary dyskinesia (PCD), 19, 90, 97, 100, 206–207, 271, 278, 375, 422
Probiotics, 103, 361–365
Proton pump inhibitors(PPI), 361–365

Q

Quality of life (QoL), 3, 9–15, 57, 158, 189–194, 268, 274, 315, 322, 334, 344, 357, 361, 364, 384, 387, 401, 403–404, 410, 413, 414, 425, 427

R

Reboot surgery, 2, 383–387, 425
Regional differences, 181, 427
Respiratory syncytial virus (RSV), 101, 133–135, 141

S

Scandinavian odor identification test (SOIT), 228, 229
Schwannomas, 250
Septoplasty, 372, 395
Serum IgE, 21, 22, 115, 168, 169, 177, 178, 345, 410, 416, 422, 423, 430
Side effects, 136, 192, 273, 306, 309, 310, 315, 318, 325, 326, 329, 346–348, 358, 417–418, 424, 428, 435
Sino-nasal epithelium, 97–103
Sinonasal inverted papilloma, 253, 254, 256
Sino-nasal outcome test-22(SNOT-22), 12, 13, 304, 326, 410
Sphenoid sinusotomy, 377–378
Staphylococcus aureus, 40, 52, 72, 100, 108–110, 112, 121–128, 135, 140, 149, 161, 162, 168, 173, 189, 204, 241, 243, 281, 330, 343, 344, 348, 362, 423
Steroid infiltrated packing materials, 325–327
Superantigens (SAgs), 40, 115, 124–128, 151, 168, 178, 189
Supra-epithelial barrier, 98–99
Surgical approaches, 177, 369, 370, 383, 424, 425

T

T helper(Th)2 cells, 2, 33, 37, 38, 99, 101, 115, 123, 140, 150, 152, 243
Transforming growth factor-beta (TGF-β), 24, 75, 82, 83, 152
Type 2 cytokines, 2, 33, 37, 39–43, 52, 59, 71, 84, 150, 163, 175, 181, 385
Type 2 immune reactions, 2, 175–179, 182, 242, 243, 370, 384, 409, 412, 416, 423

U

Uncinectomy, 213–216, 373–374, 390
Uncontrolled severe CRSwNP, 409, 422–423, 428, 430
University of Pennsylvania Smell Identification Test(UPSIT), 228–230, 232, 413, 414, 430

W

Wegener's granulomatosis (WG), 287–288

MIX
Papier aus verantwortungsvollen Quellen
Paper from responsible sources
FSC® C105338
www.fsc.org

If you have any concerns about our products,
you can contact us on
ProductSafety@springernature.com

In case Publisher is established outside the EU,
the EU authorized representative is:
Springer Nature Customer Service Center GmbH
Europaplatz 3, 69115 Heidelberg, Germany

Printed by Libri Plureos GmbH
in Hamburg, Germany